Community Health Nursing-I

for GNM Nursing Students

(As per the New Syllabus of INC for GNM)

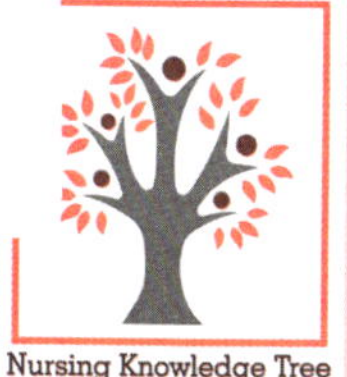

—— **Second Edition** ——

Lt. Col. KK Gill MSc (CHN), RM, RN, DNE, BSc (N) PB

Former Principal
State Institute of Nursing and Paramedical Sciences, Badal, Punjab
and
Amar Professional College of Nursing, Mohali, Punjab

CBS Publishers & Distributors Pvt Ltd

• New Delhi • Bengaluru • Chennai • Kochi • Kolkata • Lucknow • Mumbai
• Hyderabad • Jharkhand • Nagpur • Patna • Pune • Uttarakhand

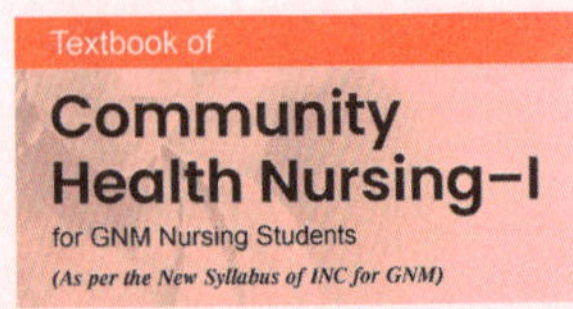

ISBN: 978-81-977500-0-7

Copyright © Publishers

Reprint: 2026

Second Edition: 2025

First Edition: 2018

Published by **Satish Kumar Jain** and produced by **Varun Jain** for

CBS Publishers and Distributors Pvt Ltd

4819/XI Prahlad Street, 24 Ansari Road, Daryaganj, New Delhi 110 002, India.
Ph: +91-11-23289259, 23266861, 23266867   Website: www.cbspd.com
Fax: 011-23243014
e-mail: delhi@cbspd.com; cbspubs@airtelmail.in.

Corporate Office: 204 FIE, Industrial Area, Patparganj, Delhi 110 092
Ph: +91-11-4934 4934   Fax: 4934 4935
e-mail: feedback@cbspd.com

Branches

- **Bengaluru:** Seema House 2975, 17th Cross, K.R. Road, Banashankari 2nd Stage, Bengaluru-560 070, Karnataka
  Ph: +91-80-26771678/79   Fax: +91-80-26771680   e-mail: bangalore@cbspd.com

- **Chennai:** 7, Subbaraya Street, Shenoy Nagar, Chennai-600 030, Tamil Nadu
  Ph: +91-44-26680620, 26681266   Fax: +91-44-42032115   e-mail: chennai@cbspd.com

- **Kochi:** 68/1534, 35, 36-Power House Road, Opp. KSEB, Cochin-682018, Kochi, Kerala
  Ph: +91-484-4059061-65   Fax: +91-484-4059065   e-mail: kochi@cbspd.com

- **Kolkata:** Hind Ceramics Compound, 1st Floor, 147, Nilganj Road, Belghoria, Kolkata-700056, West Bengal
  Ph: +91-033-2563-3055/56   e-mail: kolkata@cbspd.com

- **Lucknow:** Basement, Khushnuma Complex, 7-Meerabai Marg (Behind Jawahar Bhawan), Lucknow-226001, Uttar Pradesh
  Ph: +0522-4000032   e-mail: tiwari.lucknow@cbspd.com

- **Mumbai:** PWD Shed, Gala No. 25/26, Ramchandra Bhatt Marg, Next to J.J. Hospital Gate No. 2, Opp. Union Bank of India, Noor Baug, Mumbai-400009, Maharashtra
  Ph: +91-22-66661880/89   Fax: +91-22-24902342   e-mail: mumbai@cbspd.com

Representatives

Hyderabad	+91-9885175004	**Jharkhand**	+91-9811541605
Nagpur	+91-9421945513	**Patna**	+91-9334159340
Pune	+91-9623451994	**Uttarakhand**	+91-9716462459

Printed at : Goyal Offset Works Pvt. Ltd. Haryana

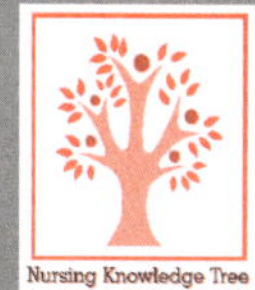

CBS Nursing Knowledge Tree

Extends its Tribute to

Florence Nightingale

For glorifying the role of women as nurses,
For holding the title of " The Lady with the Lamp,"
For working tirelessly for humanity—
Florence Nightingale will always be
remembered for her
selfless and memorable services to the
human race.

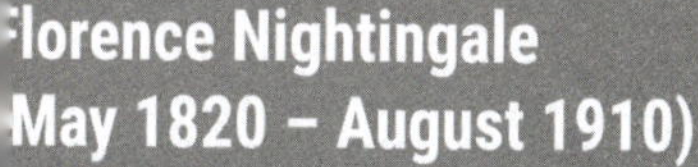

Florence Nightingale
May 1820 – August 1910)

Dedicated to

My family for their unconventional
support and constant encouragement
throughout the venture.

Preface to the Second Edition

Community Health Nursing is a rapidly growing field. According to Global Commitment of Health for All and to achieve **Millennium Development Goals** (MDGs), the Comprehensive Primary Health Care (CPHC) has been implemented through health and wellness centers (HWCs) by transforming existing Sub Centers (SCs), and Primary Health Centers (PHCs) into the basic pillars of Ayushman Bharat as a foundation of India's Health System.

The role of Accredited Social Health Activist (ASHA) has expanded. ASHA's roles now include educating and promoting health, facilitating access to health services, providing first aid, keeping records and improving sanitation. A Community Health Officer (CHO) is appointed to coordinate and accelerate the services of community health nursing team at HWC-SC and HWC-PHC.

COVID-19 has been added under the epidemiology of communicable diseases. The book is updated according to the changes made in the delivery of comprehensive primary healthcare. I hope that this edition will be useful for nursing students, teachers and other healthcare professionals to meet their requirements.

Lt. Col. KK Gill (Retd.)

Preface to the First Edition

Nurses are the frontline fighters in the battle for health and wellness of society. They are the backbone of the healthcare delivery system at all levels, be it rural or urban community, hospitals, clinics or industries. Community Health Nursing is a multidisciplinary, rapidly growing subject. The primary objective of community health nursing is to help people attain an optimal level of health through healthy lifestyle. Sound basic knowledge of community health nursing will help nursing students to assess health problems of community and take appropriate action at grassroots level.

The community health nurse needs to know about the community, its social and cultural patterns, principles of community health nursing, community diagnosis, community development, expanded health programs and roles and responsibilities of community health nurse in shaping the health-seeking behavior of the community.

It gives me immense pleasure to present this book titled *Textbook of Community Health Nursing–I for GNM Nursing Students*. This book is not only useful for students but also for the educators.

It is written in simple language according to new syllabus of GNM prescribed by the Indian Nursing Council for Community Health Nursing-I.

This book will meet the requirements of the students and will help in strengthening their basic knowledge of the subject so that they can become better equipped to provide primary healthcare to the community, thus keeping the commitment of the country to achieve 'Health for All'.

I invite constructive comments and suggestions from students, teachers and experts for the improvement of this book in future editions.

Lt. Col. KK Gill (Retd.)

Acknowledgments

First of all, I must bow my head before the Almighty God for bestowing upon me the strength, courage and wisdom to sustain myself through this endeavor. Writing a book is like undertaking a long journey of ardor and self-discovery, and without a guiding light that constantly shows the way, an author is bound to get lost in the vast sea of knowledge.

I extend my deep sense of gratitude to my children, **Dr Navneet Gill** and **Er. Kamalpreet Singh Gill.** Without their constant presence by my side, the completion of this herculean endeavor would not have been possible.

I would like to thank **Mr Satish Kumar Jain** (Chairman) and **Mr Varun Jain** (Managing Director), M/s CBS Publishers and Distributors Pvt Ltd for providing me the platform in bringing out the book.

I sincerely thank the entire CBS team for bringing out the book with utmost care and attractive presentation. I would like to thank Ms Nitasha Arora (Assistant General Manager – Publishing) and Dr Anju Dhir (Sr. Product Manager cum Commissioning Editor) for their publishing support. I would also like to extend my thanks to Ms Surbhi Gupta (Sr. Editor cum Team Lead), Mr Ashutosh Pathak (Assistant Production Manager cum TL) and all the production team members for devoting laborious hours in editing, designing and typesetting the book.

Reviewers

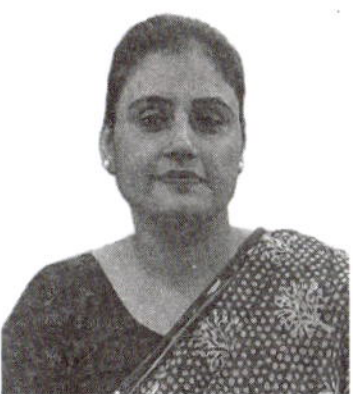

Amritpal Kaur
PhD (N), MSc (Community Health Nursing)

Professor cum Vice Principal
SGL Nursing College
Jalandhar, Punjab

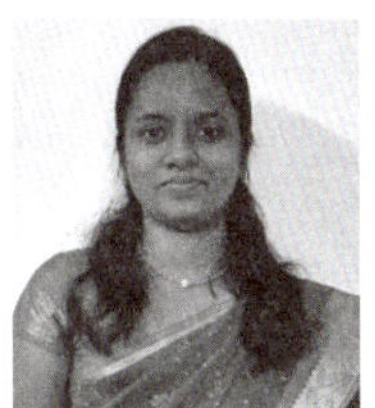

Deva Pon Pushpam
PhD Scholar, MSc (Community Health Nursing)

Professor cum HOD
BEE ENN College of Nursing
Jammu and Kashmir

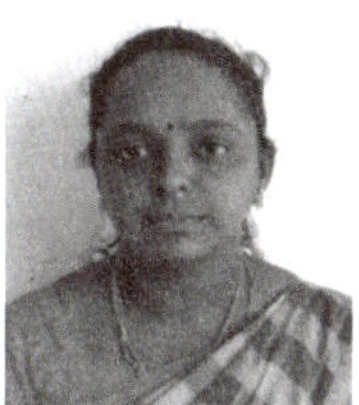

Anbumalar J
MSc (Community Health Nursing)

Vice Principal
White Memorial College of Nursing
Attoor, Veeyanoor, Tamil Nadu

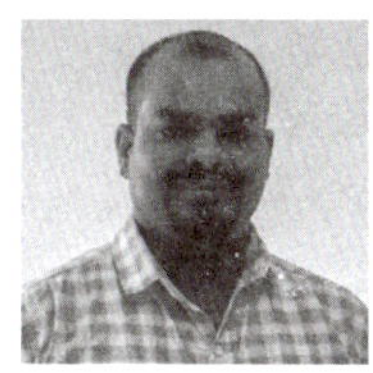

Dinesh Kumar Kachhawa
MSc (Community Health Nursing)

Professor cum Vice Principal
Sunder Devi Nursing College
Bhopal, Madhya Pradesh

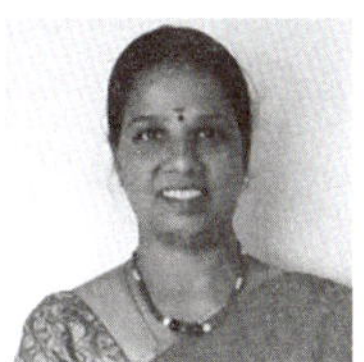

Arulmozhi Baskaran P M
PhD (N), MSc (Community Health Nursing)

Principal
PES University Institute of Nursing
Bengaluru, Karnataka

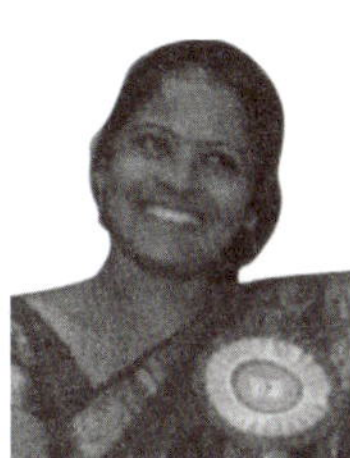

Kalpana Boddu
PhD Scholar, MSc (Community Health Nursing)

Professor
Sree Narayana Nursing College
Nellore, Andhra Pradesh

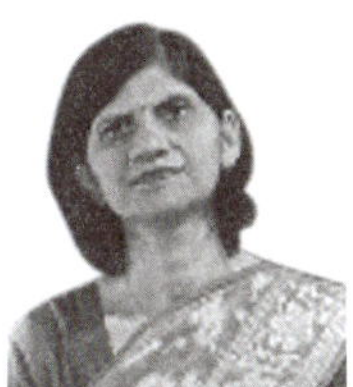

Bandana
PhD (N), MSc (Community Health Nursing)

Principal
Shri Lal Bahadur Shastri Government College of Nursing
Mandi, Himachal Pradesh

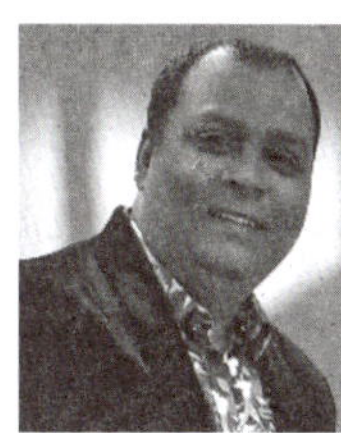

Pratul Prasann Nand
PhD (N), MSc (Community Health Nursing)

Vice Principal
Sanjivani Institute of Technology
Bilaspur, Chhattisgarh

The names of the reviewers are arranged in alphabetical order.

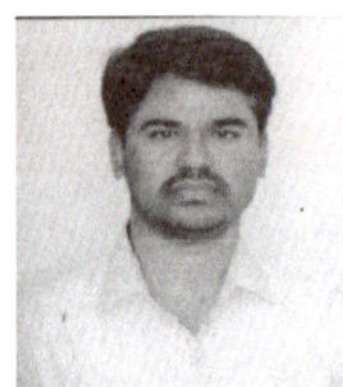

Ramakrishna Degani
MSc (Community Health Nursing)

Professor & HOD
Adesh University
Bathinda, Punjab

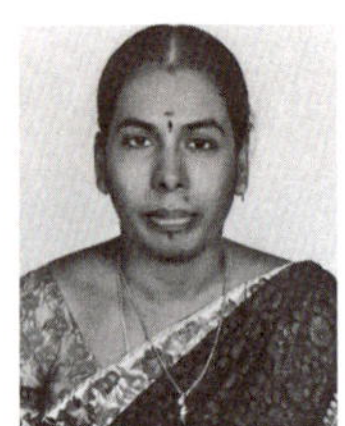

Viruthasarani K
PhD Scholar, MSc (Community Health Nursing)

Professor cum Vice Principal
Vivekanandha Nursing College
Pondicherry

The names of the reviewers are arranged in alphabetical order.

Special Features of the Book

LEARNING OBJECTIVES

After the completion of the unit, the readers will be able to:
- Discuss the concepts, goals and objectives of family health nursing care.
- Demonstrate skills in providing comprehensive nursing care to the family.
- Identify the family healthcare plan and the nursing process.
- Appreciate the roles and functions of community health nurses in family health service.

Learning Objectives given in all the units focus on the areas that a student shall gain after completing the unit.

UNIT OUTLINE

- Introduction
- Family
- Concept of Family Health
- Family Healthcare Services
- Family Healthcare Plan
- Family Health Nursing Process
- Family Health Services
- Role of Community Health Nurse in Family Health Services

Every unit starts with a **Unit Outline** that gives the glimpse of the content covered in the unit.

KEY TERMS

Family health: Health of the members of family; a state in which the family is a resource for the day-to-day living and health of its members.
Family health nursing: Nursing services provided to the family; generalized, well-balanced and integrated, comprehensive and continuous are requiring planning to accomplish its goal.
Family planning: Limiting the size of the family; the consideration of the number of children a person wishes to have, including the choice to have no children, and the age at which they wish to have them.

Important terms used in the unit are enlisted under **Key Terms**.

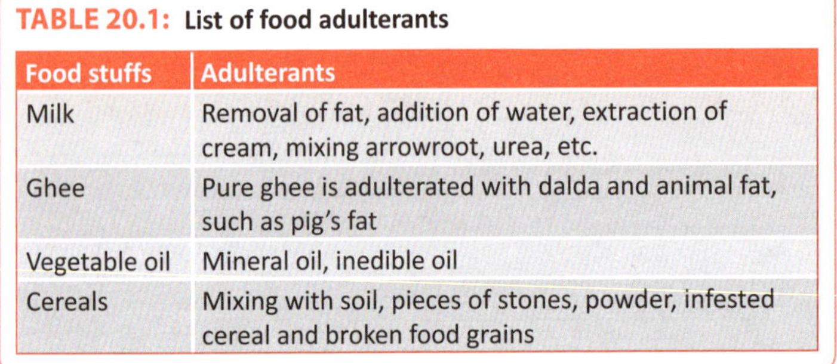

TABLE 20.1: List of food adulterants

Food stuffs	Adulterants
Milk	Removal of fat, addition of water, extraction of cream, mixing arrowroot, urea, etc.
Ghee	Pure ghee is adulterated with dalda and animal fat, such as pig's fat
Vegetable oil	Mineral oil, inedible oil
Cereals	Mixing with soil, pieces of stones, powder, infested cereal and broken food grains

Numerous Tables are used in the text to provide students with necessary data and information to supplement the text.

Several **images and diagrams** have been used at relevant places to simplify the concepts for the students.

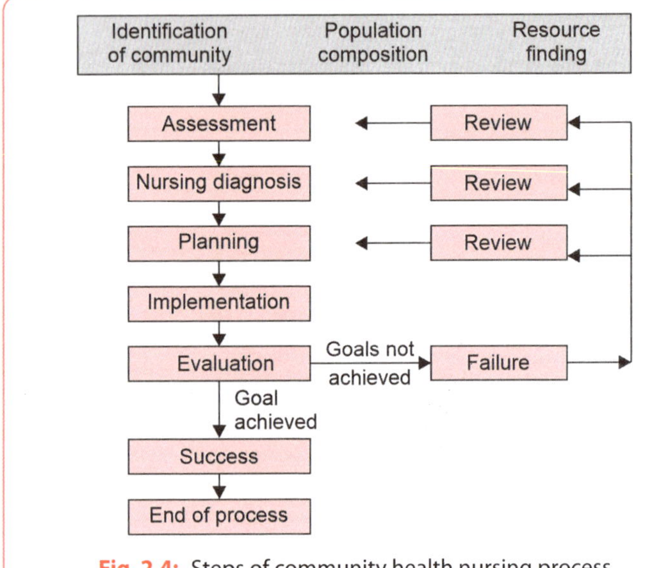

Fig. 2.4: Steps of community health nursing process

Nursing Considerations

Important Points to Remember while Immunizing
- Only disposable syringes should be used.
- Hepatitis B dose is given only within 24 hours after birth as it helps to prevent prenatal transmission of hepatitis B.
- OPV-O dose is given within 15 days after birth. OPV can be given up to 5 years of age.
- Pentavalent vaccines contain a combination of DPT, hepatitis B and Hib. Hepatitis B birth dose and booster dose of DPT will continue as before.

Nursing Considerations boxes are covered throughout the book for implementation of better clinical practices.

Recent Updates

New Stroke Prevention Guidelines (American Heart Association 2014)

Individualized Approach to Lifestyle Modifications

- Physical activity
- Diet and nutrition
- Smoking cessation
- Obesity and dyslipidemia

Prevention and Control

- Early detection and treatment of transient ischemic attack to prevent the stroke.
- **Modification of lifestyle:** Alteration in lifestyle to manage the risk factors like hypertension, diabetes and coronary heart disease, etc.
- **Healthcare facilities:** People should be made aware about the available healthcare facilities and how to make use of them.
- **Health education:** People should be educated about the prevention and control of strokes.

Recent Updates keep students aware of all the latest advances and developments in the field.

MUST KNOW

Relation between Records and Reports
Records and reports are interdependent. Reports are written based on records. Reports can also be presented as record. Records are always in written form, whereas report can be written as well as verbal. Records can be preserved, whereas verbal reports can be forgotten. In spite of being different, both seem synonymous and are interdependent. Both are important tools of communication and management in hospitals and community health centers and nursing.

Must Know boxes covering valuable facts are strategically placed to highlight critical information, ensuring readers are well-informed of key concepts and important details.

Summary

- The philosophy of community health nursing is that nursing services should be provided to all irrespective of race, religion, caste, creed and sex.
- Community health nursing is influenced by attitude of family, religion, culture, education, value, norms and beliefs of the family.
- The main goal of community health nursing is to promote the health of the individuals, families and community.
- The main principles of community health nursing include planned services according to the need and requirement of the community, maintaining good interpersonal relationship with the community, and providing services irrespective of caste, creed, color, religion, etc.

Each and every unit ends with **Summarized one-liner** for quick revision of the chapter.

Student Assignment in the form of long and short answer and multiple choice questions in each and every unit will facilitate structured learning and revision of the material provided in the respective units.

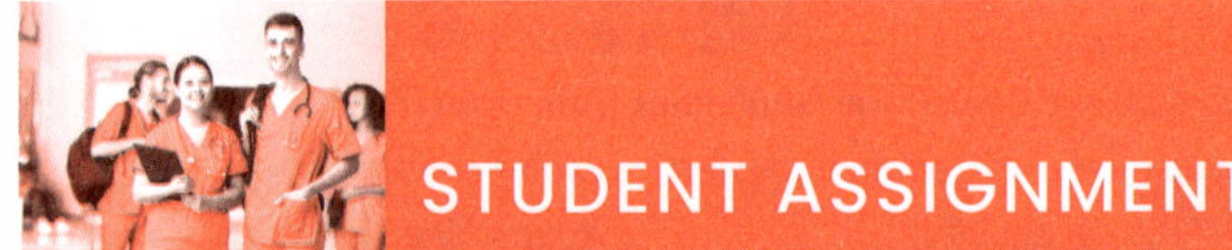

LONG ANSWER TYPE QUESTIONS

1. Describe the factors affecting environmental health.
2. Explain the environmental problems affecting human health.

SHORT ANSWER TYPE QUESTIONS

1. Define environment.
2. Enlist the components of environment.

MULTIPLE CHOICE QUESTIONS

1. **Which one of the following is not the component of physical environment?**
   a. Air
   b. Water
   c. Soil
   d. Microorganisms
2. **Which of the following is not the main component of our environment?**
   a. Physical
   b. Biological
   c. Spiritual
   d. Social

COMMUNITY HEALTH NURSING-I

Placement: First Year (GNM Nursing)   **Total Hours – 80**

Unit	Learning Objectives	Content	Hours	Teaching Learning Activities	Methods of Assessment
I.	Describe the concept of health and disease and community health.	**Introduction to Community Health** • Definitions: Community, community health, community health nursing • Concept of health and disease, dimensions and indicators of health, Health determinants • History and development of Community Health in India and its present concept • Primary health care, Millennium Development Goals • Promotion and maintenance of Health	10	Lecture cum discussions	Short answers
II.	• Explain various aspects of Community Health Nursing. • Demonstrate skills in applying nursing process in Community Health Nursing settings.	**Community Health Nursing** • Philosophy, goals, objectives and principles, Concept and importance of Community Health Nursing, - Qualities and functions of Community Health Nurse • Steps of nursing process; community identification, population composition, health and allied resources, community assessment, planning and conducting community nursing care services	14	Lecture cum discussions	• Short answers • Essay type
III.	Demonstrate skill in assessing the health status and identify deviations from normal parameters in different age groups.	**Health Assessment** • Characteristics of a healthy individual • Health assessment of infant, preschool, school going, adolescent, adult, antenatal woman, postnatal woman, adult and elderly	10	• Lecture cum discussions • Demonstration • Role Play • Videos	• Short answers • Objective type • Essay type • Return demonstration

Contd...

Unit	Learning Objectives	Content	Hours	Teaching Learning Activities	Methods of Assessment
IV.	Describe the principles of epidemiology and epidemiological methods in community health nursing practice.	**Principles of Epidemiology and Epidemiological Methods** • Definition and aims of epidemiology, communicable and noncommunicable diseases • Basic tools of measurement in epidemiology • Uses of epidemiology • Disease cycle • Spectrum of disease • Levels of prevention of disease • Disease transmission—direct and indirect • Immunizing agents, immunization and national immunization schedule • Control of infectious diseases • Disinfection	10	• Lecture cum discussions • Non-communicable disease module of government of India • Field visit	• Essay type • Short answers • Objective type
V.	Demonstrate skill in providing comprehensive nursing care to the family.	**Family Health Nursing Care** • Family as a unit of health • Concept, goals, objectives • Family health care services • Family health care plan and nursing process • Family health services—Maternal, child care and family welfare services • Roles and function of a community health nurse in family health service • Family health records	12	• Lecture cum discussions • Role play Family visit	• Essay type • Short answers
VI.	Describe the principles and techniques of family health care services at home and in clinics.	**Family Health Care Settings** Home visit: • Purposes, principles • Planning and evaluation • Bag technique Clinic: • Purposes, type of clinics and their functions • Function of Health personnel in clinics	10	• Lecture cum discussions • Demonstration • Visits—Home, health center	• Short answers • Return demonstration
VII.	Describe the referral system and community resources for referral.	**Referral System** • Levels of health care and health care settings • Referral services available—Steps in referral • Role of a nurse in referral	6	• Lecture cum discussions • Mock drill	• Short answers • Objective type

Contd...

Unit	Learning Objectives	Content	Hours	Teaching Learning Activities	Methods of Assessment
VIII.	List the records and reports used in community health nursing practice.	**Records and Reports** • Types and uses • Essential requirements of records and reports • Preparation and Maintenance	3	• Lecture cum discussions • Exhibit the records	• Short answer • Objective type
IX.	Explain the management of minor ailments.	**Minor Ailments** • Principles of management • Management as per standing instructions/orders	3	Lecture cum discussions	• Short answer • Objective type

ENVIRONMENTAL HYGIENE

Total Hours – 30

Unit	Learning Objectives	Content	Hours	Teaching Learning Activities	Methods of Assessment
I.	Explain the importance of healthy environment and its relation to health and disease.	**Introduction** • Components of environment • Importance of healthy environment	2	Lecture cum discussions	Short answer

II.	Describe the environmental factors contributing to health and illness.	**Environmental Factors Contributing to Health**
		• **Water:**
		  ■ Sources and characteristics of safe and wholesome water
		  ■ Uses of water
		  ■ Rain water harvesting
		  ■ Water pollution—natural and acquired impurities
		  ■ Water borne diseases
		  ■ Water purification-small and large scale
		• **Air:**
		  ■ Composition of air
		  ■ Airborne diseases
		  ■ Air pollution and its effect on health
		  ■ Control of air pollution and use of safety measures
			22	• Lecture cum discussions
				• Demonstration Exhibits
				• Visit to water purification plant, sewage treatment plant
					• Short answers
					• Objective type
					• Essay type

Contd...

Unit	Learning Objectives	Content	Hours	Teaching Learning Activities	Methods of Assessment
		• **Waste:** ■ Refuse—garbage, excreta and sewage ■ Health hazards ■ Waste management: Collection, transportation and disposal • **Housing:** ■ Location ■ Type ■ Characteristics of good housing ■ Basic amenities ■ Town planning • **Ventilation:** Types and standards of ventilation • **Lighting:** ■ Requirements of good lighting ■ Natural and artificial lighting ■ Use of solar energy • **Noise:** ■ Sources of noise ■ Community noise levels ■ Effects of noise pollution ■ Noise control measures • **Arthropods:** ■ Mosquitoes, housefly, sand fly, human louse, rat fleas, rodents, ticks, etc. ■ Control measures			
III.	Describe the community organization to promote environmental health.	**Community organizations to promote environmental health** • Levels and types of agencies: ■ National, state, local ■ Government, voluntary and social agencies • Legislations and acts regulating the environmental hygiene	6	Lecture cum discussions	• Short answer • Objective type

HEALTH EDUCATION AND COMMUNICATION SKILLS

Total Hours – 40

Unit	Learning Objectives	Content	Hours	Method of Teaching	Assessment Methods
I.	Describe the concept and different aspects of communication.	**Communication Skills** • Definition, process, purposes, principles, types and importance of communication • Barriers to communication • Establishment of successful communication • Observing and listening skills	8	• Lecture cum discussions • Demonstration Role play	• Short answers • Objective type • Return demonstration
II.	Describe the aims and objectives, scope, levels, approaches and principles of health education.	**Health Education** • Concept, definition, aims and objectives of health education • Principles of health education • Process of change/modification of health behavior • Levels and approaches of health education • Methods of health education • Scope and opportunities for health education in hospital and community • Nurse's role in health education	6	Lecture cum discussions	• Short answers • Objective type
III.	Demonstrate the skills of counseling.	**Counseling** • Definition, purpose, principles, scope and types • Counseling process: Steps and techniques • Qualities of a good counselor • Difference between health education and counseling • Role of nurse in counseling	8	• Lecture cum discussion • Role play	• Short answer • Essay type
IV.	• Describe the types of A-V aids. • Demonstrate skill in preparing and using different kinds of audio-visual aids.	**Methods and Media of Health Education** • Definition, purpose and types of audio-visual aids and media • Selection, preparation and use of audio-visual aids: Graphic aids, printed aids, three dimensional aids and projected aids • Advantages and limitations of different media • Preparation of health education plan	18	• Lecture cum discussions • Exhibit charts • Demonstration	• Evaluation of prepared audio visual aids • Written test

NUTRITION

Total Hours – 30

Unit	Learning Objectives	Content	Hours	Method of Teaching	Methods of Assessment
I.	Describe the relationship between nutrition and health.	**Introduction** • Meaning of food, nutrition, nutrients, etc. • Food habits and customs • Factors affecting nutrition • Changing concepts in food and nutrition • Relation of Nutrition to Health	2	• Lecture cum discussions • Explain using charts	• Short answer types • Objective type

II.	Describe the classification of food.	**Classification of food**
		• Classification by origin:
		  ▪ Food and animal origin
		  ▪ Food of plant origin
		• Classification by chemical composition and sources
		  ▪ Carbohydrates
		  ▪ Proteins
		  ▪ Fats
		  ▪ Minerals
		  ▪ Vitamins
		  ▪ Water
		• Classification by predominant functions
		  ▪ Body building food
		  ▪ Energy giving food
		  ▪ Protective food
		• Classification by nutritive value
		  ▪ Cereals and millets
		  ▪ Pulses and legumes
		  ▪ Vegetables
		  ▪ Nuts and oil seeds
		  ▪ Fruits
		  ▪ Animal food
		  ▪ Fats and oils
		  ▪ Sugar and jaggery
		  ▪ Condiments and spices
		  ▪ Miscellaneous food
			2	• Lecture cum discussions
				• Real food items
				• Exhibit charts
					• Short answers
					• Objective type
					• Essay type

III.	• Explain normal dietary requirements • Demonstrate skill in calculating normal food requirements.	**Normal Dietary Requirements** • Energy: Calorie, Measurement, Body Mass Index, Basal Metabolic Rate—determination and factors affecting	4	• Lecture cum discussions • Exhibit charts • Real food • Practical exercise	• Short answer • Objective type • Essay type

Contd...

Unit	Learning Objectives	Content	Hours	Method of Teaching	Methods of Assessment
		• Balanced Diet—nutritive value of foods, calculation for different categories of people, normal food requirement calculation. Menu plan. Combination of food affecting and enhancing the nutritive value of the diet. Budgeting for food, low cost meals, food substitutes • Diseases and disorders caused by the imbalance of nutrients • Food allergy—causes, types, diet modifications in glutein, lactose and protein intolerance, etc. • Food intolerance—inborn errors of metabolism			
IV.	Describe the principles and various methods of preparation, preservation and storage of food.	**Food Preparation, Preservation & Storage** • Principles of cooking, methods of cooking and the effect of cooking on food and various nutrients, safe food handling, health of food handlers • Methods of food preservation—household and commercial, precautions • Food storage—cooked and raw, household and commercial, ill effects of poorly stored food • Food adulteration and Acts related to it	2	• Lecture cum discussions • Field visit to food processing unit • Demonstration exhibits	• Short answer type • Objective type • Evaluation of exhibit preparation
V.	Describe the therapeutic diet.	**Therapeutic Diet** • Diet modification in relation to medical and surgical condition of the individual such as Protein Energy Malnutrition (PEM), Diabetes, Cardiovascular disease, Hepatitis, Renal, Gouts, Irritable Bowel Syndrome (IBS), Obesity, cholecystectomy, partial gastrectomy, gastrostomy, bariatric surgery and colostomy, etc. • Special diet—low sodium diet, fat free diet, diabetic diet, bland diet, high protein diet, low protein diet, low calorie diet, geriatric diet, iron rich diet, liquid diet, semi-solid diet, soft diet and high fiber diet, etc.	8	• Lecture cum discussions • Practical of planning Therapeutic diet • Demonstration • Exhibit charts	• Short answers • Objective type • Essay type

Contd...

Unit	Learning Objectives	Content	Hours	Method of Teaching	Methods of Assessment
		• Factors affecting diet acceptance, feeding the helpless patient • Health education on nutrition needs and methods in diet modification			
VI.	Describe the concept of community nutrition.	**Community Nutrition** • Nutritional problems and programs in India • Community food supply, food hygiene and commercially prepared and grown food available locally • National and international food agencies—Central Food Training Research Institute (CFTRI), Food and Agriculture Organization (FAO), National Institute of Nutrition (NIN), Food Safety and Standards Authority of India (FSSAI), Cooperative for Assistance and Relief Everywhere (CARE), National Institute of Public Cooperation and Child Development (NIPCCD), etc.	4	• Lecture cum discussions • Videos • Government of India nutrition manuals • Visit to the local food preparation/ processing agency	• Short answer • Objective type
VII.	Demonstrate skill in preparation of common food items.	**Preparation of diet/practical** • Beverages: Hot and cold, juice, shakes, soups, lassi, barley water • Egg preparation: Egg flip, scramble, omlet, poached egg • Light diet: Porridges, gruel, khichari, dahlia, kanji, boiled vegetables, salads, custards • Low cost high nutrition diets—chikki, multigrain roti	8	• Lecture cum discussions • Cookery practical	Practical evaluation

Contents

Section 1 Community Health

Unit 1 Introduction to Community Health 3–33

Unit 2 Community Health Nursing 34–54

Unit 3 Health Assessment 55–86

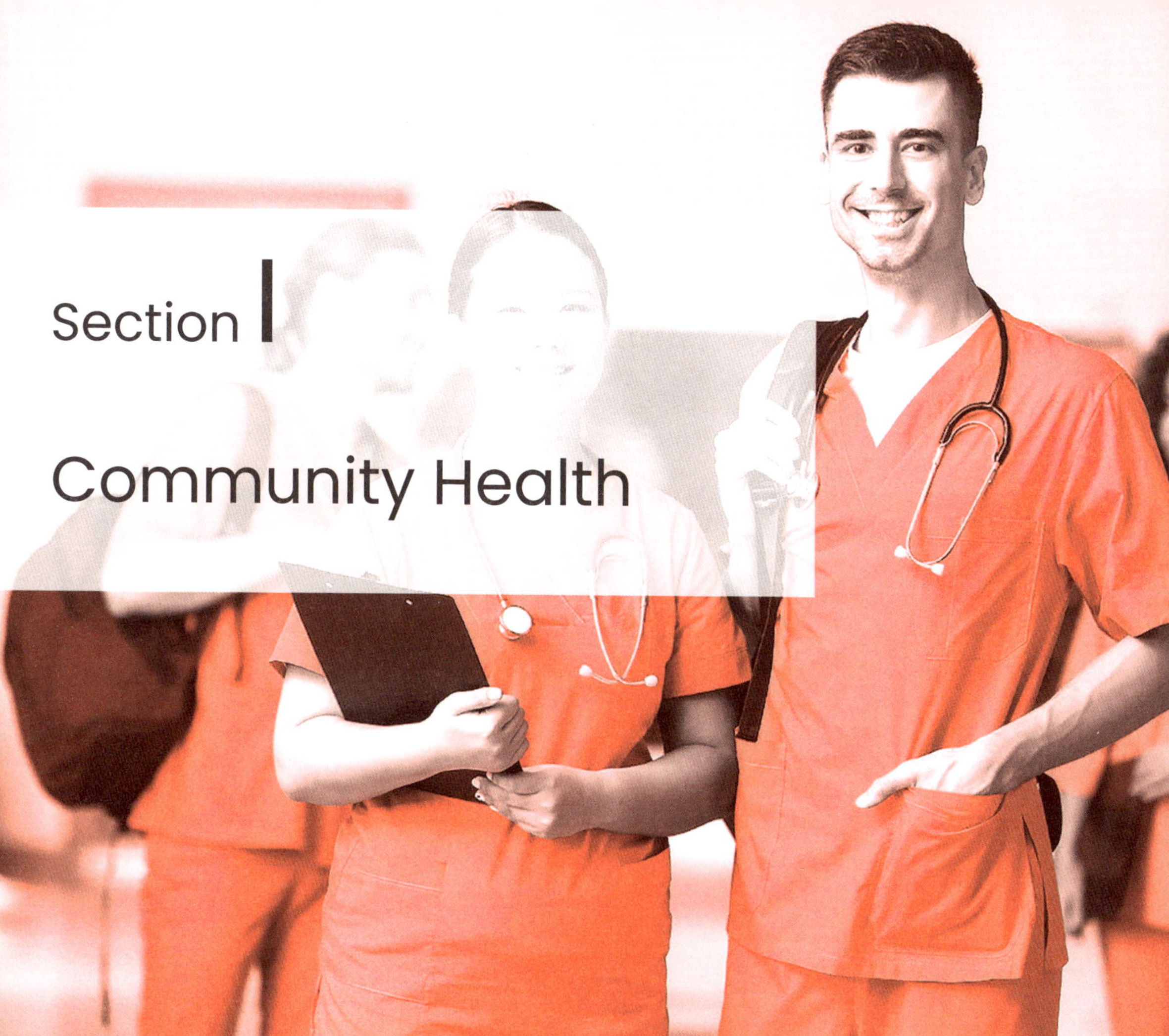

Section I

Community Health

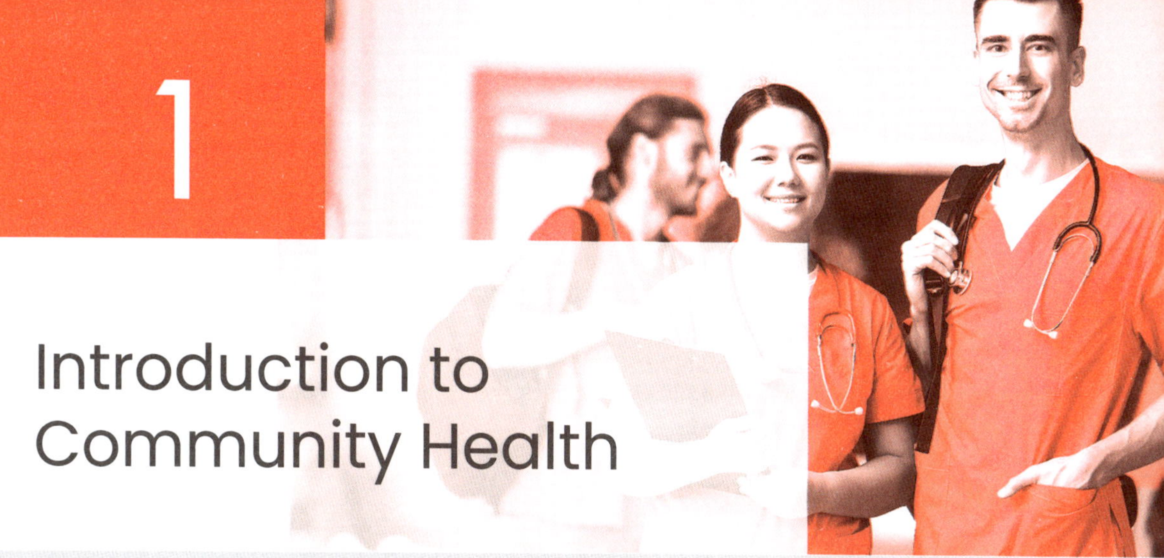

1

Introduction to Community Health

LEARNING OBJECTIVES

After the completion of the unit, the readers will be able to:
- Describe the concept of health and disease.
- Discuss the concepts of community health.
- Describe primary healthcare and Millennium Development Goals.

UNIT OUTLINE

- Introduction
- Meaning of Community
- Definitions
- Components
- Characteristics
- Types
- Functions
- Differences between Urban and Rural Communities
- Community Health
- Public Health
- Community Health: The Prevalent Concept
- Community Diagnosis
- Community Treatment
- Responsibilities for Community Health
- Community Health Nursing
- Concept of Health and Disease
- Dimensions of Health
- Health Indicators
- Determinants of Health
- History and Development of Community Health
- Development of Community Health Nursing in India
- Present Concept of Community Health
- Primary Healthcare
- Millennium Development Goals
- Promotion and Maintenance of Health
- Sustainable Development Goals

KEY TERMS

Concept: It is an abstract or generic idea generalized from particular instances.

Deleterious: This is used to describe things that are harmful in an unexpected manner and slow-acting.

Dimensions: It is a measurement of something in a particular direction, especially, its height, length, or width.

Dormant: The term suggests the inactivity of something, for example, missing of a feeling or power.

Equitable: It is a kind of dealing fairly with all concerned.

Health: A state of physical, mental, social and spiritual well-being and not merely the absence of disease or infirmity.

Indicators: Devices that provide specific information.

Synonyms: Having the same meaning.

INTRODUCTION

Community is a group of interacting organisms sharing a populated environment. The community has been described as the most useful area for improving the health of people by providing them better healthcare services. The fact is that the social, physical and cultural aspects of community influence the health status of the individual. To improve the health status and bring change in the attitude of the community toward health to avail healthcare facilities, the living standard of the community has to be improved.

MEANING OF COMMUNITY

The word "community" has been derived from the Latin word communitas ("communis" "cum", with/together + "munus", gift). The word "community" is used in many different ways in a wide variety of situations. The one element of community is identified as a "sense of place; something that could be located and described; denoting sense of boundaries". A community is an identified area or location such as city, town, village, a neighborhood or even workplace. The members of the community share their values, norms, religion, interests, worries, needs, happiness and suffering with the other members.

Other identified elements of community are "joint actions that bring people together or social ties such as family, friends and diversity".

DEFINITIONS

"A community is a social group characterized by geographical boundaries and/or common values and interests". Its members know and interact with each other. It functions within a particular social structure and exhibits and creates certain norms, values and social institutions. The individual belongs to the broader society through his family and community.

—**World Health Organization, 1974**

"A group of people who share same type of bond, who interact with each other, and who function collectively regarding common concerns".   —**Green and Anderson, 1986**

A community is defined as a "group of people, having intimacy, informal relations, common culture and living together in specific geographical boundaries".   —**Paul B Horton, 1992**

COMPONENTS

- **People:** They are the essence of community and give identity to the community. Community cannot be visualized without people. People have knowledge, values, culture, attitudes and beliefs. There are different age groups, income levels and educational levels.
- **Goals and needs:** Community has goals and needs. Nurses should help community to determine its health needs and goals to plan realistic services.
- **Environment:** Community has social, physical, biological and sociocultural environments, which influences the health needs of the people.
- **Service system:** Community has service system by which people meet their basic and specific health needs. According to Sanders (1966), the major service systems of the community are:
    - Health
    - Education
    - Governmental
    - Religious
    - Social welfare
    - Economic
    - Recreational

- **Boundaries:** Communities have boundaries, which may be concrete (definite and spatial) or conceptual (nonspatial). Definite boundaries can be seen such as mountains, deserts and political (cities and towns).

Conceptual boundaries are less definite and flexible in nature. These include boundaries, such as interest area, problem solving and service area. Boundaries of the community serve to regulate the interchange of energies between the community and its external environment.

CHARACTERISTICS

The health personnel need to know the characteristics of a community to meet its health needs and tackle its problems. The characteristics of a community are:

- **Homogeneity:** People living in a defined boundary of community have similarity in psychosocial characteristics, i.e., they have similarity in language, customs, behavior, lifestyle and traditions. Homogeneity is more common in smaller community.
- **Distinctiveness:** Each community has defined geographical boundaries having its beginning and an end. These boundaries are more remarkable in the smaller communities rather than in the larger communities.
- **Closeness:** People in community have close interaction and free communication. They participate frequently in common activities, e.g., visiting, community meals, exchanging and borrowing things.
- **Sense of belongingness:** The people in the community have community feelings and identify themselves with the community. The intensity and degree of these feeling may vary among the members of the community.
- **Sense of togetherness:** There is unity among the members of the community, which is based on their interaction and sense of belongingness.
- **Self-sufficiency:** Community provides facilities which help in meeting the basic needs of people, e.g., space to live, education, protection, security and means of livelihood.

TYPES

- **Geographic communities:** These communities refer to the communities of location. These range from neighborhood, village, town and city, region, nation or even planet as a whole.
- **Community of culture:** Culture in communities ranges from local clique, subculture, ethnic group, religious, multicultural or pluralistic civilization or the global community cultures of today.
- **Community organization:** These communities include from informal family network to more incorporated associations, political decision-making structures, economic enterprises or professional associations, health agencies, hospitals, labor unions, etc.

FUNCTIONS

The functions of community are to provide the goals and needs of members of community as accepted and supported by constitutions, formal legislation and regulations, moral and ethical codes developed by the community. Warren (1978) has described some of the functions of community as follows:

- Community provides space for housing, shelter for socialization and for recreation. Through socialization, people learn team work; how to relate to others effectively.
- Community provides opportunity for education and occupation to its members.
- It provides opportunity for employment.
- It creates and enforces norms and rules for social control for safety and security of its members.
- It provides for production, distribution and consumption of necessary goods and services for meeting the health and welfare needs of its people.
- It provides opportunities for interaction amongst members, transmits information, ideas and beliefs and provides support system.
- There are linkages with social system outside the community for meeting needs of its member.

DIFFERENCES BETWEEN URBAN AND RURAL COMMUNITIES

Differences between urban and rural communities are given in Table 1.1.

TABLE 1.1: Differences between urban and rural communities

Urban community	Rural community
Size: Geographical boundaries are large and may be >1,000 families.	The boundaries are small as size of rural community is small.
Density: With increase in size of community, the density of urban community increases.	Rural community is less dense because of low population.
Occupation: Because of more educational facilities and career opportunities, people are economically stable and lead luxurious life.	Less educational facilities and career opportunities, people are economically weak and lead hard life.
Population: Due to more educational and employment facilities, people are attracted toward urban areas of the world resulting in overcrowding.	Due to lesser number of people inhabiting the rural area, population is small and overcrowding is not there.
Health: Due to increased industrialization, the environmental pollution increases resulting in more health problems.	Pollution is less due to less industrialization, afforestation and ample space for plantation, the environmental balance is maintained.
Lifestyle: The life is fast and led lavishly.	The life is not led lavishly but people are generous and their hearts have rooms for emotions.
Satisfaction: Rise in prosperity and fast life resulted in disturbed peace.	People are not very prosperous but they live peaceful life.
Social interaction: Social interaction is less due to self-centered nature of the people. Social support is weak.	Social interaction is more and they help each other in times of need. Social support is very strong.

COMMUNITY HEALTH

The term "community health" has replaced the terms "public health", "preventive medicine" and "social medicine" because there is an element of individual responsibility and voluntary cooperation in community health. Though the meaning of community health and public health is same.

According to World Health Organization (WHO, 1971) "community health means the states of health of the members of community, problems affecting their health and health facilities available in community". It means community health is related to preventive, curative and promotional services and it focuses on health problems of community.

PUBLIC HEALTH

According to Winslow (1920), public health is "the science and art of preventing disease, prolonging life and promoting physical health and efficiency through organized state effort, by the sanitation of the environment, the control of infections, the education of the individual in principles of personal hygiene, the organization of medical and nursing service and the early diagnosis and preventive treatment of disease and the development of social machinery which will ensure to every individual a standard of living adequate for the maintenance of health, it is the organizing of these benefits in such a fashion as to enable every citizen to realize his birthright of health and longevity".

Public health is comprised of many professional disciplines like medicine, dentistry, nursing, optometry, nutrition, social work, environmental science, health education, health service, administration, behavior sciences, demography, epidemiology, biostatistics and statistics.

The mission of public health is to fulfill society's interest in ensuring condition in which people can be healthy. Public health professionals monitor and diagnose the health concern of entire communities and promote healthy practices and behaviors to ensure populations stay healthy. So, the focus of public health is to prevent rather than to treat a disease through surveillance of cases and the promotion of healthy behavior but in certain cases, treating the disease may be vital to prevent such as during the outbreak of an infectious disease. Handwashing, vaccination program and distribution of condom are examples of public health measures. Public health is typically divided into epidemiology, biostatistics and health services. Environmental, social and behavioral are its subfields. So, public health deals with preventive rather than curative aspects of health. It deals with population level rather than individual level health issues.

COMMUNITY HEALTH: THE PREVALENT CONCEPT

Community health is directly responsible for the health of the individual. It implies that all those facilities should be available in a community that are essential for providing prophylaxis, treatment and care to all members.

Community health is defined more broadly and includes the community-organized effort for maintaining, protecting and improving the health of the people. It includes preventive, promotive and curative health services. It is concerned with motivating people to change their behavior and lifestyle encouraging them to seek timely healthcare services. The aim of community health is to reduce the incidence of disease and disability in community. It is done through a team of health professionals, i.e., doctors, nurses, auxiliary nurses and midwives (ANM), female and male health workers, members of other disciplines like sociology, demography, epidemiology and statistics.

Its focus is community as a client, assessing community health needs, making community diagnosis and community treatment.

COMMUNITY DIAGNOSIS

Diagnosis is the basic necessity to treat a disease. It is the discovery of medical disease based on the signs and symptoms. Similarly, the community diagnosis refers to the problems of the community. So, intervention can be planned based on the problems of the community.

- Community diagnosis is defined as the pattern of disease in a community described in terms of important factors which influence the pattern.
- Community diagnosis is the foundation of health services which focus on finding out the health-related problems and needs of society.
- Community diagnosis is the first step in establishing health program.
- **Process of community diagnosis comprises the following steps:**
    1. Divide the population in social groups.
    2. Divide the population by age and sex.
    3. Recognition and categorization of qualitative and quantitative facts.
    4. To assess the magnanimity and epidemic nature of major disease as community diagnosis forms the basis of community treatment. It must reflect the health needs and health problems of the community. It is essential to pay attention to those social and economic factors which influence health.

COMMUNITY TREATMENT

"Community treatment refers to the steps taken in accordance with the desire of the public and the available resources to solve those health problems of the community which were ascertained through community diagnosis". It is also called the community health action. It should be acceptable, affordable, effective, safe and should involve intersectoral coordination and community participation.

Examples of community treatment are:

- Improvement in environmental sanitation
- Safe drinking water
- Health education
- Health-related laws
- Immunization
- Supply of iodized salt
- Supply of fortified foods
- Controlling of some specific diseases

Community treatment is provided at three levels:

1. Individual
2. Family
3. Community

The success of community treatment depends upon:

- Effective use of available resources
- Maintaining coordination and interrelation among other resources and agencies
- Encouraging the community to participate in health program

RESPONSIBILITIES FOR COMMUNITY HEALTH

- Individual responsibility
- Community responsibility
- National government responsibility
- International agencies responsibility

Individual Responsibility

Individuals are responsible for their own health. They should adopt healthful ways of living. They should follow the following rules:
- Related to food, exercise, rest and sleep
- Avoid smoking, drinking and drug addiction
- Avoid unhealthy habits and unhealthy lifestyle
- Immunization, regular health checkup
- Early treatment of disease

Community Responsibility

Many healthy activities can be completed with collective efforts. Cooperation and participation of community is essential. The activities of community participation include the following:
- Manpower facilities, moral agreement and funds are made available by the community for health activities.
- Active participation by the community in planning, implementation, management and evaluation of health programs.
- Maximum utilization of health services by the community.
- Understanding that fight against disease is not the sole responsibility of doctors, nurses or health workers.
- Participating actively in eradication of diseases with determination and devotion.

National Government Responsibility

The Indian Constitution has recognized health as a concurrent subject and an issue of concern to state as well as central government and placed its responsibility on both of them. India has also signed the Alma Ata declaration (1978), and Health for All by 2000; was accepted as the foundation of our health policy 1983 and new health policy has been released in September 2002 and Millennium Development Goals (MDGs) were developed and MDGs have shown the way for more Sustainable Development Goals (SDGs), the development agenda adopted in September 2015 by the United Nations General Assembly.

International Agencies Responsibility

Though health is the responsibility of individual but community, government and international organizations have an important role in it. WHO and other health institutions are shouldering this responsibility and continually working to achieve these goals. WHO is the principal body, which regulates and coordinates international health programs.

COMMUNITY HEALTH NURSING

"Community health nursing is a comprehensive branch of nursing which deals with recognition of nursing needs, nursing assessment, nursing diagnosis, planning and intervention of nursing care and its evaluation to the individual, families and community. Community health nursing is a collaborative application of nursing and public health measures within the framework of the total community health efforts".

—**Freeman, 1970**

CONCEPTS OF HEALTH AND DISEASE

Health

Health is a state when all body systems are functioning well and are in a dynamic equilibrium. It is a general condition of the person when there are no physical, mental, social or spiritual discomfort. There are many definitions of health.

"The condition of being sound in body, mind or spirit, especially freedom from disease or pain".

—**Webster English Dictionary**

"Soundness of body and mind; the condition in which its functions are duly and efficiently discharged".

—**Oxford English Dictionary**

"A state of relative equilibrium of body form and functions which result from its successful dynamic adjustment of forces tending to disturb it. It is not passive interplay between body substance and forces infringing upon it but an active response of the body forces working toward adjustment".   —**Perkins**

"A state of complete physical, mental and social well-being and not merely the absence of disease or infirmity".

—**World Health Organization, 1948**

The World Health Assembly in 1977 decided that the major social goal of government and WHO should be the attainment by all the people of the world by the year 2000 of a level of health that would permit them to lead a socially and economically productive life. "Health for All" does not mean that nobody will fall sick or there will be no disease or disability or the health workers will care for them. It means that the resources for health will be adequate, evenly distributed and essential healthcare will be accessible to all. The people will be health conscious and there will be awareness about health facilities available and they will be able to solve their health problems and needs.

Concepts of Health

The concepts of health (Fig. 1.1) have been changing with newer discoveries in the field of health, some of the changing concepts of health are:

- **Biomedical concept:** This concept is based on the principal of "Germ Theory", i.e., the disease or ill health is due to disease causing organisms. This concept is rejected as it fails to explain that many diseases are not due to

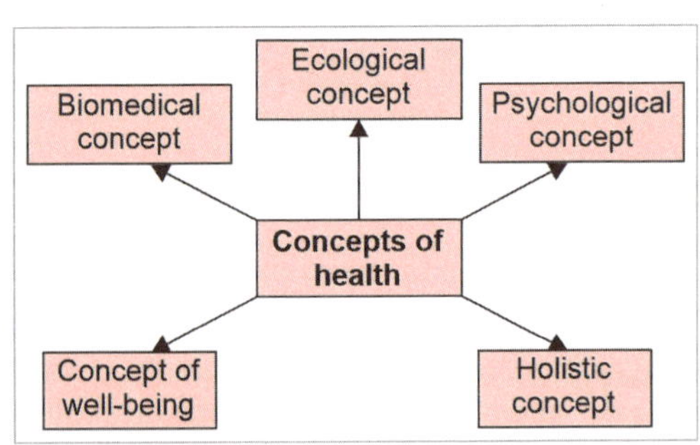

Fig. 1.1: Concepts of health

disease-causing organisms. Other factors prevalent in the environment like malnutrition, drug addiction, accidents, pollution, and mental illness are not due to disease-causing germs. This concept has been discarded.

- **Ecological concept:** According to this concept, health has been considered a dynamic equilibrium between man and his environment or an adjustment between man and his environment or balance between man and his environment. But the research could not prove that merely improving the adjustment of man and his environment, the complete goal of health can be achieved. This concept was also rejected.

- **Psychological concept:** According to social scientist, physical health and psychological well-being are inter-related. Health is influenced by one's feeling, i.e., love, affection, happiness, fear, anger, jealousy, guilt, sadness and worries. Individual's relation with his fellow may precipitate the onset of psychosocial disorders. So, health is influenced by social, psychological, economical, cultural and political factors. This concept implies that health is a biological and social issue.

- **Holistic concept:** This model is synthesis of all the aforementioned concepts. It relates to the strength of social, psychological, economical, political and environmental influence on health. All the sectors in the society like agriculture, industry, animal husbandry, education, housing, public works department, communication and political system influence health. Health is viewed as a multidimensional process involving the well-being of the whole person in the context of his biophysiological, sociological and psychological environment.

- **Concept of well-being:** This concept is based on the definition of health by WHO. "Health is a state of physical, mental and social well-being." Though the social well-being part is not clearly explained, it refers to the improvement in standard and quality of life. According to psychologists, there are subjective and objective aspects of well-being. The objective aspect includes health education, occupation, food consumption, colony housing, recreation, human right and social security. All these characteristics influence human life directly or indirectly. Among all, health component is the most important because if health is impaired, standard of living is affected.

  The subjective aspect includes individual's feeling of happiness, satisfaction or sadness about number of life concerns, i.e., the quality of life is defined as a complete measure of physical, mental and social well-being as perceived by each individual as it is experienced in such life concerns as health, marriage, family work, financial situation, educational opportunity, self-esteem, creativity, belonging and trust in others.

  So, the standard of living along with quality of life must be increased to attain a feeling of well-being.

Disease

In simple term, "Disease is a condition that is opposite to health which intervenes with the normal mental and physical functioning of body or which affects the normal functioning of different organs and systems of body.

Concept of Disease

The term "disease" is opposite to comfort. The English word "disease" actually means dis-ease which refers to the uneasiness, discomfort, distress, inconvenience and a state of being uncomfortable.

- **According to Oxford English dictionary**, "Disease is a state of body or its organs which either interferes with the functioning of the body or deranges its functions".
- **According to Ecology**, "Disease is a condition of maladjustment between the environment and organs of human body".
- **Webster defines disease** as "A condition in which body health is impaired, a departure from a state of health, an alternation of the human body interrupting the performance of vital functions".
- **Social scientists** believe that disease is a social phenomenon or condition that is found in every society.

All these definitions are considered inadequate as they neither give criteria by which to decide when a disease state confirms nor they define measurement of disease. WHO has defined health but not disease because disease has many spectrums ranging from subclinical cases to severe manifestations of illness.

Spectrum of Disease

Disease can be acute, chronic, infections, moderately severe or severe. But the clinical manifestations of the disease may be different. Some diseases commence acutely, e.g., food poisoning, and some insidiously, e.g., essential hypertension, cardiovascular diseases, rheumatoid arthritis and mental illness.

In some diseases, a carrier state occurs in which the individual remains outwardly healthy and is able to infect others, e.g., typhoid fever. In some other conditions, the same organism may cause more than one clinical manifestation. In some instances, more than one organism may cause the same disease, e.g., diarrhea. Similarly, some diseases have a short course and some others may have prolonged course.

A disease can be easily diagnosed when the signs and symptoms are well marked. But in many diseases, a border line between normal and abnormal is indistinct as in cases of mental illness, hypertension and diabetes mellitus. The outcome of a disease is variable, i.e., recovery, disability or death of the host. This variation in the presentation of signs and symptoms of the disease is called the spectrum of disease.

Spectrum of disease (Fig. 1.2) may be affected by various factors, i.e., immunity, receptivity level of the individual to infection and the external environmental factors. The spectrum of disease can be represented in Figures 1.2 and 1.3.

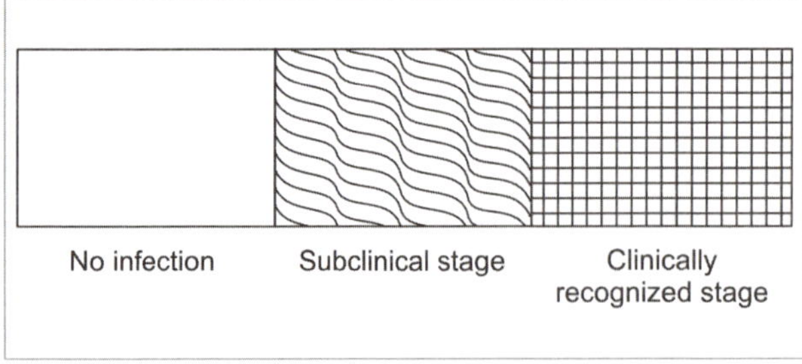

Fig. 1.2: Spectrum of disease

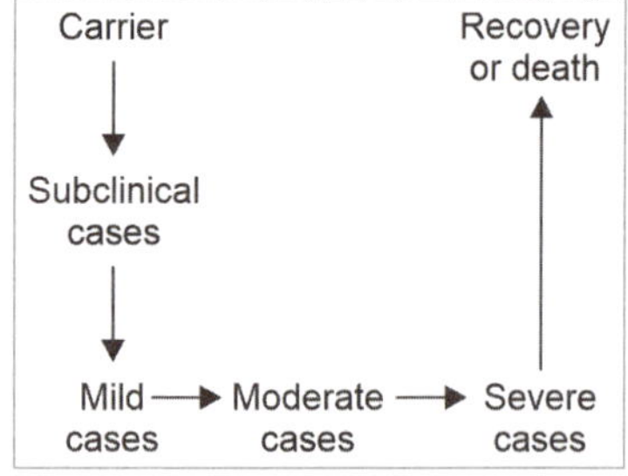

Fig. 1.3: Spectrum of disease

Synonyms of Disease

Distinction is made between the disease, illness and sickness. The word "disease" means without ease, i.e., opposite to ease or uneasiness. Illness means the presence of a specific disease and the individual's perception and behavior in response to disease as well as the impact of disease on psychosocial environment. The sickness refers to a state of social dysfunction. Susser has suggested that illness is a subjective state of the person who feels aware of not being well. Sickness is a state of social dysfunction, i.e., the role that the individual assumes when ill (sickness sole). Disease is a physiological/psychological dysfunction. A clinician sees people who are ill rather than the disease which he must diagnose and treat. In some instances, it is possible to be a victim of the disease without feeling ill and to be ill without exhibiting the signs of physical impairment. So, an adequate definition of disease is yet to be found which is satisfactory or acceptable to clinicians, epidemiologists and sociologists.

Iceberg of Disease

Only clinical cases can be diagnosed by the doctor, while the subclinical cases and the cases with primary symptoms which are usually more in number remain unrecognized and hidden in society. This condition resembles an iceberg floating in water, a very small portion of ice is visible above the surface of water—this is called the iceberg of disease (Fig. 1.4).

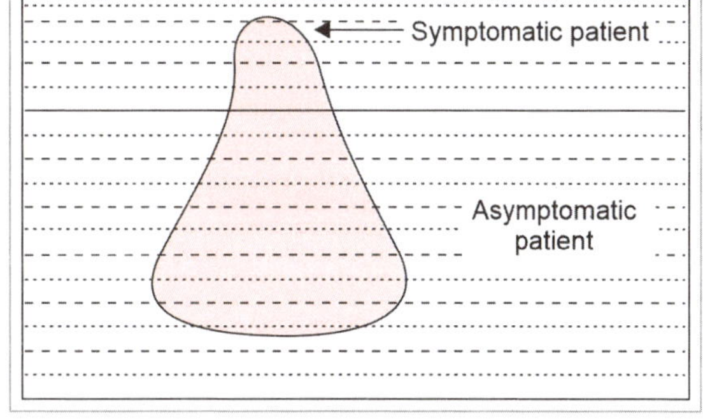

Fig. 1.4: Iceberg of disease

Concept of Causation

Various concepts of disease causation were considered up to the time of Louis Pasteur. Discoveries in microbiology brought a turning point in etiological concepts. The changing concept about "disease" can be explained on the basis of the following theories:

Germ Theory of Disease

Germ theory was propounded by Louis Pasteur. According to this theory, emphasis shifted from empirical causes to microbes as the sole cause of disease. But the pathologists consider this theory incomplete due to its stress on the "One disease one germ" concept and the other causes of disease are not considered.

Supernatural Theory

In the past, the disease was thought to be due to evil spirit, ghost, magical spell and supernatural powers. Superstitions and lack of knowledge could be the basis of this theory.

Epidemiological Triad Theory

Along with germs, host and environment are also responsible for the disease. According to the epidemiological triad theory, the germs, host and environment form a broad base for the growth of diseases and hence, they form epidemiological triad (Fig. 1.5).

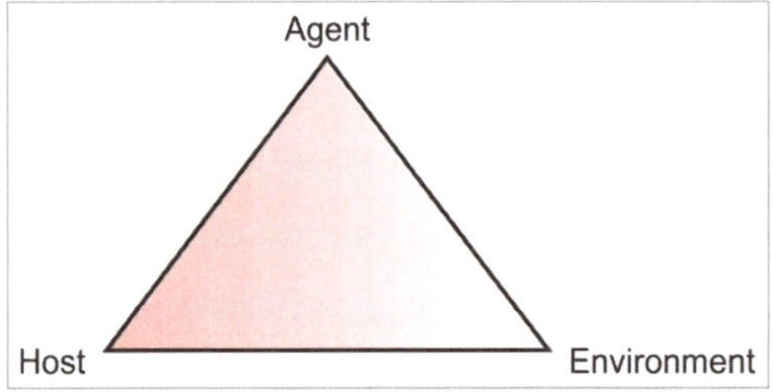

Fig. 1.5: Epidemiological triad

Multifactor Theory

According to multifactor theory, many factors are responsible for a disease. In addition to epidemiological triad and germs, the other factors like social, economic, cultural and psychological factors are also responsible for the disease. So, multifactor theory is in consideration in present day to be the origin of disease.

DIMENSIONS OF HEALTH

Health is a multidimensional subject. There are many definitions and different concepts of health. WHO definition of health implies three dimensions, i.e., physical, mental and social. Spiritual dimension is also included. There are some other nonmedical dimensions which affect the health of the individuals. Health workers working in community should have knowledge of these dimensions.

Various dimensions of health are:

- Physical dimension
- Mental dimension
- Social dimension
- Spiritual dimension
- Emotional dimension
- Vocational and economic dimension
- Educational dimension
- Nutritional dimension
- Environmental dimension

Physical Dimension

Physical dimension refers to the complete body functions. Every cell, tissue or organ of the body is functioning normally. Vital signs are in normal state, there is good appetite, sound sleep, good complexion, clear skin, eyes, normal size and functions of body organs, good coordinated movements, intact senses, regular bowel and bladder habits, and the weight is proportionate to the body size. Physical dimension can be assessed by self-assessment, questionnaires, clinical examination and laboratory investigations.

Mental Dimension

Mental dimension is considered to be a balance between man and his environment, between self and others, a state of friendly coexistence of individual with his realities, environment and other people, there is a close relationship between body and mind. Many physical ailments have psychological factors as the basis of their occurrence such as asthma, peptic ulcer and essential hypertension.

A mentally healthy person is free from internal conflicts, having self-control, recognizes his weakness and abilities. He has got ability to accept criticism and solve his problems of health, get along well with others. Of all the dimensions of health, mental dimension is very important and key to achieve optimum health.

Social Dimension

Social dimension is related to the ability of an individual to see himself as a member of the society. It includes social status, social skill, social activities, cooperation and good interpersonal relationships. The quality of family life and human environment of a person are related to his social make up and influenced by the social system of the society.

Spiritual Dimension

Spirituality helps in setting and achieving the goals of life. It involves complete submission to the supreme authority, principles, conduct and moral values. It refers to the individuals striving for finding meaning and purpose in life.

Emotional Dimension

Emotional dimension includes feelings such as joy, happiness, excitement, anger, sadness. An emotionally healthy person controls his feelings and maintains balance.

Vocational and Economic Dimension

Vocational and economic dimension is related to the job satisfaction and economic independence. It gives an individual a sense of achievement, purpose and self-realization. Economic independence gives individual self-respect, happiness and satisfaction. An unemployed individual is socially and economically dependent and is an unhappy and disintegrated personality. Similarly, financial mismanagement may destroy the health of an individual, family and even community.

Educational Dimension

Education contributes to the quality of life. An educated person obeys the health rules and inculcates good health habits. On the other hand, illiteracy leads to malnutrition, anemia, obesity due to lack of health knowledge. The physical, mental and social well-being of an individual is partly from the effect of education.

Nutritional Dimension

A well-balanced diet plays an important role in growth, development, promotion and maintenance of health. Poor nutrition causes stunted growth, delays developmental milestones and predisposes to infections. Nutrition is associated with immunity, fertility, maternal, child and family health. Culture influences health. Healthy cultural practices promote health and unhealthy ones lead to suffering. Nutritious food trends of culture maintain health, whereas faulty food trends of a culture may result in poor health.

Environmental Dimension

Environmental dimension includes the internal and external environmental dimensions. The internal refers to our body systems and their normal functioning within our body. The external environment includes the physical, biological, psychosocial and chemical environment. All these have direct impact on human well-being. So, favorable environment contributes to good health, whereas unfavorable environment may result in physical and mental ailments.

HEALTH INDICATORS

Health indicators measure the health status of a community but they also compare the health status of one country with that of another, for the assessment of healthcare needs, for monitoring and evaluation of health services, activities and health program. According to WHO, "Indicators are variables which help to measure changes, often they are used particularly when these changes cannot be measured directly, for example, health or nutritional status.

Characteristics of Health Indicators

- **Valid:** Indicators should actually measure what they are supposed to measure.
- **Reliable and objective:** Answers should be same if measured by different people in similar situation.
- **Sensitive:** Indicators should reflect the changes in the situation correctly.
- **Specific:** Indicators should correctly identify the true negative and should not give false positive results.
- **Feasible:** Indicators should have the ability to obtain required data.
- **Relevant:** Indicators should contribute to the understanding of the phenomena of interest.

Objectives of Health Indicators

- To determine community health standard
- To compare health standards with different countries
- To investigate the need of health services
- To distribute the resources properly
- To conduct research on health
- To evaluate the activities, programs and targets of health services.

Types of Health Indicators

According to various concepts of health, there are many indicators. To achieve optimum level of health, the indicators are classified into two main categories.

- **Direct or specific indicators:** These indicators are directly related to medical science and health services. These indicators include the following:
  - Mortality indicators
  - Morbidity indicators
  - Disability indicators
  - Healthcare delivery indicators
  - Health policy indicators

- **Indirect or general indicators:** These indicators influence the health directly or indirectly. They are based on nutrition, environment, economic level, politics, society, consumption level and standard of living. Some of the general indicators are:
  - Social and mental indicator
  - Socioeconomic indicators
  - Nutritional status indicators
  - Utilization rate indicators
  - Environmental indicators
  - Indicators of quality of life

Direct or Specific Indicators

Direct indicators include the following:

- **Infant mortality rate (IMR):** It is the ratio of death under 1 year of age in a given year to the total number of live births in the same year usually expressed as a rate per 1000 live births. It is one of the most universally accepted indicators of health status not only of infants but also of whole population and of the socioeconomic conditions under which they live. In addition, the infant mortality rate is a sensitive indicator of the availability, utilization and effectiveness of perinatal care.
- **Maternal mortality rate (MMR):** It refers to the total number of female deaths due to complication of pregnancy, child birth within 42 days of delivery from puerperal causes in an area during a given year per 1000 live births in the same area in the same year. It is high in developing and underdeveloped countries.
- **Crude death rate:** It indicates the number of people dying in a year for every thousand people of a country's population. A reduced crude death rate indicates the success of health services in a particular country.
- **Life expectancy:** Life expectancy at birth is "the average number of years that will be lived by those born alive into a population if the current age-specific mortality rate persists". Life expectancy at birth is influenced by infant mortality rate where that is high life expectancy at the age of 1 and life expectancy at the age of 5 excludes the influence of child mortality rate.
- **Child mortality rate:** It is defined as the number of deaths at age 1–4 years in a given year per 1000 children in that age group at the midpoint of the year.
- **Disease specific mortality rate:** It is defined as the number of deaths from a specific disease during the year per 1000 midyear population. Deaths from cancer, cardiovascular diseases, accidents, diabetes, etc. have emerged as measures of specific disease problems.
- **Proportional mortality rate:** It is the simplest measure of estimating the burden of a disease in the community. Proportional mortality rate from communicable diseases has been suggested as a useful health status indicator. It indicates the magnitude of preventable mortality.
- **Morbidity indicators:** These indicators show the health status of the population, but cannot describe the health status of the population. They cannot determine the undemonstrative subclinical conditions present in the community. The morbidity in community is assessed on the basis of the following:
  - Incidence and prevalence
  - Rate of notifying the disease
  - Attendance rates at outpatient department and health center
  - Admissions, discharge and readmission rates

- Occupancy rate and duration of stay in the hospital
- Absence from school or work
- **Disability rate:** It refers to the inability of a person to perform activities of daily living or the increase in morbidity or mortality rate. It is measured by the number of working days a person was bedridden and the restriction of movements and daily routine completion.
- **Healthcare delivery indicators:** These indicators show the availability and distribution of health services and provision of healthcare in the community. These include:
  - Doctor-population ratio
  - Doctor-nurse ratio
  - Population bed ratio
  - Population per healthcare center, sub center
  - Patient-nurse ratio
  - Population per traditional birth attendant
- **Health policy indicators:** These are the indicators of political commitment. The allocation of adequate resources, the actual and proposed expenses in the budget assigned in the health services to take care of primary health and health-related activities are the relevant health policy indicators.

Indirect or General Indicators

- **Social and mental health indicators:** These include suicide, homicide, violence, crime, road accident, juvenile delinquency, alcohol and drug abuse, smoking, consumption of tranquilizers, family violence, battered baby and battered wife syndrome, neglected and abandoned youth; all of them provide a guide to social action for improving the health of the people.
- **Socioeconomic indicators:** These indicators are the direct measure of health. These include:
  - Rate of increase of population
  - Rate of unemployment
  - Size of the family
  - Literacy rate, especially female literacy rate
  - Place of living, i.e., housing
  - Per capita income
- **National status indicators:** It is related to the birthweight of the child, height and growth chart of children which are the indicators of health status.
- **Utilization rate:** Utilization level of health services can be assessed on the basis of ratio of vaccinated children, ratio of pregnant mothers, number of people using family planning methods, hospital occupancy and discharge ratio.
- **Environmental indicators:** These reflect the quality of physical and biological environment in which people are exposed to the hazards of the polluted environment. These environment indicators include pollution of air, water, sound, radiation, solid waste, improper lighting and ventilation, exposure to toxic substances in food and water.

DETERMINANTS OF HEALTH

Health is influenced by many factors. It is a multidimensional phenomenon. In addition to the physical, mental and social factors, health is influenced by environmental factors, i.e., socioeconomic conditions, cultural patterns, the political system, behavior patterns and the healthcare delivery system. Health is determined within the individual as well as the environment in which the person lives. The important determinants are described as follows:

Biological Determinants

The heredity and genetic factors have remarkable influence on physical and mental health of the individual. The genetic endowment sets the boundaries of abilities and potential of the individual. The genetic heritage is less modifiable than other determinants. Some metabolic diseases, chromosomal abnormalities and mental retardation have genetic origin. The health worker's responsibility is to provide genetic counseling to the people who are at risk of having impaired children.

Environmental Determinants

Environmental determinants include the internal and external environment. Internal environment refers to harmonious functioning of all the body systems. The external environment is the sum total of things to which the individual is exposed, i.e., physical, biological and psychosocial factors. Environmental pollution is becoming a threat to human health. Air, water, noise, radiation, housing, waste management, etc. affect the health status and quality of life.

Political System

The political system has the power and authority to regulate the social climate in which we live. Healthcare program cannot be implemented properly without strong political will. The coordination between union and state government regarding health-related matters should be good. The sociopolitical environment, economic development, law and order are directly concerned with health and optimum level of functioning.

Behavioral Determinants

Health is the mirror of a person's lifestyle. Behavior includes lifestyle which is person's way of living, i.e., habits, attitude, social values, eating patterns, rest, sleep, exercise. Understanding and adjustment in different situations are learnt through culture, family, friends, schools, colleges and peer groups. Many health problems, such as heart disease, lung cancer, drug addiction, smoking, alcoholism and obesity, can be avoided with healthy lifestyle. Accidents can be prevented by the use of helmet or seat belt.

Socioeconomic Determinants

Socioeconomic conditions such as education, economic status, occupation, housing and nutrition have direct impact on health. Good economic and educational status can eliminate various illnesses and health hazards in the society. Female education and employment play a great role in maintaining the health of the children and family. Proper housing, occupation and economic status promote health. Unemployment leads to low socioeconomic status and low purchasing capacity for necessary requirement for health, can cause psychological and physical problems. Socioeconomic conditions of the country have to be improved for the promotion and maintenance of health.

Healthcare Delivery System

Comprehensive healthcare delivery system is required to promote and restore the health of the people. But in a large population of India, it is very difficult to provide health services at the grass root level where the health facilities are unevenly distributed. There is nonavailability of health personnel in rural areas. More importance is given to tertiary level of care. Improper referral services and lack of resources determine the health status of an individual. There is a need to improve rural health service to improve health.

Other Factors

Food and agriculture industries, roads and transport development, information technology, communication, mass media, social welfare schemes and rural electrification have positive impact on improving health of the people through socioeconomic development.

HISTORY AND DEVELOPMENT OF COMMUNITY HEALTH

The history of community health can be traced back from the earliest records of civilization. Even in the ancient times when the scientific knowledge about medicine was not developed and the primitive medicine was on trial-and-error basis, there was a practice to visit the people who were sick. The religious healers provided psychological support and offered prayers to God for healing of sick people.

The first record of visiting nursing was sponsored in 1683 by St. Vincent Depaul in Paris and carried out by the sisterhood of the Dames de Charite.

In 1617, St. Vincent Depaul organized the sisterhood of the Dames de Charity, which systematically introduced the modern principles of visiting nursing and social welfare.

Home Healthcare

Wealthy people never went to hospitals in the early modern period (1600–1800). They were provided care at home.

- **In 1747,** first visiting nurses in Canada were the Grey Nuns in Montreal.
- **In 1802,** nuns visited the poor in community for care of ill people and promoting health.
- **In 1800 to 1856,** smallpox, yellow fever, cholera, typhoid and typhus spread through immigrants in the United States of America (USA). The government of USA trained health workers to take care of those people in their homes. Later on, these health workers were known as community health nurses.

Community Health Nursing

- Community health nursing developed in the United States in the late 19th and early 20th centuries.
- In 1859, community health nursing began with William Rathbone in Liverpool, England.
- In 1860, Nightingale Training School for Nurses was established at St. Thomas Hospital in London.
- In 1866, New York Metropolitan Board of Health was established.
- In 1864, Factory Act was passed to control and treat the health problems of factory workers.
- In 1886, in Philadelphia, the first health visiting nurse society started and provided home care to the community.
- In 1910, a decision was made to take care of tuberculosis patients in their homes by nurses.
- After the 2nd World War, community health nurses visited community on foot, on bicycles and by horse-drawn buggies.

- 1931, Maternity and Child Welfare Bureau was established by the Indian Red Cross Society.
- 1935, All the health activities were grouped under the control of state and central government.
- 1937, A central advisory board of health was setup.
- 1939, Madras Public Health Act was passed. A rural health training center at Singur near Calcutta was established.
- 1940, Drug Act was passed and brought under control.
- 1943, A health survey and development committee was appointed by the Government of India under the chairmanship of Dr Joseph Bhore.
- 1946, Bhore Committee report was submitted in volumes.
- 1947, National government took up the responsibility of improving health of people.
- 1948, India joined as a member state of WHO, Employees State Insurance (ESI) Act was passed.
- 1950, Planning commission was set up by the Government of India.
- 1951, Bacillus Calmette Guérin (BCG) vaccination program was launched and first Five-Year Plan was started.
- 1959, In Pakistan, Pakistan Institute of Medical and Health Sciences Islamabad, College of Nursing Lahore, College of Nursing Jinnah Postgraduate Medical Center (JPMC) Karachi and College of Nursing **Jamshoro** are running post-basic diploma courses of community health nursing.

DEVELOPMENT OF COMMUNITY HEALTH NURSING IN INDIA

- 1918, The community health workers (earlier called public health workers) started providing health services to the community in 1918, when the Lady Reading Health School at Bara Hindu Rao, Delhi was started. It provides post basic diploma in community health nursing, post basic diploma in nursing education and administration and multipurpose health workers (female) course that was started later on.
- 1919, Public health responsibilities were transferred to an elected minister.
- 1920, Municipality and Local Boards Act was passed in several provinces.
- 1921, Provided legislation for the advancement of public health.
- 1930, At Calcutta, the All India Institute of Hygiene and Public Health was established with aid from the Rockefeller Foundation.
- 1952, Community Development Program was launched on 2nd October for overall development of the rural areas.
- 1952, India launched its National Family Planning Program.
- 1953, A Model Public Health Community was appointed.
- 1954, Central Social Welfare Board was set up.
- 1955, National Filaria Control Program was started.
- 1956, Central Health Education Bureau was established.
- 1958, National Malaria Control Program was changed to Eradication Program.
- 1959, Mudaliar Committee was appointed to review the progress of health and published its report in 1961.
- 1960, School Health Committee was appointed and pilot project in relation to smallpox eradication program was initiated.
- 1962, Central Family Planning Institute was started in Delhi.
- 1963, Applied Nutrition Program was started.

- 1964, National Institute of Health Administration and Education was started in Delhi.
- 1965, Intrauterine contraceptive device (IUCD) (Lippes loop) was introduced.
- 1966, Direct BCG vaccination without tuberculin test was introduced in India.
- 1966, A separate Department of Family Planning was established in the Ministry of Health.
- 1970, Indira Gandhi, Prime Minister of India, implemented a forced sterilization program, but failed.
- 1971, Medical Termination of Pregnancy (MTP) Act passed in Parliament and came into force in 1972.
- 1973, Minimum Needs Program was included in health services.
- 1973, Multipurpose health workers scheme was introduced by Kartar Singh Committee report.
- 1975, On July 1975, India was declared free from smallpox.
- 1976, Indian Factories Act of 1948 was amended.
- 1976, National Program for Prevention of blindness was formulated.
- 1977, International Commission declared that India has eradicated smallpox.
- 1977, National Institute of Health and Family Welfare was formed.
- 1977, Community Health Workers scheme was started by the Union Ministry of Health.
- 1977, Rural Health Scheme was introduced.
- 1978, The slogan "Health for All by 2000 AD" at Alma Ata, a declaration in the Union of Soviet Socialist Republics (USSR), underlined the primary healthcare approach.
- 1979, World Health Assembly endorsed the declaration of Alma Ata on primary healthcare.
- 1981, Air Pollution Act was passed.
- 1982, The new 20-point program was announced.
- 1982, Government of India framed National Health Policy.
- 1982, The school health services started in India on a trial basis.
- 1983, National Health Program (NHP) was approved by the Parliament.
- 1984, The ESI Amendment Bill was approved by the Parliament.
- 1985, Universal Immunization Program was launched on 19th November.
- 1987, The new 20-point program was launched.
- 1987, "Safe Motherhood" campaign was launched by the World Bank.
- 1989, Blood Safety Program was launched.
- 1992, Child Survival and Safe Motherhood Program was launched on 20th August.
- 1995, Pulse Polio Immunization Program started in January.
- 1996, Reproduction and Child Health Program was started with slight modification in Child Survival and Safe Motherhood (CSSM) Program.
- 1997, Leprosy Control Program was integrated with health services.
- 1998, National Anti-Malaria Program introduced in place of National Malaria Eradication Program (NMEP).

PRESENT CONCEPTS OF COMMUNITY HEALTH

According to WHO expert committee on community health nursing (1971), "Community Health refers to the health status of the members of the community, to the problems affecting their health and to the totality of healthcare provided to the community".

The present concept of community health is to provide curative, preventive and promotive health services to the members of community and to provide comprehensive health services to the community. The community diagnosis and community treatment has attracted the attention of the health policy makers so that the health problems of the community are dealt efficiently. As per the WHO expert committee, community health nursing comprises the skills of nursing programs for the promotion of health, the improvement of conditions in the social and physical environment, prevention of illness and disability and rehabilitation. To achieve Health for All (HFA) through primary healthcare, the community health nursing has a key role in the implementation of primary healthcare. Community health nursing includes all nursing services organized by agency to carry out nursing aspects of community health program in homes, schools, industries and health centers. Most of the health services in homes are provided by traditional birth attendants, anganwadis, community nutrition workers and ICDS program, health workers (male and female), health supervisors (male and female), ANMs and medical officers in the primary health center. Their functions are influenced by the population of that area, transport facilities, communication facilities, general health needs of the people, socioeconomic conditions, education and requirement of health workers according to the size of the population to be covered.

PRIMARY HEALTHCARE

The concept of primary healthcare was similar to the concept of basic health services in India which was proposed by Bhore Committee in 1946 and was implemented by the Government of India after independence through successive five year plans. A similar concept was also proposed by WHO and UNICEF in 1965 to provide health services uniformly through a network of infrastructures.

Primary healthcare concept was introduced at international level jointly by WHO and United Nations International Children's Emergency Fund (UNICEF), after the conference held at Alma Ata 1978, to achieve the goal of "Health for All by 2000 AD". The conference was held to form a strategy to achieve health, especially of the rural and poor people of the World's population as there were gross disparities of health services between the rural and urban, rich and poor people within the same country.

India was the signatory of the conference and was one of the first countries to recognize the merits of primary healthcare approach. So, as a commitment to achieve the social goal of HFA, the Government of India formulated National Health Policy based on primary healthcare which was approved by the Parliament in 1983. National Health Policy laid down a plan of action for shaping the existing health services to strengthen rural health infrastructure and set goals to be achieved.

Primary healthcare is the first level of contact for individuals, families and community with healthcare delivery system. It is the care given to the people, at first level contact at community level where they live and work, thereby bringing healthcare closer to the people where they live.

Definitions of Primary Healthcare

- According to WHO, "primary healthcare is essential healthcare made universally accessible to individuals and acceptable to them through their full participation and at a cost the community and country can afford.
- Alma-Ata Conference (1978) defined primary healthcare as "essential healthcare based on practical, scientifically sound and socially acceptable methods and technology made universally

accessible to individuals and families in the community through their full participation and at a cost that the community and the country can afford to maintain at every stage of their development in the spirit of self-determination."

Concept of Primary Healthcare

In the light of aforementioned definitions, the concepts of primary healthcare (Fig. 1.6) are:

- Affordable by the country and community
- Universally accessible to all citizens of country
- Available to all irrespective of rural or urban, rich or poor communities
- Socially acceptable based on practical and scientifically sound technology
- Accountable to healthcare agencies of the country.

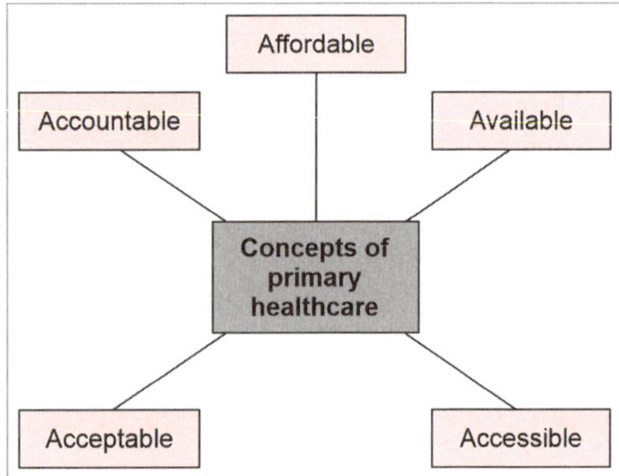

Fig. 1.6: Concepts of primary healthcare

Goals

The main goal of primary healthcare was to fulfill the global commitment of HFA by 2000 AD and to achieve an improved state of health and quality of life for all people attained through self-reliance, thereby placing people's health in people's hands.

Strategies

To strengthen the existing infrastructure of healthcare system and training of manpower to increase the strength of healthcare workers so that the health services can reach rural area at grass root level as primary healthcare is the backbone of health services delivery.

Objectives

- To reduce the incidence of communicable and noncommunicable diseases
- To sustain the population growth as per the available resources
- To reduce the mortality and morbidity rate among infants and preschool children
- To improve the level of healthcare of the community
- To maximize the contribution of other sectors for social and economic development of the community
- To extend essential health services in rural areas and underserved sectors
- To improve basic sanitation

Elements

There are eight essential elements of primary healthcare as follows:

1. **Health education:** Educate people about health, existing health problems and measures to control and prevent these health problems, make them aware of the health facilities available and make use of them when in need.

2. **Nutrition:** Good nutrition is essential for health and for the growth and development of children. Encourage people to pay attention to balanced diet and provide knowledge about preparation of food and preserving the nutrients present in diet.
3. **Water and sanitation:** Supply of safe drinking water and sanitation is necessary for good health and is an important factor in environment.
4. **Maternal and child health including family planning:** The mother and children are the most vulnerable group to health problems and account for a large percentage of population. Protection of mother and child from illness and other risks would ensure good health of family and community. The family planning services include spacing of children and adopting small family norms will check the population growth.
5. **Immunization against major infectious diseases:** Protection from major **infectious** diseases of children by providing immunization services to the children against poliomyelitis, diphtheria, tetanus, measles, tuberculosis, Hepatitis B and other vaccine preventable diseases.
6. **Prevention and control of locally endemic diseases:** To reduce morbidity rate, e.g., malaria control.
7. **Treatment:** Appropriate treatment of general diseases and injuries by using appropriate technology.
8. **Provision of essential drugs:** Ensuring easy availability of drugs.

Principles

There are five principles of primary healthcare (Fig. 1.7) given by WHO:
1. Equitable distribution
2. Community participation
3. Appropriate technology
4. Focus on prevention
5. Multisectoral coordination

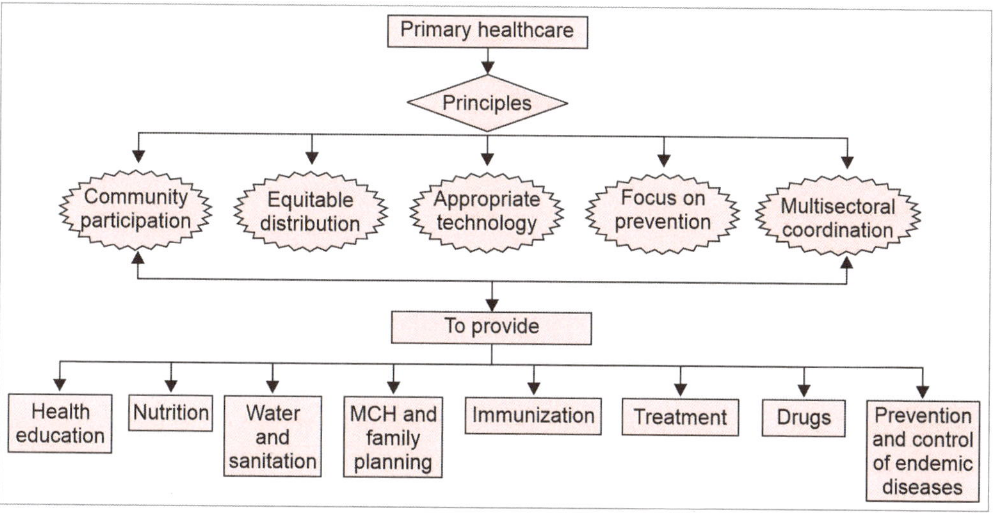

Fig. 1.7: Model of primary healthcare

The short description of these principles is as follows:

- **Equitable distribution:** The health services and resources should be equally distributed irrespective of caste, creed, gender, religion, rich, poor, urban or rural. According to this principle, primary healthcare should be available to all individuals, families and communities without any discrimination. It is based on the social justice. The people living in the rural area are the main target of primary healthcare.
- **Community participation:** Without the involvement of community, it is difficult to achieve the goal of primary healthcare. Though the responsibility of health lies with the government, the participation of community is necessary. The community should take active part in planning, execution and maintenance of primary healthcare. Primary health services are provided through village health guides, Anganwadi workers, ASHAs, TBA, male and female health workers.
- **Appropriate technology:** The technology used in primary healthcare should be scientifically sound, safe, socially acceptable, suitable to local requirement and within the financial limits and should be locally available. Use of oral rehydration solution (ORS) is an example for the treatment of diarrhea.
- **Focus on prevention:** The main focus of primary healthcare is on prevention of disease and promotion of health rather than the treatment and it is a part of all constituents of health services. Health education is also stressed by the primary healthcare.
- **Multisectoral coordination:** For the successful implementation of primary healthcare, coordination of other sectors is necessary, e.g., agriculture, sanitation, housing, nutrition, public works, communication and education. The joint efforts of all these fields are required to provide primary healthcare.

Responsibilities of Nurses in Primary Healthcare

The major responsibility of primary healthcare lies with community health nursing. So, the community health nursing system should be developed and strengthened so that nurses can effectively discharge their responsibilities related to primary healthcare. In 1984, the expert committee of WHO recommended the following responsibilities for nurses for taking care of primary health:

- Assessing the health level of individuals and community
- Ensuring the participation of community and encouraging individuals to participate
- Providing treatment in emergencies and taking care of the general health
- Referring the patients to the specialists (following the referral system)
- Keeping an eye on the epidemics
- Training and supervision of health workers
- Coordinating with other health programs
- Monitoring the progress of primary healthcare

MILLENNIUM DEVELOPMENT GOALS

In September 2000, representatives from 189 countries met at the Millennium Summit in New York to adopt the United Nations Millennium Declaration and made a commitment to address the crippling poverty and multiplying misery that grips many areas of the world.

The goals in the area of development and reducing poverty are named as Millennium Development Goals (MDGs). The health has main focus in MDGs. Out of eight goals, three are health related. Eight targets out of 18 and 18 indicators out of 48 are related to health. The member states promised to follow the strategy of MDGs and the Governments set a deadline of 2015 by which the countries would meet the following MDGs:

Goal 1: Eradicate extreme poverty and hunger

Goal 2: Achieve universal primary education

Goal 3: Promote gender equality and empower women

Goal 4: Reduce child mortality rate

Goal 5: Improve maternal health

Goal 6: Combat HIV/AIDS, malaria and other diseases

Goal 7: Ensure environmental sustainability

Goal 8: Develop a global partnership for development MDGs and health targets in India.

MDGs and Health Target in India

Goal 1: Eradicate Extreme Poverty and Hunger
Target 2: To reduce the proportion of people who suffer from hunger by half between 1990 and 2015

Goal 4: Reduce child mortality rate
Target 5: To reduce the under 5 mortality rate by two-thirds between 1990 and 2015

Goal 5: Improve maternal health
Target 6: To reduce the maternal mortality ratio by three quarters between 1990 and 2015

Goal 6: Combat HIV/AIDS, malaria and other diseases
Target 7: Have halted by 2015 and begun to reverse the spread of HIV/AIDS

PROMOTION AND MAINTENANCE OF HEALTH

Promotion of Health

Health promotion is one of the concepts of health services delivery. According to the American Journal of Health Promotion (1986), health promotion is the science and art of helping people change their lifestyle to move toward a state of optimal health. For this, the strategy is focused on informing, influencing and assisting both individuals and organization so that they accept more responsibility and become more active in matters affecting mental and physical health.

As per WHO, health promotion (2005) is "the process of enabling people to increase control over their health and its determinants, thereby improving their health". The most important methods of health promotion are self-care, mutual aid and healthy environment.

According to Ottawa Charter (1986), health promotion is not just the responsibility of the health sector, but goes beyond healthy lifestyle to well-being. It focuses on equity in health and is adapted to the local needs and responsibilities of individual countries and regions taking into account their social, cultural and economic systems. The health promotion involves all sectors, i.e., social, political, cultural, economic, behavioral and environmental to participate in the promotion of health because the prerequisites of health promotion are employment, security, quality, working conditions, sanitation and healthy environment. Health promotion can be performed in schools, work place, hospital and community.

Health Promotion in Community and Hospitals

In hospital, the main focus of the healthcare providers, mainly nurses, is on the curative aspects due to lack of time and shortage of staff. Moreover, the patients are also acutely ill and require rest. On improvement, they are shifted to subacute units for further care and then discharged. So, very little time is available to educate them on promotive aspect of health.

On the other hand, in community health nursing settings, the patients are not so ill, so it is easier to direct nursing care toward achieving greater level of health. Moreover, the community health nurse can take independent decision for care. The nurse decides with the patient, how long the care will be provided and when it will be terminated. The nurse visits the individual and community as per the needs and goals of healthcare so that the nurse gets greater opportunities to educate and motivate individuals toward promotion of health.

Maintenance of Health

A systematic program or procedure is planned to prevent illness, maintain maximum function and promote health. It is central to healthcare, especially to nursing care at all levels of care, i.e., primary, secondary and tertiary, and in all patterns, i.e., preventive, episodic, acute, chronic and catastrophic. The steps toward health maintenance (Fig. 1.8) include:

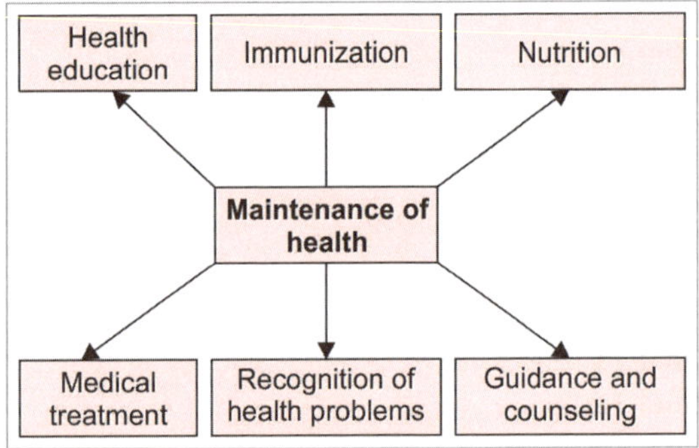

Fig. 1.8: Maintenance of health

- Health education
- Immunization
- Nutrition
- Guidance and counseling on lifestyle and physical activity
- Early recognition of health problems
- Timely seeking medical advice and appropriate treatment and follow up of the health problems

Health maintenance of the community is also one of the responsibilities of community health nurse while providing primary healthcare to the community.

SUSTAINABLE DEVELOPMENT GOALS

The Millennium Development Goals came to an end of their terms in December 2015. The United Nations General Assembly adopted new development agenda in September 2015 comprising 17 sustainable development goals and 169 targets. On January 2016, the SDGs of 2030 Agenda for sustainable development came into force. The sizeable progress of MDGs paves the way for more ambitious achievement by 2030. The 2030 Agenda comprises all three dimensions of sustainable development, i.e., economic, social and environmental. The SDGs state that eradicating poverty and inequality, developing economy and preserving the planet are deeply linked to each other and also to the health of the population. Health is centrally positioned within the 2030 Agenda with comprehensive goal—SDG-3, "Ensure healthy lives and promote well-being for all at all ages" and explicit links to many of the other goals. SDG-3 includes 13 targets covering all major health priorities.

The SDGs recognize that ending poverty will build economic growth and address social needs including education, health, social protection, raising the standard of living, job opportunities, tackling client changes and environmental protection. The 2030 agenda is designed to benefit all and universal in scope. It will require comprehensive integrated approach to sustain development as well as collective action at all levels.

There are 17 sustainable goals and 169 targets.
The sustainable development goals are as follows:

Goal 1: No poverty
Goal 2: Zero hunger
Goal 3: Ensure healthy lives and promote well-being for all at all ages
Goal 4: Quality education
Goal 5: Gender equality
Goal 6: Clean water and sanitation
Goal 7: Affordable and clean energy
Goal 8: Decent work and economic growth
Goal 9: Build resilient infrastructure, promote sustainable industrialization and foster innovation
Goal 10: Reduce inequality within and among countries
Goal 11: Sustainable cities and communities
Goal 12: Sustainable consumption and production
Goal 13: Climate action
Goal 14: Life below water. The Global Goals
Goal 15: Life on land
Goal 16: Peace, justice and strong institutions. The Global Goals
Goal 17: Partnerships for the goals

Among all the 17 SDGs, the Goal 3 is health related and includes 13 targets covering all major health priorities. The SDG-3 and its 13 targets are listed in the following table:

Sustainable Development Goal 3: Ensure healthy lives and promote well-being for all at all ages

Goals and Targets from 2030 Agenda
3.1 By 2030, reduce the global maternal mortality ratio to <70 per 100,000 live births.
3.2 By 2030, end preventable deaths of newborns and children under 5 years of age, with all countries aiming to reduce neonatal mortality to at least as low as or 12 per 1000 live births and under-5 mortality to at least as low as 25 per 1000 live births.
3.3 By 2030, end the epidemics of AIDS, tuberculosis, malaria and neglected tropical diseases and combat hepatitis, water-borne diseases and other communicable diseases.
3.4 By 2030, reduce by one third premature mortality from noncommunicable diseases through prevention and treatment and promote mental health and well-being.
3.5 Strengthen the prevention and treatment of substance abuse, including narcotic drug abuse and harmful use of alcohol.
3.6 By 2030, halve the number of global deaths and injuries from road traffic accidents.

Contd...

3.7　By 2030, ensure universal access to sexual and reproductive healthcare services, including family planning information and education, and the integration of reproductive health into national strategies and programs.

3.8　Achieve universal health coverage, including financial risk protection, access to quality essential healthcare services and access to safe, effective, quality and affordable essential medicines and vaccines for all.

3.9　By 2030, substantially reduce the number of deaths and illness from hazardous chemicals and air, water and soil pollution and contamination.

3.a　Strengthen the implementation of the World Health Organization Framework Convention on Tobacco control in all countries, as appropriate.

3.b　Support the research and development of vaccines and medicines for the communicable and noncommunicable diseases that primarily affect developing countries, provide access to affordable, essential medicines and vaccines, in accordance with the Doha Declaration on the TRIPS Agreement and Public Health, which affirms the right of developing countries to use to the full the provisions in the Agreement on Trade-Related Aspects of Intellectual Property Rights regarding flexibilities to protect public health, and, in particular, provide access to medicines for all.

3.c　Substantially increase health financing and the recruitment, development, training and retention of the health workforce in developing countries, especially in least developed countries and small island developing states.

3.d　Strengthen the capacity of all countries, in particular developing countries, for early warning, risk reduction and management of national and global health risks.

Summary

- Community is a group of people living together in a particular geographical area having common characteristics of culture, customs, language, habits, similar lifestyle and interaction among the members.
- Community health means the status of health of the members of community, problems affecting the health and healthcare facilities available in community.
- Community health is related to preventive, curative and promotive health services and it focuses on health problems of the community and means to solve these problems. It can be achieved through health education, safe environment, immunization and controlling the communicable and noncommunicable diseases.
- Community health nursing is a comprehensive branch of nursing which deals with recognition of nursing needs and intervention and evaluation of nursing care and health services provided to the community.
- Concept of health is related to biological, ecological, psychological concepts and based on the WHO definition of health. According to psychologists, there are subjective and objective aspects of health. Objective aspects are occupation, health education, nutrition, healthy environment and social security. Subjective aspects are individual's feeling of happiness, satisfaction or sadness. Both the subjective and objective aspects influence health.
- According to multifactor theory, many factors are responsible for a disease.
- Disease spectrum varies from carriers, subclinical cases, mild cases, moderate cases to severe cases.
- Dimensions of health are physical, mental, social, spiritual, emotional, vocational, nutritional and environmental.
- Indicators of healthcare are direct and indirect.
- Development of community health nursing in India started in 1918 when Lady Reading Health School was opened in Delhi to train female community health workers. It made fast progress after independence.

- The present concept of community health is to provide curative, preventive and promotive health services to the community through primary healthcare approach.
- Primary healthcare is the essential healthcare made universally accessible to the individuals and acceptable to them through their full participation and at a cost that community and country can afford.
- Responsibility of nurses in primary healthcare is to assess, diagnose, plan and provide nursing care and evaluate the care provided.
- Goals in the area of development and reducing poverty are named as Millennium Development Goals. Out of eight goals, three are health related, eight targets out of 18 and 18 indicators out of 48 are health related.
- Promotion and maintenance of health can be achieved through health education, immunization, nutrition, guidance and counseling on lifestyle and physical activities, early recognition and timely treatment of the health problems.
- The United Nations General Assembly adopted the new agenda of sustainable goals after noting the progress of MDGs. The SDGs of 2030 agenda came into force on January 1, 2016.

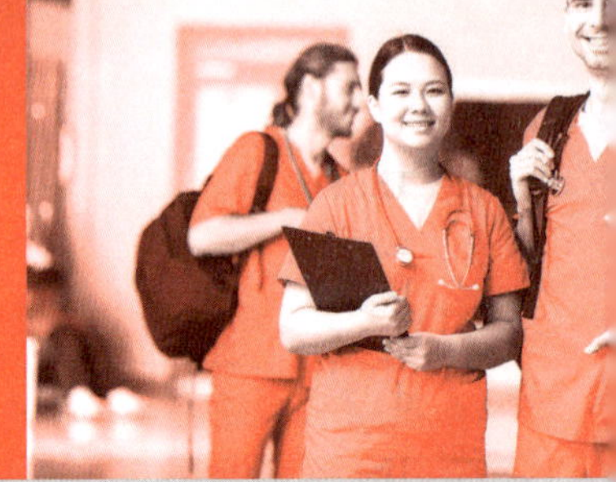

LONG ANSWER TYPE QUESTIONS

1. Explain the disease according to biomedical concept.
2. Describe the dimensions of health.
3. Define primary healthcare. What are the principles of primary healthcare?

SHORT ANSWER TYPE QUESTIONS

1. Define community, community health and community health nursing.
2. What are the responsibilities of community health nurse in primary healthcare?

MULTIPLE CHOICE QUESTIONS

1. **Which of the following factors is responsible for healthcare?**
   a. External environment
   b. Genetic inheritance
   c. Social support system
   d. All of these

2. **Community health can be achieved through:**
   a. Health education
   b. Good nutrition and immunization
   c. Safe environment and adequate healthcare facilities
   d. All of the above

3. **WHO's concept of health is:**
   a. Biological concept
   b. Social and spiritual concept
   c. Holistic concept—state of physical, mental, social and spiritual well-being
   d. Psychological and ecological concept

4. **Components of physical environment include all of the following; except:**
   a. Housing, lighting and ventilation
   b. Bacteria, viruses and spores
   c. Excreta and waste
   d. Air, water, sound and radiation

5. **The type of care provided by the institutional nurses is:**
   a. Preventive
   b. Promotive
   c. Curative
   d. All of these

6. **The emotional response of an individual to illness is:**
   a. Fear and anxiety
   b. Anger and hostility
   c. Overdependence and feeling of helplessness
   d. All of the above

7. **The aims of community health nurse are all of the following; except:**
   a. To improve standard of living of community
   b. To reduce risk factors in the community
   c. To ensure job and earn money
   d. To strengthen self-care activities of individuals

8. **Health promotion is the process to achieve health by:**
   a. Health education
   b. Immunization and nutrition
   c. Environmental sanitation
   d. All of these

9. **The nursing staff employed at community health center (CHC, PHC and SC) consists of:**
   a. Midwives and MPHW
   b. Community health nurses
   c. Lady health visitors and female health assistant
   d. All of the above

10. **Which of the following is a characteristic of community?**
    a. Different language
    b. Different lifestyle
    c. Common values, customs and culture
    d. None of the above

2

Community Health Nursing

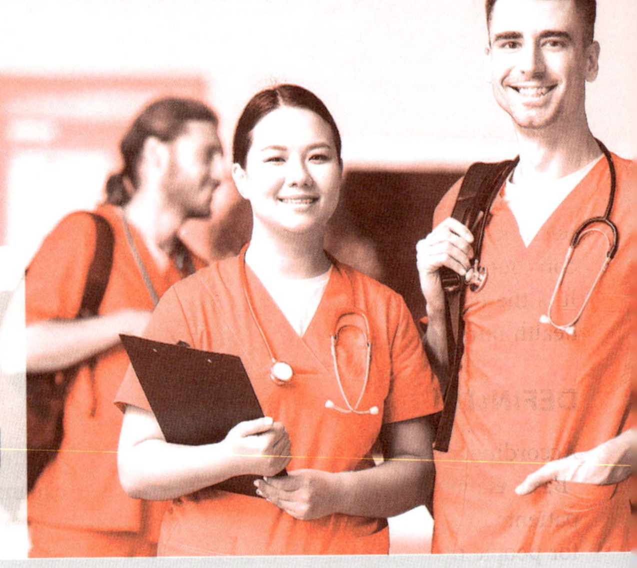

LEARNING OBJECTIVES

After the completion of the unit, the readers will be able to:
- Explain various aspects of community health nursing.
- Demonstrate skills in applying nursing process in community health nursing settings.
- Describe the philosophy, goals and objectives of community health nursing.

UNIT OUTLINE

- Introduction
- Definitions
- Philosophy
- Goals and Objectives
- Principles
- Concept and Importance
- Qualities of Community Health Nurse
- Functions of Community Health Nurse
- Nursing Process
- Community Health Nursing Process

KEY TERMS

Assessment: Precise method of collecting and interpretation of the information.

Community diagnosis: Statement of community problems based on subjective and objective data.

Data: Facts or information.

Evaluation: Outcome of the implementation.

Implementation: Putting the planned action into practice.

Planning: Deciding the line of action.

INTRODUCTION

Community health nursing implies the knowledge of the principles of general nursing, social and public health. It is a comprehensive branch of nursing, which helps in meeting health and nursing needs of the community. This is concerned with the care of healthy families and nonhospitalized sick individuals.

Community health nursing includes all nursing services organized by an agency to carry out nursing aspects of community health in homes, schools, industries and health centers. In community, the individual and family health are the building blocks of the health of the population. It is the backbone of the implementation of primary healthcare, as the main focus of community health nursing is on preventive, promotive, curative and rehabilitative services to the community.

DEFINITIONS

According to Hafden Mahler (1985), former Director of World Health Organization (WHO), "Basic element of community health nursing is expansion of primary care of health and faith of patients in nurses". According to Hafden, "As per this new perspective, nurses will be more useful for people than doctors, in the field of health."

- According to Freeman (1970), community health nursing is "a collaborative application of nursing and public health measures within the framework of the total community health efforts".
- According to the American Public Health Association (APHA, 1982), public health synthesizes "the body of knowledge from the public health science and professional nursing theories for the purpose of improving the health of the entire community".

According to the American Nurses Association (ANA, 2000), community health nursing is "a synthesis of nursing and public health practice applied to promoting and preserving the health of population, 'treat population as a whole', focus on individual, family, groups, community, utilizing health promotion, health maintenance, health education and management coordination and continuity of care for meeting population needs".

PHILOSOPHY

The philosophy implies three components, i.e., concern with knowledge, values and beliefs about existence. Community health nursing supports all three components as follows:

- Community health nursing is based on scientific knowledge and logical thinking.
- Community health nursing is governed by code of ethics (values).
- Community health nursing is committed to its own beliefs about professional practice (existence).

The philosophy of community health nursing has been derived from the basic nursing and is as follows:

- Community health nursing believes that health is a fundamental human right and every member of the community has an equal right to get healthcare in equal quantity, irrespective of color, caste, social status, area and religion.
- Community health nursing believes that prevention from disease and promotion of health is the road to achieve optimum level of health.
- Community health nursing supports the entire community as well as individual in health and during sickness.
- Community health nursing believes that advancement in science and community health has a major role in promotion of health and prolonging life.

- Community health nursing believes in honoring the social and cultural differences and values of individuals and community about health and supports the health promoting behavior in an acceptable manner.
- Community health nursing believes and supports that community-based efforts and involvement of community are essential in prevention of disease, promotion of health and prolonging life.
- Community health nursing believes and practices that health education is an important component to achieve health of the population.
- Community health nursing believes that multidisciplinary team activities and programs are essential to achieve the objectives of community health.
- Community health nursing believes that healthcare should be provided in such a way so as to develop overall growth and well-being felt and observed by the community.

GOALS AND OBJECTIVES

Goals

Goals of community health nursing are:
- To achieve the highest standard of health of the population
- To help the individuals, families and community to participate in activities in prevention of diseases and promotion of health

Objectives

Objectives of community health nursing are:
- To reduce the morbidity and mortality rate of infants and mothers
- To control and prevent communicable diseases
- To provide promotive, preventive, curative and rehabilitative services to the community
- To provide referral services at all levels of healthcare
- To increase the life expectancy
- To find the cause-and-effect relationship
- To evaluate the health programs and make future plan
- To assess the needs and priorities of vulnerable groups, pregnant mothers and children and take appropriate action
- To help other organization working in the field of community
- To enhance the standard of nursing profession through conducting nursing research, providing quality assurance in community health nursing and performing the role of nurse epidemiologist
- To provide complete well-being of the community and maintain their optimum level of functioning

PRINCIPLES

The following principles should be observed while working in the community:
- Health services should be based on the needs of individuals and community. Health programs should be planned for solving health problems. Community health nurse should have good working knowledge in the community so that she can immediately solve health problems of the people effectively.

- Health services should be planned according to the budget, resources and availability of health workers. They should be practical as well.
- There should be uniform distribution and availability of health services without any discrimination of age, sex, caste, religion, social, economic or political level.
- Family should be regarded as a unit of providing health services to its members and their active participation should be ensured.
- There should be continuity of health services without any interruption and taking care of follow up treatment is necessary.
- Health education is an integral part of community health nursing. It should be according to the needs of the families, preplanned and scientifically true and effective.
- Community health nurse should be nonpolitical in her relationship with people. She should understand and respect the values, customs, culture and religious beliefs of people and encourage them to practice the best that is in their philosophy.
- Supervision and guidance of health workers is essential for effective health services to achieve best results.
- Maintenance of records and reports is very important in community health nursing. Demographical programs and services are planned and evaluated based on records or reports. These should be carefully maintained and preserved for research purposes.
- Effective team spirit is essential for a team working in community. There should be coordination and cooperation among the members of the community health team. There should be mutual respect and sincerity irrespective of the designation and seniority to achieve the goal of community health. Community health nurse should be aware of the role of every member of the team.
- Community health authority should provide an opportunity for in-service education program and continuing education to all the members of community health team periodically to keep themselves updated.
- Community health nurse should be alert and devoted to her duties and should be responsible for professional growth.
- Community health nurse should follow professional ethics and standards in her work and behavior and should not accept any gift or money in lieu of services.
- Community health nurse should feel responsible toward the goals and philosophy of the health institution she belongs to and should have job satisfaction.
- Evaluation of services is an important factor in community health nursing. Review of community health nursing plans should be based on these evaluations to determine further plans and goals.

CONCEPT AND IMPORTANCE

The changing concept of health has made an important impact on the role of community health nursing practice. Due to changes in healthcare delivery system, community health nursing has gained much recognition in the field of health. Though the individuals are responsible for their own health, the government has got the responsibility to make health services available to the people and make them aware to avail the health facilities. Due to the limited resources of healthcare for a large population to provide equitable distribution of health services, the government as well as private institutions lay emphasis on reducing expensive institution-based care and providing home-based care by community health nursing. The community health nurse by virtue of her professional knowledge and practice of community health nursing works for the community, with the community and by the community. The members of the community are becoming more conscious about their health due to growing awareness about health through the media and taking initiative to improve their health. The community health nursing services operate within the domain of community health and help the community in meeting the health and nursing needs of community.

Community health nursing plays a challenging role in promoting and protecting the health of the community. The main emphasis of community health nursing is on prevention. There are three levels of prevention—primary, secondary and tertiary. The primary level of prevention is in the prepathogenesis phase of disease and includes all those steps taken to build up general health and well-being and protect from diseases and health problems. These steps include personal hygiene, environmental sanitation, safe drinking water, well-balanced diet, immunization, healthy habits, control of air pollution and health education. The secondary and tertiary levels of prevention are in the pathogenesis phase of the disease and include all the measures taken to arrest the disease process, control further spread, and restore health by early diagnosis, treatment and rehabilitation. In community health nursing, the top priority is given to primary level of prevention. It is an integral part of community health and provides comprehensive health and nursing care with major emphasis on promotive and preventive services and providing referral services for timely curative and rehabilitative care. Thus, the community health nursing services are of utmost importance in providing primary healthcare at the grass root level to the community and achieving the national commitment to achieve Health for All (HFA).

QUALITIES OF COMMUNITY HEALTH NURSE

- She should be polite, sympathetic and hard working.
- She should be intelligent, good observer and quick in understanding patients' physical, mental, social and behavioral problems.
- She should be sensitive to the health problems and health needs of the community.
- She should have sound professional knowledge. Her qualification, according to the new concept, should be diploma in General Nursing and Midwifery and Post Basic Diploma in Public Health or university course in nursing, i.e., BSc Nursing or Post Basic BSc nursing.
- She should be kind and should have patience to listen to clients' problems.
- She should have sound communication skills and should be a good speaker, interviewer, conversationalist and good teacher.
- She should have good interpersonal relationships with the community and with the members of community health team.
- She should be able to coordinate the services of other sectors working in the field of health.
- She should be capable of assessing the health level of individuals, families and community.
- She should have the ability to recognize the signs and symptoms of the disease.
- She should be able to take right and immediate decision according to the situation.
- She should be able to lead the health team.
- She should respect community's culture, customs and religious beliefs and should inspire the community to practice healthy culture.

- She should have knowledge of available resources and health problems of the community.
- She should understand human behavior.
- She should have managerial skills and abilities.

FUNCTIONS OF COMMUNITY HEALTH NURSE

The area of work of community health nurse is very vast. Her functions depend upon the place of her posting and designation, qualifications, experience and the organization structure. Some community health nurses work at staff level, others may function as an administrator, supervisor or instructor in health organizations. Some of the important functions of community health nurse (Fig. 2.1) are:

- **Nursing functions:**
  - Providing comprehensive nursing services to the individuals, families and community
  - Guiding the family about the care of sick at home
  - Making use of domestic appliances in the nursing work
  - Giving demonstrations on nursing procedures to the family members, e.g., washing hands, giving subcutaneous injection of insulin, urine testing and minor dressing, giving bed bath, steam inhalation, etc.
  - Assisting in the treatment and diagnosis of diseases
  - Making regular home visits
- **Educational functions:**
  - Giving health education to individuals and groups on prevention of disease and promotion of health

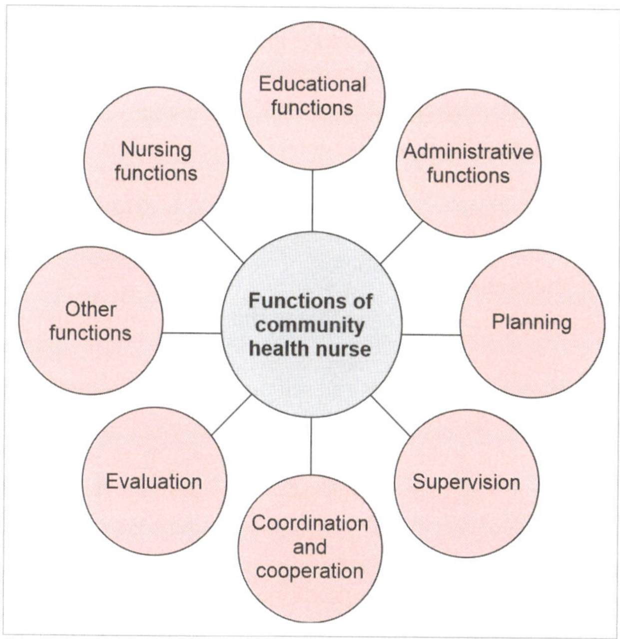

Fig. 2.1: Functions of community health nurse

- Participating in school health education programs
- Assisting in the training programs of nursing and health workers
- Preparation and intelligent use of audio-visual aids
- Providing education on improvement and development of environment
- Giving practical training about the care of patients
- Assisting in conducting surveys, demographical fact collection and presentation, etc., for research work

- **Administrative functions:**
  - Assigning duties and responsibilities to the members of health team working under her
  - Collecting information about community
  - Finding out the health problems, and determining limits and availability of resources
  - Deciding the nature and role of nursing services
  - Arranging meeting and assisting medical officers in arranging health camps in clinics and health centers
  - Epidemiological survey

- **Planning:**
  - Planning the distribution of work among the members of health team
  - Planning services in school, home and at work areas
  - Amending and improving the plans of program
  - Preparing plans to provide comprehensive nursing services to the community

- **Supervision:**
  - Supervising the work of subordinates, i.e., male and female health workers and traditional birth attendants (TBAs)
  - Inspecting the work of other health workers, e.g., health inspector, etc.
  - Supervising the care provided by members of family

- **Coordination and cooperation:**
  - Coordinating the services of all specialists concerned with patient care
  - Establishing coordination and cooperation among the members of health team
  - Procuring cooperation of the influential people of the community in health work
  - Maintaining contact with government and nongovernment organizations and other authorities
  - Participating in meetings
  - Working as a liaison officer between officers and health workers

- **Evaluation:**
  - Evaluating the work of subordinates and self on the basis of immunization, clinical services and implementation of family welfare program
  - Monthly self-assessment of the work
  - Sending the report to health authorities and agencies and receiving these back from the same.

- **Other functions:**
  - Maintenance of health records and reports and timely dispatch of reports
  - Assisting in health statistics work
  - Appropriate use of referral services

NURSING PROCESS

The term "process" indicates a series of planned actions that lead to a particular result. The word "process" when incorporated with nursing becomes "Nursing Process".

"Nursing Process is a problem-solving approach and a tool involving the science and art for the provision of quality nursing care to the individual, family and community". It can be applied at every level of care. The word "Process" is not only limited to the nursing but also applied in various fields to achieve the desired results.

Types

Nursing Process is classified into three types:

1. **Individualized nursing process:** This type of nursing process is applied to solve the individual patients' problems and most commonly used in hospital care setting.
2. **Family health nursing process:** It is applied to solve the health problems of the family and is the basic component of family health nursing.
3. **Community health nursing process:** When nursing process is applied to diagnose the health problems and meet the health needs of the community, it is known as community health nursing process.

   The goals of nursing process remain the same, i.e., to solve the health problems and meet the health needs, whether it is applied at any level of care.

Definitions

- "Nursing Process comprises systematically and scientifically planned steps of actions directed toward achieving the desired goals of nursing."
- "Nursing Process is a set of actions leading to a particular goal." **—Wolff**
- "Nursing Process is the core and essence of nursing; it is central to all nursing actions; it is applied in all settings. There is a basic theme that underlies the process; it is organized, systematic and deliberated." **—Yura and Walsh, 1983**

General Objectives

- To maintain health
- To prevent illness
- To promote recovery
- To restore health
- To provide support in peaceful death

Steps/Phases

There are five phases of nursing process (Table 2.1):
1. Assessment
2. Nursing diagnosis
3. Planning
4. Implementation
5. Evaluation

TABLE 2.1: Format of nursing care plan

Assessment	Nursing diagnosis	Planning	Implementation	Evaluation

Assessment

Assessment is an organized, systematic and ongoing process of collecting data and forms the basis for other phases. It is an independent nursing function and depends upon the skill and description of nurses. The tools of assessment include the following methods:

- Observation
- Interview
- Nursing history
- Clinical records
- Consultation
- Physical and psychological history
- Review and literature

Nursing Diagnosis

Nursing diagnosis is the result of the assessment phase. It is the statement of patients' problems derived from the systematic collection of data through the assessment phase. Steps of nursing diagnosis include:

- Analysis and interpretation of data
- Making and validating conclusion
- Comparing sign of clusters with defining characteristics
- Identifying the related factors
- Documenting the nursing diagnosis

Planning

Planning involves the action designed to prevent, correct or minimize the problems identified in the nursing diagnosis and setting priorities for nursing action. The main objective of planning is to make the best possible use of available resources to help the person achieve the desired outcome.

Objectives of Planning

- To set priorities
- To set the time schedule for outcome
- To identify nursing intervention

Implementation

Implementation means putting the plan into action according to the set priorities. It refers to the nursing activities performed to accomplish the specified goals.

Responsibilities of Nurses in Implementation of Care

- Reviewing the nursing care plan
- Scheduling the nursing actions
- Communicating the intervention
- Collaborating with other professionals
- Providing direct care
- Counseling and supervising nursing care
- Documenting nursing care

Evaluation

Evaluation refers to recording the outcome of the nursing action or the extent to which the expected outcome was achieved. It is an ongoing process in caring and related to the previous phases of nursing process. Evaluation may be formative (ongoing basis) and summative (aftercare) at the time of patient's discharge.

Steps of Evaluation

1. Identifying the outcome criteria
2. Comparing actual outcome with expected outcome
3. Summarizing the result of evaluation
4. Making corrections and modifying care plan in cases of failure in achieving the outcome
5. Documenting the evaluation process

COMMUNITY HEALTH NURSING PROCESS

The nursing process is generally applied to solve the health problems of individual patients in hospital setting. When the nursing process is used to promote community health, it becomes community health nursing process, which provides community-focused nursing care.

Definitions

- "Community health nursing process is an orderly, systematic and rational method of assessing the health problems and health needs, planning and implementing nursing care for the prevention of disease and promotion of health of the community."
- "Community health nursing process is a scientific method of assessing and solving the health problems of the community."

Objectives

- To identify actual or potential health problems/healthcare needs of the community
- To formulate the plans of nursing action to meet the assessed health needs
- To implement the plans of nursing action to solve the health problems and health needs
- To evaluate the nursing care provided to the community

Importance of Community Health Nursing Process

- Community health nursing process provides continuous and community-oriented care to the community.
- It utilizes maximum resources available in the community.
- It improves the functioning of community health team.

- There is participation of the community in each step of community health nursing process.
- It provides job satisfaction to community health nurses and other health workers working in the community.
- It contributes toward the professional growth of community health nurses.
- It provides quality assurance in community health nursing.
- It increases the community health status and makes community self-reliant.

Components of Community Health Nursing Process

- Community identification
- Knowing population composition
- Finding health and allied resources
- Applying community health nursing process in:
  - Community health nursing assessment
  - Community health nursing diagnosis
  - Planning
  - Implementation of community health nursing care services
  - Evaluation
  - Replanning

These components are sequential, progress from one phase to another, i.e., assessment phase overlaps with the diagnosis phase. From nursing diagnosis, plan of nursing care is developed stating goals and intervention to achieve the expected outcome.

Community Identification

Community identification is the first step of community health nursing process and forms the basis of the succeeding steps. Community health nurse should know the community in which community health nursing process is to be applied. Community identification refers to systematic process of knowing and exploring the defined community for assessing the health status and finding out the possible factors affecting the health of the community. There are various definitions and dimensions of the community but the following three dimensions are present in all the definitions:

- Geographical area or place
- People
- Functions of social system

Therefore, community is an aggregate of people living in a particular geographical area and social system. Every community has defined geographical area in which people live and depend for their existence.

Geographical Area or Place

Geographical area or place refers to the size, name of the area, map of the area, location, census, blocks and climate.

- **Geographical boundaries:** Politics has an important role in a particular geographical area and administration of community.
- **Means of transportation:** Buses, trains, bullock cart, Tonga horse (horse driven cart), boat, foot
- Physical environment and land use patterns, housing conditions and roads.

People

People dimension includes the social and demographic characteristics of the community. It refers to the structural characteristics of age, sex, caste, religion, education, and socioeconomic status.

Functions of Social System

Social system includes main functionaries of the community which may be different in urban and rural communities. It includes the following:

- Physical environment
- Maintenance of social control
- Education
- Employment status of the community
- Health and social services
- Production, distribution and consumption of goods and services
- Communication
- Adaptation of ongoing and expected changes
- Socialization of new members
- Provision of mutual aid and cooperation
- Recreational

Knowing Population Composition

Population composition implies all the basic information about the residents of identified community. It includes the following:

- Size and the density of the population
- Demographic characteristics such as age, sex, caste, religion, socioeconomic status, occupation and education
- Rural and urban character and dependency ratio of population
- Marital status–Single, married, divorced or widowed
- Formal groups such as families, schools, temples, gurudwaras, churches, mosques, industries, business, governmental bodies, nongovernmental organizations, voluntary social health and welfare agencies, etc.
- Informal groups such as community clubs, labor centers, friendship network, workers club, etc.
- Demographic structure of vulnerable groups, such as mother, child, handicapped, etc.
- Vital statistics, births, deaths by age

Finding Health and Allied Resources

The community health nurse should know the available health and allied resources in the community. For this, she needs help from other colleagues working with her for the community health. She should have the information about the following resources:

Health Resources

- **Health institutions**
    - Health facilities available in hospitals, teaching hospitals, dispensaries, first referral units, community health centers (CHCs), primary health centers (PHCs), subcenters (SCs),

Employees' State Insurance (ESI) hospitals, nursing homes, maternity hospitals or other special hospitals in government or private health institutions
- School and industrial health services
- Mental health services
- Traditional healers
- Voluntary health association
- National health programs
- Health-related planning and working group
- Health-related manpower such as physicians, nurses, epidemiologists, dentists, sanitary workers, social workers, etc.
- Healthcare delivery system and utilization patterns to compare the desired outcomes and available resources
- AYUSH (Ayurveda, Yoga, Naturopathy, Unani, Siddha and Homeopathy hospitals).
- **Health service resources**
  - Health services for reproductive and child health
  - Health services for elderly workers, handicapped, etc.

Allied Resources

Allied resources include the following:
- **Natural resources:** Water, land, soil and electricity
- **Financial aid services:** Health Insurance, LIC, Mediclaim, religious, and financial aid service
  - International financial support and schemes
  - Voluntary agencies working in the field of community welfare (orphanages, ashrams, etc.)
  - Transportation, education and communication resources (mass media resources)
  - Nutritional services
  - Integrated Child Development Services (ICDS) scheme
  - Employment services
  - Educational and welfare agencies
  - Social welfare agencies
- **Legal resources:** Existing public health laws such as Environmental Protection Act, Child Labor Act, Medical Termination of Pregnancy (MTP) Act and Prenatal Diagnostic Techniques Act (PNDTA), etc., along with the laws, legal aid or help forums should find out which can be helpful in implementing the community health nursing process.
- Counseling services other than the health care are available in the community
- **Professional resources:** Journals, association, etc.
- **Communication:** Newspapers, magazines, radio, TV, internet, etc.
- Recreational facilities
- Social services and public services
- Industry
- Political organization
- Community development projects

Applying Community Health Nursing Process

There are five phases of nursing process applied in community health setting.

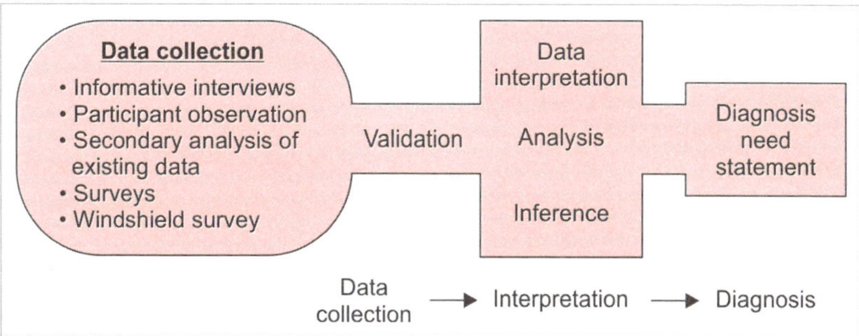

Fig. 2.2: Community health nursing assessment and diagnosis

Community Health Nursing Assessment

Community health nursing assessment (Fig. 2.2) is an organized and systematic method of assessing the health status of an identified community. Potential risk factor should be identified which may adversely affect health and the existing health problem of the community should be determined. Community health nursing assessment can be done as follows:

- **Data collection**: It is done to get information about the community and its health. It involves data gathering and data generation.
  - **Data gathering:** It is the process of obtaining existing information which is readily available from the records and reports of the health institution, and from the vital statistics. These include demographic data, e.g., age, sex, socioeconomic status, caste, racial information, infant mortality rate (IMR), maternal mortality rate (MMR), life expectancy and other morbidity and mortality data.
  - **Data generation:** Data which is not readily available but can be developed by the community health nurse or any data collector through interaction with the community members. This process of data collection is called data generation. This category of data includes values and rituals, customs, beliefs, traditions, goals and needs, community's knowledge and beliefs, norms, problem-solving process, cultural influences, leadership, caste, characters and political pressure.
- **Data interpretation:** It provides meaning to data. Interpretation of gathered and generated data is done; and the health problems of community and community resources are identified. Data interpretation is the process of analyzing the information gathered, drawing inferences and validating those inferences to determine their accuracy.
  - **Tools of data assessment and interpretation:** The following are the tools used for data assessment and interpretation.
    - **Informative interviews:** This refers to the direct conversation with the selected members of the community about community groups, members and events.
    - **Participant observation:** It is the conscious and systematic sharing in the activities and occasions for collecting data.
    - **Secondary analysis of existing data:** This is making use of previously gathered data, e.g., from records and reports or from the minutes of community meeting. These are time saving, valuable and economical also.
    - **Surveys:** These are collected from selected groups of persons. The survey sample provides data about community's health status and problems of community.

Major surveys like demographic survey, geographical, environmental survey and nutritional survey, etc. can also be used for assessment.

♦ **Windshield survey:** It refers to simple observation in which community life and environment can be carefully observed. By this type of survey, the common characteristics of street people, housing quality, rhythm of community life, common sanitary habits, community's gathering places, geographical and geopolitical dimension can be observed and related data can be collected.

This is to remember that no data collection tool is without bias. So, different tools should be used. For community health nurse, data collection or assessment is the biggest challenge as she is an outsider and represents the established healthcare system which may not be known to the people; and cooperation of the community may not be adequate.

Community Health Nursing Diagnosis

According to the North American Nursing Diagnosis Association (NANDA), "Nursing diagnosis is a clinical judgment about individual, family or community responses to actual or potential health problems/life processes. Nursing diagnosis provides the basis for selection of nursing interventions to achieve outcome for which the nurse is accountable (Figs 2.3A and B).

Community health diagnosis may be defined as "finding the pattern of health problems in a community, including factors which influence this pattern".

There is considerable overlapping in assessment and diagnosis. Community diagnosis is the scope of epidemiology and nursing from epidemiological aspect. Community diagnosis is the pattern of disease in a community described in terms of important factors which influence this pattern. This is based on the collection and interpretation of data related to demographic structure, vital statistics, incidence and prevalence of the disease in the area. On the basis of community diagnosis, community treatment is planned.

From the nursing aspect, community health nursing diagnosis is also related to the health problems of the community. It has a broader perspective and is not limited to the disease pattern. Community health nursing diagnosis requires comprehensive community health assessment. Community health nursing aims at the identification of basic health needs and existing health problems of the community. Community health nursing diagnosis is formulated on the basis of problems present in the community.

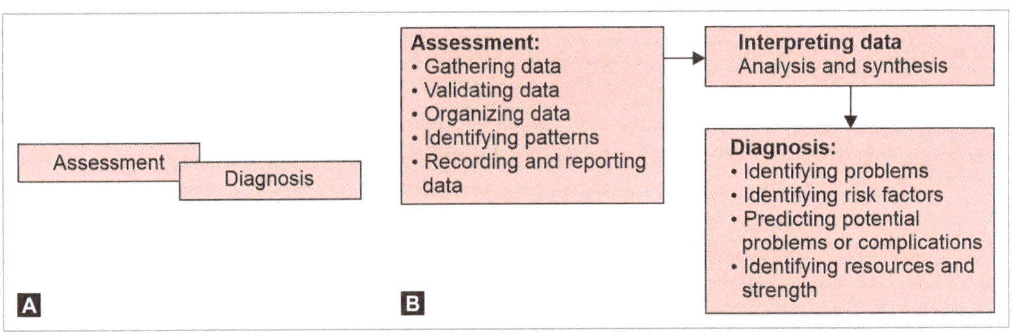

Figs 2.3A to C: **A.** Overlapping assessment and diagnosis; **B.** Assessment leading to nursing diagnosis

- **Types of problems which may be present in the community**
  - It may be directly related to health, e.g., malnutrition, malaria, diabetes mellitus, worm manifestation, etc.
  - There may be problems of health service system, i.e., lack of health institutions, lack of resources and personnel's uneven distribution of health facilities.
  - Problems related to awareness, i.e., lack of information, communication, poor transport facilities, and poor media management.
  - Low social status, i.e., illiteracy, unemployment, overcrowding community, discomfort zones, pollution of air, water, sound, poor disposal management, natural calamities, poverty, child and women abuse, lack of sex education and poor water supply.

  Thus, the community health nursing diagnosis is derived from "synthesis of assessment data that is based on the concepts of risk and health needs and situations that can be influenced by nursing intervention".

- **Community health nursing diagnosis consists of three parts:**
  1. Description of the problem
  2. Identification of factors etiologically related to the problem
  3. Signs and symptoms that are characteristics of the problem, e.g., health indicators, verifying existence of the problems

  After making community health nursing diagnosis, priorities are set.

Planning

Planning is a logical decision-making process. This refers to the designing of an orderly detailed program of action around a specific goal. This is concerned with determining how to meet the needs of individuals, families and community.

Purposes of planning are:
- To determine how to meet the community healthcare needs and solve health problems
- How to manage with limited resources for many problems of vast population
- To eliminate unnecessary expenditure

Steps of planning

Planning includes (Fig. 2.4):
- Analyzing and establishing priorities among community health problems
- Establishing goals and objectives
- Identifying intervention
  - **Analysis of problems and clarify the nature of problems:** Analysis of problems is needed for each identified problem. A team of special members (experts) in the area of problems concerned, representative of the community and the person whose organization has the capabilities to intervene, is required along with community health nurse for analysis of the problem. Once the problems are analyzed, prioritization of the problems is done. Problems are prioritized according to the severity and their impact on health. Problem prioritization criteria are determined in accordance with community awareness, community motivation to resolve the problem, nurse's ability to intervene, availability of experts to problem solution.
  - **Establishing goals and objectives:** After prioritization of the problem, the goals and objectives are established. The goals are the broad statements of the desired outcome,

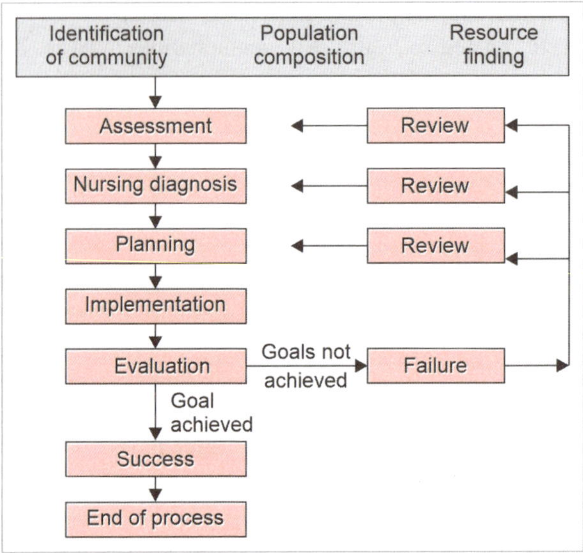

Fig. 2.4: Steps of community health nursing process

whereas objectives are the precise statements of the desired outcome. This process requires collaboration between nurse and representatives of the community groups which are related to the problems and proposed intervention.

- **Identifying intervention:** Interventions are the strategies for achieving the objectives. They describe and clarify what is to be done in what way and how it is to be done. Alternative intervention strategies must be identified and weighed with the planned ones and carefully evaluated.

Implementation of Community Health Nursing Care Services

Implementation is the process of putting the planned activities into action. The methods of implementation are the vehicles of work activities. Here, the whole community is regarded as patients. In the community health nursing process, implementation cannot be performed by a single person or community health nurse alone. It is carried out by a big group of persons or groups who have established the goals and objectives. Implementation is delegated to the people involved in the welfare of the community for solving these health needs and problems. The community health nurse is the key person in centralizing the implementation efforts.

- **Factors affecting implementation**
  - Nurse's role—she may be health educator, counselor, direct care provider, etc. affecting the community health nursing care implementation
  - Selection of the type of health problems
  - Community's readiness to participate in problem resolution
  - The characteristics of the social change process
- **Methods of intervention/implementation**
  - **Small interacting groups:** The formal groups (such as families, legislative bodies, healthcare providers, and healthcare recipients) and informal groups which include social

groups, neighborhood, etc. have a common tie. Due to this intermediate position, they can do and act, both to support and constrain change efforts at the community and individual levels. These groups play a vital role in changing the health behavior and health habits of the community. Sometimes a new small group may be needed to facilitate the change.

- **Law advisors:** They act as opinion leaders. They have higher position in the community. The village sarpanch or panch, religious persons, teachers, gram sevak, old famous body of village, mukhiyas, ward member, key informants, etc., all work as health facilitators. They are capable of bringing changes in the community.
- **Mass media:** The mass media has brought about a sizeable change in the health behavior of the people. The impact of TV, computer, CDs, videos, internet, newspaper and journals are the effective aids in intervention. For example, the use of iodized salt in prevention of goiter, ORS for the treatment of diarrhea and pulse polio immunization for polio eradication have been found effective after their advertisement on TV. The mass media is very important to communicate the health message quickly to a large number of people.
- **Health policy and public health laws:** The health policy and public health laws protect and address collective human needs and constrain individual choice for the wellness of general public health. Thus, they play a critical role in the adaptation of health for community behavior.

Evaluation

Evaluation is the process of ascertaining the outcomes against the objectives. It involves two aspects:

- Evaluation of the nurse's performance
- Evaluation of the behavioral changes in the community

  After implementing intervention, accomplishment of objectives and the effects of intervention activities are evaluated. Various tools can be used for evaluation of community health nursing process. The progress records of community-oriented health records direct the nurse to perform appraisals during the implementation. Nurses should evaluate whether the intervention activities are effective. The cost benefits are also to be evaluated. One such example of tools used for evaluation is survey:

  - **Survey:** It is performed by using following methods:
    - Questionnaire
    - Rating scales
    - Vital statistics
    - Observation (direct or indirect observation of behavior change)
    - Process recording

Replanning

If the objectives are met, community health nursing process is considered successful. In case of failure, steps of community health nursing process are again considered and the strategy is replanned.

Summary

- The philosophy of community health nursing is that nursing services should be provided to all irrespective of race, religion, caste, creed and sex.
- Community health nursing is influenced by attitude of family, religion, culture, education, value, norms and beliefs of the family.
- The main goal of community health nursing is to promote the health of the individuals, families and community.
- The main principles of community health nursing include planned services according to the need and requirement of the community, maintaining good interpersonal relationship with the community, and providing services irrespective of caste, creed, color, religion, etc.
- The community health nurse should be confident, cooperative, sincere, hardworking, good listener, intelligent, having strong professional knowledge, tactful, impartial, possessing supervisory and administrative qualities.
- Community health nursing process helps the community health nurse to prevent the occurrence of diseases in the community and helps to manage the health problems of the community intelligently, scientifically and judiciously.

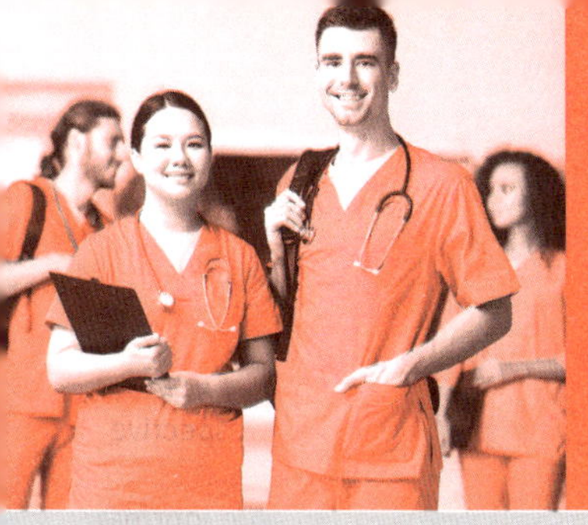

LONG ANSWER TYPE QUESTIONS

1. Define community health nursing. Explain the goals, objectives and principles of community health nursing.
2. Explain the community health nursing process.

SHORT ANSWER TYPE QUESTIONS

1. Enlist the functions of community health nursing.
2. Enumerate the steps of community health nursing process.
3. Write a short note on the following:
   a. Data collection
   b. Assessment of health problems and needs
   c. Community diagnosis
   d. Implementation of plan

MULTIPLE CHOICE QUESTIONS

1. **The environmental conditions of the community can be assessed by the:**
   a. Housing and water supply
   b. Ventilation and sanitation
   c. Disposal of waste
   d. All of the above

2. **To achieve health, the services provided by community health nurses are:**
   a. Preventive
   b. Promotive
   c. Preventive, promotive, curative and rehabilitative
   d. Curative and rehabilitative

3. **The health problems and health needs of the community can be assessed by:**
   a. Interview
   b. Survey
   c. Questionnaire
   d. All of the above

4. **After making community diagnosis, the next sequence of nursing process is:**
    a. Planning, implementation, evaluation and establishing the goals
    b. Establishing the goals, planning, implementation and evaluation
    c. Evaluation, planning, implementation and establishing the goals
    d. Planning, implementation, establishing the goals and evaluation

5. **Community health nursing diagnosis consists of:**
    a. Description of the problems
    b. Identification of etiological factors related to the problems
    c. Signs and symptoms of the problems
    d. All of the above

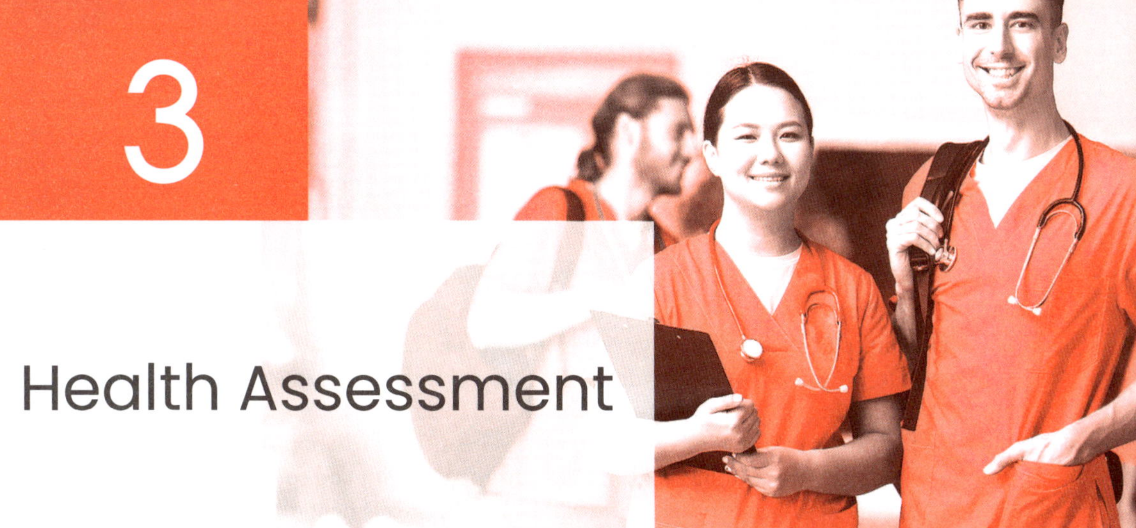

Health Assessment

LEARNING OBJECTIVES

After the completion of the unit, the readers will be able to:
- Discuss the components of health assessment.
- Identify the deviations from normal parameters in different age groups.
- Describe the technique of physical examination of the client.
- Discuss the health assessment at various stages of life.

UNIT OUTLINE

- Introduction
- Advantages of Health Assessment
- Characteristics of Healthy Individuals
- Components of Health Assessment
- Health Assessment of Infant
- Health Assessment of Preschool Child
- Health Assessment of School-Going Child
- Health Assessment of Adolescents
- Health Assessment of Antenatal Woman
- Health Assessment of Postnatal Woman
- Health Assessment of Adult
- Health Assessment of Elderly
- Collection of Specimens for Various Pathological Investigations
- Breast Examination

KEY TERMS

Assess: To make judgement about something.

Disability: Impairment; a physical, mental, cognitive, or developmental condition that impairs, interferes with or limits a person's ability to engage in certain tasks or actions or participate in typical daily activities and interactions.

Inflammation: Signs of infection with redness, heat, pain and swelling.

Interview: Formal meeting in which interviewer takes information from a person.

Kyphosis: An excessive backward curvature of dorsal spine.

Lordosis: Convex curve of the lumbar spine.

Observe: To notice or perceive (something) and register it as being significant.

Sucking in: Drawing in; to draw (something, such as liquid) into the mouth through a suction force produced by movements of the lips and tongue.

INTRODUCTION

Good health is essential to lead a successful life. Beyond being a personal responsibility, to be in good health is national and international responsibility too. It is a worldwide social goal to achieve Health for All (HFA). Spread of education and awareness have brought about a positive change in the overall attitude of individuals, government and social organizations toward health. Targets have been set to achieve optimum health for the people. Health assessment is the most important component of nursing process. It is a valuable tool to determine the health status of individuals, families and communities. Based on the health assessment, further planning, implementation, evaluation and decision regarding provision of appropriate health and social services can be made. Nurses are expected to have in-depth knowledge of the assessment skill. Health assessment is a regular and continuous process. In any setting of the health unit that focuses on health and wellness, nurses are responsible to provide primary healthcare. Hence, health assessment skill has become more critical than ever.

ADVANTAGES OF HEALTH ASSESSMENT

- Health assessment provides knowledge about the health status of an individual, family and community.
- It provides an opportunity to the community health nurses to have direct interaction with the people of different age groups of the community.
- It helps in early diagnosis of disorders or disease.
- It helps to identify the health problems of community and get information to prepare the plan.
- It helps the community health nurses to acquire knowledge about the health status of the community.
- It helps to impart health education and protection against diseases.
- It helps to develop good relations with community.

CHARACTERISTICS OF HEALTHY INDIVIDUALS

According to the World Health Organization (WHO) definition, "Health is a state of complete physical, mental and social well-being and not merely an absence of disease or infirmity". So, health does not mean to be free from illness but to attain best state of health which enables an individual to live a productive life and can be of use not only to himself but others also. So, it is our birthright to remain healthy by making use of all modern facilities.

There is no system which can describe universally acceptable characteristics of healthy individual as the characteristics are also influenced by aging process, life events and personal values. Health and disease are **subjective states**, difficult to measure. Hence, the characteristics of healthy individual are judged in accordance with health, disease, and wellness level of function.

Characteristics of healthy individual can be described under the following headings (Fig. 3.1).

- Physical
- Social
- Spiritual and cultural
- Mental

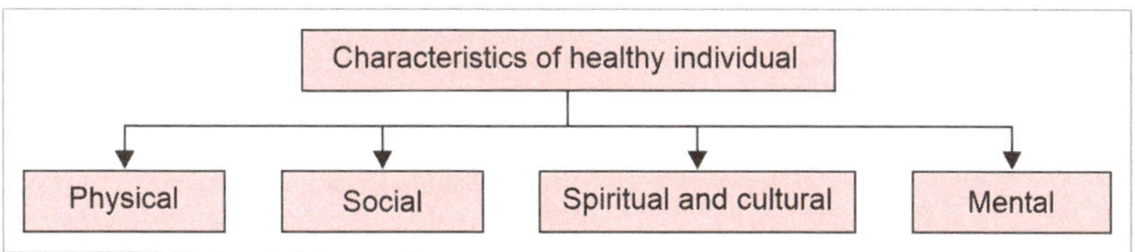

Fig. 3.1: Characteristics of healthy individuals

Physical Characteristics

Physical characteristics are related to body structure and function and can be measured from head-to-toe assessment (Fig. 3.2). These account for the major part of an individual's health and these characteristics are listed as follows:

- Healthy individual appears pleasant and cheerful. Height and weight according to the normal standard, intelligent, smiling face, friendly in nature, well dressed and good posture are some of the major characteristics.
- Healthy individual is well oriented to the person, place and time. Promptly responding to the questions, maintaining eye to eye contact, being fully conscious and having good judgment capability are some other characteristics.
- Healthy individual has clear speech, uses correct words and has good command on sentences and wordings.

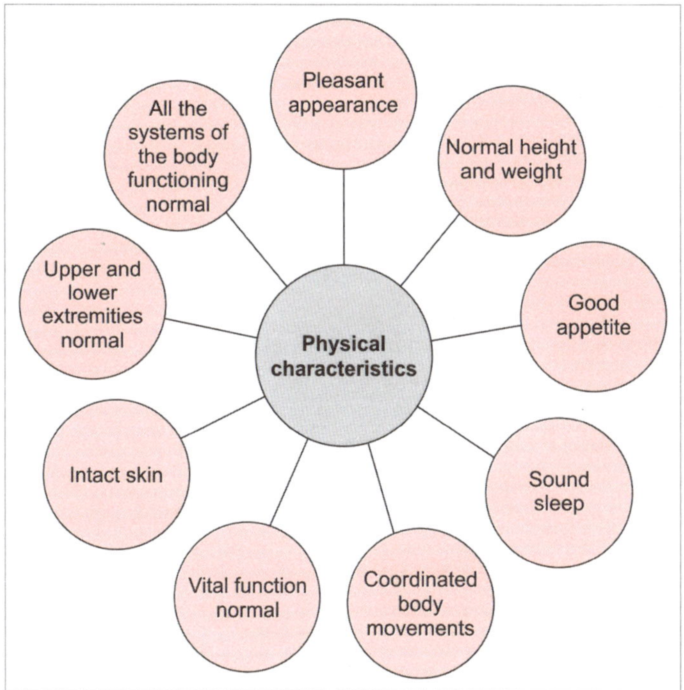

Fig. 3.2: Physical characteristics

- **Head:** Symmetrically rounded with full range of motion. Hair clean, shining, oiled, combed without dandruff scalp and skull smooth, firm symmetrical with no inflammation, **cysts, lesions** or tenderness.
- **Neck:** Symmetrical with smooth controlled movements, lymph nodes not palpable, no scar or lesions, trachea in midline.
- **Eyes:** Symmetrical and in alignment with top of ears, eyebrows with equal distribution, eyelashes evenly spaced, blinking symmetrical and involuntary. No discharge from eyes. Vision normal (6/6) with or without glasses.
- **Ears:** Normal in size and symmetrical, no deformity or discharge from ears, normal hearing
- **Nose:** Same color as face. No lesion or nodule, no discharge, nasal septum in midline, olfactory action normal.
- **Mouth:** Lips symmetrical, smooth moist, no nodule or lesion. Buccal mucosa pink, moist, without discoloration, no ulcer, gums pink and moist without erythema and cyanosis, bleeding and inflammation.
- **Teeth:** About 28–32 white in good condition, no dental caries
- **Tongue** and palate are middle, symmetrical, moist pink, with smooth movement, without nodule. Both palates in normal condition. Sweet, sour, salty, bitter and savory tastes can actually be sensed by all parts of the tongue.
- **Chest:** Symmetrical **even** and **relaxed**, respiration 16–20/min. Breathing normal without wheezing or Rhonchi. Sternum and ribs without any deformity.
- **Heart:** Apical pulse 72–76/min. regular, no extra heart sound or pulsation.
- **Breast:** Symmetrical, nontender, no lump or lesions, no discharge, Lymph nodes not palpable
- **Abdomen:** Round, soft, symmetrical. Bowel sounds audible and normal. No tenderness. Abdominal girth is less than the chest circumference.
- **Upper extremities:** Arms symmetrical, no deformities, all types of motions present. Muscle reflex normal.
- **Lower extremities:** Legs symmetrical, no lesions or bony deformity. No rashes, edema or inflammation, with full range of movements.
- **Sensory system:** Normal sensation.

All systems of body should be free from any deviation, dysfunction or problem.

Social Characteristics

A healthy individual takes an active part in overall social well-being of his society (Fig. 3.3).
- He is always positive in social interaction.
- He behaves appropriately with everyone.
- Follows the social change, socialization process and social control.
- Participates in social activities.
- Keeps good relation and harmony with members of family, society and community.

Spiritual and Cultural Characteristics

- A healthy individual should have holistic approach. He believes in his religion but respects other religions and beliefs also.
- He follows the ethics and principles and has commitment to some higher being or God.
- He should also respect the cultural values of self, society, as well as should give respect to others' cultural norms and values.

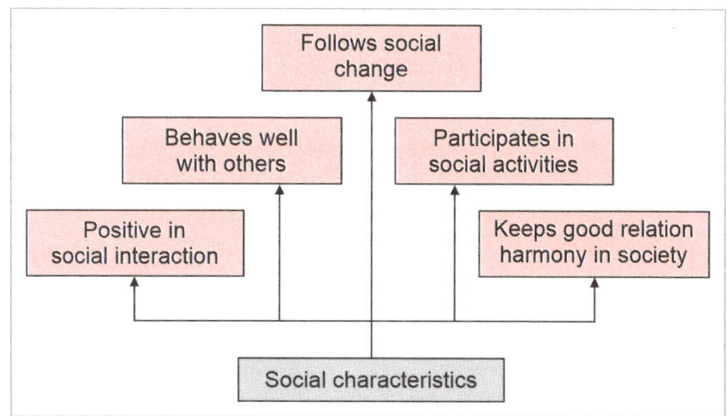

Fig. 3.3: Social characteristics

Mental Characteristics

Mental health is also a state like physical health. It relates to the mind and refers to the normal functioning of the mind and not merely the absence of mental illness. Some of the characteristics of mentally healthy individual are:

- Mentally healthy individual is well-adjusted with himself and the society.
- Aware of his limits, knows his strength and weakness.
- Free from mental conflicts and tension.
- Lives in a world of reality and not in fantasy.
- Self-confident, has self-identity and strong sense of self-esteem.
- Ability to give and receive love.
- Able to meet the demands of his life, able to solve his problems.
- Makes adjustment with new situations with minimum discomfort.
- Behaves in a responsible manner and expresses his feelings and thoughts clearly.
- Has a variety of interests and lives well-balanced life of work, rest and recreation.
- Able to think himself and takes his own decisions.
- Mentally healthy individual is able to accomplish all works of life in natural and mature manner without any problems.
- Maintains good social relation with people of the society.
- Satisfied with his job and occupation.
- He has ability to bear the stress and strain of life and keeps the ability to adjust as per the situation.
- Maintains balance in every aspect of life, work and behavior. He is responsible for his own actions.

COMPONENTS OF HEALTH ASSESSMENT

There are two main components of health assessment (Fig. 3.4):

1. History taking
2. Physical examination

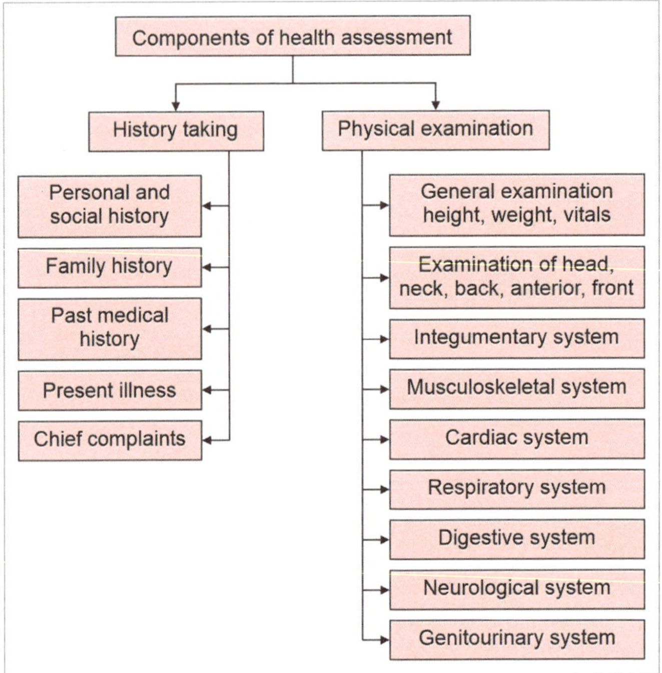

Fig. 3.4: Components of health assessment

History Taking

History taking is a tool of collecting information about the individual, his family, socioeconomic background, nutrition status, previous medical and surgical history and present complaints. It helps to get information about the person's previous health status and present problems. By history taking, we can gain patient's confidence and establish rapport.

Responsibility of Community Health Nurse in History Taking

- Introduce yourself to the patient and tell the purpose of taking history.
- Address the patient very respectfully.
- Make the patient (to sit if he can) comfortable while taking history and sit near him.
- Listen to the patient patiently, never show hurry.
- Give shape, form to the present problems.
- Concentrate on the main complaints.
- Collect data about personal, family, previous treatment, emotional aspect and social background.
- Respect the patient's beliefs and culture.
- Never criticize any habit or attitude of the patient.
- Always maintain privacy, secrecy and confidentiality of the patient.
- Never hesitate to ask essential questions.
- Show your concern about the patient's problems.
- Use the language that patient can understand.

Components of History

- Personal and social history
- Family history
- Past medical history
- Present illness
- Chief complaints

Personal and Social History

Personal and social history includes:
- Name
- Sex
- Age
- Address and Phone no.
- Education
- Occupation: Type of work, duration of employment and hours of work
- Monthly Income
- Religion
- Habits: Rest, sleep, recreation, etc.
- Nutritional status
- Marital status
- Number of family members
- History of taking drugs, alcohol or smoking, etc., urinary and bowel activity, sexual activity

Family History

- Type of family
- Number of members in the family
- Any significant illness in the family
- Health history of the family members, family income

Past Medical History

- Any illness in the childhood
- Immunization
- H/O Allergy
- Medical illness in the past
- Serious accident and injuries
- **Surgical history:** Any operation, hospitalization if any (type and duration), history of blood transfusion

Present Illness

Onset of disease, its duration, symptoms and location, precipitating factors, associated symptoms, treatment taken, current medication and its prescriptions, side effect of medication, if any.

Chief Complaints

- Present complaints
- Onset, duration
- Medication

Physical Examination

- **General survey:** In this, the general appearance of the client, his age, sex, gait, body movement, body type, personal hygiene, speech, mood and manner of dressing are noted.
- **Vital signs:** Temperature, pulse, respiration and blood pressure are checked.
- **Height** and weight are recorded.
- **Physical examination** of all structures, organs and body system is done.

Preparation for Physical Examination

- Keep all the required equipment like blood pressure instrument, stethoscope, tongue depressor, clinical thermometer, knee hammer, needles and pins, salt, sugar, hot and cold water, etc. to check the sensations.
- Prepare the examination table with clean top and bottom sheet.
- Screen the examination table to provide privacy.
- Introduce yourself to the client.
- Provide comfortable environment, free from distractions and disturbances.
- There should be good light to make observations.
- Explain the purpose of conducting physical examination to the client.
- Ask the patient to empty the bladder before starting physical examination.
- Keep your hands warm before starting physical examination.
- Record the height and weight of the client.
- Make the client lie down on the examination table comfortably.
- Record temperature, pulse, respiration and blood pressure.
- Cover the patient with top sheet and expose the area to be examined only.
- Maintain the dignity and privacy of the patient.
- Avoid unnecessary touch and handling.
- Be polite and gentle while making physical examination.
- Be very careful while examining the sensitive areas like breast and genitalia.

Techniques of Physical Examination

There are four basic techniques used in physical assessment:

1. **Inspection:** Inspection is the most frequently used technique of physical assessment. The area to be observed should be fully exposed and observed in good light. By this method, we can note the color, size, shape, symmetry and position of the body organs or any lesion, if present. Inspection can be direct relying on the sight like observing appearance, color, gait, look, body type, etc. By indirect inspection, we can use tongue depressor to examine the throat and tonsils; and nasal speculum, vaginal speculum, otoscope and ophthalmoscope are used to examine nasal cavity, vagina, ear and eyes respectively. Inspection also includes asking the patient to take deep breath and exhale against pursed lips, and involves touch to note the pitting edema or pressing thumb nail and assessing blood return, any impairment of function, if present, is noted, maintain objectivity while inspecting.

2. **Palpation:** This technique is used to gather data by touching. Finger tips are used lightly to feel the pulsations or vibrations or to elicit pain. Touch may be used deeply to palpate enlarged liver or spleen or to note the size of any swelling or nodule.

3. **Percussion:** In this technique, the quick, sharp tapping of the fingers or hands is used against body surface (chest and abdomen) to produce sounds to detect tenderness or assess the reflexes.

4. **Auscultation:** This method involves listening to the sounds within the body like sound produced by the lungs, heart, stomach and intestines. Most sound is indirect, and involves the use of stethoscope. Direct sound is listened by ears to identify crepitus or asthmatic wheeze. The diaphragm of stethoscope is used to listen to the sound of lungs, heart and bowels. The bell of stethoscope is used to listen to the vascular sound.

Nursing Considerations

Sequence of Physical Examination

- **General overview:** General appearance, built, gait, coordination, balance, speech, cognition, mental status, interaction, height, weight, vital signs, temperature, pulse, respiration and blood pressure recorded.
- **Skin:** Inspect and palpate all visible skin surface.
  - Inspect nails and hair
  - Evaluate lesions, if any
- **Head:** Inspect and palpate cranium, eyes, ears, nose, sinuses, mouth and throat.
- **Neck:** Inspect, palpate thyroid gland, lymph nodes, carotid pulses, jugular vein, range of motions
- **Back:** Inspect and palpate the symmetry, spinal alignment, scoliosis, lordosis, costovertebral angle, tenderness, mobility of the spine.
- **Anterior trunk:** Inspect breast, palpate any lump or nodule, palpate axillary and epitrochlear lymph nodes.
  Auscultate breath sounds, heart sounds, palpate carotid pulses, auscultate apical pulse, palpate brachial pulses. Assess the range of motion of upper extremities. Auscultate apex for murmur with patient leaning on left side, inspect the respiratory movements.
- **Abdomen:** Inspect the color, contour and diaphragmatic movements. Palpate the abdomen for any lump, tenderness, any enlargement of the liver, spleen, inguinal nodes, femoral pulses. Auscultate over abdominal aorta, renal artery, percuss the abdomen for any fluid thrill, palpate or percuss for bladder distension.
- **Musculoskeletal system:** Assess the gait, posture, weight bearing, check extremities for edema. Inspect and palpate upper and lower extremities and joints for tenderness, heat or crepitus. Check the muscle tone, wasting of muscles, symmetry, check the range of motion of lower extremities and check edema. Palpate popliteal, dorsalis pedis and posterior popliteal arteries.
- **Neurological system**
  - Test the reflexes—biceps, triceps brachioradialis, patellar, achilles and plantar reflex
  - Test the balance and fine motor movement
  - Test cranial nerves and sensory perception
  Assess color, warmth, strength, range of motion, gait and gross motor movements.
- **Genitourinary system**
  - Examine external genitalia for any discharge, growth or any abnormality
  - Rectal and vaginal examination, if indicated
  - Prostate examination, if indicated

HEALTH ASSESSMENT OF INFANT

Children below the age of 1 year are called infants. Health history and important information about infant's health are collected from the mother. In the absence of mother, the information is obtained from the caretaker of the infant. Health assessment of the infant is described under the following points.

Personal Data

- Name of the child
- Age
- Parents name, address and telephone number.

Past Health History

- Mother's health before pregnancy, mother's health during pregnancy.
- Age of the mother.
- Any drugs taken during pregnancy, prescribed or nonprescribed, smoking, alcohol, illegal drugs whether pregnancy was planned, normal or high-risk pregnancy, complications of pregnancy, if any.
- Any other illness.
- Exposure to toxins, chemicals, radiations or any other hazards.

Natal History

- Period of gestation at the time of delivery, place of birth whether hospital delivery or home delivery.
- **Type of delivery:** Spontaneous vaginal delivery or operative delivery like forceps or cesarean section.
- APGAR score.
- Birthweight, length, head and chest circumference of the baby, complications, if any.

Neonatal History

- Condition of the baby at birth.
- Whether oxygen, ventilator or incubator care given, estimation of gestational age, congenital anomalies, if any.
- **Problems:** Feeding, respiratory distress or jaundice.
- Age at discharge from the hospital.
- Weight at discharge from the hospital.
- **First month of life:** Family adaptations.

Feeding History

Breastfeeding, duration, supplements started, type, amount, weight gain, age at which solid foods started, type of foods, infant's response to the foods, parent's response to feeding their infant, weaning, food preferences, current feeding, type, schedule.

Developmental History

- Height and weight at different ages, head, chest and mid arm circumference at different ages.
- At what age (month) child started holding head, rolled from back to stomach and back, sitting with support and without support, walking with support and without support, speaking words.
- Eruption of first tooth.
- Reached for toys.
- Toilet training.

Immunization History

Immunization received date-wise, any reaction, allergy, etc.

Family History

- Parents relationship with each other.
- Employment of parents.
- Educational and nutritional condition in the family.
- Any consanguinity in the family.
- Parents illness.
- Adequacy of food, clothing, sleep arrangements and transportation.
- Sibling relationship to one another.
- Sibling illness.

Safety History

- Protection from electric points, detergents, poisons, medications or matches by proper storage.
- Protection from access to staircase, fire, ponds and pools.
- Infant sleeping on back or side not on abdomen.
- **Past illness:** History of hospitalization, operation, etc.

Present Illness and Chief Complaints

- History of present illness is obtained from the parents.
- **Review of systems:** Detailed checkup is done of all the systems of infant. Special attention is paid to the following:
  - Skin disease.
  - Ear disease.
  - Excessive running of nose.
  - Breathing from mouth or other allergic conditions, nutritional pattern of the infant.
  - For health assessment of infant, the community health nurse is required to have special skills. Active support of the mother or guardian is required.

HEALTH ASSESSMENT OF PRESCHOOL CHILD

Preschool going age is the age between 1 to 4 years. This is the period of intense growth and development. Children are more likely to suffer from malnutrition, infections, diarrhea and dehydration. Immunization is almost complete during this period.

Health assessment of preschool going child is discussed as follows:

Personal Data

- Name
- Sex and age
- Parents name, address and telephone number whether the child attending crèche or play way school.
- The duration of stay at crèche/play way school
- Whether the child likes to attend play way school or not

Past Medical History

- General health and strength of the child.
- History of any communicable disease/accident or hospitalization for any reason.
- If the child was hospitalized, the reason and duration of hospitalization and the treatment undergone.
- The reaction of child to illness and hospitalization.

Family History

- Type of family
- Number of members in the family
- Significant illness in the family
- Socioeconomic status of the family
- Number of children in the family

Immunization History

Immunization history can be recorded from the immunization card of the child. It determines whether the child is immunized against all vaccine preventable diseases or not.

Nutritional/Dietetic History

- The age child started eating normal food.
- The kind of foods being given to the child and the interval of providing food. Whether these foods fulfill the nutritional requirement of the child.
- Types of food being prepared for the child.
- Ability to feed self.
- Any history of allergy to any type of food.
- Weight gain.

Developmental History

- History of weight and height at different ages, head, chest and mid arm circumference at different ages.
- At what age child started walking, started talking in one word, two-word sentences, used toilet.
- Dressed self, dressed with help, started running, climbing **stairs**, **engaged** in solitary play, walked down stairs with alternate foot, followed commands.
- Recognized colors, sleep patterns.
- Habits—nail biting, thumb sucking.

Present Condition of Health and Major Health Problems

- Child's general appearance
- Level of nourishment
- Child's complaints
- Parents complaints about child's health
- The duration of onset of complaints noted

Physical Examination

- General appearance, weight, height, posture, nature, level of intelligence as per the age are noted, vital signs recorded.
- Whether the child is oriented to place, person and time, gives prompt answers to the questions, speech, mental status and gait. Coordination and balance are noted.
- Skin color, any rash, pigmentation texture of skin noted.
- Head, scalp for dandruff, pediculosis, color and texture of hair noted.
- **Eye:** For any infections, discharge, eyesight.
- **Nose:** Rhinitis or deviated nasal septum.
- **Mouth:** Tongue, buccal mucosa noted.
- **Teeth:** If any caries or malocclusion.
- **Throat:** Inspected for adenoids or enlarged tonsils.
- **Ear:** Any discharge present.
- **Neck:** Lymph nodes palpated. Observed for any abnormality.
- **Back:** Symmetry, spinal alignment noted.
- **Anterior trunk:** Chest inspected for any evidence of rickets, heart sound, lung sounds noted or enlarged abdomen or any abnormality is observed.
- **Musculoskeletal system:** Inspected for gait and posture, knock knee looked for evidence of rickets. Bowels and bladder habits are noted. Based on the history and physical examination, the provisional diagnosis is made to plan care.

HEALTH ASSESSMENT OF SCHOOL-GOING CHILD

Health assessment of school-going child is a part of school health services. Other than community health nurse, the teacher and physician are also involved as they are the members of school health team. The components of health assessment of school-going children are:

- **Periodic checkup of children:** It includes:
  - Checkup at the time of admission
  - Health checkup of children every year or more frequently
  - Checkup at the time of leaving school
- **Health checkup at the time of school admission:** It includes:
  - **Measurement of height:** Weight, dental checkup, eye checkup, hearing test speech. Routine examination of stool, urine and blood are done, child's health card is made and after every routine medical checkup, the entries are made in the card.
  - **Nutritional assessment:** Height, weight, appearance, built give an idea about the nutritional status of the child. Information about the diet child gets at home and supplementary meals given at school suffice the requirement of calories and nutrients required for proper growth and development of the child. If the food child gets at home is not sufficient and deficient in essential nutrients, the parents are given education to improve the child's diet at home.
- **Daily examination:** Daily examination of the child is conducted by the teachers. The teachers are required to be given training about diagnosing the minor ailments of the children and are supposed to give treatment as per the requirement like treatment for cold, cough, fever, headache, dehydration, skin disease. They are also expected to note that whether the child is able to see blackboard properly to diagnosis early disorders of vision, and to note down any discharge from the ear for otitis media or appearance of rash on the body for detection of communicable diseases to refer the child accordingly.

Personal and Family History

Personal and family history is collected at the time of admission of the child by the school health nurse from parents or parent-teacher meeting if not collected at the time of admission.

Past Medical History

Past medical history is collected from the parents while making child's health card at the time of admission.

The health assessment of the school going child is collective responsibility of the parents, teachers, community health nurse, doctors; and cooperation of other local bodies like municipality, panchayat, municipal corporation and voluntary organizations is also required.

HEALTH ASSESSMENT OF ADOLESCENTS

An adolescent is a young person in the process of developing from a child into an adult. The children between the age group of 13 and 18 years are called adolescent children. Up to the age of 18 years, complete physical development and stability is achieved. According to WHO, the adolescent period from the age of 10–19 years is divided into three stages:

1. **Early adolescent:** 10–13 years
2. **Middle adolescent:** 14–16 years
3. **Late adolescent:** 17–20 years

Personal Biodata

- Name
- Age
- Sex
- Parents name and address and telephone number
- Educational qualification
- Hobbies and interests
- Whether the adolescent adult is independent, depends on parents for financial support
- If independent, the type of employment and income
- History of taking drugs, tobacco, alcohol, etc.
- **Nutritional pattern:** Appetite, types of food preferred, fluid intake, interval between meals, quantity of essential nutrients and caloric requirement, exercise and recreation, bowel and bladder habits.

Past Medical History

History of any medical or surgical disorder, operation, hospitalization, duration and treatment taken.

Family History

Type of family:
- Number of members in the family and their educational qualification
- Any consanguinity in family
- Employment status of the family, family income, parent's relation with each other
- Adequacy of food, clothing and transportation, sibling relation to one another, sibling illness

Immunization History

Immunization time, date, complete, incomplete can be recorded from the health card/immunization card.

Sexual Development

- Age of voice change and pubic hair growth (boys)
- Age of breast development and menarche (girls)
- Social relation with same and opposite gender, curiosity about gender
- Parent's response and instructions to the child about sexuality and dating

Social History

- Sleep pattern, problems, terrors, speech clear, stuttering, delays, stress and its level
- **Discipline used:** Type, frequency, effectiveness, attitude, response of parents to temper tantrum.
- **School:** School, grade, attendance, failure, performance level, problems
- **Social behavior:** Relationship with peers, parents, teachers, type of pear group, level of independence and spiritual practices.

Present Illness

- The onset, duration and treatment taken are noted.
- **Chief complaints:** Main complaints are noted by asking questions and special attention is paid to those complaints while planning care.

Physical Examination

- General appearance, gait, built, level of nourishment, speech, mental status, height, weight and temperature, pulse, respiration, blood pressure are recorded. Complete physical examination from head to toe is performed to detect any abnormalities.

  Special attention is paid to major health problems of adolescent period, such as:
  - **Nutritional problems:** May be undernutrition or over nutrition or anemic. Adolescent children neglect their meals; especially girls suffer from anemia. Anemia may be due to worms or due to heavy blood loss during menstruation. Some girls may suffer from anorexia nervosa.
  - **Sexuality related problems:** The boys and girls get attracted toward each other as they get mature and may indulge in pre-marital sex relations resulting in illegitimate pregnancies and associated social problems. Malicious sexual practices can result in HIV/AIDS, STD and hepatitis B.
  - **Alcohol and drug abuse:** In peer group, adolescents easily become prey to the use of alcohol, drugs and smoking habits resulting in social problem and their personal health problem and family problems.
  - **Self-esteem related problems:** Adolescents want self-respect and identity among friends and society. They try their best to fulfill the desire of admirations. If they fail to achieve, they may feel unworthy and can lose mental balance resulting in depression.
  - **Depression:** It may result from fatigue, boredom, restlessness, failure to achieve their goals, difficulty in concentration. Professional help is required in such condition. These health problems are specific to the adolescent period viewed seriously. Professional help, guidance and counseling are required with the involvement of parents.

HEALTH ASSESSMENT OF ANTENATAL WOMAN

Health assessment of antenatal woman begins from the time of confirmation of pregnancy.

Aim

Aim of antenatal health assessment is to ensure delivery of a healthy baby to a healthy mother at the end of pregnancy.

Objectives

- To promote, protect and maintain the health of pregnant mothers
- To detect high-risk pregnancy and manage it appropriately
- To reduce maternal and neonatal morbidity and mortality rate
- To foresee complications and prevent them
- To teach the mother about elements of child care, nutrition and personal hygiene
- To educate the mother about the need of family planning

Components

- Taking medical history
- Physical examination
- Laboratory examination
- Monitoring the growth and development of the embryo
- Detection of high-risk pregnancy

History Taking

Personal Data

- Name
- Age
- Address and telephone number

Past Medical History

Any previous medical or surgical/hospitalization history for any reason.

Menstrual History

- Age at menarche
- Menstrual cycle
- Regularity, flow, amount and interval, complication regarding menstruation, if any
- Date of last menstrual period (LMP). Expected date of delivery (EDD) is calculated by adding nine months and seven days to the LMP.

Obstetrical History

- Number of pregnancies
- Previous pregnancy
- Place of delivery, i.e., Home/Hospital delivery
- Date and time of delivery
- Type of delivery, i.e., normal or operative
- Sex and weight of the child
- Health condition of the child at present
- **Present pregnancy:** Planned/unplanned, signs and symptoms of pregnancy

Personal and Family History

- Marital and sexual history, educational standard of the woman and her husband
- Occupation and income of the pregnant woman and her husband.

Social History

- Habits related to rest, sleep, exercise, food, recreation and elimination
- Minor disorder of pregnancy, if any
- General status of health
- Any significant disease in the family
- Type of family, number of family members, education and employment status and monthly income.

Physical Examination

General examination: Weight and height, appearance and built, nourishment, jaundice, anemia are noted. Vital signs, i.e., temperature, pulse, blood pressure, respiration are also noted. Pulse oximetry and head-to-toe examination are performed.

Obstetrical Examination

- **Examination of the breast:** Breast is examined for inverted/cracked nipples or any other abnormality.
- **Examination of the abdomen:** Examination of the abdomen on inspection, shape, contour, presence of striae gravidarum, scar of previous operation, if any.
- **Palpation:** Fundal height, presentation and position noted.
- **Auscultation:** Recording of fetal heart sound.
- **Vaginal examination:** If necessary, during the first visit to diagnose pregnancy, and after 37 weeks of gestation in case of primi for pelvic assessment.

Laboratory Examination

At the first visit to the antenatal clinic, the following investigations are done:
- Hemoglobin estimation, TLC and DLC
- Blood group and Rh factor
- Blood sugar, STD screening
- Urine for albumin and sugar and microscopic examination
- PAP smear
- Stool test for worm infestations
- Ultrasonography
- X-ray chest, if necessary

Monitoring the Growth and Development of the Embryo

The growth and development of the embryo is recorded during antenatal visits. The pregnant woman is advised to visit antenatal clinic:
- Once in a month till 30th week of pregnancy (she can visit any time if any problem comes)
- Once in 15 days from 30 to 36 weeks
- Once in a week after 36 weeks till labor pain starts.

During antenatal visit, fetal growth and development is recorded from maternal weight gain, fundal height corresponding to the gestational age. Date of quickening is noted and fetal movements are recorded. Fetal heart sound is checked.

Mother's health is also monitored; and BP, edema and Hb% are checked. Any serious sign is noted and treated.

Detection of High-Risk Pregnancy

- Elderly primi >30 years of age or very young primi <15 years of age.
- Grand multipara undergone more than four deliveries.

- Anemia, hemoglobin <10 g%.
- Malpresentation.
- Antepartum hemorrhage.
- Bad obstetric history.
- Multiple pregnancy.
- Hydramnios.
- Previous cesarean section.
- Preeclampsia and eclampsia.
- Post maturity.
- Pregnancy with hypertension, diabetes mellitus, renal diseases, tuberculosis, heart disease.
- Pregnancy with fibroids or ovarian cyst.
- Short statured woman, height <140 cm.
- History of previous stillbirth.

If a pregnant woman is detected as high-risk case, appropriate care is taken throughout pregnancy and she is booked for hospital delivery.

HEALTH ASSESSMENT OF POSTNATAL WOMAN

Postnatal period is the time after delivery of the baby till 6 weeks. During this period, generative organs return to their prepregnant stage.

Aims

- To provide care to the mother and child and bring back mother to optimum health as early as possible.
- To protect the mother and child from complications during the postnatal period.
- To assist the mother for early breastfeeding to avoid engorgement of breast and protecting the baby from physiological jaundice and dehydration.
- To provide health education to the mother regarding personal hygiene, care of breast, perineum and nutritional education.
- To teach postnatal exercises to the mother.
- To provide family planning services.
- To teach care of the newborn baby.

During postnatal health assessment, the baby's health is also assessed along with the mother's health. To provide psychological support, her fear and worries are to be relieved by showing concern toward the health of mother and her baby before starting the health assessment.

Main Components of Postnatal Health Assessment

- Physical examination
- Laboratory examination
- Examination of psychological responses

Physical Examination

Objectives of postnatal physical examination are:

- To collect the data regarding involution of the uterus.
- To assess the needs of the lactating mother.
- To provide health education.

Physical examination includes:

- **General observation:** Mother's general appearance, posture, facial expression are noted.
- **Recording the vital signs:** Temperature initially falls because a lot of heat is lost from the body, she may have shivering immediately after delivery. During this phase, warmth is provided.

  Pulse rate may fall. Blood pressure is checked. If blood pressure is low, foot end of bed is raised. Quick examination is made for evidence of excessive blood loss. Meanwhile resuscitative measures are taken. Respiration is usually normal.

- **Abdominal examination:** Abdomen is palpated. Uterus should be felt hard and contracted. After delivery, its size is 2.5 cm above the umbilicus and then starts decreasing 1.25–2.5 cm/day. If uterus is felt soft, that means some membranes or placental pieces are left inside the uterus. Uterus is massaged and stimulated to contract. If necessary, vaginal examination is done to remove it.

- **Bladder examination:** Abdomen is also observed for bladder distension. After the removal of placenta, the antidiuretic hormone falls in blood; so, diuresis starts and bladder may be felt full. Sometimes mother may not feel the urge to pass urine. This is because of minor injury or bruises on urethral muscle or temporary paralysis of urethral muscle due to excessive compression during the delivery of baby. Mother is encouraged to pass urine. If she is not able to pass urine, the bladder should be catheterized. After few hours, she will be able to pass herself but needs to be encouraged. Otherwise full bladder results in poor uterine contraction and causes bleeding per vagina from the opened uterine sinuses.

- **Breast examination:** Mother is usually exhausted after delivery. Her breast may be heavy due to lactation. Breast should be cleaned and she is helped to breastfeed the baby.

  Sometimes there may be cracks on the nipple which are very painful when the baby sucks, she may be afraid to give breastfeed. Cracked nipples are to be treated by applying soft antiseptic cream. But nipples should be cleaned before giving feed to the baby. The leftover milk after baby's feed should be expressed and thrown to avoid breast engorgement.

- **Examination of the uterus:** Uterus is felt for its consistency. It should be hard and palpable. Fundal height is checked every day for uterine involution, size of the uterus should decrease 2.5 cm every day and by 13th day, it should not be palpable above the symphysis pubis.

- **Examination of the perineum and vagina:** The perineum and vagina are inspected for any tear, laceration or episiotomy wound. Decidua forms layers inside the uterus in 1–2 days. The outer layer secretes lochia, it is red for first 2–3 days and then changes to pink for 4–7 days and then creamy white. The color, quantity and smell of lochia are noted. During this postnatal period, the uterus, cervix, vagina and perineum regain their tone.

- **Pelvic examination:** Pelvic examination is performed after 6 weeks to know the involution of the pelvic organs.

Laboratory Examination

Blood hemoglobin is estimated after 3rd day of delivery. Then at the end of puerperium, urine is tested for routine examination, and ultrasonography is performed, if considered necessary.

Examination of Psychological Responses

Developmental Approach

- Acceptance of the baby
  - Taking care of the newborn baby
  - Feeding the baby
  - Feeling relief from discomfort of pregnancy, labor pains and delivery
  - Regarding physical and mental strength
  - Establishing family relationship with baby

Dependent Phase

After a few days of delivery, the women need help for taking care of baby and herself. Also, for how long she remains dependent on others depends on her mental makeup, willpower and physical stamina. Emotional ups and downs may be observed during this period.

- **Bonding with infant:** Mother loves her baby holding it close to her body. Father and other family members also assist in care of the baby and find satisfaction by touching and holding the baby.
- **Adverse responses:** In case of unwanted pregnancy or child is born out of some compulsion, mother may show rejection. This type of situation should be tackled carefully by counseling the mother and all family members to help mother accept the baby.
- **Health education:** During the process of making health assessment or while taking care of postnatal woman, the health education regarding rest, sleep, nutrition, excretion, personal hygiene related to care of the baby, cord care, eye care skin care and breastfeeding is given.
- **Postnatal visits:** The community health nurse can make as many visits as required according to the type of delivery and requirement of the visits, but for normal delivery a minimum of four visits should be made. The first visit should be within 24 hours after delivery or after discharge from hospital. Second visit is made during 3rd day of delivery when there is chance of breast engorgement, to note physiological jaundice of the newborn and 3rd visit on 5th day of delivery and 4th visit after 7–10 days. Visits can be increased according to the requirement. After 6 weeks, lady should attend postnatal clinic along with baby.

HEALTH ASSESSMENT OF ADULT

Health assessment of adult includes the following steps:

Personal Biodata

- Name
- Sex
- Age
- Address and phone number
- Religion, nationality
- Educational qualification
- Occupation, type and working hours
- Monthly income

- Marital status
- Age of the spouse
- Education of the spouse and occupation
- Number of children and their age

History of Present Illness

- Chief complaints
- Onset, duration
- Location of symptoms
- Treatment taken and its response
- Current medication

Past Health History

- Childhood illness, dates, type of medication or surgical disease, accident, operation, hospitalization, duration and response to the treatment.
- Immunization history.
- History of allergy to the drug, food or any other.

Family Health History

- **Type of family:** Number of members in the family, educational level and employment status of the family members, family income. Any significant illness in the family.
- **Personal habits** and patterns of living, rest and sleep, how many hours of rest, type of sleep sound, disturbed.
- **Employment:** Duration, type, working hours and working environment.
- **Stress:** At home in the family, at work place or with relatives and friends.
- **Exercise:** Type and duration.
- Recreation, leisure, types of hobbies.
- **Nutritional status:** Types of food, vegetarian/nonvegetarian, intervals between the meals. Any change in appetite, taking special diet for any reason, bowel and bladder habits.
- **Psychosocial history:** Client's relationship with family members, friends, neighbors, coworkers, with spouse, religious group, social and civic organization in the community, satisfaction with employment, occupation and household responsibilities, recreational activities, leisure, time and sports enjoyed.
- **Spiritual history:** Believes and practices spirituality, concept of God, values placed on religious practices and spiritual adviser.

Physical Examination

- **General overview:** General appearance healthy or sick looking, nourishment, body type normal, well built, thin built, height, weight, personality, gait, balance, speech, mental status, vital signs, temperature, pulse, respiration and blood pressure recorded.
- **Examination of skin:** Color, rash, dryness, presence of lesions.
- **Head:** Inspect and palpate cranium, scalp hair and its texture, color, dandruff, pediculosis.
- **Eyes:** Vision with or without glasses, discharge, infection, any other abnormality.
- **Ears:** Discharge, hearing capacity. Nose, mouth, throat inspected; preauricular, postauricular and occipital nodes palpated.
- **Neck:** Inspect and palpate thyroid gland, lymph nodes. Feel for carotid pulsation and jugular vein, and note the range of motions.

- **Back:** Symmetry and spinal alignment, evidence of scoliosis or lordosis, mobility.
- **Anterior trunk:** Inspect the breast and chest. Watch out for expansion during respiratory movements, auscultate breath sound, heart sound and apical pulse, palpate the auxiliary glands.
- **Abdomen:** Observe for the presence of any scar, and shape of abdomen; palpate liver, spleen, inguinal nodes; observe femoral pulses, presence of free fluid in abdominal cavity; auscultate bowel sound.
- **Musculoskeletal system:** Examine upper and lower extremities, joints, note the range of motion, swelling or tenderness of the joints.
- **Neurological system:** Assess any tenderness, color, warmth, strength, range of motion, gait, gross motor movements; test reflexes, balance, fine motor movements; test cranial nerve, test sensory perception.

Genitourinary System

- Inspect external genitalia for any discharge or infection.
- Rectal examination, if indicated.
- Prostate examination, if indicated.
- Vaginal examination and PAP smear in case of female, if indicated.
- Depending upon the history and physical examination, care is planned for adult.

HEALTH ASSESSMENT OF ELDERLY

The age of 60 years has been accepted as cut off age for elderly in most developing countries including India. The aged population is increasing fast because of the availability of better health facilities, education and awareness. Aging is inevitable and irreversible. It is slow and gradual process spread over last 20–30 years of life. As the individual grows old, various changes take place with time under the influence of biological factors within the individual and external factors in the environment and the kind of lifestyle. Many of the changes can be delayed by modifying various factors such as diet, exercise, lifestyle, support system and early management of expected problems that may occur due to aging. As per the WHO, theme of the year 1999 was "Active aging makes the difference". So, the health assessment of elderly contributes to active aging.

Objectives

- To maintain and protect the health of elderlies so that they can live disability-free life.
- To help them retain physical, physiological, psychological and social fitness to its maximum so that they can live normal life like earlier days.
- To help them cope well with the physical, mental, social and spiritual activities.
- To help them live productive life as long as possible and contribute to family and community.
- Health assessment of elderly includes history taking and complete physical examination of the aged people.
  The following points should be kept in mind while making health assessment of elderly:
  - Old people may suffer from more than one health problems. Loneliness, lack of social and financial independence and negligence aggravate the problem.
  - The symptoms of disease may not be well marked in the aged people.

- They may become used to live with the disease as they believe that there is no remedy or they may be afraid of complaining because others may ignore it.
- Behavior of the family plays an important role in the health assessment of aged people.

Personal Biodata

- Name
- Sex
- Age
- Home address and telephone number
- Place of birth
- Education
- Socioeconomic status
- Domestic environment
- Married, divorcee or widow
- Cultural background
- Position of the family
- Interest and hobbies
- Other aspects of general life, religion, belief

Family History

- Type of family
- Number of family members
- Attitude of family members towards the health of elderly
- Support system
- Any significant disease in the family

Past Medical History

- General health and strength, diseases of childhood and youth like measles, chickenpox, diphtheria, polio, etc. in childhood and jaundice, hypertension, heart disease and diabetes or any other disease in adult life. Any operation or accident, allergy or any emotional or behavior problem, treatment taken, if any.
- **Assessment of disabilities:** Elderly person may experience problems while sitting, walking, getting up, climbing the stairs, holding things and maintaining balance. They may have problems in cooking, domestic work, washing clothes, shopping, taking medicine and managing money and in activities of daily living like going to toilet, bathing, changing clothes. They may be suffering from psychological and social disabilities, making use of some devices like walking sticks, walker, wheelchair, spectacles or hearing aids, dentures, etc. They become dependent on others. So, there is need of social protection and support.
- **Nutritional status:** Different aspects such as appetite, types of food, number of meals, menu, availability of food items, difficulties faced with regard to money, availability, etc. are considered. Other aspects that are considered are whether taking any special diet like diabetic diet, low salt, low fat and high fiber diet, associated health problems interfering with ingestion, digestion and absorption of food and stability of weight.

- **Social aspects:** These include whether living with family or alone; if living with family, different aspects such as family size, composition, their general health, occupation, activities and status of elderly in the family, his involvement in household activities and family support are considered.
- If living alone, the reasons for living alone, the type of support from relatives, friends, neighbors and social workers are taken into consideration.
- **Housing conditions:** These include aspects such as own house/rented, the number of rooms and facilities available to the elderly.
- **Activities of daily living:** Personal hygiene, washing, cleaning the house, shopping, preparing food, dressing, grooming, medication, administration, paying bills, etc., are being managed independently by the patient or with other's help.

Social Support

Family/Friends

- Community involvement, member of any religious organization.
- **Living arrangement:** Living with family, alone or in nursing home.
- **Community services:** Whether uses daycare center, home healthcare or rehabilitation services.
- **Present illness:** The duration and onset of the disease, treatment taken, individual's response to the treatment.
- **Chief complaints:** The main chief complaints like pains and aches, difficulty in breathing, loss of appetite, constipation, incontinence of urine, chronic cough, temperature, imbalance of body, inability to move, etc. are noted to decide about the implementation of the care.
- **Substance abuse:** Information must be obtained regarding the use of alcohol and its effects or taking drugs, etc.
- **Cognition:** Memory, orientation to the time, place and persons, ability to retain information, ability to understand and explain the concept, judgment, follow commands are noted.

Physical Examination

- **General appearance:** Body type, nourishment, look, gait, personality, balance, speech, mental status, height, weight and vital signs such as temperature, pulse, respiration, blood pressure are recorded.
- **Integumentary system:** Skin color, pigmentation, rash, dryness, texture and any lesions.
- **Head:** Examine scalp for dandruff, pediculosis, scar or any other lesion, etc.
- **Eyes:** Vision, discharge from eyes or infection if wearing spectacles, whether it is comfortable or needs change.
- **Ears:** Hearing test using hearing aid feels comfortable or any discomfort felt with the use of hearing aid.
- **Teeth:** If using denture, inspect mouth, tongue and buccal mucosa for any injury.
- **Mouth and tongue:** Inspected for any infection and lesions.
- **Neck:** Trachea in midline, palpate for enlarged lymph nodes.
- **Chest:** Watch out for expansion during respiratory movements, any wheezing sound during expiration, auscultate breath sounds, heart sounds and apical pulse.

- **Abdomen:** Presence of any scar, shape of abdomen, any distension, accumulation of free fluid in the abdominal/peritoneal cavity, palpate liver, spine, inguinal node, femoral pulses. Auscultate bowel sounds, feel bladder for any distension.
- **Back:** Symmetry, spinal alignment, presence of scoliosis and lordosis are noted.
- **Musculoskeletal system:** Examine upper and lower extremities for muscle wasting, range of motion, swelling and tenderness of joints, if present.
- **Neurological system:** Assess any tenderness, color, warmth, strength, range of motion, gait, gross motor movements, test reflexes, balance, fine motor movements. Test cranial nerves and sensory perception.
- **Genitourinary system:** Examine external genitalia, enlarged prostate gland, urine, any difficulty in passing urine, retention or incontinence of urine. In females, prolapsed uterus and bladder, etc., are noted.

Depending upon history and physical examination, care is planned and implemented.

COLLECTION OF SPECIMENS FOR VARIOUS PATHOLOGICAL INVESTIGATIONS

Collection of specimens is a part of client's health assessment. The exact treatment is usually started after the availability of the laboratory test. The cure of the disease depends upon the reliability, accuracy and standard of laboratory investigation reports. There may be laboratory personnel for collection of specimens but in community setup, the community health nurse is involved in collection of specimens and also performance of some simple tests like testing urine for sugar, albumin and ketone bodies, making blood smear for malaria parasites or filaria or testing hemoglobin and blood sugar level.

Community health nurse is responsible for collecting and transporting specimen to laboratory. Thorough knowledge of collecting and transporting the specimens to the laboratory is very important. Any type of negligence in collecting or transporting specimen is a serious crime and against the code of ethics. So, all specimens should be collected religiously in accurate manner and technique so as to get the correct report. Appropriate treatment can be started to the client for his speedy recovery.

Specimens can be collected in the hospitals or in community setting.

- **In hospital setting:**
  - In outdoor patient department (OPD). Nowadays, most of the investigations are performed in OPD.
  - Patients unit, i.e., indoor patients
  - In special lab and diagnostic room
- **In community setting:**
  - In homes, during home visits
  - Health camps/clinics
  - Health centers (SC, PHC, CHC)
  - In epidemic conditions in affected area
- **Points to be remembered and kept in mind while collecting specimens in community health:**
  - Community health nurse should have thorough knowledge of the technique of collecting specimens.
  - Proper container should be provided to the patient while collecting urine, stool or sputum specimens; and technique of collecting the sample should be explained to the patients.
  - Specimen container should be labeled correctly with patient's name, number and address.

- Specimen should be transported to laboratory immediately after its collection; otherwise it will start decomposing.
- Laboratory test reports should be kept strictly confidential and only authorized persons are told about the results. Reports about positive **HIV/AIDS, STD,** cancer test should be disclosed by the doctor to the patients or relatives.
- It is to be kept in mind that laboratory test reports help in making diagnosis. A positive report may not be final one, and a negative report also does not guarantee that person is free from disease. In both cases, all matters should be taken into consideration before giving final results.
- **While taking samples, special attention should be given to the following:**
  - Specimen should be collected in proper clean container (Sterile containers are indicated for culture and antibiotic sensitivity test).
  - Specimen should be taken from the most infected source.
  - Specimen should not get contaminated from any external material.
  - Specimen should have proper and clear label.
  - Specimen should be sent to the place of examination without any delay.

Collection of Samples for Specific Examination

- Making blood smear for malaria parasite (MP) or filaria.
  - **Articles required:** Spirit swab, sterile pricking needle, clean blood slides, clean and dry paper.
  - **Procedure:** Community health nurse should wash her hands. Take spirit swab and clean the patient's finger at the distal top and press it for a few seconds. Take sterile pricking needle and prick the finger top gently. Take one drop of blood on the sides of two slides. Keep spirit swab on the pricked area and ask patient to press it till bleeding stops. Keep the slides on the table on paper blood dropped on right side, hold slide with left hand. Take another slide in the right hand and touch it on the blood drop in such a way that it spreads up to the side, hold the slide in slanting position and move the slide from left to right in such a way that a thin uniform film of the blood is formed. Prepare the smear on the other slide also and allow the blood to dry up. Send the slides to laboratory for examination, wash hands.
- **Collecting smear for filaria:** In this case, a thick smear is taken, i.e., the blood dropped on a slide is covered with cover slip of thin glass. Allow it to dry and then send to laboratory.
- **Collecting sputum specimen:** Sputum AFB examination is required in case of tuberculosis and sometime for culture in other infectious conditions of respiratory tract. Early morning specimen of sputum is collected. A wide-mouthed container with cover is provided to the patient. Patient is told to rinse the mouth with water and then cough forcefully to bring out the sputum which is collected in the container. It is covered, labeled and sent to the laboratory.
- **Collection of stool specimen:** Examination of stool is done in cases of intestinal parasites, enteritis, intestinal infections and in case of cholera. Some specimens are collected for culture and some are examined directly. For collection of stool specimen, patient is provided with wide-mouthed containers with lid and a spatula or small stick. Patient is instructed to keep a small quantity of stool in the provided container with the help of wooden spatula and cover the container. Container is labeled properly and sent to laboratory with the lab forms or requisition form needed for test.

- **Collection of urine specimen:** Urine sample is collected during home visit by community health nurse while making health assessment of diabetic client or pregnant woman for testing sugar, albumin, ketone bodies. Client is asked to clean the genitalia and pass some urine and then collect in wide mouth container or test tube provided to the client/patient for collection and then pass the remaining urine, i.e., midstream urine is collected, labeled and sent to laboratory with requisition form or it may be tested by the community health nurse right at the place of collection with the help of Clinistix, Urostix or Multistix for sugar, albumin or for pregnancy test, whereas culture specimen is sent to laboratory immediately after collection.
- **Collecting the specimen for blood sugar:** Patient is asked to wash hands with soap and water. Tip of any finger is cleaned with spirit swab after pressing and then pricked with sharp sterile pricking needle. A drop of blood is taken on a specified place of sticks and after specified time, color is compared according to printed instructions.

  Blood sugar test is also done with the help of glucometer. Patient is also taught about the use of glucometer for sugar testing.
- Other specimens like throat swab for culture, eye swab, pus swab, vaginal swab for culture are also collected by the community health nurse and sent to laboratory immediately.

BREAST EXAMINATION

Breast examination is a part of health assessment not only in women but also in men. They should be taught breast self-examination. Breast lumps are common but not always cancerous.

Time

- At the time of general health checkup at least once in a year.
- If there is history of breast cancer in the family twice in a year.
- During menopause, breast self-examination should be done once in a month.
- During reproductive age, once in a month, one week after the menses.

Components

- Physical examination by palpation and inspection.
- Laboratory examination if secretions are there.
- Biopsy if any lump or nodule present.
- Mammography is radiographic examination of the breast.

Technique

Inspection: Can be done in sitting position with hands above the head or hand on the waist or leaning toward front.

Palpation: It is done in supine position.

Points of Breast Examination

- **Breast size and symmetry:** Normal breasts are round and of the same size. Slight difference may be noticed in the size of left and right breasts.
- **Color of the skin and areola:** Skin is usually of the same color as that of the abdomen, plain, smooth and elastic. Any change in the color and inflammation indicate infection or cancer. It should be viewed seriously for further investigation.

- **Nipple size and shape:** Nipples are erect and pointing to the front and of the same size. Inversion of nipples toward inside, becoming flat or broad is suspicious of cancer. Secretions from the nipples do not indicate cancer. Presence of rash or wound should be checked.
- **Color of areola:** Its color changes during pregnancy, i.e., becomes pinkish in fair colored women and darker in black or brown colored women.
- **Breast palpation:**
    - Women should lie down in supine position.
    - Both the breasts should be palpated gently.
    - Surrounding area of the breast, i.e., base and axilla should be palpated for the presence of any lump.
    - With the help of finger pads, the parts all around the breast and breast tissues are palpated circularly.
    - If a lady complains of lump in one breast, the other breast should be palpated first to know the difference.
    - If any lump, mass or nodule is detected, its shape, size, mobility and consistency are noted.
    - In addition to the breast, the under arms and axilla should also be examined for the presence of any lump.
    - Nipple and areola are pressed to check the presence of secretions.

Breast Self-Examination by a Female

Breast self-examination should be done after menses. It can be done in standing in front of mirror in dressing room or bathroom or in bedroom.

Steps

1. Stand in front of the mirror. Inspect both the breasts for any change in size or shape. Examine the nipples for any discharge, dimpling, scaling of the skin or flattening of the nipple (Fig. 3.5, Step I).
2. Clasp your hands behind head and press your hands forward and watch the shape and contour of breast in the mirror (Fig. 3.5, Step II).
3. Press your hands on the hips and lean slightly toward the mirror and note any change in shape and size of the breast (Fig. 3.5, Step III).
4. Raise your left arm, and use the pads of three middle fingers of your right hand, examine the left breast by palpating with the finger pads in circular movements so that the entire breast is examined. Gradually work toward the nipples. Pay special attention to the area between the breast and under arm and feel for any unusual mass or lump (Fig. 3.5, Step IV).
5. Gently squeeze the nipple; if any discharge is present, consult the doctor (Fig. 3.5, Step V).
6. Repeat the steps IV and V for examining the right breast.
7. If any abnormality is found, consult your doctor.

Breast Self-Examination by a Male

Males should also examine their breast for any lump, nodule, any tenderness or color change from time to time.

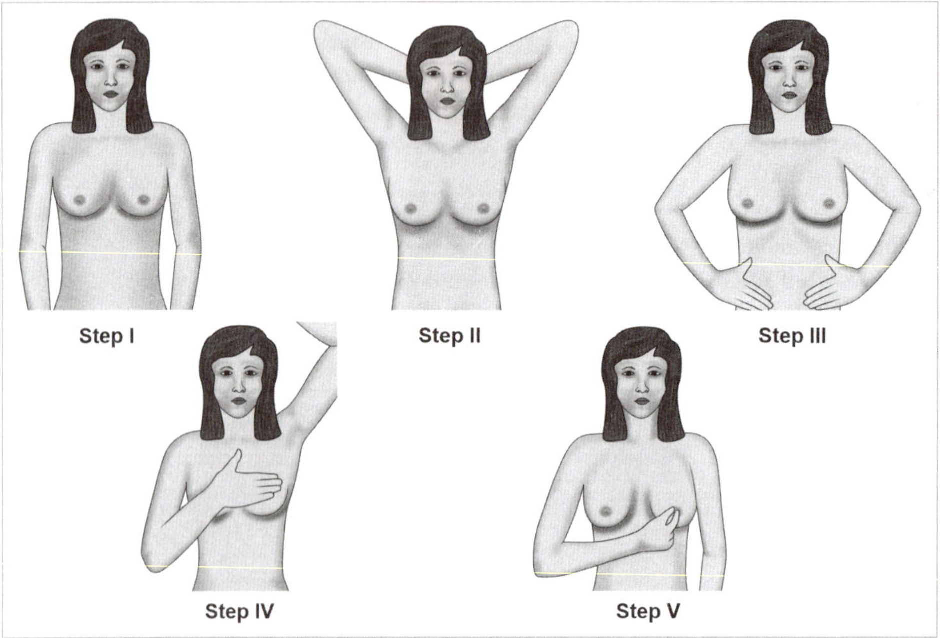

Fig. 3.5: Breast self-examination

Summary

- Health assessment is a systematic process of collecting, analyzing and interpreting data to identify the health status, needs and concerns of patients, as well as to develop appropriate nursing interventions.
- The characteristics of a healthy individual are pleasant appearance, appropriate weight and height, intelligent, smiling face, friendly in nature, well-balanced (mentally and emotionally), well-groomed and having good posture.
- Health assessment differs according to age groups, i.e., infants, preschool and school going children, adolescents, adults, aged persons and pregnant women. But in general, it includes family history, past medical history, personal history, present illness and chief complaints, assessment of development in infants, review of systems and head-to-toe examination.
- Assessment of pregnant women includes history taking, antenatal examination, laboratory examination, monitoring growth and development of the fetus and detecting high-risk pregnancy.
- Health assessment of postnatal women includes postnatal examination, i.e., examination of breast, abdomen, perineum and vagina and laboratory examination.
- Specimens can be collected in community setting, in hospitals in OPD or in health clinics.
- The community health nurse should teach the steps of breast self-examination as a part of health education. It can help in early detection and treatment of breast cancer.

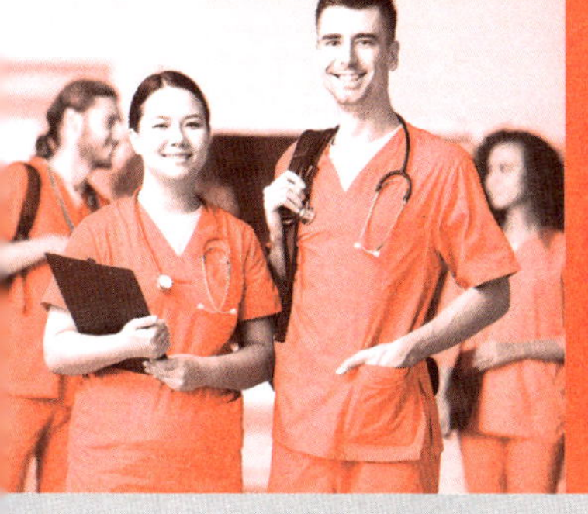

STUDENT ASSIGNMENT

LONG ANSWER TYPE QUESTIONS

1. What are the components of health assessment? Describe the method of physical examination.
2. Describe the characteristics of healthy individuals.

SHORT ANSWER TYPE QUESTIONS

1. Define health assessment and enlist the advantages of health assessment.
2. Enlist the body parts that are examined during head-to-toe examination.
3. Write a short note on:
     i. Health assessment
    ii. Breast self-examination
   iii. Nurses' responsibility in collection of specimens

MULTIPLE CHOICE QUESTIONS

1. **The methods used in physical examinations are:**
   a. Palpation
   b. Auscultation
   c. Percussion
   d. All of these

2. **Health assessment of school child includes:**
   a. Checkup related to the growth and development
   b. Immunization status of the child
   c. Nutrition level of the child and his eating habits
   d. All of the above

3. **Which of the following test is not done during the assessment of a pregnant woman?**
   a. Urine and stool test
   b. X-rays chest and abdomen
   c. Blood sugar and WBC count
   d. Hg%, blood group and pH faction

4. **Which of the following disability is required to be assessed in aged persons?**
   a. Physical
   b. Psychological
   c. Sexual
   d. All of these

5. **Yellow color of the skin and eye may result from:**
   a. Jaundice
   b. Cirrhosis of liver
   c. Amoebic abscess
   d. All of these

6. **Which of the following is not a healthy sign?**
    a. Face—shining, no abnormal marks or movements
    b. Lips—symmetrical, smooth and moist
    c. Heart—irregular pulse
    d. Abdomen—soft, round symmetrical, audible bowel sound

7. **Which of the following is high-risk pregnancy?**
    a. Malpresentation
    b. Multiple pregnancy and anemia
    c. Elderly primi, intrapartum hemorrhage
    d. All of the above

4

Principles of Epidemiology and Epidemiological Methods

LEARNING OBJECTIVES

After the completion of the unit, the readers will be able to:
- Describe the principles of epidemiology.
- Describe communicable and noncommunicable diseases.
- Explain the basic tools and methods used in epidemiology.
- Discuss the levels of transmission and prevention of disease.
- Explain the methods of control of infectious diseases.
- Define disinfection and describe various methods of disinfection.

UNIT OUTLINE

- Introduction
- Epidemiology
- Epidemiological Differences between Communicable and Noncommunicable Diseases
- Communicable Diseases
- Noncommunicable Diseases
- Epidemiological Investigations
- Basic Tools of Measurement in Epidemiology
- Applications of Epidemiology
- Course of Disease
- Spectrum of Disease
- Levels of Prevention
- Disease Transmission
- Immunity
- Immunizing Agents
- Immunization
- National Immunization Schedule
- Cold Chain
- Potency Test
- Control of Infectious Diseases

KEY TERMS

Anemia: Decreased level of hemoglobin which is <10 g%.

Azoospermia: Absence of sperms.

Bactericidal drugs: Drugs which kill the bacteria *in vivo*.

Bacteriostatic: Drugs which inhibit the multiplication of bacteria.

Carditis: Inflammation of heart.

Centrifugal: From periphery toward center.

Chemoprophylaxis: Administration of drugs to those exposed to a case.

Convalescent stage: Recovery stage.

Disinfectant: An agent which kills infectious agents outside the body by direct exposure to the chemical.

Endemic: The constant presence of a disease or infection within a geographical area relatively at low level.

Epidemic: An outbreak of disease in a community in excess of normal expectation and derived from a common or propagated source.

Epidemiological triad: Complex interaction between host, agent and environment.

Epidemiology: The study of distribution and determinants of disease in human population.

Fomites: Inanimate objects.

Hyperglycemia: Increased blood sugar level, i.e., >140 mg%.

Immunity: Host defense against infection; the state of being insusceptible or resistant to a noxious agent or process, especially a pathogen or infectious disease.

Immunizing agents: Agents used to provide immunity.

Incubation period: Begins from the time of entry of an infectious agent into the body till the appearance of first signs and symptoms of disease.

Ischemic heart disease: Impairment of heart function due to inadequate blood supply to heart muscles either due to blockage or narrowing of coronary arteries.

Koplik spot: Bluish spot with red base.

Malnutrition: Relative or absolute deficiency or excess of nutrients in human body.

Pandemic: An epidemic which spreads from country to country over the whole world.

Pathogenesis: Diseased condition; the process by which a disease or disorder develops.

Polyuria: Increased excretion of urine than normal.

Prepathogenesis: Process in the environment before the onset of disease.

Primary hypertension: High blood pressure without involvement of primary disease process.

Prodromal period: Short period of 1–4 days from entry of pathogenic agent to the appearance of vague symptoms.

Secondary hypertension: High blood pressure due to involvement of some other disease.

Sporadic: The incidence of a single scattered case of disease.

Subcutaneous nodules: Presence of nodules in subcutaneous area.

Transmission: Movements of infectious agent from one host to new host.

INTRODUCTION

In a broader sense, epidemiology is the study of occurrence, distribution and causes of diseases in mankind. Epidemiology focuses on population and community to measure the distribution and determinants of disease for the purpose of preventing disease and promoting health. Historically, epidemiology has been applied to the study of epidemics, pandemics and the infectious diseases but the modern epidemiology has entered the most exciting phase of its evolution. By identifying the risk factors and evaluating treatment modalities and health services; new opportunities for prevention, treatment, planning and improving efficiency of health services are provided.

EPIDEMIOLOGY

Epidemiology is the basic science of preventive and social medicine. The word "epidemiology" is derived from the word "epidemic" which is very old word dating back to the 3rd century. Literally the word "epidemiology" is a combination of three Greek words:

Epi = Among

Demos = People

Logos = Study of science

It means epidemiology is the study of events that occur among people. Though the concept of epidemiology became popular from the 19th century, it has evolved rapidly during the past three decades.

Epidemiology is not only applied to infectious diseases, but also today it is concerned with noninfectious diseases also. Epidemiology has given many new branches in the modern era such as infectious disease epidemiology, chronic disease epidemiology, clinical epidemiology, serological epidemiology, cancer epidemiology, malaria epidemiology, neuroepidemiology, genetic epidemiology, occupational epidemiology and psychological epidemiology. So, it includes all diseases that affect the human population. These include cancer, heart disease, metabolic disorders, mental illness, drug addiction, accidents, pregnancy, growth and development, poisoning, alcoholism, mental retardation, family life, family planning and environmental factors. Current epidemiological investigations are involved in determining the environmental relationships as sociocultural factors are also responsible for an individual's health status.

Definitions of Epidemiology

There are many definitions of epidemiology but the main components of definitions are same which include:
- Study of the frequency of the disease
- Study of the distribution of disease
- Study of the causes of disease

Common definitions of epidemiology are as follows:
- Study of the distribution and determinants of health-related states or events in specified population, and the application of this study to the control of health problems.

  —Johan M Last, 1988
- Branch of medical science which treats epidemics.   **—Parkin, 1973**
- It is the study of distribution and determination of disease and health-related events in human population with a view to ensure that health services are planned rationally, disease surveillance is affected and that preventive and control measures are undertaken.

  —Accepted by WHO, 1981
- Epidemiology is the study of occurrence, causes and distribution of infectious diseases as it occurs in humans.   **—Historical approach**
- The study of the distribution and determinants of disease frequency in humans.

  —Mac Mohan, 1960
- Broadly, epidemiology is a field of science which is concerned with various factors and conditions that determine the occurrence and distribution of health, disease, defect, disability and death among individuals and groups.   **—Leavell and Clark, 1965**

There is no single definition to which all epidemiologists agree, but three components are common to most of them:
1. Study of disease frequency
2. Study of distribution
3. Study of determinants

The subject matter of epidemiology is continuously changing. The current scope of epidemiology is the study of health-related conditions, events and factual life of population along with infectious disease. Today epidemiology focuses not only on those factors in environment that have a negative effect on our health status, but also focuses on the factors present in the environment that have positive or protective effects on our health.

Aims

The International Epidemiological Association (IEA) has laid down three main aims:

1. To describe the distribution and magnitude (degree of size) of health and disease problems among individuals and groups (human population)
2. To identify etiological factors (risk factors) in the pathogenesis of disease
3. To provide data for planning, implementation and evaluation of services for the prevention, control and treatment of disease and for setting up of priorities among those services.

In order to fulfill these aims, different classes of epidemiological studies may be used, i.e., descriptive studies, analytical studies, experimental and interventional studies. The ultimate aim of epidemiology is to lead to the effective action as follows:

- To eliminate or reduce the health problems and their complications
- To promote health and well-being of the community as a whole

EPIDEMIOLOGICAL DIFFERENCES BETWEEN COMMUNICABLE AND NONCOMMUNICABLE DISEASES

The epidemiological difference between communicable and noncommunicable diseases is the time factor. Communicable diseases have a shorter incubation period as compared to the noncommunicable diseases. The frequency of noncommunicable diseases is low, but the occurrence and distribution take place in similar fashion as that of communicable diseases.

Noncommunicable diseases such as coronary heart disease, hypertension and cancer have a longer incubation period. Many factors such as diet, exercise, obesity, cigarette smoking, alcoholism and sedentary lifestyle contribute to disease development overtime creating a more complex situation for determining web of causation or cause-effect relationship. The epidemiological investigations remain the same for the study of these diseases, the hypothesis testing step becomes the main focus of investigation with more than one factor often being studied simultaneously. In cases of chronic noncommunicable diseases, where disease agent is not exactly known and disease is caused due to interaction of multiple factors, this is called the web causation. The web causation is considered by all predisposing factors which contribute toward the causation of disease.

Natural History of Disease

Disease usually occurs in two phases:

1. **Prepathogenic phase:** This is the period before occurrence of disease. The disease producing organisms or agents are present in the environment but disease does not occur unless the disease agent is brought closer to human by interaction of agent, host and environmental factors. These three factors are known as **epidemiological triad** (Fig. 4.1).

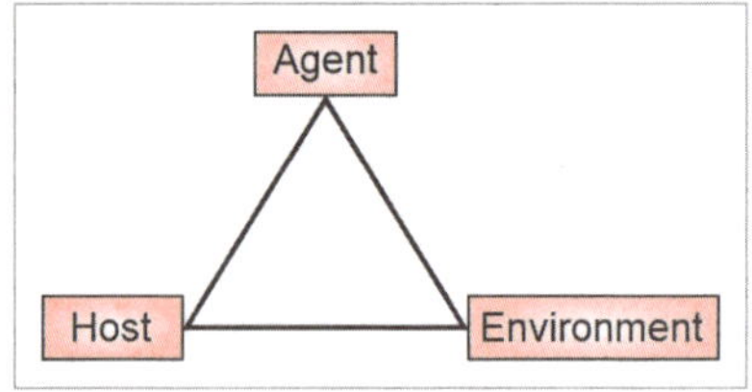

Fig. 4.1: Epidemiological triad

Interaction between these factors results in disease which may be seen as one case or an epidemic. For example, the typhoid bacilli are present in the feces or urine of cases or carrier, contaminated water or food. It may enter the human host through orofecal route either directly or indirectly. Poor personal hygiene, lack of knowledge and low standard of food may lower the resistance of the body to infection and facilitate the entry of organism, thereby causing infection. Similarly, disobeying the traffic rules can predispose to accidents; so, the interaction of host, agent and environment can initiate the disease.

2. **Pathogenic phase:** This phase includes the following stages:
    - **Incubation period:** It is characterized by multiplication of the disease agent and pathophysiological changes.
    - **Early pathogenesis:** It is characterized by the appearance of clinical stage, i.e., vague signs and symptoms. Clinical diagnosis is not possible.
    - **Late pathogenesis:** There are marked signs and symptoms of the disease. Patient is confined to bed. Clinical diagnosis is possible. Patient may recover completely or may develop disability. Stage of recovery is known as convalescence.

In noncommunicable diseases, the early pathogenic phase may not show clear signs and symptoms of the disease and this stage is known as **presymptomatic stage,** example of this stage is hypertension or cancer. Later the disease shows signs and symptoms; and the disease is much advanced. Pathogenesis phase may be altered by primary, secondary or tertiary levels of prevention. Steps taken at primary prevention include immunization, health promotion and specific protection which can prevent communicable as well as noncommunicable diseases. Measures at secondary prevention include early diagnosis and treatment. Tertiary prevention includes measures to rehabilitate and limit the disability.

Epidemiological Triad

The epidemiological triad, also known as the epidemiological triangle, is comprised of agent, host, environment.

- **Agent factors (Fig. 4.2):** The agent is a substance that may be living or nonliving or a force which is responsible for initiating the disease. The disease producing agents are classified as biological, physical, chemical, nutrients, mechanical, and social agents.

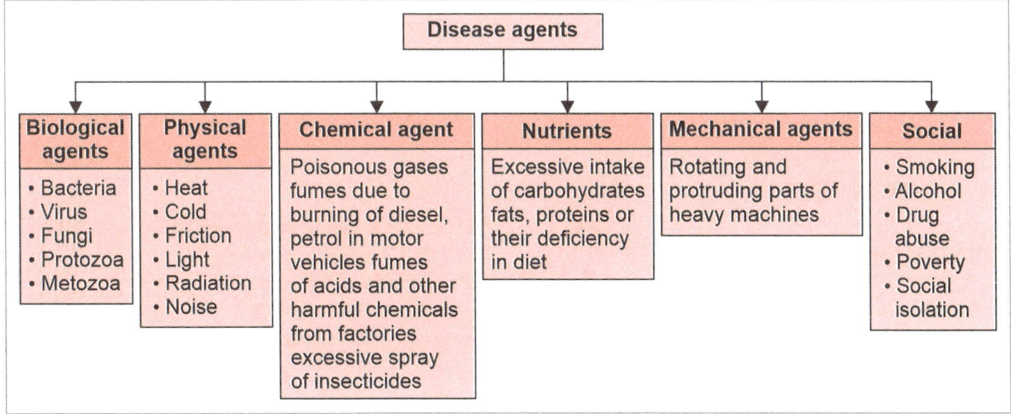

Fig. 4.2: Types of disease agents

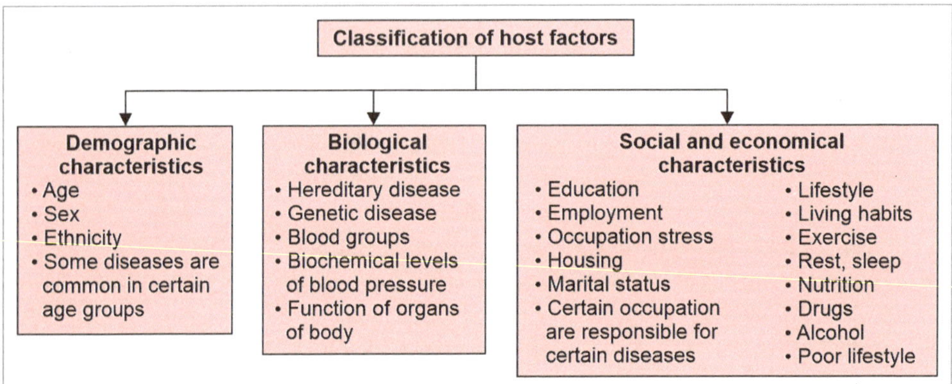

Fig. 4.3: Classification of host factors

- **Host factors (Fig. 4.3):** The human beings or animals who come in contact with the agents, when the resistance of the host is low, the agents succeed in producing disease. The susceptibility of the host to cause disease again depends upon lifestyle, demographic characteristics, biological, social and economic characteristics.

- **Environmental factors:** These factors play an important role in the individual's health. As long as there is harmonious equilibrium between the man and the environment, he lives a healthy life. But when there is maladjustment of the man with the environment, deviation from the optimum health occurs depending upon the degree of maladjustment. Environmental factors include internal environment and external environment. The internal environment refers to the harmonious functions of tissues, organs and body system. The external environment includes air, water, food, housing, other living and nonliving objects around him, etc., with which he is in constant interaction. Disease occurs due to maladjustment of the man to his total environment.

Classification of environment:

- **Physical environment:** All physical factors such as air, water, food, housing, heat, cold, noise, light radiation, friction, etc.

- **Biological environment:** All living things around man, i.e., microorganisms, insects, rodents, animals and plants. All of them work for their existence but some of them act as disease-producing agents.

- **Psychosocial environment:** It includes the lifestyle, culture, habits, attitude toward health, religion, beliefs, customs, values, and psychological makeup of the individuals. The structure and social functions of the social groups, parents love and affection help the child grow well mentally and physically, whereas negligence and criticism will lead to retarded physical and mental growth.

COMMUNICABLE DISEASES

Diseases which may be transmitted from one person to another directly or indirectly or due to a specific infectious agent or its poisonous products through transmission in an individual or community are known as communicable diseases.

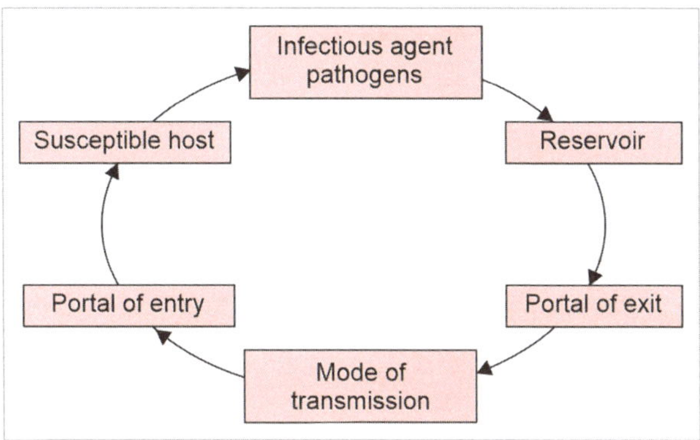

Fig. 4.4: Chain of communicable diseases

The chain of communicable diseases (Fig. 4.4): Communicable diseases have a chain of links. The spread of communicable disease can be arrested by breaking the chain at any point.

- **The infectious agent:** It includes bacteria, virus, protozoa, rickettsia.
- **Reservoir:** Human beings, animals and environment.
- **Portals of exit:** Respiratory tract, intestinal tract, mosquito bite, dog bite, insect bite, rodents, etc.
- **Mode of transmission:** Direct or indirect.
- **Portals of entry:** Respiratory, intestinal or any other system of body.
- **Susceptible host:** Low immunity and impaired physical and mental health, nutritional status and age of the individual.

Common communicable diseases are discussed in the subsequent sections.

Measles (Rubeola)

Measles is also known as Khasra and Rubeola which means red spot (Fig. 4.5). The disease is endemic in all parts of the world but in India, it spreads more between January and April.

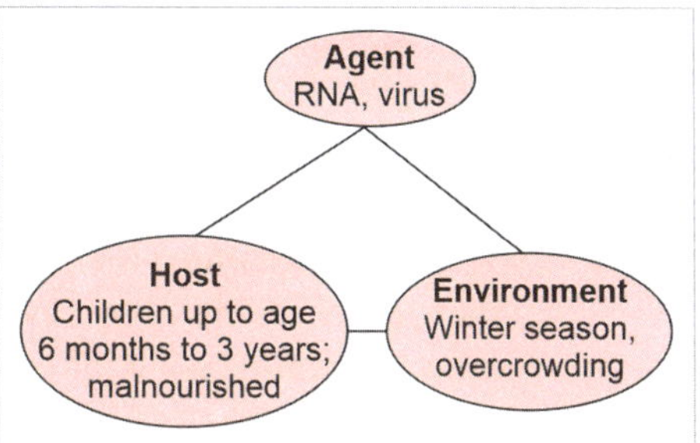

Fig. 4.5: Epidemiological triad of measles

- **Epidemiological triad:**
  - **Causative agent:** RNA virus of paramyxo-virus family
  - **Susceptible host:**
    - Children between age group of 6 months to 3 years.
    - Malnourished children are affected severely
    - Incidence is equal in male and female children.
  - **Environmental factors:**
    - Low socioeconomic conditions
    - Overcrowding residents
- **Modes of transmission:**
  - Direct contact during the period of infectivity, i.e., 4 days before appearance of rash and 5 days after appearance of rash.

- ■ Droplet infections as the virus is present in respiratory secretions
- ■ Droplet nuclei
- **Portal of entry:** Respiratory tract
- **Incubation period:** 10–14 days

Clinical Manifestations

Measles consists of two stages, namely pre-eruptive stage and eruptive stage.

1. **Pre-eruptive stage:** Onset is abrupt and resembles the following:
   - ■ Severe cold
   - ■ Moderate fever (102°F)
   - ■ Cough
   - ■ Sneezing
   - ■ Watering of eyes and nose
   - ■ Eyes become red and sensitive to light
   - ■ Hoarseness of voice due to laryngitis
   - ■ Appearance of Koplik spot on the mucous membrane of mouth and inner surface of lips seen opposite the lower molar in good light.
2. **Eruptive stage:**
   - ■ On 4th day, there is an increase in the severity of symptoms.
   - ■ Bronchitis is well marked.
   - ■ Eye lids become puffy and swollen.
   - ■ Rash appears on forehead, temples and behind the ears, face, trunk and limbs as slightly raised dusky spots as macules.
   - ■ Eruption lasts for 3–4 days followed by straining of the skin.
   - ■ Temperature remains high for 1–2 days and then gradually subsides in the absence of complications.

Management

Management of measles includes the following steps:

- **Prevention:** It comprises:
  - ■ **Active immunization:** Can be achieved by giving measles vaccine 0.5 mL subcutaneously at the age of 9 months or by MMR vaccine.
  - ■ **Passive immunization:** Immunoglobulin 0.25 mL/kg body weight can be given during the incubation period, i.e., after 3–4 days of exposure to protect the child from disease.
- **Isolation:** Child should be isolated for 7 days after the onset of the rash to prevent spread of infection.
- Notification of the disease to the concerned authorities.
- **Diagnosis** is confirmed from the appearance of Koplik spots and distribution and type of rash.
- **Treatment:**
  - ■ Rest in bed
  - ■ Reduce fever by antipyretics
  - ■ Adequate fluids and feeds
  - ■ Antibiotics to prevent complication
- Take care of the eyes

- Immunization at the beginning of an epidemic helps to control the disease.
- **Disinfection:** Proper disinfection of articles and linen used by the child including toys and furniture.

Complications

- Bronchitis
- Pneumonia
- Conjunctivitis
- Otitis media
- Encephalitis
- Febrile convulsions
- Diarrhea

Influenza

Influenza is an acute respiratory tract infection of short duration due to influenza virus. This virus has three categories, i.e., type A, B and C. Influenza A and influenza B affect humans (Fig. 4.6). The infection is worldwide epidemic.

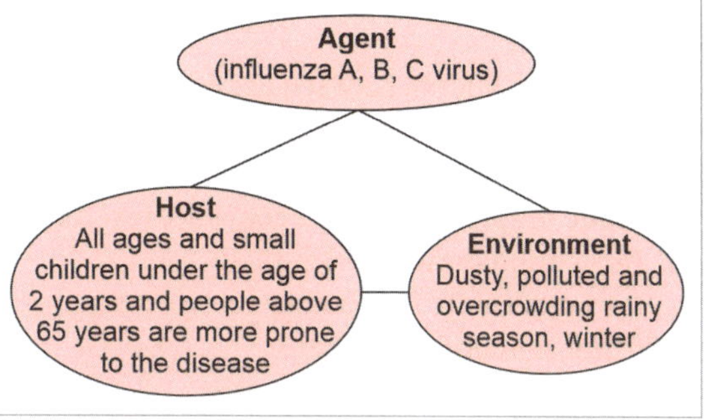

Fig. 4.6: Epidemiological triad of influenza

- **Causative agent:** Influenza virus (A and B).
- **Mode of spread:** Droplet infection, droplet nucleic and personal contact.
- **Incubation period:** 1–3 days
- **Portal of entry:** Respiratory tract
- **Clinical manifestations:**
  - Influenza starts with cold and cough
  - Fever starts after 1–4 days of cold and cough and patient feels cold and chills
  - Body aches, dry cough, blockage of nose
  - Running nose, headache, sore throat
  - Generalized weakness, loss of appetite
- **Diagnosis:**
  - By clinical signs and symptoms.
  - By laboratory investigations, serological examination, virus is detected by indirect fluorescent antibody technique.
- **Prevention:** By giving influenza vaccine but the immunity is short lived up to 6 months.
- **Control:**
  - Avoid overcrowded places
  - Good housing and ventilation
  - Covering face and nose while coughing and sneezing with handkerchief
  - Isolation of infected cases
- **Management:**
  - There is no specific treatment, only symptomatic treatment to protect from complications.
  - Isolation and rest in bed in well-ventilated room.
  - To control fever by antipyretics.

- To control cough and cold by giving steam inhalation and cough expectorant.
- Antibiotics to prevent secondary infection, maintain adequate caloric requirement and build up general resistance to infection.
- Antiviral drugs like amantadine or rimantadine 100 mg BD for 3–5 days may be given.
- **Complications:**
    - Pneumonia
    - Bronchitis
    - Pleurisy

German Measles or Rubella

Rubella is an acute infectious disease of children. It is also called 3-day measles.

- **Epidemiological factors:**
    - **Causative agent:** Rubella virus. This is RNA virus of toga virus family.
    - **Host:**
        - Children between age of 3 and 10 years are affected
        - Pregnant mothers may be affected and infections may induce abortions or congenital defects or birth defects
- **Mode of spread:** Personal contact, droplet infection, droplet nucleus
- **Incubation period:** 2–3 weeks
- **Portal of entry:** Respiratory tract
- **Clinical manifestations:**
    - Low grade fever, throat pain
    - Cough, conjunctivitis
    - **Lymphadenopathy:** The enlargement of postauricular and posterior cervical lymph nodes.
    - On 2nd day of fever, pinkish rash appears on skin; it may be macular or papular stage and may disappear after 3rd day.
- **Diagnosis:**
    - Clinical signs and symptoms
    - Serological examinations
    - Throat swab for culture and ABST
- **Prevention:** By giving MMR vaccine to children at the age of 9 months
    - Vaccine is contraindicated in pregnancy
    - Women are advised not to conceive within 3 months after getting the vaccine.
- **Management and control:**
    - Isolation
    - Notification
    - Early diagnosis
    - Rest in bed
    - Symptomatic treatment
- **Complications:**
    - Arthralgia
    - Thrombocytopenic purpura

Mumps (Infective Parotitis)

Mumps is a highly infectious disease which occurs due to viral infections and causes inflammation of parotid glands. It occurs throughout the world. Morbidity is high and mortality is negligible. It occurs more during winter and spring season.

- **Epidemiological triad:** The epidemiological triad of mumps is given in Figure 4.7.
  - **Causative agent:** RNA virus of paramyxovirus family
  - **Environment:** Common in children between 5 and 15 years of age but it also occurs in adults in severe forms. One-time infection produces life time immunity.
  - **Host:** Children 5–15 years, adult also get infection
- **Mode of spread:** Personal contact, droplet, nuclei
- **Incubation period:** 2–3 weeks
- **Clinical manifestations:**
  - Swelling of one or both the parotid glands
  - Fever
  - Pain over the swollen glands
  - Stiffness in opening mouth
  - Pain during mastication and swallowing fluids
  - Body ache and restlessness
  - May be earache on affected side
  - Headache
  - Swelling remains for a week; other symptoms may disappear
- **Clinical diagnosis:**
  - By signs and symptoms
  - By palpating the swelling behind and below the ear
- **Prevention:** By vaccinating children with combined vaccination of MMR at the age of 9 months
- **Control and management:**
  - Early diagnosis
  - Isolation
  - Disinfection of the fomites and secretions
  - Notification
  - Surveillance
  - Management further includes:
    - Rest in bed and isolation
    - Treatment of fever
    - Plenty of oral fluids, soft and nourishing diet
    - Frequent mouth wash with antiseptic solutions
    - General care
- **Complications:** Otitis media, orchitis in males, oophoritis in females, pancreatitis, myocarditis, encephalitis.

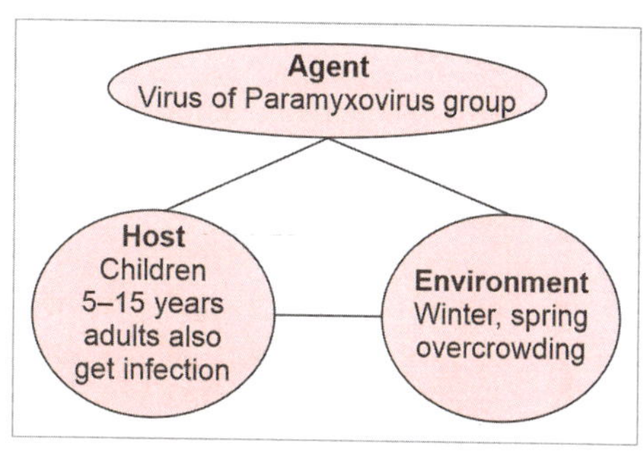

Fig. 4.7: Epidemiological triad of mumps

Chickenpox

Chickenpox is an acute infectious disease which occurs in epidemic and endemic throughout the world. In India, it is also called "chhoti mata".

- **Epidemiological triad:** The epidemiological triad of chickenpox is given in Figure 4.8.
    - **Environment:** Disease is more common in winter season and overcrowded residential areas. One attack produces immunity; second attacks are very rare.
    - **Causative agent:** Varicella zoster virus
    - **Host:** Children under the age of 10 years; adults are also affected
- **Mode of transmission:** Direct contact, droplet infection, droplet nuclei.
- **Portal of entry:** Respiratory tract
- **Incubation period:** 7–21 days
- **Clinical signs and symptoms:** It varies from mild illness to severe illness. The clinical course has two stages.
    i. **Pre-eruptive stage:**
        - At the onset of the disease, low to moderate fever accompanied by shivering and malaise.
        - Backache, restlessness. This stage lasts for 24 hours.
    ii. **Eruptive stage:** Rash starts appearing on the body with onset of fever, itching of the skin. Rash appears symmetrically in the body. First on the trunk and then on the face, axilla, arms and legs. Rash is more on the body, i.e., centripetal distribution.
        - Different stages of rashes are seen together, i.e., macule, papule, vesicles and scabs, i.e., pleomorphism.
        - This stage lasts for 4–7 days. Rashes do not occur on the palms and soles.
- **Diagnosis:** The characteristics of rashes, i.e., appearance of all stages together is diagnostic in chickenpox.
- **Prevention:** Varicella zoster immunoglobulin can be given within 7 hours of exposure.
- **Control of chickenpox:** It includes:
    - Isolation
    - Notification
    - Early diagnosis
    - Treatment is symptomatic
    - Rest in bed
    - Antipyretics to reduce fever
    - Antiseptic soothing lotions can be applied on the skin
    - Plenty of oral fluids and soft diet
    - Disinfection of the articles used for patient

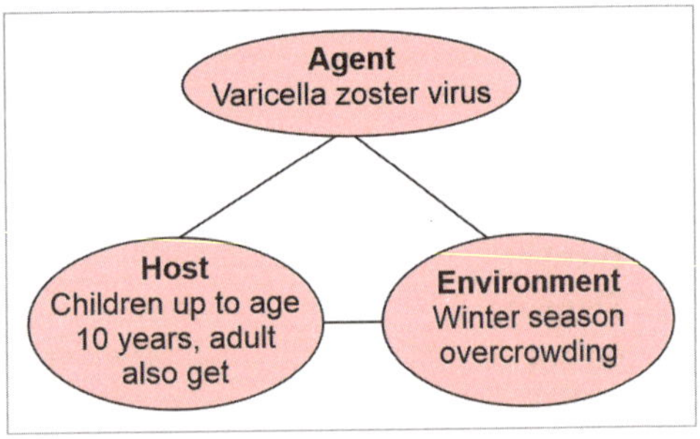

Fig. 4.8: Epidemiological triad of chickenpox

- **Complications:** Complications are rare. But in certain cases, it may cause:
  - Pneumonia
  - Hemorrhages
  - Encephalitis
  - Reye's syndrome

Smallpox

- Smallpox is caused by variola virus.
- It is highly infectious and characterized by high fever, headache, backache, vomiting and convulsions. Appearance of rash occurs in centrifugal distribution.
- **Incubation period:** 12 days.
- **Signs and symptoms:** Sudden onset of fever with headache, backache, vomiting. Rashes appear on 3rd day of fever, and passes through successive stages of macule, papule, vesicle, pustule, and scab. Distribution of rash is centrifugal type. On 8th May 1980, WHO declared that the disease had been eradicated totally from the world and since 1982, all member nations of WHO stopped smallpox vaccination. India is also a smallpox free country.

Diphtheria

Diphtheria is an acute highly infectious disease caused by bacterial infection. The bacteria remain in the throat and produce highly poisonous exotoxins which affect the heart and nervous system. The disease is transmitted through the secretions of patient's nose and throat and infected material. The disease is endemic in developing and underdeveloped communities where the vaccination against diphtheria is not done properly.

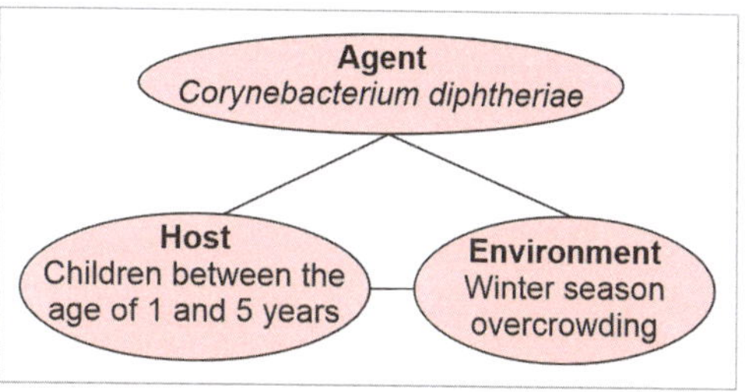

Fig. 4.9: Epidemiological triad of diphtheria

- **Epidemiological triad (Fig. 4.9)**
  - **The causative agent:** *Corynebacterium diphtheriae* present in nasopharyngeal secretions, discharge of skin lessons and contaminated fomites of the infected host.
  - **Environment:** It occurs in all seasons but it is more common in winter.
  - **Host:** Children between age group of 1–5 years are affected, both males and females are affected.
- **Incubation period:** 2–6 days. The period of infectivity is 14–28 days from the onset of disease.
  - **Mode of spread:** Droplet nuclei, infected skin, lesion, fomites, skin cuts and wounds.
  - **Portal of entry:** Respiratory route, cuts and wounds.
- **Clinical features:** Diphtheria affects ear, nose, and throat. Its types and characteristics are:
  - i. **Pharyngotonsillar diphtheria:**
    - Sore throat
    - Difficulty in swallowing
    - Restlessness and fever
    - A whitish membrane is found on the tonsils. This can be easily wiped off. Later it becomes thick blue-white to gray and difficult to remove if tried and results in bleeding.
    - Lymph glands around neck get swollen and give "Bull neck appearance".

   ◆ Edema of submandibular area
   ◆ Mucosal edema around the membrane
ii. **Laryngotracheal diphtheria:**
   ◆ Breathing difficulty
   ◆ Hoarseness of voice
   ◆ Severe irritating cough
   ◆ Infection may spread into the respiratory tract and can cause serious conditions.
iii. **Nasal diphtheria:**
   ◆ Mucus and blood come from nose.
   ◆ One side nostril may be blocked.
   ◆ If membrane is formed, difficulty in inhaling occurs.

- **Diagnosis:**
  - Diagnosis is made from clinical signs and symptoms.
  - Examination of nose and throat and presence of diphtheria membrane.
  - Laboratory test includes examination of nose and throat secretions.
  - Schick test is done to know whether the individual is susceptible to *Corynebacterium diphtheriae* toxins.
- **Control and prevention:**
  - Early detection, hospitalization and isolation.
  - Notification of the disease to the concerned authorities.
- **Management:**
  - Diphtheria antitoxins 10,000–80,000 units should be given IM or IV depending upon the severity of the disease.
  - Antibiotics injection sodium penicillin 2.5 lac QID for 5 days or injection erythromycin 250 mg QID.
  - In case of laryngotracheal diphtheria if respiratory stridor is present, tracheostomy may be required.
  - Care of tracheostomy tube
  - General care of the patient
- **Prevention:** Immunization by triple vaccination. Three doses of diphtheria, pertussis and tetanus (DPT) after birth at the age of 6 weeks, 10 weeks, 14 weeks and then booster doses as follows:

At 6 weeks	DPT I	0.5 mL	IM anterolateral side of mid-thigh
10 weeks	DPT II	0.5 mL	IM anterolateral side of mid-thigh
14 weeks	DPT III	0.5 mL	IM anterolateral side of mid-thigh
At 18 months	DTP (booster dose I)	0.5 mL	IM anterolateral side of mid-thigh
5–6 years	DT (booster dose II)	0.5 mL	IM anterolateral side of mid-thigh

DPT provides immunity against diphtheria, whooping cough and tetanus.

- **Complications:**
  - Pneumonia
  - Nephritis
  - Laryngitis
  - Myocarditis
  - Peripheral neuritis

Poliomyelitis

Poliomyelitis is a highly infectious disease caused by polio virus. The disease affects the nervous tissues and causes paralysis and deformities.

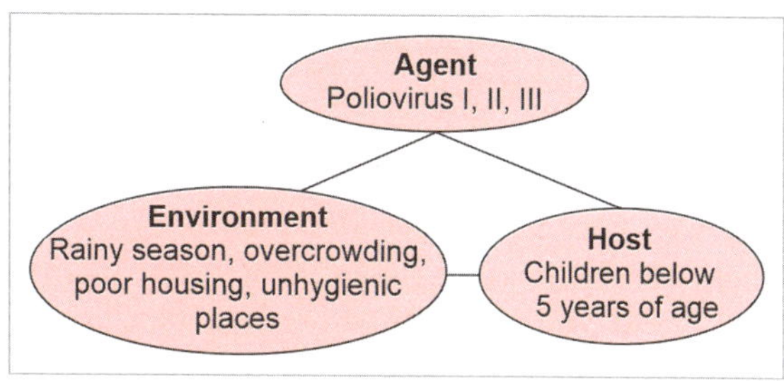

Fig. 4.10: Epidemiological triad of poliomyelitis

- **Epidemiological factors (Fig. 4.10):**
  - **Agent:** Causative organisms are polio virus I, II and III.
  - **Host:** It attacks children below the age of 5 years.
  - **Environment:** Infection is more in unhygienic places, overcrowded and dirty places where personal hygiene is neglected. Polio is more common during rainy season.
- **Sources of infection:** Contaminated water, food, milk. The consumption of contaminated food water, milk results in entry of infection in the digestive tract
- **Mode of spread:** Orofecal route, flies play an important role in spreading infection as virus remains in the stool of infected person for three months
- **Incubation period:** 7–14 days
- **Clinical signs and symptoms:**
  - Fever
  - Headache
  - Vomiting
  - Diarrhea
  - Fatigue
  - Cough and cold
  - Muscular weakness
  - Stiffness in the back and neck are the warning signs of paralysis. Paralysis may occur in legs, face, larynx and esophagus.
  - Paralysis is common in lower parts of body; patient becomes permanently handicapped.
- **Diagnosis:** Made from signs and symptoms
- **Complications:** Paralysis and permanent deformity; if respiratory muscles are involved, death may occur.
- **Management:**
  - No specific treatment
  - Symptomatic care
  - Physiotherapy of the affected limbs to minimize deformity
  - Disinfection of the secretions and articles used for patient
- **Prevention and control:**
  - Notification of cases
  - Active immunization with polio vaccines
  - The success of Pulse Polio Program in India is attaining near 100% coverage. On January 13, 2023, India has completed 12 polio-free years.

> **Recent Updates**
>
> As of August 22, 2024, India has not reported any cases of wild polio. However, there was a case of vaccine-derived polio in a two-year-old child in Meghalaya's West Garo Hills district. The World Health Organization (WHO) is investigating the case to determine if it's a new strain of polio.

Whooping Cough (Pertussis)

Whooping cough is a highly infectious disease of children. The cough produces long noisy inspiration which ends in a special voice called whoop.

Whooping cough occurs in all the countries endemically and epidemically. One attack produces sufficient immunity. Because of the awareness of vaccination, the attack of this disease has reduced remarkably and mortality has reduced.

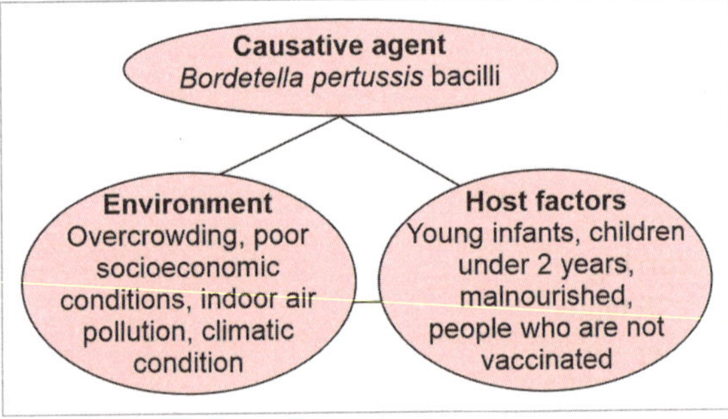

Fig. 4.11: Epidemiological triad of whooping cough

- **Epidemiological factors (Fig. 4.11):**
  - **Causative agent:** *Bordetella pertussis* bacilli.
  - **Susceptible host:** Infants and children under the age of two years who are not vaccinated are affected
  - **Environment:** Winter season, poor socioeconomic status, spring season and overcrowding favor the disease
- **Mode of spread:** Droplet infection, droplet nuclei and direct contact
- **Incubation period:** 7–14 days
- **Clinical manifestations:** Whooping cough has three stages:
  - i. **First or catarrhal stage:** This stage is accompanied by:
    - Sneezing
    - Watering from eyes and nose
    - Mild fever
    - Loss of appetite
    - Hacking and nocturnal cough
    - This stage lasts for 10 days
  - ii. **Second and paroxysmal stage:**
    - Bouts of cough occur and each bout ends in a specific inspirational noise resembling kho kho.
    - Because of mucus blockage, vomiting may occur. Child's face becomes red during the bout.
    - This stage lasts for 2–3 weeks.
  - iii. **Third or convalescent stage:**
    - Bouts of cough and vomiting become less but the ordinary respiratory infection can bring about attacks of cough.
- **Diagnosis:** It is made with typical types of coughs.
  Throat and nasal swabs and sputum for culture and ABST can show the growth of B. pertussis.
- **Control and management:**
  - Whooping cough can be controlled by active immunization with DPT vaccination.
- **Management includes:**
  - Admission in the hospital
  - Isolation
  - Antibiotics to control infection
  - Cough syrup
  - Antipyretic syrup
  - Oxygen therapy, if indicated
  - Plenty of oral fluids and nourishing diet
  - Disinfection of secretion and fomites

- **Complications:**
  - Pneumonia
  - Bronchitis
  - Encephalitis
  - Hernia
  - Bleeding from eyes and nose

Tetanus

Tetanus is an acute infectious disease. It is more common in developing countries. Tetanus occurring in newborn is known as tetanus neonatorum.

Tetanus occurs in unvaccinated individuals. Newborns and infants infected with tetanus have higher mortality rate. Rural population is affected more than urban. Infection spreads in more unhygienic environment and when aseptic precautions are not taken during delivery.

- **Epidemiological factors (Fig. 4.12):**
  - **Causative agent:** Tetanus is caused by anaerobic spore forming bacteria called *Clostridium tetani.*
  - **Host:** All ages are affected. Farmers, people engaged in mines and those involved with soil and dust for their wages are affected more. Disease is transmitted when cuts, wounds, surgical incision and burns come in contact with contaminated material or dust.

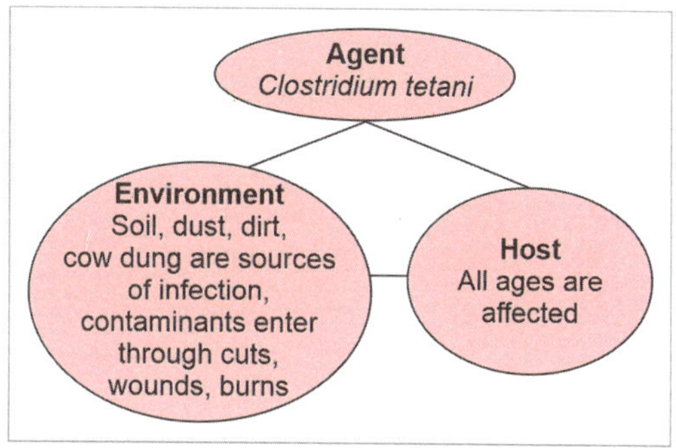

Fig. 4.12: Epidemiological triad of tetanus

  - **Environment:** Soil, dust, cow dung and dirt are the sources of infection.
- **Incubation period:** 3–21 days
- **Mode of spread:** Open wound with contaminated material
- **Clinical manifestations:** The exotoxins produced by the clostridium tetani enter the blood circulation and lymphatic system and affect the central nervous system and produce the following symptoms:
  - Fever, tachycardia, restlessness, sweating
  - Spasm of muscles and irritability
  - Difficulty in opening the mouth (Lock jaw)
  - Particular type of facial appearance known as sardonic smile
  - Bowing of the back (opisthotonos)
  - Repeated convulsions
  - Involuntary contraction of muscles
  - Severe pain
  - Immediate death may occur if there is spasm of respiratory muscles
- **Diagnosis:** History of injury and from the signs and symptoms
- **Complications:**
  - Pneumonia
  - Atelectasis
  - Respiratory emboli
  - Severe stomach ulcer
  - Arrhythmia
  - Death may occur, if proper treatment is not implemented

- **Control measures:**
  - To prevent tetanus neonatorum, mothers are immunized against tetanus during antenatal period by giving two doses of injection T.T. 0.5 mL IM during pregnancy at intervals of 4 weeks.
  - All children are immunized against tetanus as per the National Immunization Schedule
  - During any injury, cut and open wound, it is to be cleaned with antiseptic lotion and injection T.T. 0.5 mL IM to be given within 72 hours.
  - Aseptic technique to be practiced during surgical procedure and delivery.
- **Management:**
  - Hospital admission
  - Isolation
  - Tetanus antitoxins to neutralize the bacterial toxin
  - Muscle relaxant to control spasm
  - Sedatives and anticonvulsant drugs
  - Care of open wound
  - Antibiotics
  - General care of patient
  - Nutrition to be maintained
  - Proper disinfection of all soiled linen and equipment.

Tuberculosis

Tuberculosis is a public health problem of the entire world including the developing and developed countries. It mainly affects the lungs (about 80%), but any part of the body can be affected.

- **Epidemiological factors:**
  - Tuberculosis is an infectious disease and affects all age groups, both sexes, rich and poor, rural and urban. Dr Robert Koch first discovered tuberculosis bacilli which cause the disease.
  - India accounted for 27% of total global TB burden in 2023 with 1.8 million dying due to TB every year.
  - Tuberculosis affects women more in reproductive age group; and it is estimated that 1/3rd of the total infertility of females in India is caused by tuberculosis.
  - The most affected age group is 15–54 years which is economically productive age; and 70% of TB cases occur in low socioeconomic groups due to poverty, illiteracy, crowded environment and lack of personal hygiene.
    - Tuberculosis is one of the six killer diseases.
    - Tuberculosis of animals is known as bovine tuberculosis.
    - People suffering from HIV infection are more prone to get tuberculosis.
- **Epidemiological triad (Fig. 4.13):**
  - **Causative agent:** *Mycobacterium tuberculosis*
  - **Environment:** Overcrowding, poor housing, illiteracy, low socioeconomic, status, poor personal hygiene.
  - **Susceptible host:** All age groups. Malnourished and persons suffering from HIV/AIDS are more prone to the disease.

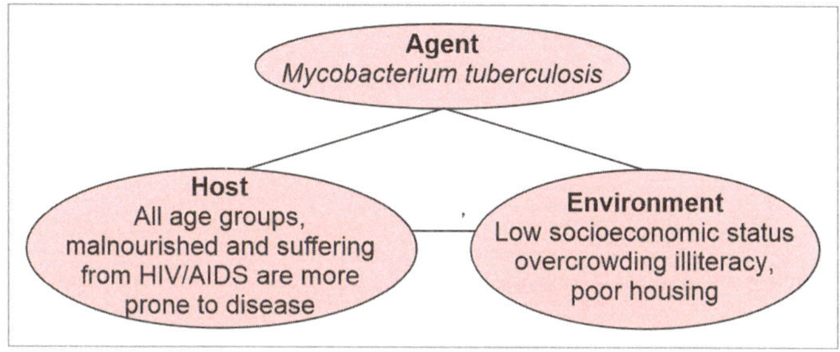

Fig. 4.13: Epidemiological triad of tuberculosis

- **Incubation period:** 4–8 weeks
- **Mode of spread:** Droplet infection and droplet nuclei, direct contact
- **Portal of entry:** Respiratory tract
- **Clinical manifestations:**
  - Low grade fever which increases in the evening
  - Loss of weight
  - Loss of appetite
  - Sweating at night
  - Cough for 3 weeks or more
  - Fatigue and general weakness
  - Chest pain, breathing difficulty and blood with sputum (hemoptysis) may be coughed out
  - Enlargement of lymph nodes

Miliary Tuberculosis (TB)

Miliary TB can affect lymph glands, brain, bones, joints, kidneys and intestine.

- **Clinical findings:**
  - Weight loss
  - Fever
  - Night sweats
  - Swelling of the glands, joints pain in the affected area
  - Enlargement of glands
- **Diagnosis:**
  - From clinical signs and symptoms
  - Microscopic examination of sputum for acid fast bacilli
  - Chest X-ray
  - Tuberculin test and FNAC
  - Tissue biopsy
- **Complications:**
  - Physical disability
  - Danger of AIDS attack
  - Death

- **Prevention and control**
  - Early diagnosis
    - Sputum examination
    - Radiography
    - Tuberculin test
  - **Prevention:** Case finding, active immunization by Bacillus Calmette-Guérin (BCG) vaccination

Treatment of Detected Cases

Chemotherapy includes:

- Antitubercular drugs:
  - **First line drugs:** First line drugs are given during intensive phase. They are given for initial 1–3 months to control acute symptoms and reduce infectiousness. During this phase, a combination of 3 or 4 drugs is given.
    - Bactericidal—isonex, rifampicin, streptomycin, and pyrazinamide
    - Bacteriostatic—ethambutol, thiacetazone (thioacetazone)
    - **Bactericidal drugs**
      - **Tab rifampicin** 10–12 mg/kg body weight given on empty stomach for better absorption. Side effects are gastritis, hepatotoxicity, nephrotoxicity and thrombocytopenia.
      - **INH (isonex)** 4–5 mg/kg body weight. Maximum dose 300 mg/OD.
        Side effects of isonex are peripheral neuritis, gastritis, intestinal disturbance, hepatitis.
        Tab pyridoxine (Vitamin B_6) 10–20 mg is given once a day to prevent peripheral neuritis.
      - **Injection streptomycin:** Dose 0.75–1 g once a day intramuscularly. It is toxic to VIII cranial nerve and causes deafness, giddiness and ataxia.
        Note: If the patient complains of ringing in the ears, injection streptomycin should be stopped.
      - **Pyrazinamide:** Dose 30 mg/kg body weight in divided doses of 2–3 per day. Side effects include arthralgia, hepatitis.
    - **Bacteriostatic drugs:** Bacteriostatic drugs are given during continuation phase after intensive phase. These are given for 4–6 months after bactericidal combination of 2 or 3 drugs has already been given.
      - Tab. ethambutol 15 mg/kg body weight (800 mg/day) in divided doses.
        Side effects are blurring of vision and retrobulbar neuritis.
      - Thioacetazone: Dose 2 mg/kg body weight (150 mg/day).
        Side effects are GIT disturbances and blurring of vision.
  - **Second line drugs:** Second line drugs are used when the first line drugs are not responding or cannot be used for some reasons. These include ethionamide (or prothionamide), cycloserine, kanamycin, viomycin, ofloxacin and capreomycin.
- **DOTS or directly observed treatment short course:** This course was developed by WHO to control the spread of disease and avoid the development of multidrug resistance. The patients are given short course chemotherapy under the supervision of health workers during the intensive phase.

During the continuation phase, the first dose is swallowed by the patient in the presence of health worker and is provided medicine in multi-blister combipack for one week. After one week, patient is asked to bring the empty multi-blister combipack by which the health worker comes to know that patient has taken the medicine.

DOTS chemotherapy includes three types of cases, which are divided into three categories:

Category I:

Type of patient	Treatment regimen
• New sputum smear positive • Seriously ill, new sputum smear negative • Seriously ill, new extra pulmonary	$2H_3R_3Z_3E_3 + 4H_3R_3$

Category II:

Type of patient	Treatment regimen
• Sputum smear positive relapse • Sputum smear positive failure • Sputum smear positive treatment after default • If sputum smear is positive at the end of the intensive phase, additional month of intensive treatment should be given	$2H_3R_3Z_3E_3S_3 + 1H_3R_3E_3 + 5H_3R_3E_3$

Category III:

Type of patient	Treatment regimen
• New sputum smear negative • Not seriously ill • New extra pulmonary	$2H_3R_3Z_3 + 4H_3R_3$

Note: *Interpretation of the numbers and letters placed in regimen.*

The numbers before letters refer to the number of months of treatment. The suffix numbers of letter refer to the frequency of administration in a week.

R—stands for rifampicin
H—for isoniazid
S—for streptomycin
Z—for pyrazinamide
E—for ethambutol

No suffix means given daily.

Revised National Tuberculosis Program

In the year 1992, Government of India, WHO and World Bank together reviewed the National Tuberculosis Program (NTP). After the revision, it is referred to as Revised National Tuberculosis Control Program (RNTCP). The main objectives of RNTCP:

- To achieve the cure rate of not <85% through short course chemotherapy
- To detect 70% of the estimated cases through sputum smears
- To involve nongovernmental organization
- To use DOTS as community-based treatment

WHO Stop TB Strategy

WHO recommends all countries and public and private healthcare providers functioning at national and local levels to implement the following to bring down the burden of TB:

- Practice high quality of 'DOTS' expansion and enhancement
- Ensure early detection of cases and diagnosis and maintain quality
- Provide standardized treatment with suitable supervision and patient support
- Ensure effective drug supply and management
- Strengthen the health system
- Engage all care providers
- Empower patients and communities
- Pay attention to TB-HIV, MDR-TB and the needs of vulnerable population
- Take necessary steps to improve and enhance research

> **MUST KNOW**
>
> **Main components which contributed to the success of DOTS:**
> - Political determination
> - Diagnosis through microscopic examination of sputum
> - Standardized short-term medical treatment
> - Regular supply of drugs
> - Good monitoring system including the right recording and reporting of the data of treatment

Meningococcal Meningitis

Meningococcal meningitis is a bacterial infection of meningeal layers of the brain and spinal cord. It occurs in sporadic form in small outbreaks in most parts of the world. About 10–20% of the people carry *Neisseria meningitidis* in their throat. Mortality rate is 23 per lakh population. In 2018, about 3382 cases were reported and 152 deaths occurred in India.

Meningococcal meningitis affects both the sexes. About 5–30% of normal population carries organism in nasopharynx. Immunity is acquired by subclinical infections. During the epidemic, the percentage of carriers goes up to 70–80%.

- **Epidemiological Triad (Fig. 4.14):**
    - **Causative agent:** *Neisseria meningitidis.* There are 12 serogroups of N. meningitides, six of which can cause epidemics. These are group A, B, C, W, X and Y.
    - **Environment:** Overcrowding, poor housing, low socioeconomic people, illiteracy, dry and cold months of the year.
    - **Susceptible host:** Children and young adults of all age groups but younger age group is more prone to the disease.

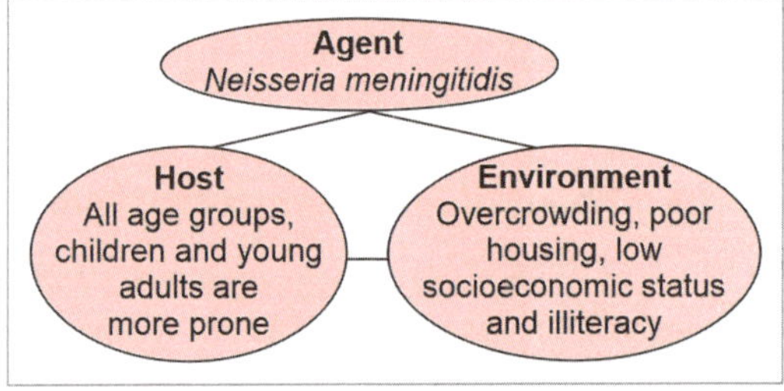

Fig. 4.14: Epidemiological triad of meningococcal meningitis

- **Mode of transmission:** From person to person through droplets and throat secretions from the carriers.
- **Portal of entry:** Nasopharynx of respiratory system
- **Incubation period:** 2–10 days. Normally, it is 4 days
- **Signs and symptoms:**
  - Fever ranging from 103°F to 105°F
  - Tachycardia
  - Stiffness of neck
  - Headache
  - Vomiting
  - Sensitivity to light
- **Diagnosis:**
  - Examination of cerebrospinal fluid
  - Positive Kernig's sign
  - Blood culture
  - Clinical signs and symptoms of the disease
- **Prevention and control:**
  - Isolation
  - Early diagnosis
- **Immunization:** Meningococcal polysaccharide vaccines prepared from purified group A, C; group A, C and Y; group A, C, Y and W, help to control the disease. They should not be given to children under 2 years and infants.
- **Treatment:** The drug of choice is penicillin for carriers. Chloramphenicol is the alternative drug for patients who are sensitive to penicillin. For contacts, sulfadiazine 1 g BD for 2 days; and those who are sensitive to sulfadiazine, rifampicin 600 mg BD is given for 2 days.
  - Symptomatic treatment for fever
  - Patient to be nursed in semi dark room
  - Care of the eyes
  - In acute stage, usually the patients are semiconscious; nasogastric feeds are given taking care of caloric requirement and nutrients
  - General care of the patient
  - Disinfection of the infected material.
  - **Mass treatment:** It should be done under close medical supervision. It causes immediate drop in the incidence rate of cases and in proportion to carriers.
- **Environmental sanitation:**
  - Prevention of overcrowding
  - Good housing and ventilation
  - To prevent close contact during infectivity period with cases and carriers covering the nose and mouth during sneezing and coughing.
- **Complications:**
  - Brain damage
  - Hearing loss
  - Meningococcal septicemia
  - Learning disability
  - Hemorrhagic rash
  - Circulatory collapse

Dengue

Dengue infection is caused by dengue virus which is spread in human beings by the mosquito *Aedes aegypti* and *Aedes albopictus*. The fever caused by the dengue infection is called dengue fever. Dengue is a worldwide health problem. In India, according to the reports of 1996, a total of 16531 cases were detected, 545 deaths were notified. Due to increasing awareness and proper treatment, the incidence rate and death rate have reduced in the subsequent years. During 2019, about 157,996 cases were reported with 253 deaths. It has been recorded that cases are increasing year after year. In 2022, 2.3 lakh cases and 303 deaths were reported. In 2023, 2.89 lakh cases and 485 deaths were reported.

- **Epidemiological Triad:** The epidemiological triad of dengue is given in Figure 4.15.

  - **Causative agent:** Dengue virus is transmitted by *Aedes aegypti* and *Aedes albopictus* vector. The causative agents of dengue are dengue virus types—DENV-1, DENV-2, DENV-3 and DENV-4.

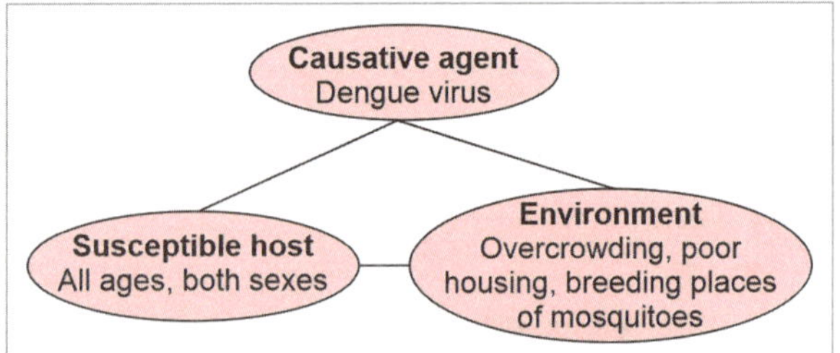

Fig. 4.15: Epidemiological triad of dengue

  - **Environment:** Hot and humid regions, overcrowding, poor housing, poor sanitation, stagnant water favor the disease. Epidemic and endemic both may occur.
  - **Susceptible host:** All age groups and both sexes are affected.
- **Mode of spread:** By the bite of mosquito *Aedes aegypti* which carries the dengue virus
- **Incubation period:** 4–6 days
- **Clinical manifestations:** Dengue infection occurs in three forms:
  i. **Dengue fever:**
     - High grade fever
     - Weakness, fatigue
     - Pain at the back of eyes
     - Severe pain in forehead
     - Loss of appetite, nausea, vomiting
     - Pain in the muscles and joints
     - Small rashes may appear on chest and arms.
  ii. **Dengue hemorrhagic fever:**
     - High fever which is continuous and it may continue for 2–7 days
     - Purpura, epistaxis, hematemesis and melena may occur
     - Thrombocytopenia, platelet count may fall below 50,000/mm^3
     - Hemoconcentration and hemoglobin level may increase 20% above the normal
  iii. **Dengue shock syndrome:**
     - All signs and symptoms of dengue fever and dengue hemorrhage
     - Bradycardia
     - BP falls by 20 mm Hg
     - Cold skin
     - Confusion and imbalanced mind

- **Diagnosis:**
    - Physical examination and noting the clinical signs and symptoms
    - Serological test
    - Platelet count
- **Management:**
    - Complete bed rest
    - Antipyretics to reduce fever but no aspirin or ibuprofen
    - Hydrotherapy
    - Plenty of oral fluids. If vomiting is there, give intravenous fluids
    - Blood transfusion, if platelet count is abnormally low
    - General care of the patient
- **Control and prevention:**
    - Early diagnosis and management
    - Notification
    - Control of mosquitoes and their breeding places
    - Health education of the people by informing them to:
        - Use mosquito net at night
        - Use mosquito repellents
        - Destroy the breeding places of mosquitoes
        - Remove stagnant water from drains, coolers and flower pots, etc.
        - Watch out for signs and symptoms and treat dengue infection
- **Immunity:**
    - No vaccine has been developed so far
    - Single attack of dengue produces resistance

Acute Respiratory Infections

Acute respiratory tract infections are most common health problems in developing countries. They are more common among children under the age of 5 years and elder people. In India, pneumonia is found to be responsible for 13–16% of all deaths occurring in children. Statistics have shown that 3.5% of global burden of disease is caused by acute respiratory infection (ARI). In India, during 2023, about 100 million cases of ARI were reported with 1 million people dying yearly.

Acute respiratory tract infections are divided into:

- **Upper respiratory tract infections:**
    - Common cold
    - Pharyngitis
    - Otitis media
- **Lower respiratory tract infections:**
    - Epiglottitis
    - Laryngitis
    - Laryngotracheitis
    - Bronchitis
    - Bronchiolitis
    - Pneumonia

It has been estimated that 3.9 million deaths occur worldwide due to ARIs; and ARI deaths due to pneumonia have been estimated about 90%. Children below the age of 5 years suffer about 5 episodes of ARI per year.

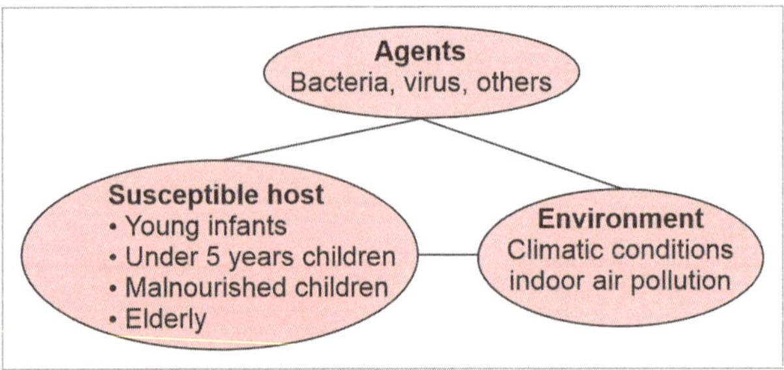

Fig. 4.16: Epidemiological triad of acute respiratory infections

- **Epidemiological triad:** Refer to Figure 4.16 to understand the epidemiological triad of acute respiratory infections.
  - **Causative agents (Fig. 4.17):** Bacterial agents, virus, others
  - **Environment:**
    - Incidence is higher in cold weather, in autumn and spring season
    - Overcrowding
    - Poor housing and ventilation
    - Indoor air pollution, i.e., smoke pollution in the house
    - Industrialization and urbanization
  - **Host:** Infants, young children under the age of 5 years, fatality rate is higher in malnourished children. Elderly people are affected due to low immunity.
- **Mode of spread:** Airborne, face to face contact.
- **Clinical symptoms:**
  - Fever
  - Cough
  - Sore throat
  - Rhinitis
  - Irregular breathing, fast respiration
  - General malaise
  - Unable to drink
- **Diagnosis:** From clinical signs and symptoms and history. The assessment of acute respiratory infections is done from respiratory rate, type of breathing, temperature, nutritional status and age of the child.

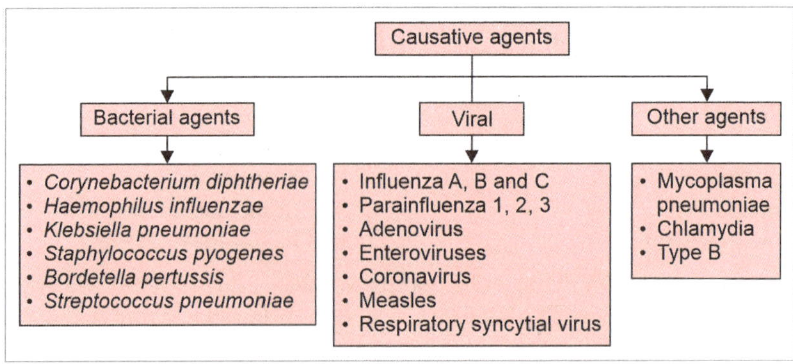

Fig. 4.17: Causative agents in respiratory infections

Assessment of Acute Respiratory Infections

The assessment of acute respiratory infections is summarized in Table 4.1.

Pneumonia is graded based on the aforementioned assessment and managed accordingly.

Dangerous signs of serious illness in case of <2-month-old infants:

- Not taking feeds
- Drowsy
- Wheezing sound of respiration
- Stridor when calm
- Either having fever or subnormal temperature

Prevention and control of acute respiratory infections:

- Improve living condition
- Provide clothing to the child according to the season
- Maintain good nutrition
- Avoid indoor smoking pollution
- Promote and maintain maternal and child healthcare
- Strictly follow the national immunization schedule
- Provide health education to the mothers regarding care of the child and recognize early signs of acute respiratory disease
- Conduct health promotional activities in vulnerable areas
- In India, Acute Respiratory Infections Control Program is being practiced under Child Survival and Safe Motherhood (CSSM) Program since 1992.

TABLE 4.1: Acute respiratory infections in children and their evaluation

Respiratory rate	Age of child	Evaluation
60 breaths/min	<2 months	Fast breathing
50 breaths/min	2–12 months	Fast breathing
40 breaths/min	12 months to 5 years	Fast breathing
Chest indrawing (While breathing, lower chest walls go in)	If present	Effort required is more
Look, listen for stridor	Harsh noise when breathing in	Narrowing of air passage
Look for wheeze	Soft whistling noise	Narrowing of passage
Alertness	Abnormally sleepy	Awake and abort
Temperature	Check temperature	Assess record
Malnutrition	Drawing in of chest wall cannot be elicited	Manage carefully
Cyanosis	Signs of hypoxia	Check in good light

Severe Acute Respiratory Syndrome

Severe acute respiratory syndrome (SARS) is a communicable disease caused by virus called coronavirus. SARS was reported in February 2003 in Asia. SARS is associated with flu-like syndrome which may progress into pneumonia, respiratory failure and even death.

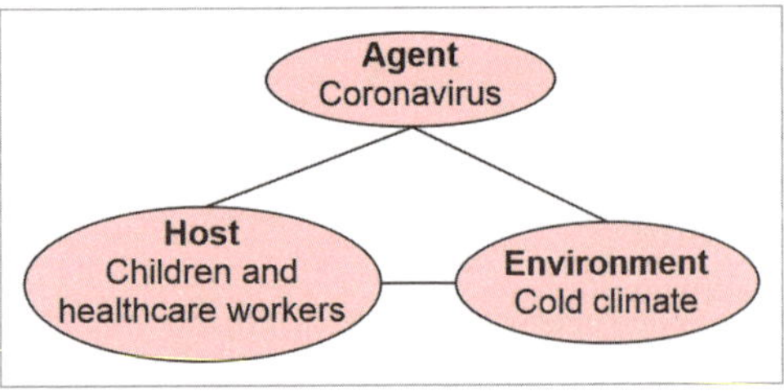

Fig. 4.18: Epidemiological triads of SARS

- **Epidemiological triad (Fig. 4.18):**
    - **Causative agent:** SARS is caused by coronavirus present in infective material of eyes, nose and mouth, urine and stool of infected cases. Coronavirus is thought to be an animal virus from uncertain animal reservoir perhaps bats that spread to other animals.
    - **Host:**
        - Healthcare workers are affected more due to their involvement in procedures which generate aerosols
        - Men are affected more
        - Infants are rarely affected
    - **Environment:**
        - SARS is an airborne disease.
        - The virus can survive for a longer period during cold.
        - It can survive for hours in external environment.
- **Incubation period:** 2–7 days
- **Modes of transmission:**
    - Close contact with patient
    - Infectious respiratory secretion
- **Clinical signs/symptoms:**
    - Fever
    - Running nose
    - Chills
    - Sore throat
    - Malaise
    - Myalgia
- **Prevention and control of SARS:**
    - **Identification** of cases suffering from SARS based on clinical signs and symptoms.
    - **Notification:** Cases of SARS should be notified to the local authorities.
    - **Isolation:** Patients should be isolated during the period when maximum excretion of virus occurs during illness which is about 10 days in a case.
        - Doors of the rooms should be closed.
        - Visitors should be restricted.
        - Rooms should be well-ventilated.
        - Concurrent disinfection of the infected materials
    - **Personal protective measures:**
        - Respiratory protection by using mask
        - Protection of eyes with goggles
        - Use of gowns and gloves
        - Hand washing after every contact
        - No aerosol therapy
- **Treatment:** Antiviral agents such as Ribavirin along with corticosteroids are given intravenously.

Coronavirus Disease-19

Coronavirus disease 2019 (COVID-19) is an acute highly infectious respiratory disease caused by newly identified coronavirus named SARS-CoV-2. The virus was detected in Wuhan in China in December 2019. It is a single stranded RNA virus with crown-like appearance under an electronic microscope. It is about 60–140 nm in diameter. High temperature decreases its replication but the virus can resist the cold temperature. The coronavirus is sensitive to ultraviolet rays but gets inactivated by lipid solvents such as ether, ethanol, chloroform, chlorine containing disinfectants peroxyacetic acid except chlorhexidine. The origin of the virus is not known exactly but speculated to be of an animal origin.

COVID-19 became a global health problem that was spread over 200 countries and territories. WHO declared COVID-19 as pandemic on March 11, 2020. On December 14, 2020, a new strain of COVID-19 was reported from UK, which was highly contagious, 70% more transmissible than the old variant. The mortality and morbidity were very high and this was fatal as compared to the coronavirus of December 2019. On February 14, 2021, about 11.08 crore cases were reported globally with 24,53,582 deaths. About 8.58 crore of people were recovered and recovery was 77.4%.

Age above 60 years and underlying noncommunicable diseases such as hypertension, heart disease, diabetes, chronic lung disease, cerebrovascular diseases and kidney diseases, immunosuppression and cancer are associated with higher morbidity.

In India: India's cases of coronavirus per million population were lowest as compared to the global cases of coronavirus in the world. The first case of coronavirus in India was reported from Kerala on January 30, 2020. In India, per day cases peaked in mid-September 2020 with about 90,000 cases per day and after that it declined to about 12,000 cases per day in February 2021. An epidemic outbreak of the disease was declared and Epidemic Diseases Act, 1897 was evoked leading to temporary closure of all educational, religious, entertainment and commercial establishments. All tourist visas were suspended in March 2020. The worst hit states were Maharashtra, Delhi, Kerala, Andhra Pradesh, Karnataka and Tamil Nadu. Due to the closure of commercial establishments, people lost their jobs and the worst affected were the daily wagers. By February 19, 2021, about 10.1 million persons had received vaccination in India. As on first July 2022, about 93% of eligible population got fully vaccinated.

- **Epidemiological Triad of COVID-19**
  - **Causative agent:** COVID-19 is caused by SARS-CoV-2 (Fig. 4.19). The virus is single stranded RNA virus, is a beta coronavirus closely linked to SARS virus. The virus can become inactivated at high temperature. Temperature of 65°–70°C can kill the virus.
  - **Host:** The disease affects all ages and both sexes. There is no existing human immunity against COVID-19.

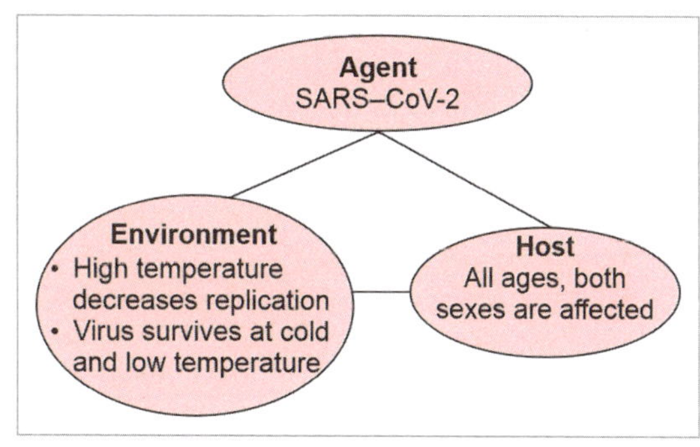

Fig. 4.19: Epidemiological triad of COVID-19

- **Environment:**
  - High temperature decreases the replication of the virus.
  - The virus can resist cold temperature. The virus is sensitive to ultraviolet rays.
  - Virus is inactivated by lipid solvents.
- **Mode of Transmission:**
  - The transmission of SARS-CoV-2 is airborne and can occur by droplet infection.
  - It can be by direct contact with an infected person.
  - By indirect contact through fomites or surfaces which have been contaminated with secretions of the infected person. The respiratory droplets are >5–10 μm in diameter, whereas droplets <5 μm in diameter are droplet nuclei or aerosols.
  - The respiratory transmission can occur when the person is in contact with the infected person at a distance of one meter.
- **Period of communicability:** As per the research, it has been suggested that COVID-19 can be detected in people 1–3 days prior to the appearance of symptoms. The highest viral load as measured by RT-PCR test is observed around the day of symptoms, onset followed by a gradual decline over time. The RT-PCR test remains positive for 1–2 weeks in asymptomatic patients and up to 3 weeks or more in patients with mild to moderate disease.
- **Incubation period:** It is 2–14 days.
- **Clinical features:** The spectrum of the disease ranges from asymptomatic to severe illness, ranging from mild symptoms to severe illness. The symptoms may appear within 2–14 days after exposure to the virus.
- **Symptoms:** Onset starts with mild irritation of throat to severe throat pain which is very discomforting and it remains for 3–4 days then declines accompanied by the following symptoms:
  - Fever with chills
  - Headache
  - Fatigue
  - Dry cough
  - Congestion and running nose
  - Shortness of breath or difficulty in breathing
  - Nausea and vomiting in some cases
  - Diarrhea may be found in certain cases
  - Loss of taste or smell
  - In a small proportion of cases, patients may progress to more severe and systemic disease characterized by acute respiratory distress syndrome (ARDS), sepsis and septic shock, multiorgan failure and cardiac injury.
- **Diagnosis:** It is made by the following means:
  - History of exposure to infected case
  - Presence of clinical signs and symptoms
  - Laboratory investigation
- **Laboratory diagnosis:**
  - **Molecular test:** Respiratory samples are collected, i.e., nasopharyngeal and oropharyngeal swabs are collected for rapid test and RT-PCR test.
    - **Rapid diagnostic test (RDS):** It is cheap, quick and gives report within half an hour. The test can detect only high viral load, so this test can miss many people with lower

levels of the SARS-CoV-2 virus. But it is useful to quickly detect the pandemic and identify most contagious people who might pass on infections to others unknowingly. So, by this test, appropriate measures can be taken to control pandemic. The negative test does not rule out the infection. Therefore, the confirmatory test is to be done, i.e., RT-PCR test.

- ◆ **Reverse transcriptase polymerase chain reaction (RT-PCR):** This test is the most widely used laboratory method for detecting COVID-19 virus. This test remains the gold standard for detecting current SARS-CoV-2 infection even when the viral load is low.

- **Chest X-rays:** In early stage, it shows negative finding, i.e., no involvement but in more advanced stage, it shows bilateral multifocal alveolar opacities, which tend to confluence up to complete opacity of lung-pleural effusion.

- **Computed tomography (CT) of chest:** This test can detect pneumonia even in early stage; and nonspecific finding can be detected. Most common is the multifocal bilateral "ground glass" (GG) areas associated with consolidation areas with patch distribution mainly peripheral and sub-pleural and with greater involvement of posterior regions and lower lobes.

- **Management of COVID-19:**

The aim of management is to:

- Break the chain of transmission
- Provide symptomatic treatment in early stage of the disease
- Provide hydration therapy to remove the viral toxins from the body
- Improve ventilation by breathing exercise and provide prone position for better oxygen intake.
- Maintain nutrition of the patient
- Prevent the complications

Steps of management are:

1. Isolate the patient either in home or in COVID care centers, i.e., first referral units, community health centers, sub-district hospitals, district hospitals or medical college hospitals.
2. Take clinical history of the patient including comorbidities.
3. Record vital signs, i.e., temperature, pulse, respiration, blood pressure and oxygen saturation. If there is any deviation from normal, patient may require urgent referral for life support measures
4. Patients with comorbidities are monitored more carefully for deterioration of conditions such as mental confusion, difficulty in breathing, persistent pain or pressure in the chest, agnosia, dehydration, decreased urine output, etc. Such patients should be immediately transferred to dedicated COVID care hospitals.
5. Symptomatic treatment for fever and body ache is provided.
6. Steam inhalation and hot saline gargling to relieve sore throat and chest congestion
7. Diet should contain 5–6 L of fluids including fruit juices, coconut water, soup and soft easily digestible diet.
8. Deep breathing exercises and chest physiotherapy to prevent chest congestion
9. Psychological support to relieve fear and anxiety

10. Patients are advised to rest in prone position for better oxygenation
11. Hospital attendants must wear mask, gown and cap while attending the patients
12. The clothes and linen used by patients should be disinfected in antiseptic lotion as the virus can be easily destroyed by lipid solvents.
13. Patients are kept in isolation in COVID care centers for about 14 days or till 2 samples of RT-PCR test are negative.

- **Management of moderate and severe cases of COVID-19 positive:** Patients with moderate and severe COVID infections are kept in dedicated COVID hospitals with all life support and ventilator facilities. The management of such patients includes:
  - Isolation
  - Psychological support to relieve fear and anxiety
  - Monitoring vital signs and oxygen saturation if it goes below 90% oxygen inhalation at the rate of 4 L/min.
  - Awake proning position may be given to patients who continue to have hypoxemia despite oxygen inhalation.
  - Corticosteroids: Methylprednisolone 0.5–1 mg/kg body weight or dexamethasone 0.1–0.2 mg/kg body weight for 3–5 days.
  - Antiviral drugs: The HCQ 400 mg BD for one day, 400 mg OD for 4 days; if no contraindication and after assessment of ECG for QT interval, CRP D-Dimer and ferritin every 48–72 hours.
  - CBC with differential count
  - Injection remdesivir 200 mg intravenously on day-1, followed by 100 mg daily intravenously for the next 4 days, i.e., total 5 days in moderate to severe disease on oxygen or mechanical ventilation in early disease onset.
  - Use of convalescent plasma 200 mg single dose may be repeated after 24 hours.
  - Injection tocilizumab 8 mg/kg body weight, maximum dose 800 mg once. Usual dose 400 mg may be considered in moderate to severe cases.
- **Prevention of complications:**
  - Prevention of secondary infection
  - Reduce incidence of ventilator-associated pneumonia
  - Prevent catheter-related bloodstream infection
  - Reduce days of invasive mechanical ventilation
  - Prevent development of adverse drug effects
  - Adequate hydration
  - Proper disposal of infected material and cleaning of articles and linens
  - Well-ventilated room promotes early recovery
  - Patients are advised to:
    - Wear mask and keep 1 meter distance while going out
    - Avoid crowded places
    - Take plenty of oral fluids
    - Perform light physical exercises and daily yoga and breathing exercises, saline gargling, steam inhalation.
    - Have balanced nutrition
    - Take adequate rest and sleep

- Avoid smoking and alcohol
- Perform self-health monitoring at home and take regular medication as advised.
- Seek medical advice in case of high fever, persistent cough, breathlessness and oxygen saturation <90%.

Home Isolation: Only mild cases are suggested for home isolation. They are advised to have separate rooms and articles to be used by them. Family members or other people residing in same home are advised to wear mask and take precautions while providing food or other necessities to patient while taking care and disinfect articles used by patient.

- Medication is explained to patients
- Rest of the care is same, i.e., hydration, nutrition, mild exercises, deep breathing exercises, personal care.
- Patient is isolated for 2 weeks and then medical treatment and advice are reviewed.
- **Prevention and Control of COVID-19:** Although 89% of India's eligible population has been vaccinated, appropriate COVID behavior should be strictly maintained as follows:
  - Wear mask in public places
  - Hand washing. Avoid touching face, eyes, nose while outdoor
  - Maintain physical distance about 6 feet while going out or in public places. Follow the slogan of "Do Gaj Ki Doori, Mask Hai Jaruri".
  - Cover nose and mouth while coughing and sneezing

Vaccination: Two types of vaccination are used in India:

- Covishield—this is manufactured by Serum Institute of India, Pune.
- Bharat Biotech's COVID Vaccine "Covaxin".
- Injections are given in two doses at an interval of 28 days to individuals above the age of 18 years; and booster dose is given to people who are above 60 years of age, to healthcare workers and people having other comorbidities.

Contraindications: Injection should not be given below the age of 18 years, to pregnant and lactating women.

- Those with allergic reactions to vaccine, plasma-derived products and notable food allergies
- Patients with immunodeficiency such as in HIV patients
- Patients who are on immunosuppressants due to any condition

Side-effects: Injection site pain, fever, myalgia, lethargy, discomfort, nausea, very rare complications

Public health surveillance: The aim of national surveillance of COVID-19 is to reduce the transmission of infection and minimize morbidity and mortality due to coronavirus infection.

The objectives of COVID-19 surveillance are:

- Rapid detection testing, isolation and management
- Detect and contain clusters and outbreaks among vulnerable population
- Identify, follow up and quarantine contacts
- Guide the implementation and adjustment of targeted control measures
- Evaluate the impact of pandemic on healthcare system and society
- Monitor long-term epidemiological trends and evolution of SARS-CoV-2 virus and monitor trends in COVID-19 deaths.

- Contribute to the understanding of the cocirculation of SARS-CoV-2 virus, influenza and other respiratory viruses and other pathogens.
- Monitor mortality and morbidity of healthcare workers
- Assess the impact of control measures

NONCOMMUNICABLE DISEASES

Noncommunicable diseases (NCDs) such as coronary heart disease, hypertension, cancer have a longer incubation period. Factors such as diet, exercise, cigarette smoking, alcoholism and sedentary lifestyle contribute to the development of the disease. NCDs are global health problems in developed and developing countries. In India, there is rapid transition with rising burden of NCDs. Some of the noncommunicable diseases are discussed ahead.

Hypertension

Hypertension is a global health problem; 1.3 billion people suffer from hypertension globally as estimated in 2019 and out of that, about 2/3rd people are from the developing countries. As per March 10, 2023 data, 1.4 billion people have hypertension. The incidence of the disease is increasing and it is estimated that up to year 2025, about 1.56 billion people will be suffering from hypertension. About 50% of heart diseases are followed by hypertension and 40% of death due to diabetes mellitus are also resulting from hypertension. WHO has graded the blood pressure in different classes (Table 4.2). The incidence is higher in urban population as compared to rural population due to sedentary lifestyle.

TABLE 4.2: Grading of hypertension as per WHO/blood pressure classification

Stages	Systolic (mm Hg)	Diastolic (mm Hg)
Normal	<130	<85
Grade I	140–159	90–99
Grade II	160–179	100–109
Grade III	>180	>110

Classification

- **Primary or essential hypertension:** The causes are unknown. The contributing factors such as aging, obesity, lack of exercise, dietary habits, i.e., excessive intake of fat and sedentary lifestyle. Stress and heredity play important role in the development of the disease.
- **Secondary hypertension:** This results due to some other disease process such as chronic glomerulonephritis.

Epidemiological Triad

Agent

- High intake of alcohol is associated with increased risk of high blood pressure.
- Excessive smoking is also linked with an increase in blood pressure.
- High intake of salt (7–8 g/day) increases blood pressure.
- Increased intake of saturated fat results in high blood pressure.
- Lack of fiber in the diet increases the risk of hypertension.
- Oral contraceptives cause hypertension

- Lack of physical exercise and obesity have direct effect on increasing blood pressure
- Genetic factors are also associated with an increase in blood pressure.

Environment

Psychological factors such as stress, worries, anxiety, family burden, poor job satisfaction (Fig. 4.20).

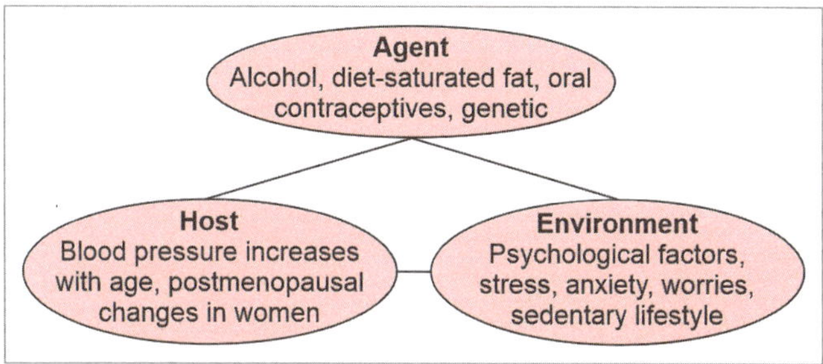

Fig. 4.20: Epidemiological triad of hypertension

Host

- Blood pressure increases with advancing age due to pathological changes in the blood vessels, dietary pattern of the family and lack of exercise.
- Excessive intake of sodium in diet.

Prevention and Control

- **Early detection of case and treatment:** This can be done by regular health checkup. Then awareness about health checkup can be created by providing health education and changing their health behavior. Once the cases are detected, the treatment is started which is lifelong; but it can prevent the incidence of strokes, coronary artery disease, diabetes mellitus and renal diseases.
- **Health promotion:** It includes all the measures to reduce the incidence of disease by reducing the risk of onset.
- **Nutrition:** Education on nutrition to bring changes in the food habits of people. It includes:
  - Reduction in the intake of saturated fat in diet
  - Reduction in salt intake, i.e. not >5 g/day in normal cases
  - Increase in the fiber intake of food
  - Avoiding intake of fast foods
- **Weight reduction:** Increased body weight is associated with increased blood pressure. Body weight has to be brought to the desired standard by decreasing the calorie intake and by doing regular physical activities.
- **Physical activity and regular exercise:** The regular exercises help in controlling weight and bringing blood pressure and blood lipids to the normal level.
- **Changes in the lifestyle:** Regular physical exercise such as walking for 30 minutes daily, practicing yoga, meditation, etc., relaxes the muscles and reduces stress which helps to prevent hypertension.

- Balanced diet should include fresh fruits and vegetables that provide essential minerals and fibers, which helps in maintaining normal blood pressure.
- **Health education:** People should be educated related to the risk of hypertension, modification of lifestyle to prevent the risk factors.

Cerebrovascular Accidents (Stroke)

Stroke is caused by an obstruction or blockage of blood vessels supplying the brain. As a result, the part of the brain supplied by that blood vessel does not get oxygen and nutrients. This results in hypoxia and death of the cells.

Definition

The World Health Organization (WHO) defines strokes as "rapidly developing clinical signs of focal disturbance of cerebral function, with symptoms lasting 24 hours or longer or leading to death, with no apparent cause other than of vascular origin".

Stroke is one of the leading causes of death and disability throughout the world. According to WHO estimates, about 15 million people suffer from stroke worldwide every year, of these 5 million die within three weeks and another 5 million are permanently disabled. With reduction in smoking rate, the developed countries have shown a decline in strokes. The mean age of stroke is 73 years in developed countries. In India, 0.706 million people died of strokes in 2016, crude death rate was about 54.2 per 100,000 population. The current prevalence rate varies from 44.54 to 150 per 100,000 population.

Risk Factors

- Hereditary
- Cigarette smoking
- Alcoholism, drug abuse
- High blood pressure
- Atherosclerosis
- Coronary heart disease
- Diabetes mellitus
- Increased level of blood cholesterol
- History of prior strokes
- Transient ischemic heart disease

Host Factors

- Stroke can affect at any age
- Around 1/5th of all strokes take place in the age group of 40 years
- Incidence is higher in males as compared to females
- It occurs as a result of complication of heart disease, hypertension and diabetes mellitus

Warning Signs of Stroke

- All of a sudden weakness occurs on the face, arm or leg particularly on one side of the body.
- Sudden confusion, difficulty in understanding and speaking
- Unexpected vision problems in one or both eyes
- Lack of coordination, poor balance and difficulty in walking
- Severe headache of unknown cause in case of hemorrhagic stroke.

Rheumatic Heart Disease

Rheumatic heart disease (RHD) is a complication of rheumatic fever which is caused by beta hemolytic streptococci affecting connective tissues particularly of the joints and heart. About 15.6 million people are estimated to be currently affected by rheumatic heart disease globally. RHD accounts for 12–65% of all cases of cardiovascular diseases admitted to the hospital. In India, prevalence of RHD is 5–7 per thousand in 5–15 years, age group and there are 1 million RHD cases in India.

Epidemiological Triad

- **Agent:** RHD is followed by rheumatic fever which is caused by beta hemolytic streptococci.
- **Host:** Rheumatic fever and rheumatic heart disease are diseases of childhood and adolescents between 5 and 15 years of age.
  - It affects both sexes equally.
  - Low socioeconomic group is at higher risk.
- **Environment (Fig. 4.21):** The environmental factors which lead to rheumatic fever and rheumatic heart disease are:
  - Low socioeconomic status
  - Poor housing
  - Overcrowding
  - Inadequate health services
  - Illiteracy

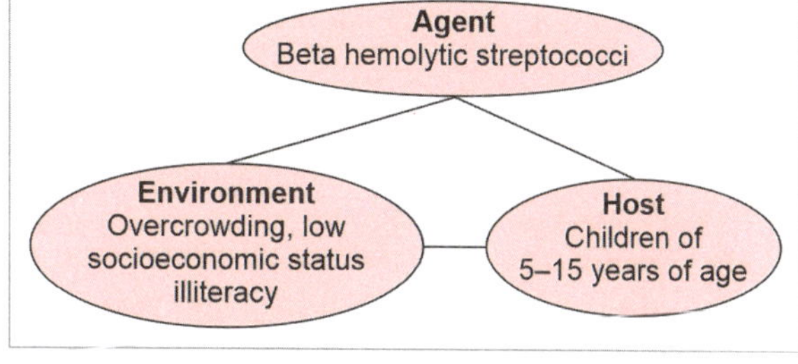

Fig. 4.21: Epidemiological triad of rheumatic heart disease

Clinical Signs and Symptoms

- **Fever**
- **Sore throat:** It is caused by streptococcal infection.
- **Polyarthritis:** Child will have painful swollen and red joint, i.e., larger joints like knee, elbow or shoulder are affected and swelling subsides within 2–3 days.

- **Carditis:** All the layers of the heart are involved and manifested by:
  - Tachycardia
  - Cardiac murmur
  - Cardiac enlargement
  - Pericarditis
  - Heart failure
- **Subcutaneous nodule:** Small painless, non-tender nodules tend to appear below the skin 4 weeks after the onset of rheumatic fever.
- **Erythema marginatum:** Skin rashes occur as a circular pattern of bright pink macules or papules on the trunk and extremities.
- **Chorea:** Jerky, uncoordinated movements of hands, feet, face and tongue occur but disappear during the sleep.

Diagnosis

Diagnosis is made based on clinical manifestations, i.e., minor and major criteria.

Major criteria
- Polyarthritis
- Chorea
- Erythema marginatum
- Subcutaneous nodules

Minor criteria
- Polyarthritis
- Fever

Laboratory Investigation

- Raised ESR
- Leukocytosis
- Throat swab shows positive β hemolytic streptococci and ECG shows prolonged P–R interval.

Prevention and Control

- **Primary prevention includes:**
  - Identification of high-risk groups such as school children.
  - Swab culture is taken for sore throat.
  - Inj. benzathine penicillin 1–2 mega units of adults IM after sensitivity test and 600,000 units for children or oral penicillin V or G for 10 days.
  - Erythromycin is given to those who are sensitive to penicillin.
- **Secondary prevention:**
  - Identify the cases of rheumatic fever.
  - Treatment of cases with benzathine penicillin—1.2 million units for adults and 600,000 units for children, once in three weeks for 5 years in case of children and for 10 years in case of adults.
- **Health education:** Improving the living standard of people, providing adequate information on rheumatic fever and its prevention.

Coronary Heart Disease

Coronary heart disease is due to inadequate blood supply to the muscles of the heart which results in blockage of coronary artery. It is a worldwide health problem. In developed countries, highest coronary disease mortality is seen. An estimated 17 million people die of cardiovascular diseases and strokes every year.

Risk Factors

- **Nonmodifiable factors:** Age, sex, family history, genetic factors
- **Modifiable factors:** Cigarette, smoking, high blood pressure, obesity, diabetes, elevated cholesterol level, excessive intake of alcohol, stress, sedentary lifestyle, high intake of saturated fats, lack of physical activities.
- **Others:** Hormones, oral contraceptive.

Prevention

- **Early diagnosis and treatment:** Screening of high risk cases and early treatment of diagnosed cases by medication, surgery, modifying behavior in relation to nutrition, exercise and changing the lifestyle.
- **Modification of diet:** The WHO expert committee has recommended the following dietary changes:
  - Limited consumption of saturated fats
  - Reduction of dietary cholesterol
  - Reduction in fat intake 20–30% of total energy intake
  - Avoidance of alcohol
  - Reduction of salt intake to 5 g daily or less
  - An increase in complex carbohydrates
- **Physical activity and exercise promotion:** Physical activity such as daily walk for 30 minutes improves circulation and decreases the chances of coronary artery disease.
- **Monitoring of blood pressure:** Blood pressure should be maintained at normal level by regular health checkup. Individuals who are suffering or at risk should be treated with medicines as well as other factors which help in maintaining blood pressure:
  - Regular physical activity
  - Reduction in salt intake
  - Reduction in weight
  - Reduction of saturated fat in diet
  - Avoiding stress factors
  - Modifying lifestyle
- **Health education:** People should be taught about risk factors involved in coronary heart disease and its complications. Emphasis should be given on prevention as well as controlling the occurrence of coronary heart disease.
- **Prevention of coronary heart disease as recommended by WHO:**
  - **Population strategy:** Mass approach is used to focus on the underlying risk factors in whole population. The complete community education should be provided on lifestyle modification to prevent coronary heart disease. Team work and community involvement are the basic factors. The recommended strategies are:
  - **Specific interventions:**
    - **Dietary changes:**
      - Reduction of salt intake—5 g/day or less
      - Reduction of fat intake—20–30% of total intake
      - Reduction of saturated fat
      - Reduction of dietary cholesterol

- ◆ Avoidance of alcohol consumption
- ◆ Smoking prohibition and making area smoke free
- ◆ Regular physical activity
- ◆ Maintaining blood pressure
  - ■ **Primordial prevention:** It involves all the preventive measures adopted to prevent the emergence and spread of coronary heart disease risk factors and lifestyles that have not yet appeared.
- **High-risk strategy:** This involves identifying high risk individuals having history of smoking, alcoholism, obesity, diabetes, and hypertension, etc. and providing them specific advice to take action against all the identified risk factors.
- **Secondary prevention:** The aim of secondary prevention is to prevent the occurrence and progression of coronary heart disease. The disease can be controlled by early diagnosis and prompt treatment with drugs. Surgery is advised, if indicated.

Cancer

Caner is becoming a worldwide health problem and it is one of the major causes of death among the developing countries. 19.292 million new cases of cancer were found in 2020; out of that 9.958 million people died. In 2022, 20 million new cases were found and out of that, 9.7 million deaths occurred. Cancer incidence is higher in females as compared to males. About 80–90% of cancer is due to environmental and lifestyle factors such as consumption of alcohol, tobacco, and dietary habits. About 30% of cancer causes are preventable by adopting healthy lifestyle, which includes low intake of fat, avoiding obesity, increasing physical activities and avoiding tobacco and alcohol intake, increasing the intake of vegetable and fruits in diet. The most common types of cancer among males in India are: Cancer of mouth, tongue, esophagus, stomach, trachea, bronchus and lungs. In females, the cancer of cervix, breast, mouth, and esophagus are the most common. The breast cancer is associated with late marriage, birth of first child at later age and shorter period of breastfeeding. Breast cancer is found more in urban women as compared to rural.

Causes

Cancer is a multifactorial disease. There are many predisposing factors.

Environmental factors influencing cancer are:

- **Tobacco consumption:** Chewing of tobacco causes cancer of mouth. Smoking causes cancer of lungs, larynx, pharynx, esophagus, pancreas, gallbladder and kidney.
- **Alcohol:** It causes liver cancer.
- **Diet:** Diet containing high fat influences breast and gallbladder cancer, whereas eating red meat for a longer duration is responsible for bowel cancer.
- **Chemical agents:** People working in chemical industries are exposed to chemicals for a longer period, which makes them more prone to cancer.
- **Indoor pollution:** Burning of solid fuels in the house creates smoke which may induce cancer.
- **Viruses:** Hepatitis 'B' and 'C' viruses cause hepatocellular carcinoma.
- **Genetic factors:** They also play a role in causing cancers.

Prevention and Control

Primary Prevention

- Control of tobacco and alcohol consumption. This will help to reduce the incidence of tobacco and alcohol-induced cancer.
- Avoid exposure to radiation and industrial carcinogen
- Maintain personal hygiene to prevent cervical cancer
- Control air pollution
- Liver cancer and cervical cancer can be prevented by vaccines
- Foods, drugs and cosmetics should be tested for carcinogens
- **Legislation:** Legislative measures can go a long way to prevent cancer by banning smoking, alcohol and controlling air pollution.
- **Education on cancer:** Community must be educated on preventive measures of cancer and its early detection by equipping people with adequate knowledge about the warning signs of cancer.

MUST KNOW

Warning signs of cancer: The common acronym used all over the world for warning signs of cancer is "CAUTION"

C: Change in bowel or bladder habit usually seen in colorectal cancer.

A: A sore that does not heal on time. Any sore on the skin or in mouth that does not heal by taking adequate treatment may be suspected as skin or oral cancer.

U: Unusual bleeding or discharge from vagina, rectum, bladder may indicate cervical, colorectal or prostate cancer.

T: Thickening of breast tissue and lump can be a sign of cancer. A lump developed on a testicle can mean testicular cancer.

I: Indigestion or difficulty in swallowing can be a symptom of throat, stomach, esophagus or mouth cancer.

O: Obvious changes to moles or warts are the most common signs of skin cancer.

N: Nagging cough—a cough that lasts for four weeks and longer can be indication of lung cancer.

Secondary Prevention-Cancer Registration

Cancer registration is necessary to know the magnitude of the problem and for planning the necessary services.

Types of Cancer Registration

Major types of cancer registration are:

- **Hospital-based registration:** This includes all indoor and outdoor treated patients by a particular hospital. The register should collect a minimum set of data as mentioned in "WHO handbook for standardized cancer registries".
- **Population-based registers:** The hospital registry is extended to the population. The major aim of this is to bring in the information related to the entire cancer situation of the area.

Diagnosis and Treatment

- **Early diagnosis and treatment:** Educating the public about early signs and symptoms of cancer helps in early detection and treatment of cancer. This brings better outcome.

- **Treatment of cancer:** Every cancer type has specific treatment regimen depending upon the staging. It may involve one or more approaches like surgery, radiotherapy and chemotherapy.
- **Palliative care:** It can be referred to terminal care in case when the clients report to the hospital at final stage either due to ignorance or financial constraints. Palliative care provides symptomatic treatment, i.e., relief from pain, providing comfort and peace and helping them to have a dignified death.

MUST KNOW

Screening Tests for Some Cancers

- Mammography screening for breast cancer
- Breast self-examination for breast cancer
- Testicular self-examination
- Cervical pap smear test for detecting cervical cancer
- Human papilloma virus (HPV) testing for cervical cancer
- Visual inspection with acetic acid for cervical cancer

Diabetes Mellitus

Diabetes mellitus is a chronic noncommunicable disease found all over the world. This occurs due to failure of cells of pancreas to produce sufficient insulin or the insulin produced is having defective action. According to WHO (2014), the number of diabetes mellitus patients is estimated to be about 422 million worldwide. About 80% of diabetes deaths occur in low-middle income countries. From the recent estimates, it has been found that diabetes is responsible as a direct cause for 1.6 million deaths in the year 2016 and 0.5 million deaths in the year 2022.

In India, the incidence in urban population is from 10.9 to 14.2% as compared to rural with incidence from 3.7 to 7.87. The increasing incidence is associated with industrialization and socioeconomic factors.

Types

- **Type-I or IDDM:** This is insulin-dependent diabetes mellitus in which the beta cells of pancreas are unable to produce insulin, which is vital to life. It is common in children and adolescents.
- **Type-II or NIDDM:** This is noninsulin-dependent diabetes mellitus in which the body cells cannot utilize the insulin produced by the pancreas. This occurs in case of adults. It accounts for 90% of all diabetic cases worldwide.
- **Gestational diabetes:** This type of diabetes occurs during pregnancy with blood glucose level above the normal values and shows impaired glucose tolerance.

Epidemiological Triad

Agent Factors

- Cystic fibrosis
- Neoplasm of pancreas
- Viral infections
- Autoimmunity
- Genetic defects in insulin genes
- Chemical agents
- Fault in secretion of insulin
- Pancreatitis

Host Factors

- Diabetes mellitus occurs equally in both sexes.
- It can occur at any age but prevalence rises with age.

- Obese people are at higher risk.
- Defective immunological mechanism results in self-destruction of body's own insulin-producing cells.
- Children of diabetic pregnancies are at risk of developing type II diabetes.

Environmental Factors

- Lack of exercise
- Sedentary lifestyle
- Intake of high saturated fat in diet
- Malnutrition
- Excessive intake of alcohol
- Viral infections
- Surgical removal of pancreas
- Low fiber diet
- Socioeconomic factors and stress

Prevention and Control of Diabetes

Primordial Prevention

Primordial prevention includes the prevention of development of risk factors in the population which have not yet appeared. It aims at preventing the adoption of harmful lifestyle from childhood. Parents have got major role in this aspect. This type of prevention involves preventing malnutrition, taking low intake of saturated fats, high fiber diet, inculcating habits of physical exercise and educating children about harmful effects of alcohol.

Primary Prevention

Primary prevention involves the action taken prior to the onset of diabetes mellitus. It has two types of strategies.

1. **Population strategy:** It is for noninsulin-dependent diabetes mellitus. It is based on the elimination of the following factors which are responsible for causing diabetes:
   - Prevention of malnutrition
   - Low saturated fats in diet
   - High fiber diet
   - Physical exercise
   - Maintaining normal body weight
   - Avoiding intake of alcohol and sweets
   - Healthy eating habits
   - Eliminating food toxins
2. **High-risk strategy:** It is aimed at finding the high-risk population and taking appropriate action to prevent the occurrence of diabetes mellitus in them. It involves guiding, counseling and educating people on prevention of diabetes mellitus.

Secondary Prevention

Secondary prevention includes early diagnosis and treatment. Early diagnosis is made by testing fasting blood glucose level and postprandial level, i.e., 2 hours after meal and by glucose tolerance test (GTT). In this, fasting blood sugar is taken and then 75 g of glucose is given in lime juice and blood samples are taken at half an hour interval for 2 hours.

The sample taken 2 hours after glucose ingestion should not have value >180 mg% and fasting sample should not have >120 mg% in normal cases. If the values are more, treatment is started.

- **Treatment:** Oral antidiabetic drugs are advised depending upon the level of GTT values. Treatment has three approaches:
  i. Diet and physical exercises alone
  ii. Diet, drugs and physical exercises
  iii. Diet and insulin

- **Routine checkup:**
  - Daily weight recording
  - Monitoring blood sugar
  - Urine for protein and ketone bodies
  - Visual acuity test
  - Regular examination of feet to assess blood circulation, loss of sensation and health of the skin
  - Glycosylated hemoglobin estimation at half-yearly interval.
- **Self-care:**
  - To take medication regularly in time
  - Self-testing of urine and blood sugar
  - Self-administration of insulin
  - Care of feet to prevent any injury leading to infection
  - Regular physical activities and weight control
  - Stop alcohol
  - Report any hypoglycemia and glycosuria
  - To carry some candies or sweets
  - To carry a diabetic card that includes details of treatment, name and address and phone number

Tertiary Prevention

Tertiary prevention is aimed at preventing complications like wound, infection and gangrene, blindness, kidney failure, coronary thrombosis, etc.

- **Health education:** Health education is to be provided on:
  - Diet and medication
  - Physical exercise
  - Avoid alcohol
- **Signs and symptoms of hypoglycemia and their management:** Hypoglycemia occurs when the blood glucose level falls below 60 mg/dL. Signs of hypoglycemia include sweating, nausea, confusion and pallor. Symptoms include feeling extremely hungry, trembling, palpitation and feeling faint. When the client experiences such signs and symptoms he should quickly take some sweets or candies which he is instructed to carry with him always and take some rest. Once the patient is stabilized, he should seek medical advice.

EPIDEMIOLOGICAL INVESTIGATIONS

Steps of Epidemiological Investigation

There are six steps of epidemiological investigations that are applicable to both communicable as well as noncommunicable diseases. These are as listed as follows:

1. Establishing the occurrence of a problem
2. Verifying the diagnosis
3. Collecting related data
4. Describing the occurrence in terms of person, place and time
5. Formulating hypothesis
6. Testing the hypothesis

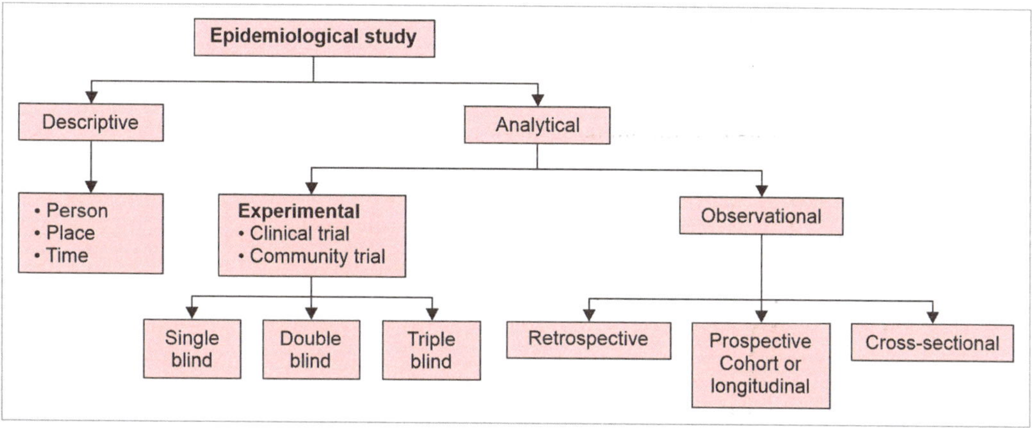

Fig. 4.22: Methods of epidemiological study

Methods of Epidemiological Investigations

Methods of epidemiological study (Fig. 4.22): are applied to know the disease etiology. Various epidemiological study methods are applied to find out the occurrence of a disease in people who may be involved in the process of spreading the disease. In community health nursing, the following study methods are applied to the cause and effect of a disease: (1) Descriptive method, (2) Analytical study method.

Descriptive Method

This method is concerned with the amount and distribution of a disease in the population to provide data required to formulate hypothesis to be tested. The descriptive study design describes the disease occurrence in relation to person, place and time. The main objectives of this method are as follows:

- To provide a database for planning, providing and evaluating health services
- To evaluate the trends in health sector and provide a basis for comparison among groups
- To identify problems for further analysis

  In descriptive study, the three things are important, i.e., person, place and time.

  i. **Person:** Here the various demographic and social characteristics of the person are studied, for example, age, sex, marital status, religion, occupation and socioeconomic status. All these characteristics have relation with the occurrence and distribution of disease.

  ii. **Place:** The nature and occurrence of disease are seen in different ways in developed, developing and underdeveloped countries. For example, tuberculosis is more common in poor countries, whereas cardiovascular diseases are more common in developed countries.

  iii. **Time:** It is the third important characteristic of descriptive study in relation to the occurrence of disease. There may be long-term variation, cyclic or periodic changes in the occurrence of a disease or short-term fluctuations which may occur with epidemics, for example, influenza most frequently occurs during December to March months and diarrhea is more common in spring season.

Analytical Study Method

By this method, the formulated hypothesis from the data gathered from the descriptive method is tested. This method is concerned with finding the reasons for the frequency of occurrence of a disease in a particular population. It demonstrates the hypothesized association between disease occurrence and certain pointed out demographic variables. Analytical method has two approaches:

1. **Experimental approach:** This approach is used for testing the hypothesis of scientific researches and confined to only treatment of diseases. To determine the cause-effect relationship, one factor is controlled, i.e., independent variable and the subsequent effect on dependent variable is measured. In clinical area, it is used to test the effectiveness and efficiency or side effect of a drug. But in community, it is used to test the efficiency of procedures on a group of individuals, for example, evaluation of dental disorders in community with or without fluoride added to the drinking water. There may be a chance of bias on the part of investigator in the experiment method. To eliminate this, single blind (subjects are not aware about experiment), double blind (neither subjects nor investigator know to which group the subject belongs) and triple blind (subjects, investigator and data analyzer do not know group assignment) methods are used.

2. **Observational approach:** This approach is more commonly applied in epidemiology. The subject of interest is the individual within the population and object is the test hypothesis. The investigator observes the occurrence of disease in individuals who are grouped on the basis of particular characteristics, experiences or exposure. Observation approach is of three types:

    i. **Retrospective or case control:** Retrospective study includes two population, i.e., cases and control. It compares the individuals who have been diagnosed or have a particular disease called cases with individuals who do not have the disease called control. Study determines whether there is any difference between the groups in exposure to one or more antecedent factors.

    ii. **Prospective or cohort studies:** This study is carried out after identification of possible disease-causing factors through retrospective study. Cohort study confirms the previously observed association between suspected cause and disease. It gives more definitive information about disease etiology.

    The main steps of cohort study include:
    - Selection of the subject under study
    - Obtaining data about exposure
    - Selection of comparison groups
    - Follow-up and analysis of data in terms of incidence rates of disease
    - Estimation of risk
        - **Disadvantage of cohort study:** It requires more time to complete and is expensive.
        - **Advantages of cohort study:**
        - It provides measurement of relative risk of actually developing disease.
        - Less likely to be biased since the group is identified before the disease develops.
        - May provide information about etiology of additional diseases other than the one under study.

    iii. **Cross-sectional studies:** It has common elements of both retrospective and cohort studies. It examines the presence or absence of relationship between identified factors and already existing disease at single point of time. The cohort is divided in subgroups according to previous exposure to a particular factor and then, these subgroups are examined to find out the presence or absence of a disease. The study provides data on the relationship of previous exposure or pre-existing factors and the present existence of a particular disease.

BASIC TOOLS OF MEASUREMENT IN EPIDEMIOLOGY

Biostatistics is considered a fundamental tool of epidemiology. After the completion of epidemiological studies, the gathered raw material or data are organized and categorized to compare and evaluate study results.

The basic tools of measurement in epidemiology are as follows:
- Rates
- Ratio
- Proportion
- Distribution

Rates

The rate is the primary measurement in descriptive epidemiology. Rate may be defined as measurement of a specific event, condition or disease in a given population within a specific time period.

Rate can be expressed in a formula as:

$$\text{Rate} = \frac{\text{Number of people affected in given time period}}{\text{Total population in a same area}}$$

Rates may be used for the comparison between groups. Specific rates are concerned with specific events, time period, causes or specific groups. By using rates, it is possible to compare events that occur at different time and places, and the different people. Rates present demographic data and morbidity data.

- **Demographic rates:** When the demographic data are converted into rates, they become very meaningful for the assessment of community health status. The rate consists of two parts, a numerator and a denominator. The numerator is composed of the number of conditions or events of interest occurred within a specified period of time.

  Denominator is the total population at risk during the same period of time. If the time period is long, the population at risk is estimated at mid-period such as mid-year.

- **General principles of calculation of rate:**
  - Numerator must include all of the events that are being measured, such as deaths of cases and each of those must be in the denominator.
  - Everyone in the denominator must be at risk for the event in the numerator because rate is a fraction or a proportion.
  - It is necessary to multiply by a base which is usually a multiple of ten. The procedure removes the decimal points and makes composition of the rates easier.
  - Any base multiple of ten may be chosen that results in the rate above the volume of one. The rate should be reasonable size, not a fraction.

$$\text{Rate} = \frac{\text{No. of events occurring in a period of time}}{\text{Population at risk during the same period of time}} \times 1000$$

Rate can be expressed per 1,000, 10,000 or 100,000 accordingly to avoid decimals.

Some important rates which represent the demographic data are as follows:

- Crude birth rate (CBR)
- Crude death rate (CDR)
- Infant mortality rate (IMR)
- Maternal mortality rate (MMR)
- Neonatal mortality rate (NMR)
- Total fertility rate (TFR)
- Age specific death rate
- **Crude birth rate:** This is expressed as the ratio of the number of live births per thousand to estimated mid-year population in a given year.

$$\text{Crude birth rate} = \frac{\text{No. of live birth during a year}}{\text{Estimated mid-year population}} \times 1000$$

- **Crude death rate:** This is expressed as the ratio of the number of deaths (from all causes) per thousand to estimated mid-year population in one year in a given place.

$$\text{Crude death rate (CDR)} = \frac{\text{No. of deaths during the year}}{\text{Estimated mid-year population in same year}} \times 1000$$

- **Infant mortality rate:** This expresses the ratio of infant deaths registered in a given year to the total number of live births in the same year, usually expressed as a rate per 1000 live births.

$$\text{Infant mortality rate (IMR)} = \frac{\text{No. of deaths of infants in a year}}{\text{No of total live birth in the same year}} \times 1000$$

- **Maternal mortality rate:** According to WHO, "maternal mortality rate expresses the death of a women while pregnant or within 42 days of termination of pregnancy, irrespective of the duration and site of pregnancy from any cause related to or aggravated by the pregnancy or its management but not from accidental or incidental causes".

$$\text{Maternal mortality rate (MMR)} = \frac{\begin{array}{c}\text{Total number of female deaths due} \\ \text{to complications of pregnancy, childbirth or} \\ \text{within 42 days of delivery from} \\ \text{puerperal causes during the given year}\end{array}}{\begin{array}{c}\text{Total number of live births in the} \\ \text{same area and year}\end{array}} \times 1000$$

- **Neonatal mortality rate:** This expresses the number of neonatal deaths (infant <28 days) in a given year per thousand live births in that year.

$$\text{Neonatal mortality rate} = \frac{\text{Number of deaths of children <28 days of age in a year}}{\text{Total live birth in the same year}} \times 1000$$

- **Total fertility rate:** It represents the average number of children a woman would have if she were to pass through her reproductive years bearing children at the same rate as the women now in each age groups. It is computed by summing the age-specific fertility rate for all ages.
- **Age specific death rate:** This represents the ratio of total number of deaths of a specific age group to the total number of people of the same age group in the same year in a specified area.

- **Morbidity rates:** Morbidity is the state of departure from physiological well-being. Two most commonly used morbidity rates are incidence rate and prevalence rate.
- **Incidence rate:** It indicates the number of new cases of a particular disease in a defined population during a specific period of time. Incidence rates provide a direct measure of the rate at which new cases occur in a given population. It serves as a valuable tool for the study of the causes of disease. It may be expressed as (Incidence only new cases):

$$\text{Incidence rate (Only new cases)} = \frac{\text{Number of new cases of a disease specific illness in a defined period}}{\text{Mid-year population at risk during the same period}} \times 1000$$

Incidence rates are more useful in assessing the risk of acute disease. Examples of incidence rates are hospital admission rate, case rate or attack rate, secondary attack rate, etc.

Attack rate: It is similar to the incidence rate and represents the incidence of illness among the exposed population during a specified time period and expressed as a percent.

$$\text{Attack rate} = \frac{\text{Number of new cases of specified diseases occurring in a particular place during the specified time interval}}{\text{Total population at risk during the same time interval}} \times 100$$

- **Prevalence rate (for all new and old cases):** It indicates the number of existing cases (new and old) of disease in the total population at a particular point of time. Prevalence rate is ratio rather than rate. It is of two types.

$$\text{i. Point prevalence} = \frac{\text{Number of all current cases (old + new) of specified disease during a particular period of time interval}}{\text{Total population at the same point of time}} \times 100$$

$$\text{ii. Period prevalence} = \frac{\text{Number of existing cases (old and new) of a specified disease during a particular period of time interval}}{\text{Estimated mid interval population at risk}} \times 100$$

Prevalence rate may be affected by treatment. As the disease is cured, prevalence rate may be decreased. Prevalence rates are useful in:
- Planning the disease control program
- Administration of hospital
- Treatment and rehabilitation

Ratio

It is defined as the relationship in size between two random quantities. In ratio, the numerator is not a component of the denominator. Ratio is the result of dividing one quantity by another. It is expressed in the form of:

$$P : q = \frac{P}{q}$$

Examples of ratio are nurse patient ratio, doctor patient ratio, bed patient ratio, teacher student ratio, etc.

Proportion

It is defined as a ratio which indicates the relationship in magnitude (intensity) of a part to the whole. Numerator is always included in the denominator. It is calculated in percentage.

$$\text{Proportion} = \frac{\text{Number of children with ARI}}{\text{Total number of children in the community in defined time period}} \times 100$$

Distribution

It indicates the number of individuals found to have each value or each small range of value. Frequency distribution demonstrates the qualitative characteristics such as height, weight or investigation values, etc. Frequency distribution is another way of organizing data. The rates, ratio, proportion and distribution serve as basic tools for the community health nurse in assessing and evaluating the community health needs.

APPLICATIONS OF EPIDEMIOLOGY

The main purpose of epidemiological approach in working with communities is disease prevention and early intervention for maintenance and promotion of health.

Morris and other epidemiologists have given the use of epidemiology as follows:

- **Study of the history of disease:** Epidemiology provides time trends and disease profiles in the population. It measures the fluctuations between the health and diseases. The trend of disease helps in prediction of future health problems.
- **Planning:** Epidemiological studies and information help in planning for the medical care facilities and preventive services. It can also be used for research planning.
- **Community diagnosis:** Epidemiology identifies the health problems prevailing in the community. After making the community diagnosis, healthcare therapies can be provided according to the needs of population. Thus, epidemiology investigates the disease and health status of the community.
- **Assessment of individuals' risk:** Epidemiology helps in determining the risk factors and their degree in the population. Epidemiologists try to find the relative risk and attributable risk which may be the cause of a disease. For example, prostitution is a risk for the HIV infection among women.
- **Identification of syndrome:** Epidemiological studies are used to define various disease syndromes. Along with the identification, they also reject the wrong associations, misconceptions about the existing disease syndrome and modify accordingly.
- **Completion of the clinical picture of chronic disease:** Epidemiology indicates the complete clinical picture of chronic disease. It provides spectrum of disease in population. Modern epidemiologists are studying the data about chronic disease and fill the gap in the epidemiological triad, if any exist.
- **Searching for causes:** Finding the cause-and-effect relationship is the central point of epidemiology. But epidemiologists are also paying attention to the search for causes and risk factors, which can produce the new disease or may increase the chronic diseases.
- **Evaluation:** Epidemiology provides important tools and information for the evaluation of health measures or programs. Evaluation of control methods or preventive measures can be performed easily on the basis of epidemiological studies. Through this, epidemiology helps in cost analysis.

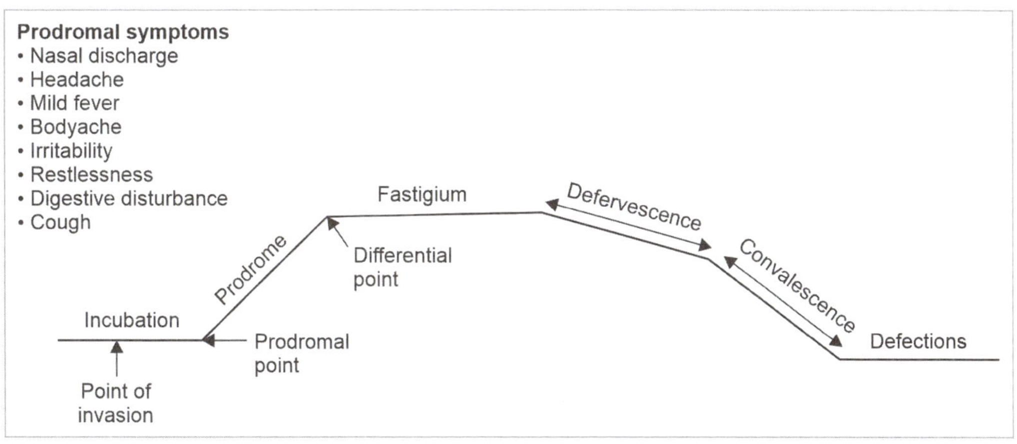

Fig. 4.23: Course of disease

COURSE OF DISEASE

The course of most communicable diseases (Fig. 4.23) is marked by certain stages starting from the entry of infection to the stage of recovery. These stages are listed as follows:

- **Incubation period:** This is the time interval between the entry of the disease agent in the body and manifestation of clinical signs and symptoms of the disease.
- **Prodromal period:** This is a short period ranging from 1 to 4 days and is marked by vague signs and symptoms. Clinical diagnosis is usually not possible.
- **Fastigium stage:** This period represents height of the disease. Signs and symptoms are clear-cut. The patient is confined to bed. Clinical diagnosis is possible.
- **Defervescence:** In this stage, patient begins to feel better because the body defense (immunity) begins to work or respond to the pathogens.
- **Convalescence:** The patient's recovery is established. This condition improves fast but still it may continue to be infective in others.
- **Defection:** The patient recovers totally from the illness but may continue to harbor the disease agent for varying period.

SPECTRUM OF DISEASE

The term "spectrum of disease" is a graphic representation of the disease (Fig. 4.24). The disease that occurs in the community is identical to the spectrum of light where the colors of rainbow vary from one end to the other but difficult to determine where one color ends and the other begins. Similarly, in disease the one stage ends and the other begins, but it is difficult to pin point where one stage ends and the other begins on the spectrum of disease. One end of the spectrum is subclinical or unapparent infections which are not ordinarily identified; and on the other end is the serious illness and in between one stage progresses to another and so on. In the middle, it may be mild to severe. This variation in the presentation of signs and symptoms of disease is called **spectrum of disease**. It may be affected by various factors and generally represents the immunity and receptivity level of the individual to infection.

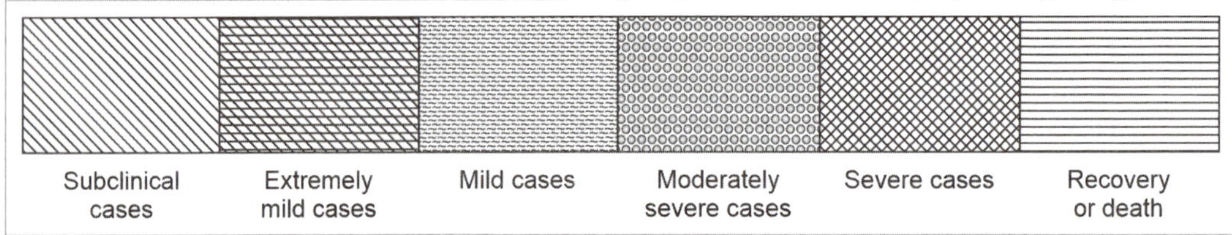

| Subclinical cases | Extremely mild cases | Mild cases | Moderately severe cases | Severe cases | Recovery or death |

Fig. 4.24: Spectrum of disease

LEVELS OF PREVENTION

The aim of community health is prevention of disease and promotion of health. Successful prevention from diseases depends upon the knowledge of causation, dynamics of transmission, identification of risk factors and groups, availability of prophylactic measures, early detection, treatment measures, and effective organization for applying these preventive measures to appropriate groups.

The natural history of disease provides the basis for community health intervention. Leavell HR and Clark EG in 1965 proposed three level model of prevention:

1. Primary prevention
2. Secondary prevention
3. Tertiary prevention

The modern concept of prevention is defined at four levels. WHO recommended the primordial prevention besides the aforementioned three levels of prevention. All four levels of prevention are discussed as follows.

1. Primordial Prevention

This is the new concept of preventing the development of risk factors in a chronic disease. In this, prevention efforts are directed toward discouraging from adopting harmful lifestyle through individuals and mass education. Primordial prevention is concerned with helping people to develop healthy lifestyle such as eating healthy food, having adequate rest and sleep, regular exercises, avoiding the use of tobacco, alcohol and drugs so that they do not develop health problems like obesity, heart disease, hypertension, cancer, etc.

2. Primary Prevention

Primary prevention can be defined as "action taken prior to the onset of disease, which removes the possibility that a disease will ever occur". It is aimed at intervention before pathological changes have begun. The specific interventions are as follows:

- **Health promotion:** By promoting the health of individuals and community, the number of diseases such as typhoid, fever, tuberculosis, cholera and nutritional deficiencies can be prevented. Health promotion is the process of enabling people to increase control over, and to improve their health. The following measures may be adopted to promote health:
  - Health education
  - Personal hygiene
  - Environmental sanitation: Provision of safe water supply, facilities for the safe disposal of human excreta and other wastes, control of insects and rodents, etc.
  - Adequate rest, sleep and regular exercise

- Good nutritional intake, i.e., balanced diet, healthy food habits and drinking plenty of water
- Provision of adequate housing, healthy and safe working conditions
- Attention to personality development and recreation
- Periodic health screening and selective examination
- Marriage counseling and sex education
- Genetic counseling

- **Specific protection:** It refers to those measures which are directed to intercept causative agents of a particular disease or group of diseases before these agents can cause disease in population. In developed countries, a large part of the budget is spent on protection against diseases. The following measures are a part of specific protection:
  - Specific immunization
  - Use of specific nutrients to prevent deficiency diseases
  - Protection against industrial and other accidents (road accidents, etc.)
  - Protection from environmental and occupational hazards
  - Controlling air and sound pollution
  - Protection from allergens
  - Protection from carcinogens
  - Use of prophylactic and supportive drugs
  - Control of quality and safety of food
  - Chemoprophylaxis

3. Secondary Prevention

It may be defined as "action which halts the progress of disease at its incipient stage and prevents complication". The secondary prevention focuses on individuals who are experiencing health problems and are at risk of developing complications or worsening the disease. The aims of secondary prevention are early diagnosis and prompt treatment.

- **Early diagnosis:**
  - Case finding measures
  - Screening surveys
  - Periodic examination and selective examination
- **Prompt treatment:** The aims of prompt treatment are:
  - To arrest the disease process and shorten the duration
  - To prevent the complications
  - To help to reduce morbidity and mortality in certain diseases.

4. Tertiary Prevention

It is the third level of prevention. It may be defined as, "all measures available to reduce or limit impairments and disabilities, minimize suffering caused by existing departure from good health and to promote the patient's adjustment to irremediable conditions." Tertiary prevention activities focus on the later phase of clinical disease when irreversible pathological damage produces disability. It is due to either primary and secondary preventive measures which are not effective or not known. Tertiary prevention aims to achieve the following:

- **Limiting the disability:** Disability interventions are applied in the late pathogenesis phase to minimize suffering and to promote the patient's adjustment to untreatable conditions. The objective of disability limitation is to prevent further advancement of the disease process from impairment to handicap. Disability interventions are often social or environmental as well as medical.

- **Rehabilitation of the case:** It is defined as "combined and coordinated efforts of medical, social, educational and vocational measures for training and retraining the individuals to the higher possible level of functional ability. It aims at social integration of the disabled and handicapped. Measures included in rehabilitation are physical medicine or physiotherapy, occupational therapy, speech therapy, social work and vocational guidance and replacement services. Areas of rehabilitation are as follows:
  - Medical rehabilitation—restoration of functions
  - Vocational rehabilitation—restoration of professional and economic capabilities
  - Social rehabilitation—restoration of family and social relationship
  - Psychological rehabilitation—restoration of personal dignity and confidence

DISEASE TRANSMISSION

Communicable diseases are transmitted from the reservoir or source of infection to the susceptible host (Fig. 4.25). There are three links in the chain of transmission as follows:

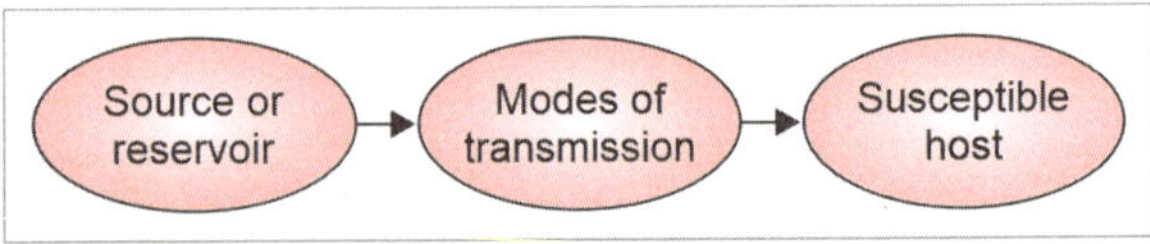

Fig. 4.25: Chain of infection in disease transmission

1. Source or reservoir
2. Modes of transmission of diseases
3. Susceptible host

1. Source or Reservoir

The **source** is defined as "the person, animal, object or substance from which an infectious agent passes or is disseminated to the host". A **reservoir** is defined as "any person, animal, arthropod, plant or substance in which an infectious agent lives and multiplies and on which it depends primarily for survival and can be transmitted to a host." The reservoir is the natural habitat in which it metabolizes and replicates. For example, in case of hookworm infection, man is the reservoir and soil is the source of infection which is contaminated with infective larvae, but in some diseases the source and reservoir may be the same, e.g., tetanus.

The reservoir may be of the following types:

Human Reservoir

Man is the most important source or reservoir of infection. He may be a case or carrier.

- **Case:** It is defined as "a person in the population group identified as having a particular disease, health disorder or condition under investigation." The presence of infection in a host may be subclinical or latent. These variations in the manifestations of disease are known as spectrum of diseases. Clinical cases show the clear-cut manifestation of the disease. Clinical cases may be mild, moderate, severe or fatal depending upon the virulence of the disease, but mild and ambulatory cases spread infection wherever they go. The severe cases are confined to bed and can spread infection only to those who come in contact or care givers if they do not take proper precautions.
  - **Subclinical cases:** They do not show the signs and symptoms of the disease. The disease agent multiplies in the host. It is eliminated from host and contaminates the environment. Subclinical infection is detected only by laboratory tests.

- ■ **Latent cases:** In latent infection, the host does not shed infectious agent which lies dormant within the host, without symptoms and not detected by laboratory investigation in blood, tissues or body secretions.
- ● **Carriers:** In some diseases, the disease agent is not completely eliminated leading to a carrier state. A carrier is defined as an infected person or animal that harbors specific infectious agents in the absence of discernible clinical disease and serves as a potential source of infection to others. Epidemiologically, carriers are more dangerous though less infectious. They are not documented and continue to infect the susceptible individuals over a larger area and larger period of time under favorable condition. Carriers are classified into three categories:
  - i. *By type:*
    - ◆ **Incubatory carriers:** They shed the infectious disease during the last few days of the incubation period, e.g., measles, mumps, polio, diphtheria, influenza, pertussis and hepatitis B.
    - ◆ **Convalescent carriers:** They continue to shed the disease agents during the period of convalescence, e.g., typhoid, cholera, diphtheria, whooping cough. They can infect the unprotected household members. In case of typhoid fever, Typhoid bacilli are excreted up to 6 months after the clinical recovery.
    - ◆ **Healthy carriers:** They are victims of subclinical state and do not show the signs and symptoms of the disease but are shedding the disease agent, e.g., poliomyelitis, cholera, meningococcal meningitis, salmonella and diphtheria. Persons in subclinical state may or may not be carriers. On the other hand, persons with positive tuberculin test in case of tuberculosis do not disseminate tubercular bacilli and are not the carriers.
  - ii. *By duration:*
    - ◆ **Temporary carriers:** They shed the disease agent for a short time.
    - ◆ **Chronic carriers:** They excrete the infectious agent for a longer time, e.g., typhoid fever, hepatitis B, dysentery, cerebrospinal fever, malaria, gonorrhea, etc. The longer the carrier state, the greater the risk to the community.
  - iii. *By portal of exit:* According to the portal of exit, the carriers are urinary carriers, intestinal carriers, respiratory carriers, nasal carriers, skin eruptions, open wound and blood.

Animal Reservoir

The diseases and infections are also transmitted to man through the animals and birds. There are >100 diseases which may be conveyed to man from animals and birds, e.g., rabies, yellow fever, influenza.

Reservoir in Nonliving Things

The soil and inanimate matter can act as reservoirs of infections, e.g., soil may have agents that cause tetanus, anthrax, coccidioidomycosis and hookworm infestation.

2. Modes of Disease Transmission

Disease may be transmitted from the reservoir or source of infection to the susceptible host in many different modes depending upon the infectious agent, portal of entry and the local ecological condition (Fig. 4.26).

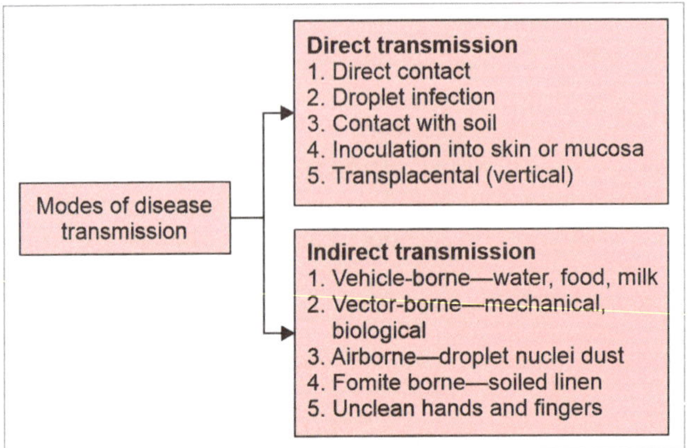

Fig. 4.26: Modes of disease transmission

Direct Transmission

- **Direct contact:** Infection may be transmitted by direct contact from skin to skin, mucosa to mucosa or mucosa to skin of the same person or another person. This is the direct and immediate transfer of infectious agent from the reservoir or source to a susceptible individual without an intermediate agency, e.g., skin to skin contact, by touching, kissing or sexual intercourse or continued close contact. Sexually transmitted disease (STD), acquired immune deficiency syndrome (AIDS), leprosy, skin and eye infections are transmitted by direct contact.

- **Droplet infection:** Small droplets of saliva and nasopharyngeal secretions can get sprayed into the surrounding atmosphere during coughing, sneezing, talking and spitting. These sprayed droplets may be inhaled by another person or they may directly impinge on the conjunctiva or respiratory mucosa or skin of a close contact. Particles with a diameter of 10 mm or greater are filtered off by nose, whereas particles with a diameter of 5 mm or smaller can penetrate deeply and reach the alveoli. The spread droplets are limited to a distance of 30–60 cm between the source of infection and others. When a healthy susceptible person comes within this range, he is likely to inhale some of these infected droplets and acquire infection. These tiny droplets may contain millions of bacteria and viruses which cause infection. Diseases transmitted through droplets are respiratory tract infections, i.e., diphtheria, whooping cough, tuberculosis, meningococcal meningitis and infections of nervous system. Overcrowding, lack of ventilation and close proximity favor droplet infection.

- **Contact with soil:** When the susceptible tissue of body comes in contact with disease agent present in the soil, compost or decaying vegetable matter in which disease agents lead a saprophytic existence, the infection is carried to the body tissue directly from the soil, e.g., tetanus, hookworm larvae, mycosis, etc.

- **Inoculation into skin or mucosa:** Disease agents may be directly inoculated into the skin or mucosa, e.g., rabies virus by dog bite, hepatitis B by infected needles and syringes, etc.

- **Transplacental:** Disease agents may be transmitted transplacentally from mother to the fetus. Example includes TORCH:

TO : Toxoplasma gondii

 R : Rubella virus

 C : Cytomegalovirus

 H : Herpes virus

Other examples are hepatitis B, AIDS, syphilis and varicella virus. Some of the nonliving agents can also be transmitted transplacentally, e.g., thalidomide, diethylstilbestrol and produce malformation of the embryo by disturbing its development.

Indirect Transmission

When the pathogenic organisms can survive outside the human host without losing their pathogenicity and virulence and can cause infection in the new host when they get entry into the new host, this is called indirect transmission. The infection in the new host depends upon the characteristics of the organism, the inanimate objects and influence of the environmental factors like temperature and humidity. Indirect infection can occur in the following ways:

- **Common source transmission:** The common sources of transmission of infection are:
  - **Vehicle based transmission:** Contaminated food, water, i.e., milk, milk products, raw vegetables, fruits, blood and its components play the role of vehicle for the transmission of diseases. Some of the vehicle-borne diseases are:

Vehicle	Diseases
1. Food, milk and milk products, raw vegetables and fluid, water	Diarrhea, cholera, polio, intestinal infections, hepatitis A, typhoid, food poisoning
2. Blood	Hepatitis B, syphilis, AIDS, malaria, brucellosis, etc.

  - **Fomites:** They are the nonliving agents which transmit infection. They include linen, books, soiled clothes, dressings, utensils, stationery material, toys, furniture, phones, mobile causing eye, ear, and skin infections, hepatitis A, diarrhea and dysentery.
  - **Hands:** Unclean hands of the care giver, doctors, nurses, paramedical staff and patients are the main sources of transmission of infection. Gastrointestinal tract (GIT) infections, intestinal parasites, hepatitis A, typhoid are transmitted by unclean hands.
- **Airborne transmission:** This is the major source of hospital acquired (nosocomial infection) infection. The air carries droplet nuclei which are the small residue of the evaporated fluid from droplets, coughed or sneezed by infected person. These droplet nuclei remain suspended in air for a long time. The large droplet may become a part of the dust and may survive on furniture, clothes and bedding. Both the suspended air droplets and dust droplets carrying the pathogenic organism transmit the infection. Mainly respiratory tract infections, tuberculosis, measles, COVID-19, chickenpox and influenza are transmitted by air.
- **Vector-borne transmission:** Any living thing or arthropod carries infection to the susceptible host and transmits infection. This method of transmission of infection is called vector-borne transmission. The vectors include flies, mosquitoes, rodents and fleas. Vector-borne transmission is of two types:
  - i. **Mechanical:** This method involves simply carrying the pathogenic organism by feet, crawling, flying insects carrying infective material through soiling of its feet or proboscis

or passage of organism through gastrointestinal tract. There is no development or the multiplication of the organisms by the vectors.

ii. **Biological:** Cyclic development and multiplication of the organism take place on the arthropod before transmitting the infection to man. Transmission may be by saliva, biting, regurgitation or deposition on the skin, or feces or other material capable of penetrating subsequently through bite, wound or through the area of trauma from scratching or rubbing.

IMMUNITY

Immunity is the resistance offered by the host to fight against the harmful effects of pathogenic microbial infection. Types of immunity are shown in Figure 4.27.

Components of Immunity

There are two important components of immunity:
1. Humoral immunity
2. Cellular immunity

Humoral Immunity

Humoral immunity is concerned with the production of specific antibodies. The B cells produce specific antibodies after antigen enters the body. The antibodies produced are of five types of immunoglobulins, i.e., IgG, IgM, IgA, IgD and IgE. These antibodies circulate in the blood and neutralize the microbes or toxins. These immunoglobulins have different functions to neutralize different antigens. All antibodies are immunoglobulins. Different types of immunoglobulins are:

- **IgG:** It consists of 75% of the total serum immunoglobulin and is a major immunoglobulin. It has smaller molecular weight, can pass through placenta and can diffuse into the interstitial fluid. Antibodies found in IgG are against gram-positive bacteria, virus and toxins of bacilli.
- **IgM:** Antibodies are formed with exposure to antigen. IgM antibodies are found in recent infections. They form 10% of the serum immunoglobulin. They have high agglutinating and fixing ability.
- **IgA:** It forms around 15% of the total serum immunoglobulin. It provides protection against local infections. IgA is found in large quantities in body secretions, i.e., saliva, milk, colostrum,

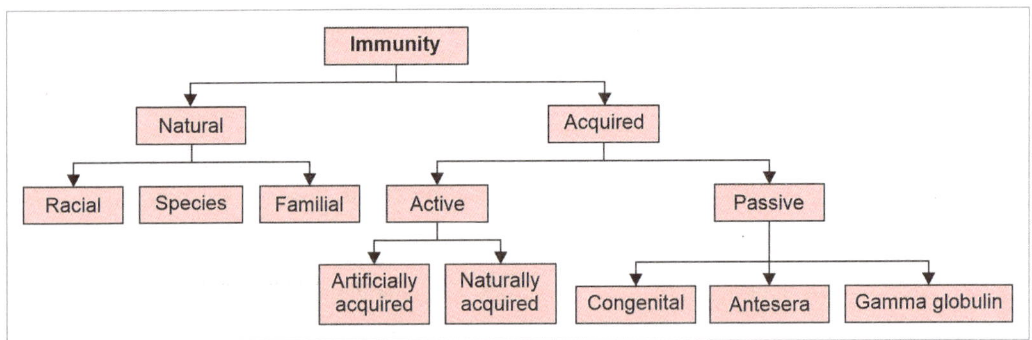

Fig. 4.27: Types of immunity

tears, bronchial secretions, nasal secretions, vaginal secretions and intestinal secretions. IgA antibodies destroy the bacterial and viral infections.

- **IgD:** Its quantity is very limited in the serum. Its functions are not well-known.
- **IgE:** It is concentrated in submucous tissue and its major antibody response is for immediate anaphylactic reactions.

Cellular Immunity

Cellular immunity is associated with T cells, a type of white blood cells. It does not produce antibodies but can recognize antigens and initiate the response, i.e., activating macrophages, release of cytotoxin. Cellular immunity is responsible for immunity against many diseases, e.g., tuberculosis, brucellosis and for body's reaction to foreign materials like skin grafting. Both the humoral immunity and cellular immunity are complementary to each other and help the individual in resisting the infection and disease.

- **Antigen:** Any substance or bacteria that stimulate the production of antibodies under favorable conditions is called antigen.
- **Antibody:** A special type of blood protein which is produced by lymphocytes and is capable of resisting the antigens or toxins is called antibody. Antibodies are produced by the reaction of antigen and react specifically to that antigen only.

Therefore, immunity is the ability of the body to recognize, segregate and destroy the antigen (bacteria, viruses and foreign protein).

Classification of Immunity

Immunity is classified into:
- Natural immunity
- Acquired immunity

Natural Immunity

Natural immunity is acquired through genetic structure. Certain cases are more likely to suffer from some specific diseases. Some diseases are found only in animals, e.g., animal plague, while some other diseases attack only humans like typhoid fever. Monkeys do not get syphilis and goats do not get tuberculosis (TB). White horses are more likely to develop leprosy.

Acquired Immunity

The immunity which an individual develops during life time is called acquired immunity. It can be of the following types:
- **Active immunity:**
    - **Naturally acquired immunity:** This type of immunity develops in a person after the attack of a disease. Immunity develops after the attack of measles, diphtheria and yellow fever. Immunity can develop in cases of mild attack of the disease or even in subclinical cases.
    - **Artificially acquired immunity:** The immunity that develops as a result of immunization. This type of immunity is acquired against polio, diphtheria, tetanus, measles, mumps, rubella and TB.

- **Passive immunity:** The body does not develop this type of immunity. The person depends upon readymade antibodies. In cases of emergency, the readymade antibodies are given to fight against disease. The impact of this type of immunity is short lived. It can be acquired as mentioned ahead:
  - **Congenital immunity:** Child acquires antibodies present in mother's serum through the placenta or breastfeeding.
  - **Antiserum injections:** After the attack of tetanus, antitetanus serum (ATS) is given; antidiphtheria serum (ADS) injection is given in case of diphtheria, and anti-snake venom is given in case of snakebite.
  - **Gamma globulin:** These are the antibodies acquired from human gamma globulin. These are prepared from multiple donors who are immunized or have recovered from some specific diseases. This type of gamma globulin is used to fight against diseases. But this type of immunity is temporary. The gamma globulin called immunoglobulin is given against hepatitis, tetanus and measles.
  - **Herd immunity:** The term "herd immunity" means that a large number of individuals in a community are immune to pathogens. There is overall level of immunity in a community. Population with low grade immunity are susceptible to diseases.

IMMUNIZING AGENTS

Immunizing agents are those substances which when introduced into the body produce immunity or substances which when introduced into the body prepare antibodies.

Classification

Immunizing agents are classified as follows:
- Vaccines
- Immunoglobulins
- Antisera or antitoxins

Vaccines

There are 5 types of vaccines (Fig. 4.28).

1. **Live vaccines:** These are prepared from live attenuated microorganisms. These are more potent than the killed vaccines and cannot activate the disease. After entering the host, they multiply resulting in large antigenic dose. They have all major and minor antigenic components. Due to their reaction, body receives a large quantity of active antibodies. Vaccines of BCG, measles

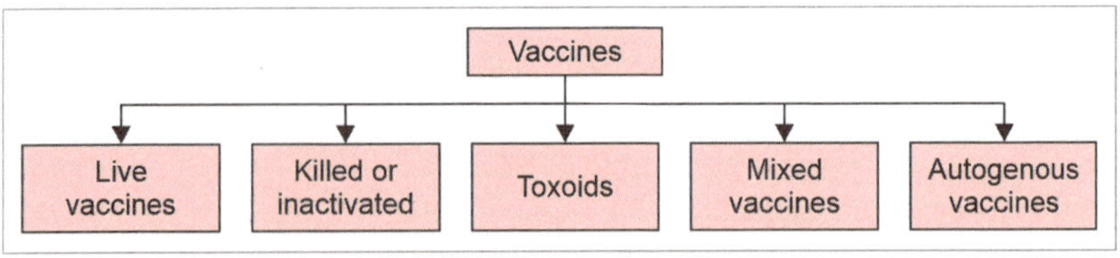

Fig. 4.28: Types of vaccines

and polio are included in this category. Usually, single dose produces antibodies, except polio where three or more doses are required. Persons with poor immunity such as leukemia, lymphoma, malignancy, pregnancy and immunodeficiency disease should not be administered with these vaccines.

2. **Killed or inactivated vaccines:** These are prepared from the organisms killed by heat or chemicals. They produce active immunity. Their effectiveness is less than the live vaccines. Killed vaccines are administered subcutaneously or intramuscularly and are safe. Two to three primary doses are required to produce adequate antibody response. Cholera and typhoid vaccines are examples of killed vaccines. Cholera vaccine offers only 50% effectiveness.

3. **Toxoids:** These are prepared by detoxicating the exotoxins produced by certain organisms. Antibodies produced by these toxoids neutralize the toxic effects generated by the infection rather than acting on the bacteria. Toxoids of tetanus and diphtheria are used in cases of tetanus and diphtheria to neutralize the toxic effects of infection.

4. **Mixed vaccines:** Vaccines prepared with combination of more than one immunizing agent are called mixed vaccines. Examples of mixed vaccines are DPT (against diphtheria, pertussis and tetanus), DT (against diphtheria and tetanus), DP (against diphtheria and pertussis) and MMR (against measles, mumps and rubella).

   Advantages of mixed vaccines are:
   - They are low cost
   - Single prick
   - Save time
   - Less inconvenient to use

5. **Autogenous vaccines:** These vaccines are prepared from the extracted cellular fraction from the bacteria of the same patient to whom the vaccine is to be administered. These vaccines are more effective than the normal vaccines. Adjuvants are added to enhance their potency. Examples of this kind of vaccines are meningococcal vaccine from the polysaccharide antigen of the cell wall, pneumococcal vaccine from polysaccharides from the capsule of organism.

Immunoglobulins

Immunoglobulins are prepared from the donors who have recovered from the disease or are immunized against infectious diseases. There are various types of immunoglobulins used to resist different types of antigens but two types of immunoglobulin preparations are used for vaccination. Immunity acquired is passive and temporary.

- Normal human immunoglobulin is used against measles and hepatitis B.
- Specific hyperimmune human immunoglobulin is used for prophylaxis of tetanus and rabies, and replacement of antibodies in immunodeficient patients. Vaccines of immunoglobulins are administered intramuscularly. They produce more antibodies and desired prophylaxis; local or systemic reaction may occur occasionally.

Antisera or Antitoxins

Antiserum is prepared from blood of animals, usually of horse. The serum equipped with antibodies is made to act against a disease. The immunity produced by antiserum is passive. The common antisera used are Antidiphtheria serum, Antirabies serum and anti-gas gangrene serum. Anti-snake venom is given in case of snakebite. Administration of these sera may give rise to serum sickness or anaphylactic shock due to abnormal sensitivity of recipient.

TABLE 4.3: Immunizing agents used against various infectious diseases

Immunizing agents (Types of vaccines)	Vaccines against infectious diseases	Prepared from
Live attenuated vaccines	BCG, typhoid, Oral polio, measles, mumps, rubella, influenza and yellow fever	Bacteria Virus
Killed or inactivated vaccines	Typhoid, cholera, pertussis, meningitis, plague, Rabies, Salk (polio) influenza, hepatitis B, Japanese encephalitis	Bacteria Virus
Toxoids	Diphtheria, tetanus	Bacteria
Immunoglobulins	Hepatitis A, measles, rabies, tetanus, mumps, Hepatitis B, varicella, diphtheria	Humans normally Ig Humans specifically Ig
Antisera	Diphtheria, Tetanus, gas gangrene, botulism, rabies	Bacteria, virus

The immunizing agents used against various infectious diseases are given in Table 4.3.

IMMUNIZATION

Infectious diseases can be prevented by effective immunization. Immunization programs are the most important and integral part of health activities in every country of the world.

Definition

Immunization is defined as the means of providing immunity against some communicable diseases through specially made immunizing agents or it can be defined as the mechanism of building immunity through artificial means.

Objectives

- To reduce the infant mortality rate by providing immunization against six killer diseases of children (polio, diphtheria, whooping cough, tetanus, measles and TB).
- To reduce maternal mortality rate by immunizing the pregnant mothers against tetanus.
- To increase the health status and life expectancy of the people by taking prophylactic measures against diseases.
- To control infectious diseases and their carriers.
- To develop sufficient capacity and technique to manufacture vaccines.

NATIONAL IMMUNIZATION SCHEDULE

Immunization program in India was introduced in 1978 as expanded program of immunization. In 1985, it became universal immunization. In 1992, it became a part of Child Survival and Safe Motherhood (CSSM) Program. Since 1997, it has been an important component of reproductive and child health (RCH). Universal immunization became one of the important components of National Rural Health Mission (NRHM) in 2005. National Immunization Schedule is given in Table 4.4.

TABLE 4.4: National Immunization Schedule for infants, children and pregnant women

	Vaccination	When to give	Maximum age	Dose	Route	Site
For infants	BCG	At birth or as early as possible	Till one year of age	0.1 mL (0.05 mL until 1 month of age)	Intradermal	Left upper arm
	Hepatitis B birth dose	At birth or as early as possible	Within 24 hours	0.5 mL	Intra-muscular	Anterolateral side of mid-thigh left
	OPV-O	At birth or as early as possible	Within first 15 days	2 drops	Oral	–
	OPV-1, 2 and 3	At 6, 10 and 14 weeks	Till 5 years of age	2 drops	Oral	–
	Rota virus vaccine	At 6, 10 and 14 weeks	Till 1 year of age	5 drops	Oral	–
	Inactivated polio vaccine (IPV)	At 14 weeks	Up to 1 year of age	0.5 mL	Intra-muscular	Anterolateral side of mid-thigh right
	Pentavalent 1, 2 and 3	At 6, 10 and 14 weeks	Till 1 year of age	0.5 mL	Intra-muscular	Anterolateral side of mid-thigh left
	Measles 1st dose	9–12 completed months	Given till 5 years of age	0.5 mL	Sub-cutaneous	Right upper arm
	Japanese encephalitis 1st dose	9–12 completed months	Till 15 years of age	0.5 mL	Sub-cutaneous	Left upper arm
	Vitamin A 1st dose	At 9 completed months with measles	Till 5 years of age	1 mL (1 Lakh IU)	Oral	–
For children	DPT Booster-1	16–24 months	7 years	0.5 mL	Intra-muscular	Antero-lateral side of mid-thigh (left)
	Measles 2nd dose	16–24 months	Till 5 years of age	0.5 mL	Sub-cutaneous	Right upper arm
	OPV Booster	16–24 months	Till 5 years of age	2 drops	Oral	–
	Japanese encephalitis 2nd dose	16–24 months	–	0.5 mL	Sub-cutaneous	Left upper arm
	Vitamin A (2nd to 9th dose)	16 months then one dose every 6 months	Till 5 years of age	2 mL (2 Lakh IU)	Oral	–

Contd...

	Vaccination	When to give	Maximum age	Dose	Route	Site
	DPT Booster-2	5–6 years	7 years	0.5 mL	Intra-muscular	Upper arm (left)
	TT	10 years and 16 years	–	0.5 mL	Intra-muscular	Upper arm
For pregnant women	TT-1	Early in pregnancy	–	0.5 mL	Intra-muscular	Upper arm
	TT-2	4 weeks after TT-1	–	0.5 mL	Intra-muscular	Upper arm
	TT-Booster	If received TT doses in a pregnancy within the last 3 years	–	0.5 mL	Intra-muscular	Upper arm

Nursing Considerations

Important Points to Remember while Immunizing
- Only disposable syringes should be used.
- Hepatitis B dose is given only within 24 hours after birth as it helps to prevent prenatal transmission of hepatitis B.
- OPV-O dose is given within 15 days after birth. OPV can be given up to 5 years of age.
- Pentavalent vaccines contain a combination of DPT, hepatitis B and Hib. Hepatitis B birth dose and booster dose of DPT will continue as before.
- Interval between 2 doses of pentavalent, OPV and hepatitis B should not be less than one month.
- There is no restriction of vaccination in case of minor cough, cold and minor fever.

Hazards of Immunization

- **Local reaction:** At the site of vaccination, there may be swelling, redness and pain which disappears after 48 hours.
- **General reaction:** It includes nausea, vomiting, fever, headache, uneasiness. If these signs appear, these should be reported to the doctor.
- **Allergic reactions:** These are due to hypersensitivity of person toward immunizing agents. In case of anaphylactic shock, it can be life-threatening reaction. It can be immediate or delayed. Symptoms of anaphylactic reaction are tachycardia, dyspnea, cold and clammy skin, itching, rashes on the skin, fainting and low blood pressure. The symptom should be noted and immediate intervention is required. Symptoms of serum sickness are fever, rashes on the skin, swelling and pain in joints that develops after 7–12 days after vaccination.
- Abscess formation at the site of vaccination due to technical errors, due to defective sterilization or technique not following the cold chain.

Responsibilities of Community Health Nurse in Immunization

- Nurse should have thorough knowledge and practice of immunization schedule.
- Nurse should supervise the work of health team engaged in immunization.
- The hazards of vaccination should be prevented by accurate technique and precautions.
- Children or people with normal health should be vaccinated only.
- Vaccination should be postponed in case of children suffering from high fever, acute respiratory tract infection, seizure or any severe illness.
- Malnourished children should be vaccinated but their parents should be advised regarding proper nutrition.
- Before the administration of antitoxin or antiserum, allergy test should be done.
- Emergency medicine, equipment, oxygen and all antianaphylactic drugs should be ready at hand to handle emergency. All health workers dealing with immunization should have thorough practice for the management of anaphylaxis.
- Only disposable syringes and needles should be used.
- Cold chain should be maintained.
- Restraints can be used for vaccinating children.
- During pregnancy, precautions should be taken while administering vaccines other than tetanus toxoid.
- Follow the six rights of medication, right patient, right drug, right dose, right route, right time and right person.
- Reassure children and mothers. Inform about next immunization sessions.

COLD CHAIN

"Cold chain" implies a system of storage and transport of vaccines at low temperature from the place of manufacturer to the actual vaccination site. Cold chain is necessary to prevent vaccines from getting denatured and to prevent vaccine failure. The term C4 that is, "complete care cold chain" is also in vogue in maintenance of cold chain of vaccine. All vaccines must be stored under the recommended conditions of the manufacturer in the literature accompanying the vaccines otherwise they become denatured and ineffective. Vaccines that should be kept in freezer compartment are polio and measles as polio is most sensitive to heat and must be stored at −20°C. Vaccines of typhoid, DPT, TT, DT, and BCG and diluents are stored in the cold part but never allowed to freeze.

Importance of Cold Chain and Maintenance of Potency of Vaccination

- All vaccines must be stored at a temperature suggested by the manufacturer.
- Vaccines should be protected from sun light and antiseptics.
- Opened multidose vials which have not been fully used should be reused for subsequent sessions up to 28 days subject to meeting certain conditions under open vial policy.
- Cold chain is essential for obtaining the vaccines from manufacturer.
- For storing and transporting the vaccine.
- There should be uninterrupted supply of electricity to maintain cold chain.
- Essential equipment should be there to maintain cold chain.

- Cold chain is important in maintaining the potency of vaccines and preventing the vaccines from getting denatured or ineffective.

Components of Cold Chain

The major components of cold chain system are as follows:

- **Apparatus:** Two categories of apparatus are required. The temperature of first category is kept at 4°–8°C to keep the vaccines. The temperature of second category is maintained to freeze the vaccines. The size varies from a small cooler to a walk-in cooler.
- **Supplies:** These include the vaccines and solvents. These are kept at low temperature. Vaccines of polio, TB and measles are kept in frozen conditions. Vaccines of DPT, DT and TT lose their potency if kept in frozen condition. These are kept at 4°–8°C.
- **Manual efforts:** Persons engaged in manufacturing vaccines, equipment, supplies, transportation and communication should be properly trained in the process of maintaining cold chain. Health officers, health workers and those storing and transporting the vaccination should work together to maintain the cold chain.
- **Transportation:** Rapid means of transportation should be used to maintain the potency of vaccines. Heat resistant equipment should be used in the journey. Refrigerators should be arranged in tracks. Airplanes can be used to save time.
- **Communication:** All information, instructions and orders concerned with cold chain should be immediately and clearly sent, received and followed. A reliable and effective communication system must be maintained for cold chain.

Equipment of Cold Chain

- **Vaccine carriers:** These are meant for carrying vaccines to health subcenters, villages, schools, industries, satellite towns and small towns. These are made of heat-resistant material and light in weight so that they can be carried easily in hands or on shoulder. Four packs of ice are kept along four sides of the containers. If the ice packs are completely frozen and lid is tightly closed, the vaccines can be kept at low temperature for a few days despite the outside temperature being 32°–43°C. Vaccine carrier should be properly cleaned from inside and the lid should be properly closed.
- **Cold packs:** These are flat bottles of plastic which are filled with water and used in vaccine carriers after freezing their water. These are kept in deep freezers for a minimum of 6 hours to freeze the water inside these. Some of these bottles are sealed. Some are having caps which can be opened.
- **Day carrier:** This equipment is used to keep the vaccine safe for a day. Thermocol boxes and thermos flask are included in day carriers. Cold packs can be used in thermocol boxes.
- **Refrigerator:** This is an important equipment of cold chain. Polio, measles and TB vaccines are kept in freezer. DPT, DT, TT and typhoid vaccines are kept in cold part at 4°–8°C. Deep freezer, small deep freezer and ice lined refrigerator are used for making cold or ice packs and storing vaccines.
- **Walk-in cooler:** This is the refrigerator of the size of a room 10' × 10' in which all types of vaccines can be kept safe. At district health centers, vaccines are stored in walk-in coolers only. These coolers have the arrangement to keep the vaccines at appropriate temperature for long hours even if electricity supply is interrupted.

Methods of Controlling Cold Chain

- Vaccines should be kept at appropriate temperature as per the instructions of manufacturer.
- All cold chain precautions should be followed while transporting vaccines.
- Temperature of storage place should be recorded and maintained.
- Communication system should be effective and up to date.
- All health workers engaged in maintaining cold chain should be properly trained with up-to-date knowledge.
- The equipment and components of cold chain should be kept properly functioning at all times and potency of vaccination should be maintained.

POTENCY TEST

Potency test is a method of investigating the effectiveness of vaccines. It is conducted to ensure that vaccines do not lose their potency. Open vial policy (OVP) is used as quality indicator for this test. Lack of potency makes the vaccines ineffective as they will not generate immunity. The following methods are used to check the potency of vaccines.

Open Vial Policy

The open vial policy is implemented to prevent the wastage of multidose vaccine vials. According to this policy, the partially used multidose vials of vaccine can be reused under the universal immunization program in subsequent sessions up to 28 days subject to meeting certain conditions.

Nursing Considerations

The open vial policy is only applicable to the following vaccines:
- DPT
- TT
- Hepatitis B
- Oral polio vaccine (OPV)
- Liquid pentavalent

The open vial policy is not applicable to the following vaccines:
- Measles
- BCG
- Japanese encephalitis

Vaccine vials opened in session site can be used in more than one immunization session up to four weeks provided the following conditions are fulfilled:

- The expiry date has not passed.
- Vaccines are stored at appropriate temperature range strictly both during transportation and at cold chain point.
- Vaccine vial septum has not been submerged in water or contaminated in any way.
- Strict aseptic technique has been used to withdraw all doses from the vial.
- Vaccine vial monitor has not reached discard point.
- Open vial should never be submerged in water as it increases the risk of contamination of the vial septum.
- Ensure all open vials have recorded date and time of opening.
- At the end of the session, all open vials should be returned to cold chain point.

- At cold chain point, open vials should be segregated into reusable and nonreusable open vials.
  - The reusable open vials of DPT, TT, hepatitis B and pentavalent vaccine vials fulfilling the abovementioned criteria.
  - Nonreusable open vials of measles, BCG and JE
- All open vials of measles, BCG and JE should be destroyed after 48 hours or before next session whichever is earlier.
- In case of any report of adverse events following immunization (AEFI), all open vials (usable and nonusable) should not be discarded or used. All open vials should be stored under proper cold chain till investigation is complete.
- All vials (open or unopened) should be transported in a zipper bag in the vaccine carrier and recorded in the stock register.
- Well-sealed conditioned ice packs should be used in vaccine carriers; and water should not be allowed to accumulate where vaccine vials and diluents are stored.

Vaccine Vial Monitors

Vaccine vial monitor (VVM) is a chemical indicator label attached to the vaccine vial container, i.e., vial, ampule or dropper, by the vaccine manufacture to check the potency of the vial as shown in Figure 4.29. On exposure to heat, VVM starts changing its color as shown in Figures 4.30A to D.

As the vaccine container moves through the supply chain, the VVM records the cumulative heat exposure through a gradual change in color.

If the color of the inner square is the same color or darker than the outer circle, the vaccine has been exposed to too much

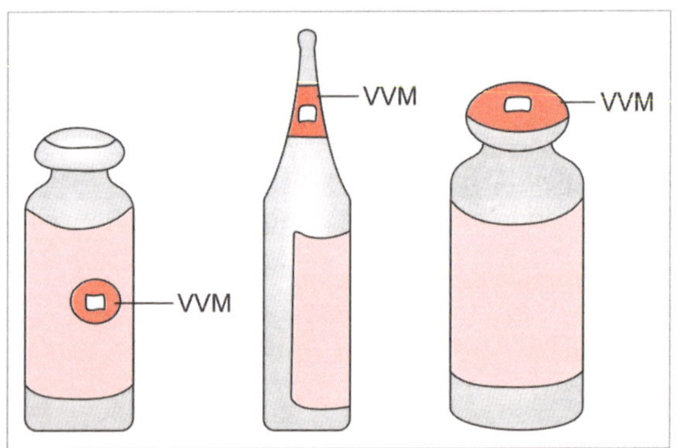

Fig. 4.29: Position of vaccine vial monitor shown on vials and ampule
Abbreviation: VVM, Vaccine vial monitor

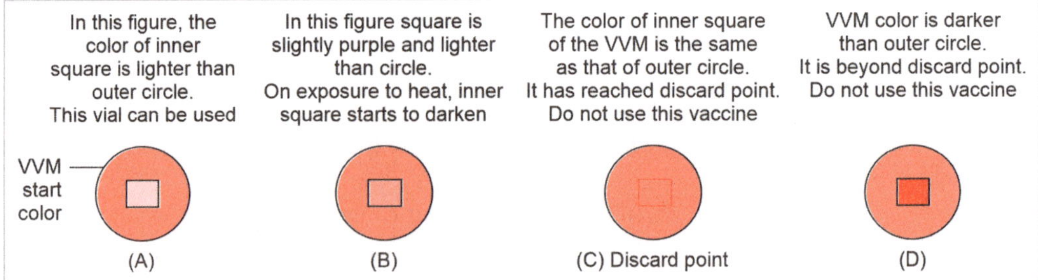

Figs 4.30A to D: Vaccine vial monitor showing the potency of vials after exposure to heat: **A.** Before exposure to heat; **B.** After exposure, the color of inner square is changed but lighter than outer circle, the vial can be used; **C.** The color of outer circle and inner square are same; it cannot be used as it has reached discard point; **D.** The color of inner square (VVM) is darker than outer circle, it is beyond the discard point. It cannot be used.

heat and should be discarded. To match the heat sensitivity, there are four types of VVM. These are VVM2, VVM7, VVM14 and VVM30. The VVM number is the time in days that it takes for the inner square to reach the color indicating discard point.

There are two different locations for VVMs and each is associated with specific guidance for handling opened multidose vials of vaccine.

- WHO prequalified vaccines where the VVM is attached on the label of the vaccine; the vaccine vial once opened can be kept for subsequent immunization session up to 28 days regardless of the formulation of the product (liquid or freeze dried)
- WHO prequalified vaccine where the VVM is attached in a location other than on the label, e.g., cap or neck of the ampule. In this case, the vaccine vial once opened must be discarded at the end of the immunization session or within six hours of opening whichever comes first. This is regardless of the formulation of the product (liquid or freeze-dried).
- **Freeze damage to the vaccine:** Freeze-sensitive vaccines get spoiled if they are frozen and cannot be used. The causes of vaccine freezing are:
  - Improper storage in ice lined refrigerator (ILR)
  - Cold climates; and if ambient temperature is <0°C
  - Storage and transport with nonconditioned frozen ice packs
  - Defective ILR
  - Innocent thermostat adjustment
  - Improperly trained or untrained staff handling vaccine/cold chain

To check whether the freeze-sensitive vaccines have been damaged by exposure to temperature below 0°C, The shake test is used after the frozen vaccine vial has thawed and does not have the appearance of a cloudy liquid, but tends to form flakes that settle down at the bottom of the vial.

Shake Test

To check the freeze damage of the vaccine vial, the shake test (Fig. 4.31) is conducted in the following way:

- Take a vaccine vial you suspect that may have been frozen is the 'Test Vial'
- **Frozen control vial**
  - Take a vaccine vial of the same antigen, same manufacturer and same batch number as the suspect vaccine vial which is to be tested.
  - Freeze solid the vial at –20°C overnight in the DF and this is the 'frozen control' vial and label it accordingly to avoid its use.
  - Let it thaw. DO NOT heat it.
  - Hold the control and test vial together between thumb and forefinger. Shake the vials vigorously for 10–15 seconds.
  - Place both vials to rest on flat surface; and observe them side by side for 30 minutes.
  - Compare the rate of sedimentation.
  - If the sedimentation in the test vial is slower than that in the "frozen control vial", the vaccine has not been damaged, and it has passed the shake test. Use vaccine vial, it is not damaged.
  - If the sedimentation is similar in both vials or if sedimentation is faster in "Test" vial than that in the "frozen control vial", the vaccine is damaged. It failed the shake test. DO NOT use this vial. Notify the superior.

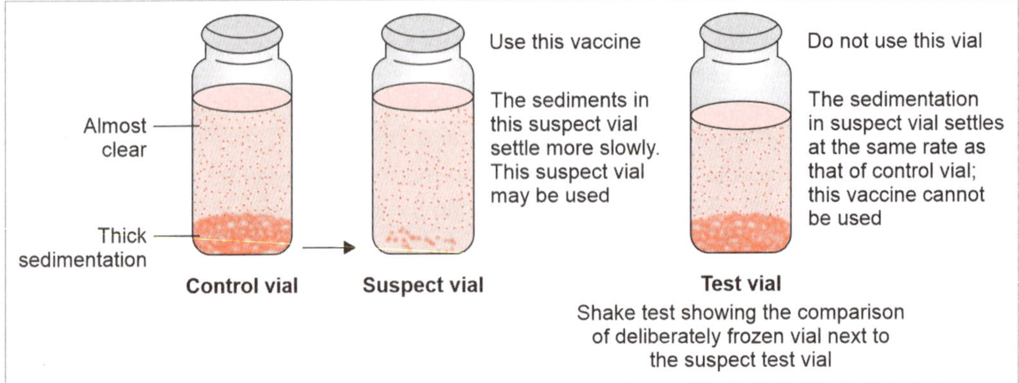

Fig. 4.31: Shake test showing the comparison of deliberately frozen vial next to the suspect test vial

CONTROL OF INFECTIOUS DISEASES

The control of infectious diseases mainly refers to prevention of diseases. It includes primary and secondary prevention. The disease control is a continuous process.

The main objectives of disease control include the following:

- To reduce the occurrence of disease by proper immunization and prophylaxis
- To reduce the transmission of disease by isolation and practicing universal precautions
- To decrease the duration of disease by early diagnosis and treatment
- To decrease the possible complications
- To reduce the financial burden on the population
- To decrease the morbidity and mortality rates

So, the disease control involves all the measures designed to prevent or reduce the incidence, prevalence and consequences of diseases as much as possible. This includes community participation, political support and intersectoral coordination. The following measures help in controlling the disease.

Controlling the Reservoir

- **Early diagnosis:** To find out the source of infection, to study the distribution of disease and apply control measures.
- **Notification:** As soon as an infectious disease is diagnosed; it should be notified to the local health authorities so that the control measures can be implemented. Notification can be done by the physician, community leader or even by a family member.
- **Epidemiological investigation:** It is done to identify the source of infection and other factors such as climate, sociocultural and behavioral factors related to the spread of infection.
- **Isolation:** Separation or segregation of infected persons or animals for a period of communicability from others to such places so as to prevent or limit direct or indirect transmission of infectious agents from those infected to those who are susceptible or who may spread the agents to others in case of diphtheria, cholera, plague, etc.
- **Early treatment of the disease:** By using effective drugs, limit the disease and cut short the duration of the disease and interrupt transmission of the disease.

- **Quarantine**: By limiting the freedom of movements of such well persons or domestic animals exposed to communicable diseases for a period not longer than the longest usual incubation period of the disease in such a manner to prevent effective contact with those who are not so exposed to the disease.
- **Interruption of disease transmission:** Breaking the chain of transmission of disease helps in controlling the communicable diseases. It consists of preventing the entry of infective agents in susceptible hosts. Measures taken for interruption of disease include safe water supply and control of insects and rodents. Malaria, filaria, dengue, yellow fever, Japanese encephalitis can be prevented by controlling the breeding places of mosquitoes. Typhoid, cholera and dysentery can be prevented by supplying purified water.
- **Immunization of the susceptible host:** Immunization strengthens the immunity of the susceptible host and breaks the chain of transmission of communicable diseases.
- **Chemoprophylaxis:** Protection from diseases occur using chemotherapeutics. Certain diseases can be prevented by chemotherapy, such as prevention of clinical symptoms of cholera by tetracycline or furazolidone for household contacts.
- **Nonspecific measures:** Measures taken to improve general sanitation, nutritional status and education have an important role in controlling and preventing disease.

Disinfection

Disinfection is defined as the destruction of pathogenic microorganisms by physical, chemical or other means. The control of microbial growth can be achieved by two ways, i.e., by killing or destroying the microorganisms and inhibiting their growth. To control the growth of microorganisms, various methods and agents are used. The terminology applied for various methods of disinfection is given as follows:

- **Concurrent disinfection** implies the destruction of infectious agents as soon as they are released from the body. It is the disposal of contaminated material or equipment as early as possible.
- **Terminal disinfection** implies the destruction of infectious material or cleaning the room, furniture, bedding, etc. after the discharge or transfer or death of the patient from the hospital, health center or recovery at home.
- **Sterilization:** It refers to destruction of all forms of microorganisms including the spores. It is the complete destruction of all pathogenic and nonpathogenic microorganisms and viruses or elimination of all viable organisms.
- **Disinfectant:** It refers to a substance that destroys harmful microorganisms but not necessarily their spores. Disinfectants are only suitable to use on inanimate objects.
- **Antiseptics:** They refer to substances that destroy or inhibit the growth of microorganisms. They are less strong and are safe enough to be used on living tissues.
- **Deodorant:** It refers to a substance (e.g., body sprays, creams, etc.) that suppresses or neutralizes bad odors.
- **Detergent:** It refers to a surface cleaning substance that acts by lowering surface tension, e.g., detergent soaps and powders.
- **Cleaning:** It refers to removing all visible dust, soil and other foreign materials. Routine cleaning is necessary to reduce the number of microorganisms on environmental surfaces and also for aesthetic reason.

Methods/Agents for Disinfection

Methods of disinfection are classified into the following types:

- **Natural methods/agents:** Sunlight, air, cold.
- **Physical methods/agents:**
  - Heat
    - Dry heat: Burning, flaming, hot air
    - Moist heat: Boiling, autoclaving
  - Radiation
- **Chemical methods/agents**
  - Alcohol
  - Aldehyde
  - Halogens
  - Oxidizing agents
  - Phenol and related compounds
  - Quaternary ammonium group
- **Miscellaneous methods**

Natural Methods/Agents

Nature tries to help in controlling the pathogenic microbes and thus maintains the ecological balance. But nowadays these methods are limited to domestic use.

- **Sunlight:** Many disease-producing organisms are destroyed by direct and continuous exposure to sunlight. The ultraviolet rays of sunlight destroy the bacteria and virus when the material to be disinfected is exposed to sunlight for several hours for 2–3 days. Linen, bedding, furniture, etc. can be disinfected by sunlight.
- **Air:** Exposure to open air dries or evaporates moisture which is lethal to most bacteria. Airing also helps in water purification.
- **Cold:** Cold prevents multiplication of bacteria and low temperature also delays the microbial activity. Microorganisms causing meningitis and gonorrhea may be killed by cold. Cold storages are used for the preservation of food stuff. Domestic fridge also prevents food decomposition.

Physical Methods/Agents

Heat

Heat is the most common and economical method of disinfection. It coagulates the albumin and destroys the valuable enzymes of the organism resulting in their destruction. The effect of heat to disinfect materials depends upon the kind and quantity of heat, characteristics of microorganism, time of exposure and the method of heat application used. Dry heat and moist heat are the two types of heat, which have been explained as follows:

Dry heat:

- **Burning or incineration:** It is safe, cheap, easy and effective method of disinfection. This method is used in hospitals and comes under hospital waste management. The contaminated dressing, swabs, rags and placenta are disposed of by burning. Burning should not be done in open air. It is to be done in an incinerator. Feces can also be disposed of by burning. The combustible material such as kerosene, dust, paper aid in burning; so, they can be added to the disposable material while burning.
- **Flaming:** Contaminated noninflammable articles like metallic wire (platinum and copper) needles, points of forceps, probes, incubatory wires, etc. are disinfected by this method.

The objects are held near the flame till they become red hot. This is a quick method and can be used in emergency.

- **Hot air:** Hot air oven is used for hot air disinfection and sterilization. Hot air is very useful for sterilizing articles such as glassware, syringes, swabs, dressings. The temperature of hot air is maintained between 160°C and 180°C for one hour. It can destroy microbes including their spores. The drawback of hot air is that it has no penetrating power and is not suitable for bulky items. The plastic, rubber and other delicate substances cannot be disinfected by this method.

Moist heat

Boiling: This is the simplest, oldest, economical and most commonly used method for destruction of microorganisms. Boiling for 5–10 minutes will kill the bacteria but not spores or viruses. Boilers provide temperature above 90°C in an atmosphere of steam which is exposed to open air. For complete destruction of the spores, temperature should be above 100°C which cannot be achieved in boilers. Boiling is suitable for the material which is not used for subcutaneous insertion. Boiling for 30 minutes is adequate for disinfection of small instruments, tools, stainless steel utensils, linen, rubber goods, kidney trays, urinals and bed pans.

Autoclaving (Steam under pressure): Sterilizers which operate at a high temperature above 100°C and high pressure are called autoclaves. They generate steam under pressure (saturated steam) which is the most effective sterilizing agent. With increased pressure, temperature of water can be raised and the steam generated has the penetration power to sterilize all the articles and destroy all types of organisms including the spores. It works on the principle of domestic pressure cooker. It is widely used in hospitals and laboratories. Temperature and pressure are adjusted according to various categories of articles to be used.

Radiation

Ionizing radiation (gamma rays and cathode ray, X-rays, etc.) and nonionizing radiation (infrared, ultraviolet rays) can be used for disinfection and sterilization. The articles to be sterilized are placed in plastic bags before radiation and remain sterile until opened. Dressings, bandages, surgical instruments are sterilized. Ionizing radiation has great penetrating power with no heating effect. This method is very effective but expensive.

Chemical Methods/Agents

Chemical methods of disinfection are used for those articles which cannot be sterilized by boiling or autoclaving. They are immersed in chemical disinfectants. Chemical agents are also used for disinfection of urine and feces. Chemical agents perform their microbial activity in the following ways:

- By destroying the enzymes
- By denaturing the proteins
- By oxidation/reduction, etc.

Some of the commonly used antiseptics and disinfectants are:

- **Alcohol:** It is the most commonly used disinfectant in the hospitals and healthcare settings. It is used in 70% concentration. Methylated spirit (industrial form of ethyl alcohol) is used for skin disinfection and hand washing. Skin disinfection before inoculation destroys all types of nonspore-forming bacteria.

- **Aldehyde:** It is bactericidal and sporicidal. Most common aldehydes used are available in gas, solid and liquid forms.
  - **Formaldehyde:** It is used for disinfection of linen, blankets, books, beds, instruments, furniture, etc. Paraformaldehyde powder is used for disinfecting room; and by fumigation room is disinfected.
  - **Formalin solution:** It is used for disinfection of rooms, walls, furniture, etc., in 2–3% strength by spraying. Specimens are preserved in formalin solution.
- **Halogens and their compounds**
  - **Bleaching powder:** This is chlorinated lime, white amorphous powder with pungent smell of chlorine. Bleaching powder is widely used for disinfection of water, feces and urine. Drawback of this compound is that it is unstable and loses its chlorine content on storage. 5% solution is suitable for disinfection of feces and urine allowing a period of one hour for disinfection.
  - **Sodium hypochlorite:** It acts like bleaching powder but is stronger and contains 80,000 to 1,80,000 ppm of available chlorine. It is used to sterilize infant feeding bottles. It is widely used in hospitals, healthcare agencies under the hospital waste management system.
  - **Halogen tablets:** These are chlorine tablets; one tablet contains 4 mg of halogen sufficient to disinfect 1 L of water from half an hour to one hour period.
  - **Iodine:** It is the oldest and most effective bactericidal skin antiseptic. It is an alcoholic solution popularly known as tincture iodine. Only 1–2% of iodine is applicable. Higher concentration may cause skin irritation.
  - **Povidone:** It is an iodophorus compound commonly known as betadine (brand name), but does not cause skin irritation, though it has same effect as iodine.
- **Oxidizing agents (KMO_4):** Potassium permanganate in a very low concentration is used as antiseptic for skin infection. 1:5000 solution is used for mouthwash.
- **Hydrogen peroxide (H_2O_2):** It is useful in cleaning the wound, killing microorganisms and protecting the wound from further infection.
- **Phenol and related compounds:** This group is concerned with hydroxyl and chloro compounds.
  - **Phenol:** Pure phenol or carbolic acid is a good germicide. Pure form is not used. Crude phenol 3–5% solution is used for sterilization of instruments, mopping the floors, furniture, etc.
  - **Cresol:** 5–10% of the solution is used for disinfection of feces, urine, etc. Cresol emulsion (Lysol) is also used for disinfection.
  - **Dettol (Chloroxylenol):** It is a commonly used antiseptic available in the form of soaps, emulsions, solutions, etc., 5% concentration of Dettol solution is appropriate for disinfection of instruments, thermometers and plastic material.
- **Quaternary ammonium group:** It includes cetrimide and Savlon.
  - **Cetrimide:** It is a bactericidal antiseptic agent used in 1–2% concentration; commonly known as Cetavlon.
  - **Savlon:** It is a combination of cetrimide + chlorhexidine (Hibitane). It has good bactericidal effect when applied with spirit.

Miscellaneous Methods

In miscellaneous methods, some agents inhibit the growth of organisms, some reduce the number and some are germicidal. Some methods are also mentioned that preserve the food and check the activities of microorganisms.

- **Acids:** Acetic acid is used for the preservation of food, whereas boric acid has an antiseptic effect.
- **Alkalies:** Lime and sodium hydroxide act as powerful bactericidal agents.
- **Dyes:** They destroy the reproductive capacity of microorganisms, e.g., gentian violet (GV paint), Mercurochrome, acriflavine, crystal violet are useful and cheap antiseptics.
- **Filtration:** Filtration reduces the number of organisms. Different types of filters are used for filtration of biological liquids, animal serum or solutions of vitamins, enzymes, antibiotics, etc.
- **Sound vibrations:** Rapid vibrations of sound or ultrasound may kill the bacteria, but this method is not having practical use.
- **Gases:** Some gases serve the purpose of sterilization. Ethylene oxide kills all types of microorganisms including their spores and viruses. It is used in 3% concentration and sterilizes metal, glass, paper, plastic materials, catheters, books, etc. Mechanical aeration is essential after sterilization to avoid toxic effects of ethylene oxide.

Summary

- Epidemiology is the study of diseases in population. It means epidemiology is the study of the spread of diseases within and between population.
- Aims of epidemiology are to determine frequency distribution, to identify etiology and to provide data for planning implementation and evaluation of services for prevention, control and treatment of diseases.
- Basic tools of measurement are rates, ratio, proportion and distribution.
- Uses of epidemiology include determination of origin of a disease with known causes, investigation and control of unknown diseases, studying ecology and natural history of diseases, planning and monitoring disease control program and assessment of economic aspects of diseases.
- Epidemiological triad means interaction between man, agent and environment. It means three links are there in chain transmission.
- Communicable diseases are transmitted from the source of infection to the susceptible host by three links in the chain of transmission, i.e., host, environment and an agent.
- The ratio, proportion and rates are used to describe three aspects of human condition, i.e., morbidity, mortality and natality. Four levels of prevention correspond to different phases in the development of diseases.
- A disease is transmitted from the reservoir to the susceptible host either directly or indirectly by single or several routes.
- Immunity is the host defense against infection. It is of two types; active immunity that develops as a result of infection and passive immunity that develops through administration of immunizing agents.
- The immunizing agents used are vaccines, immunoglobulins and antisera.
- Two types of immunity are produced: active and passive immunity. Infectious diseases can be controlled by controlling the reservoir, interruption of disease transmission and strengthening the susceptible host.
- Disinfectants are the agents which kill the infectious agents. Methods of disinfection are of three types, namely concurrent, terminal and prophylactic disinfectants.

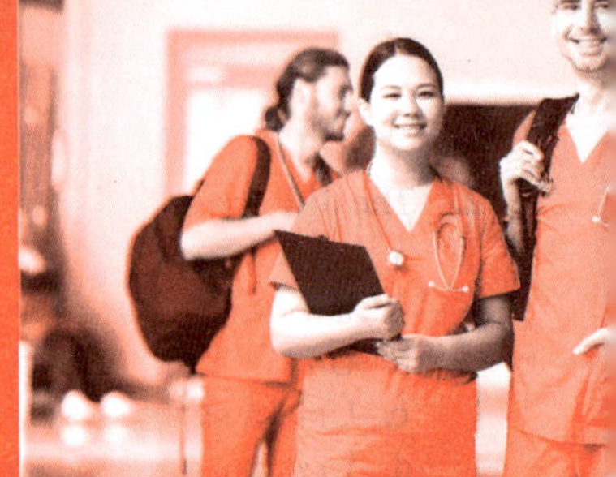

LONG ANSWER TYPE QUESTIONS

1. Describe the methods of epidemiological study.
2. Define communicable diseases. Describe in detail various modes of transmission of communicable diseases.
3. What is specific protection? Describe the National Immunization Schedule in India.

SHORT ANSWER TYPE QUESTIONS

1. Write short notes on:
   a. Epidemiological triad
   b. Carriers
   c. Natural history of the disease
   d. Levels of prevention
   e. Uses of epidemiology
2. Define the following:
   a. Epidemiology
   b. Carriers
   c. Infection
   d. Infestation
   e. Incubation period
   f. Incidence and prevalence
   g. Epidemic and endemic
   h. Pandemic and sporadic
   i. Rates, ratio and proportion
3. List the purposes of epidemiology.
4. Name four vaccines and disease(s) against which they are given.

MULTIPLE CHOICE QUESTIONS

1. **The measurements of epidemiology include:**
   a. Measurement of frequency of diseases
   b. Measurement of distribution of diseases
   c. Measurement of determinants of disease
   d. All of the above

2. **The difference between clinical medicine and epidemiology is:**
   a. In clinical medicine, unit of study is case and in epidemiology, the unit of study is population at risk.
   b. Unit of study in clinical medicine is population at risk and in epidemiology, it is a case.
   c. Unit of study in clinical medicine and epidemiology is population at risk.
   d. Unit of study in clinical medicine and epidemiology is carrier.

3. **Primary prevention means measures taken to prevent the occurrence of disease:**
   a. Before the occurrence of disease
   b. After the initiation of disease
   c. After the disease becomes complicated
   d. None of the above

4. **Person characteristics of epidemiology include all of the following; except:**
   a. Age
   b. Education
   c. Population
   d. Parity

5. **Quantitative measures of health status include:**
   a. Proportions
   b. Rates
   c. Ratio
   d. All of these

6. **Important characteristics of descriptive epidemiology include:**
   a. Pattern, disease, time
   b. Person, place, time
   c. Resource, time, disease
   d. None of these

7. **Descriptive epidemiology is one of the methods of epidemiology. It includes:**
   a. Description of the occurrence of disease in population
   b. Relationship between health status and other variables
   c. The alteration in the program of disease
   d. None of the above

8. **Primary prevention includes:**
   a. Health promotion and specific protection
   b. Early diagnosis and treatment
   c. Disability limitation
   d. All of the above

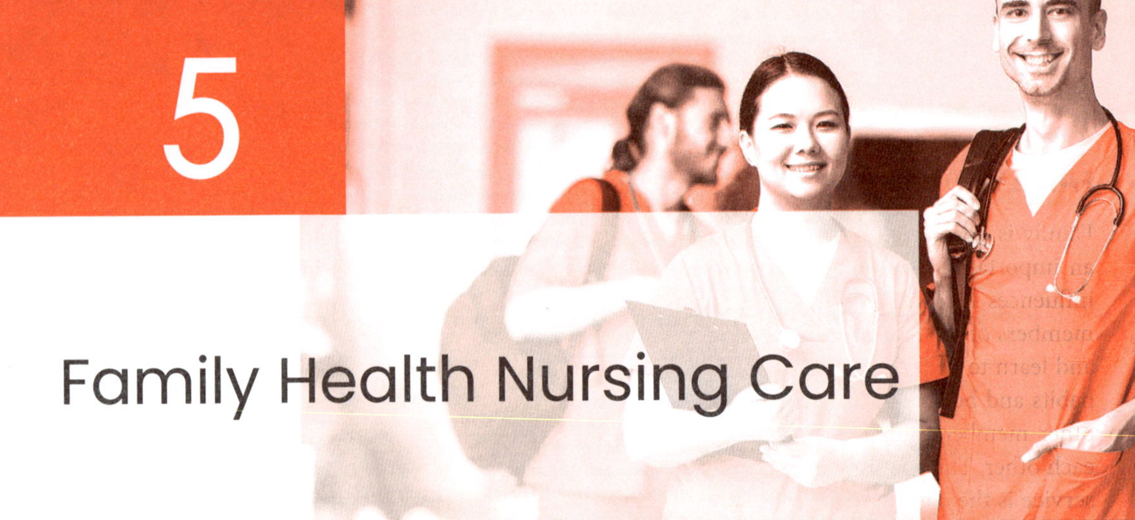

Family Health Nursing Care

INTRODUCTION

Family health nursing is generalized, well balanced and integrated comprehensive and continuous are requiring comprehensive planning to accomplish its goal. The goals of the family health nursing include optimal functioning for the individual and for the family as a unit." The concept of family health nursing includes the caregiver's partnership with the family and the involvement of the whole family in the care of the family member.

FAMILY

Family is considered a natural and fundamental unit of society. In a family, every individual has an important influence. There is an interactive communication network in which every member influences the entire system and in turn the individual is also influenced by the system. The members of the family grow, develop, mature, learn culture, customs, traditions, beliefs and habits and learn to help each other. Family helps in developing health knowledge, values, attitude, health habits and behavior of its members. The health problem of one member in the family affects the other members of the family emotionally, socially and physically as they are interdependent on each other. The health of an individual is the outcome of family's group dynamic, so family health service is the control point of health services. It is an important component of "Health for All" as it is the unit of service in all community health programs.

Definitions of Family

"Family is a group of persons united by the ties of marriage, blood or adoption; consisting of a single household, interacting and intercommunicating with each other in their respective social roles of husband and wife, mother and father, son and daughter, brother and sister creating a common culture."   **—Burgers and Locke**

"Family is a group of two or more persons related by birth, marriage adoption and residing together in a household."   **—U S Bureau**

"Family involves people who are related in a traditional or nontraditional sense by marriage, blood, adoption or friendship."   **—Jarris L**

Types of Family

There are four types of families:
1. **Nuclear family:** The family consists of a husband, wife and their natural or adopted children.
2. **Extended or joint family:** This consists of a nuclear family; in addition to other who are blood-related or marriage-related. There are grandparents, aunts, uncles and cousins in this type of family.
3. **Blended family:** This includes married couples; one or both of them have been married previously and had children from the previous marriage and the couple has their own children as well.
4. **Single parent:** A single parent either male or female who lives alone with his or her child or children. They may be naturally born or adopted children.

Characteristics of Family

- **Family changes according to time and place:** The organization and societal task are varying with the social change, increasing urbanization and industrialization. The size of the family also reflects the social and economic condition. The socioeconomic condition of the family may fall in good or bad days.
- **Family develops its own life cycle:** Each family has its own culture, behavior, style, administration, rules and regulation, decision making, power, dominance of one over another and division of work for example in some families, mother makes decisions about home management and in case of the children, whereas father decides the economic aspects of the family.

- ▪ In some of the joint families, the head of the family keeps the power of decision making regarding his children or grandchildren.
- ▪ In some families, children are permitted to make their own decisions about them.
- **Family operates as a group:** For decision making to solve the problem the whole family puts froth their views. All the members of family share their ideas, think over and then decide. In that way, the whole family is involved. But in certain families, the one member usually the head of the family takes the decision to solve the problems.
- **Family accommodates to the needs of the individual:** In a family, every member is considered an individual. Sometimes the family needs and individual needs do not match resulting in conflicts in the family. There must be some adjustment between the two different needs.
- **Family related to the community:** Family utilizes community institutions and contributes to the community whatever it can do for the betterment of the family. Some families may have responsibility for the community development, whereas other families may not show their concern.

Factors Affecting the Health of Family

- **Family composition:** Health of a family depends on the number of family members. If there are small children and elder people who are dependent and need more care and attention and the working people are few maybe one or two. They may not be able to pay much attention toward the large number of dependents. On the other hand, if one or two children along with one or two elders, are looked after easily by paying special attention.
- **Literacy of the family:** The educated family will understand the importance of good health and will be health conscious, whereas a lack of education leads to superstitions and lack of the attitude to follow health rules.
- **Family income:** Family income is directly proportional to the health. Family with good incomes has some budget for health and will seek health services for maintenance of health, whereas family with low incomes struggles to meet both ends and are not able to avail of health services.
- **Standard of living:** Good housing, personal hygiene, healthy habits, good living conditions contribute to good health.
- **Nutrition:** Nutrition is related to promotive, preventive and curative aspects of health. The knowledge of nutritional values of food, food fads, liking and disliking of certain foods and the family's budget for food affects the health of the family members.
- **Environmental factors:** These factors like air, water, sanitation, lighting, sound, temperature, housing and waste disposal affect the health status of the family.
- **Cultural values of the family:** The family's customs, beliefs, traditions and rituals and their behaviors and attitude toward the care of children, aged and women influences the welfare of the family members.
- **Health goals:** Family's awareness of health, health values, beliefs and attitudes toward health contribute to achieving health.
- **Role of family in health and illness:** As the members of the family are interdependent and they are concerned with health and health needs of each other. If a member of the family falls sick other members provide care and support to the sick.
- **Coping and support system of the family:** The family is capable of maintaining a home environment conducive to personal development and health promotion, recognizing health

needs and health problems. Provide care to the sick and disabled and make decisions of other family problems and take appropriate action. This coping ability of the family varies. Some families can deal with problems as they come whereas some other families seek help.

- **Availability of health services:** To make use of available health services, the quality, quantity and specialization of community health services also affect the health of a family.

Family as a Unit of Health

Family health nursing is a nursing aspect of organized family health services which are focused, on the family as the unit of care with 'health as a goal.' Family health is the basic unit of healthcare. Family is a basic unit of health. As the individual grows in family, his health behavior including health values, health habits and health perceptions are developed, organized and performed within the family.

His attitude toward illness is influenced by the other members of the family as the members are socially and emotionally interdependent and interlocked. The genetic factors, socialization, personal health, family economy, emotional aspects and social security surrounding the family are closely related to healthcare services.

Family healthcare is the building block of healthcare services as community health services are provided through family healthcare or family being the basic unit of any healthcare system.

Family is considered a unit of healthcare on the following facts:

- Family provides conducive environmental support for its members to develop healthy attitude, good health habits and health practices, values and positive health behavior. The members of the family interact with common physical, social and environmental forces which influence their health.
- Family members have interpersonal relationships and interdependency with each other which creates awareness about health among family members.
- Family is considered a natural and fundamental unit of society. The family size, structure, educational standard, family income and culture, customs and health habits and environment affect the health standard of the family.
- Family as a group generates, prevents and corrects health problems. Its support in healthcare needs plays an important role.
- Illness of one family member affects the health of other family members as the health problems of the family are interlocking.
- Individual health problems can be tackled and solved easily through family healthcare.
- Comprehensive healthcare can be delivered to the community through family healthcare services.
- The successful family life can be achieved by family healthcare services.

CONCEPT OF FAMILY HEALTH

The concept of family health is based on health of family as an integrated unit and is concerned with the health of all family members. Family health services aim at overall welfare of family. Many kinds of services are needed to assist family members in dealing with their problems. In a family variety of health problems are detected. There may be aged people, handicapped, small children, pregnant women and lactating mothers. The health problems of each group will be different so, all these problems can be tackled within the family during the home visit by the community health nurse, and other healthcare providers and keeping each family healthy and the targets of health goal can be achieved.

Goals of Family Health Nursing Services

The goal of family health services is to achieve the highest level of Health for All the members of the family through health services. The major goals of these services include:

- To promote the health of the family and prevent diseases by developing self-reliance and ability to manage their own health problems both existing and anticipated but at the same time preserving family functioning.
- To reduce the maternal and infant mortality and morbidity rate.
- To provide family planning services and motivating for small family norms.
- To provide health education to the family to solve their health problems.
- To conserve and strengthen community services for the healthcare of the family and community.

Objectives of Family Health Nursing Services

The main objectives of family health nursing services are:

- To identify the health problems and health needs of each family by combining community health nursing efforts with other health workers.
- To ensure family's understanding and acceptance of these needs and problems.
- To provide need-based healthcare to each member of the family.
- To plan and provide health and nursing services with the active participation of family members.
- To help families develop the abilities and competence of each family member to deal with their health needs and health problems, and become independent in tackling the health situation.
- To contribute to the personal and social development of the family.
- To provide health education, guidance and counseling to family members to cultivate good health status, practice safe cultural practices and maintain congenial, physical, social, psychological and spiritual environment.
- To help families make use of promotive, preventive, therapeutic and rehabilitative health and allied facilities and services available in the community.

Principles of Family Health Nursing Services

- Community health nurses should maintain good working relations with the family to gain confidence and faith so that they cooperate in assessing the health needs and implementing the care.
- Family health nursing is a part of family healthcare services so the community health nurse should know the family healthcare policies, goals, objectives and the nature of family healthcare services as she needs to plan and provide family health nursing services with the active participation of family members.
- Family health nursing is family-focused. It is very important for the community health nurse to know about family composition, education, occupation, income, customs, tradition, environmental factors, health and medical history of family members.

- Family health nursing should be realistic in terms of resources available, so proper estimation of health needs, health problems and priorities in terms of money, material, manpower and time is required.
- Problems should be discussed with the family members. To find the solution to the problems, guidance to the family members should be provided to make them independent for making decision and taking action in healthcare.
- Cooperation of family members should be taken to implement desired plan of action.
- Health education, guidance and supervision are integral parts of family health nursing because these help the family to improve knowledge, develop competence, create interest and become self- dependent.
- Provide preventive, promotive and need-based support and services to the family to improve their health status.
- Continuous services are more effective. Community health nurse provides care not only when the family member is sick but also must provide continuous contact to promote and maintain health and prevent diseases.
- Proper health messages to be communicated to the family during every contact to help the family members take care of their health needs intelligently.
- Effective system of records and reports of family health nursing services should be maintained as it is an effective means of continuous care, evaluation and further planning.
- Periodic and continuous appraisal and evaluation should be done. Family is dynamic. It grows and develops with time and changes with place. Health needs and problems keep changing from time to time. These changes have to be assessed as the family grows and develops through various stages of development. This helps in meeting changing needs of the family.
- Family health nursing should be rendered to all families without any discrimination. Every family has a right to attain optimum health and an environment conducive to healthy living to lead a productive and useful life.

Setting of Family Health Nursing

Family health nursing can be rendered directly at family setting, i.e., home, clinic, school and workplace. Each setting has its own advantages, disadvantages and limitations. No one setting is complete by itself in fulfilling the objectives of family health nursing but all the settings are utilized according to the feasibility in some proportion to achieve the objectives.

FAMILY HEALTHCARE SERVICES

Family health services include maternal health, child health, family planning, immunization, nutrition, environmental sanitation and geriatric care. When these services are provided as integrated into a total package of family healthcare, family health is greatly improved and the mortality rate is reduced. For providing integrated family healthcare services "community health nurse has to plan carefully and exercise her leadership qualities as she has to procure active cooperation of all the members of the health team, i.e., male and female health workers, Traditional Birth Attendant (TBA), Accredited Social Health Activist (ASHA) and others".

The target of every member of health team is to "keep the family healthy". The areas of integrated family health services are as follows:

- Mother and child health
- Family planning
- Nutrition of the family
- Immunization services
- Family life, education of parents
- Care of the sick, aged and handicapped in the home
- Prevention and control of communicable diseases

FAMILY HEALTHCARE PLAN

Family health refers to the health status of members of the family, the problems affecting their health and the totality of healthcare provided to the family. Family health fluctuates from optimal health to illness or total disability under the influence of various factors from within the family and its environment and the community to which it belongs. Family health is an art and science of preventing disease and promoting health and efficiency through organized family efforts for the safe family environment by educating the family members on personal and environmental hygiene and seeking medical advice for early diagnosis and treatment of the health problem. Family health nursing is the synthesis of nursing care and healthcare. It helps to develop self-care abilities of the family to promote, protect and maintain health.

FAMILY HEALTH NURSING PROCESS

Family health nursing process is a series of planned steps and interventions directed to help families to develop and strengthen their capabilities to meet their healthcare needs and solve health problems. The family health nursing process is the same as that of the patient but here the focus is on the family and its environment. Family health nursing process is closely related to the community health nursing process. Family health nursing process is a problem-solving approach and is systematically planned to analyze health problems and finding their solutions, it is a tool that can be implemented at primary, secondary and tertiary levels of care. The main components of the family health nursing process are as follows:

- Family health nursing assessment
- Nursing diagnosis
- Planning
- Implementation
- Evaluation

These components are interdependent and many times overlap when the process is in action. During the assessment phase, certain situations may arise which require immediate intervention, e.g., a child with minor injuries or an adult with high fever. Similarly, when the planned care is implemented, there may be new emerging situations that need to be explored and assessed. These components or phases do not only overlap but also go on continuously.

Family Health Nursing Assessment

Family health nursing assessment is a continuous process that becomes more accurate as the knowledge of the people deepens. It provides baseline data for formulating family nursing diagnoses and family nursing care plans.

In fact, "Nursing assessment is a continuous, systematic, critical, orderly, analyzing and interpreting information about physical, psychological and social needs of a person, the nature of self-care deficit and other factors influencing condition and care".

Steps of Assessment Process

It includes:

1. Data collection of the family
2. Analyzing and interpretation of family data to identify family health needs and problems. Data is also analyzed to estimate the capability of the family to perform health tasks with respect to the identified health problem and needs.
3. **Aspects of collecting family data:** Data is collected on the following aspects:
   - **Family structure:** Number of family members, age, sex, marital status, type of the family and role and relationship.
   - **Family environment:** Type of houses, water supply, sanitation, kitchen, pet animals, excreta disposal, transportation, communication facilities, neighborhood and community.
   - **Socioeconomic and cultural factors:** Data regarding culture, religion, education, occupation, family income from all sources, dietary habits, leisure time activities, social relationship with community, belief and values about health, illness, health services, superstitions and attitude toward health.
   - **Family process:** Communication patterns, decision making and problem solving.
   - **Family coping:** Life changes, conflicts, family satisfaction.
   - **Support system:** Support groups, relatives, friends, financial institutions, nongovernmental organizations (NGOs).
   - **Family health status:** The past medical history and present illness, duration, physical health assessment, nutritional status, height, weight, vital signs, lifestyle assessment, i.e., sleep, rest, exercise, habits (drugs/alcohol/smoking) stress, recreational and diversional activities.
4. **Analysis and interpretation of the data:** It includes:
   - Analysis of the information gathered
   - Conclusion drawn from the data
   - Validating conclusions to determine their accuracy
   - While making a family health assessment, professional skill is required for:
     - Making judgment
     - Effective communication
     - Investigation and measurements
5. **Tools for family health assessment:**
   - Observation
   - Questionnaires (structured and nonstructured)
   - Conversation, discussion
   - Examination
   - Investigations
   - Anecdotal reports
   - Review of family health records

After data collection, all the gathered information is analyzed and interpreted for making the nursing diagnosis.

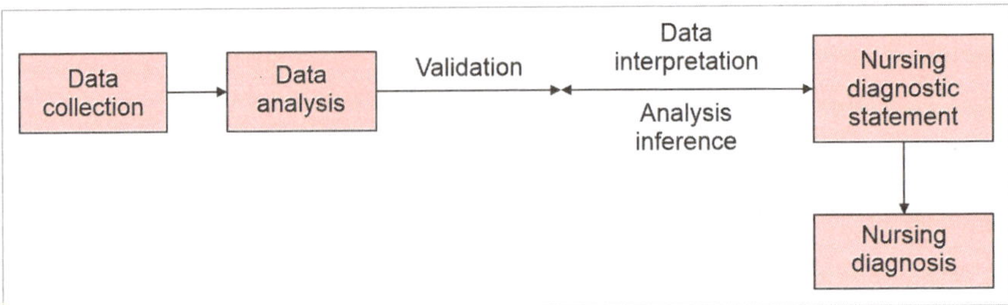

Fig. 5.1: Health assessment and nursing diagnosis

Nursing Diagnosis

Nursing diagnosis is the clinical judgment about a family's actual or potential health problems based upon the data obtained from family health assessment (Fig. 5.1). Nursing diagnosis should be clearly and concisely stated, for example:

- Knowledge deficit related to the complication of hypertension or diabetes mellitus
- Self-care deficit related to helpless individual
- Health-seeking behavior regarding immunization. Health assessment and nursing diagnosis is an ongoing process.

Steps in formulating nursing diagnosis:

1. Data analysis
2. Deriving conclusion
3. Formulating nursing diagnosis statement

Planning

Planning is a logical decision-making process desired for the purpose of intervention around the specific goals and objectives to resolve family's healthcare needs and problems based on the nursing diagnosis.

Steps in Planning

1. Listing health problems and needs in order of priority.
2. Formulating goals and objectives.
3. Selecting the best possible line of action among the available actions.
4. Selecting the appropriate nursing intervention.
5. Identifying appropriate nursing intervention.
6. Identifying appropriate resources for care.
7. Documenting the plan.

After listing the family problems, priorities are set on the basis of the following criteria:

- Family awareness of the problem.
- Motivation of family about problem solving.
- Ability of the nurse to influence the solution of the problem.
- Severity of the consequences (in case the problem remains unresolved).

- Time factor during which the resolution of the problems has to be achieved
- Type of family, high risk, moderate risk, low risk

After problem prioritization, objectives are set, nursing actions are planned and family nursing care is prepared.

Implementation

Implementation is the process of putting the formulated nursing care plan into action. It is the foundation of nursing practice. Implementation in the case of family health nursing care is not just nursing intervention but a collaborative action taken by the nurse and the family members. The primary goal of family health nursing service is to increase the capability of the family to help themselves toward the optimum level of health. To achieve the goal of family healthcare, the nurse must involve the family members in the deliberate process and encourage their sense of responsibility and autonomy.

The activities to be carried out while implementing family nursing care are as follows:

- Identify the required knowledge and skills to be developed by the family.
- Designate the responsibility for implementation. The person who is designated should have the knowledge and skills to implement the plan and care.
- The technical and complex part of the planned activities should be carried out by the nurse unless designated person has acquired the requisite knowledge and skill.
- Provide information, education and communication to the members who are involved in implementation of care plan.
- Provide comfortable environment for implementation, i.e., providing privacy, safety of the client, adequate rest period in between the activities, allow for physical and mental comfort. Allow verbal expression of clients' concerns related to cost, physical disability or sensory deficit, etc.
- Discuss the behavior of the family members that demonstrate functional and dysfunctional areas of coping.
- Provide compassionate support throughout the nurse-patient and nurse-family relationships.
- Emphasize the ways family members can contribute to the individual and family health.
- Carry out the planned activities:
  - Motivate and involve client/family member
  - Prepare the client to receive care and communicate with the client to build up trust and positive attitude
  - Monitor the action taken
  - Document the care implemented for family progress notes
  - Evaluate the care given against the stated objective
  - Modify the plan of care if necessary

Barriers in Implementation

- Poor planning
- Lack of resources (material, manpower and money)
- Lack of support from family, authorities and other agencies
- Family not understanding the importance of change in behavior

- **Sociocultural pattern:** Family culture might interfere in providing family healthcare. Nurse must study the cultural and social patterns to remove the barriers
    - Poor participation and cooperation of the family members
    - Families with multiple problems and disorganized families
- **Language:** The rural population may not understand language of the community health nurse so the nurse can involve local leaders within the community and help in making the people understand.

Evaluation

Evaluation is the process of measuring the extent to which goals and objectives of family care have been met. The effectiveness of implementation is ascertained by noting family response and examining the outcome by the following methods:

- **Direct observation:** Changes in the physical health status by using precision instruments, i.e., by use of clinical thermometers, BP instruments, stethoscopes, weighing machines.
- **Records:** By reviewing the records such as immunization reports, diagnostic lab tests.
- **Interview or questionnaire:** Behavior modification, broad and complex attitudes by interviewing or questionnaire method.

Evaluation can be done during the implementation phase, i.e., formative evolution, at the end of implementation phase, i.e., summative evaluation. Comprehensive evaluation cannot be made at each visit but the nurse should end each visit with clarification of goals for next visit. The result of evaluation, success or failure are utilized for further family health nursing process. In case of failure, future modification is done in strategies of nursing intervention.

FAMILY HEALTH SERVICES

Maternal Health Services

Maternal health services are one of the most important components of family health services. Mother is the foundation of the family. She has got vital role in the family function. The husband, children and other dependent members of the family are dependent on the mother. The mother performs the managerial services in the family. She prepares food, provides clean clothes, maintains a clean and comfortable home environment for resting, sleeping, working and provides emotional support in bringing up children in healthy culture and inculcating healthy habits. She is a backbone of the family, suppose if the mother falls sick, the family life gets disturbed. The maternal health is one of the priorities of the community health program and a part of primary healthcare.

Goals of Maternal Health Services

- To reduce the maternal morbidity and mortality rate
- To have 100% deliveries conducted by trained personnel

Components of Maternal Health Services

Antenatal care

Antenatal care is the care given to the expectant mother right from conception till the delivery of the baby.

- **Objectives of antenatal care:**
  - To ensure the birth of a mature, life and healthy baby to a healthy mother.
  - To promote, protect and maintain the health of mother throughout pregnancy.
  - To screen high-risk mothers and give appropriate treatment to prevent complications.
  - To reduce the maternal and neonatal mortality rate.
  - To detect and treat any abnormality found in pregnancy as early as possible.
  - To educate mother how to care for herself during pregnancy and prepare her for care of baby and early breastfeeding.
  - To sensitize the mother for small family norms.
- **Components of antenatal care:**
  - **Registration of pregnant women:** The pregnant mother should get registered as soon as she misses her period at health subcenter, primary health center, hospital or clinic. Thorough physical and obstetrical examination is done to screen risk factors.
  - **Antenatal visits:** Ideally the woman should visit antenatal clinic once a month during first 6 months, twice in a month during 7th and 8th months of pregnancy and once a week during the 9th month. But if not possible, then at least a minimum of three visits are must.
    - 1st visit during the first 20 weeks or earlier
    - 2nd visit at 32 weeks of pregnancy
    - 3rd visit at 36 weeks of pregnancy

    These visits are for normal pregnancy but in case of high-risk pregnancy or complications, more visits are required as guided by the obstetrician.

    Care during the first visit or contact includes:
    - **Health history:** Past medical history, obstetrical history, socioeconomic history, the personal biodata including last menstrual period are noted.
    - **Physical examination:** Height, weight, blood pressure, pulse, temperature, respiration and general examination from head to toe is made.
    - **General medical examination:** Systemic examination is done of all systems of the body.
    - **Obstetrical examination:** Includes examination of the breast to detect any abnormality.
    - **Abdominal examination:** Includes inspection, palpation and auscultation to assess the size of the uterus, palpate fetal parts and hear fetal heart sounds. Vaginal examination is done if necessary.
    - **Laboratory examination:** Blood grouping is done for both, i.e., pregnant woman and her husband to know the Rh factor. Serological tests are also done for the couple to rule out sexually transmitted diseases (STDs). For lady Hb%, total leukocyte count (TLC), differential leukocyte count (DLC), BT CT, blood sugar random, urine analysis and stool examination are done.
    - **During the subsequent visits:** Weight, blood pressure, abdominal examination, blood for Hb% and urine for albumin and sugar are done. After the completion of 3 months, iron and folic acid tablets are given to prevent anemia. All these examinations are entered in the registration card made during the first visit. Antenatal advice is given by the auxiliary nurse and midwife (ANM), health supervisors or doctor in the clinic.

- **Immunization against tetanus:** Injection of tetanus toxoid; two doses are given between 16 and 36 weeks of pregnancy at an interval of 1 month. The second dose should be given 1 month before expected date of delivery
- **Supplementary iron folic acid, Vitamin A and D:** During pregnancy, especially after mid- pregnancy, the growth of the fetus is fast as the fetus has to draw his requirements from maternal blood. Mothers are likely to be anemic if their diet is deficient in iron and folic acid. As preventive measure supplementary iron and folic acid tablets containing 60 mg of iron and 500 mcg folic acid one tablet twice in a day is given as preventive measure against anemia.
- **Health education** on personal hygiene, diet, rest, sleep, exercises, smoking, drinking, drugs, traveling and sexual activities.
- **Personal hygiene:** Advised to have daily bath, cleaning breast, nipples, private parts, wearing clean and comfortable clothes, for regular bowel habits and wearing flat shoes. Extra care of gums and teeth as bleeding gums during pregnancy is often noticed.
- **Diet:** The caloric requirement is increased, i.e., 300 kcal above the normal. Protein 2 g/kg body weight, extra iron, calcium and vitamin C are required, so food with high content of iron, folic acid, vitamin C and calcium is advised.
- **Rest and sleep:** She should have 8 hours of sleep during night and 2 hours of rest in bed during day to promote normal growth of the fetus.
- **Exercise and fresh air:** Antenatal exercises are advised and fresh air walk is recommended. Smoking and drinking are harmful to the growing fetus as it causes growth retardation. It should be avoided.
- **Drugs:** Pregnant women should not take any drug other than the one prescribed by the obstetrician or physician as some drugs may cause fetal abnormalities.
- **Traveling:** Traveling on a bike or other vehicles which causes jerky movements should be avoided as it can induce abortion or premature labor.
- Sexual activities should be avoided during the first trimester and the last 2 months of pregnancy.
- Lady is instructed to report immediately to health personnel if she experiences the following:
  - Swelling of feet, hands and face
  - Headache, dizziness and blurred vision
  - Not feeling the fetal movements
  - Bleeding from the vagina or pain in the abdomen.
- **Education regarding the care of newborn:** Advised about the care of baby, bath hygiene, breastfeeding, immunization, wearing clothes and care of minor disorders.
- **Follow-up visit:** Instructed to follow the schedule of visits and follow the instructions of the doctor.
- **Preparing for delivery:** The pregnant woman should be prepared about the process of normal labor as well as for the anticipated operative delivery, by explaining to her in simple language the need for hospital delivery. The psychosocial support to the lady and her family members is to be provided.
- **Family planning:** She is explained about spacing of children by contraceptive method if it is first pregnancy. If multigravida, she is motivated for family planning.

Intranatal Care

- Encouraging institutional delivery and preparing the place for delivery.
- Arranging the required equipment and sterilized supply for the delivery.
- Assessing the maternal and fetal parameters:
    - Providing psychological support.
    - Preparing the mother for labor.
    - Asserting presentation, position, level of presenting part, effacement of cervix and dilatation of OS and presence or absence of the membranes.
    - Checking the fetal heart sounds.
    - Noting the intensity and duration of uterine contractions and watching bladder for distension.
    - Recording general condition of the mother at the time of membranes ruptured.
    - Ensuring safe delivery by observing the principle of maintaining asepsis. Examining umbilical cord and noting abnormalities.
    - Taking the help of a doctor or referring if required. Taking care of newborn and mother after delivery. Noting Apgar score and correct time of birth of the baby.
    - Maintaining thorough asepsis during delivery.

Postnatal Care

Postnatal care is the care given to the mother after delivery for up to 6 weeks. It is the time starts immediately after the delivery of the placenta up to 6 weeks during which the genital organs return to their pregravid state.

- **Objectives of postnatal care:**
    - To restore, promote and maintain the health of the mother and baby.
    - To prevent complications.
    - To promote breastfeeding and establish good nutrition for the baby.
    - To prevent infection.
    - To support and strengthen the confidence of the mother to take care of herself and the baby.
    - To educate mother and family on various aspects of mother and child care.
    - To motivate for small family norms.
- **Postnatal care requirements:**
    - Check the vital parameters of the mother immediately after delivery and then half hourly up to 2 hours.
    - Watch for bleeding from vagina.
    - Inspect the perineum for any tear or laceration.
    - The uterus should be well contracted, if not contracted, make it to contract by massaging gently.
    - Watch for bladder distension. If present, encourage the mother to pass urine. If she is not able to pass catheterize the bladder.
    - Maintain temperature by applying warmth as the lady may feel cold or shivering as she has lost so much heat from the body, i.e., amniotic fluid lost, placenta and baby out.
    - Give some stimulating drinks like coffee or tea. Food should be given after shifting from labor room.
    - Daily care of the mother includes nutrition, personal hygiene, postnatal exercises.

- Perineal care has to be given when she goes to toilet. She is educated to clean perineum with antiseptic lotion, dry it and apply sterile pad.
- Color and quantity of lochia to be observed.
- Breast care: She should start breastfeed as soon as she is able to sit.
- Watch for breast engorgement, cracked or inverted nipples and treat accordingly.
- Watch and protect from postpartum hemorrhage, urinary incontinence, urinary retention, thrombophlebitis and puerperal sepsis.
- Protect from postpartum psychosis.
- Record fundal height and check the involution of the uterus.
- During postnatal period, the health worker should make 3 visits. 1st after 12 hours of delivery, 2nd visit within 3–4 days and 3rd visit on 5th day of delivery. Visits can be increased depending upon the requirement. The 4th visit in 7–10 days. After 6 weeks she should attend the postnatal clinic.
- Counsel the mother for family planning
- Maintain proper records

Neonatal Care

Immediate care of the baby after delivery is to help the newborn baby to adjust to a new environment.

- **Objectives of neonatal care**:
  - To establish clear airway and maintain respiration.
  - To maintain body temperature by maintaining adequate room temperature and keeping baby warm.
  - To prevent infection.
  - To detect any congenital anomalies.
- **Neonatal care requirements:**
  - Identify the baby
  - Clean the eyes with wet saline swabs
  - Keep the airway clear by cleaning the mouth with wet gauze or by gentle suctioning or with mucus sucker
  - Maintain body temperature by wrapping the baby in blanket and keeping the room temperature adequate
  - Assess the physical condition of the body by noting the APGAR score
  - Resuscitate if the APGAR score is low
  - Watch for visible congenital anomalies
  - Give injection of vitamin K 1 mg, intramuscularly (IM)
  - Record birth weight
    - Help the mother to give breastfeed to the baby
    - Observe the cry, watch for urination and meconium, sleep and feeding pattern of newborn and give care accordingly

Child Care Services

Child care refers to the care of children from inception to birth and after birth till the age of 5 years. Child health services are part of maternal health services and are an important component of family health services. Children below the age of 15 years constitute 40% of the Indian population.

Their health is very important as they are the future of the country. According to the belief of economists, "safe life of a child is the investment of the future". According to WHO, 15 lakh children die before attaining the age of 1 month in developing countries, the infant mortality rate is very high. So, by paying attention to the health of the children, the country/nation can imagine strong and pleasant future for the country.

- **Importance of child care in India can be explained from the following facts:**
  - The infant mortality rate in India was estimated at 57/1000 live births by National Family Health Survey (NFHS) III (2006) and 55/1000 live births Ministry of Health and Family Welfare (MoHFW, 2008–2009). It is very high compared to USA 6.3/1000 and Japan 3–2/1000 live births.
  - 15.42% of children below age of 6 years according to *Census* 2001.
  - 40% of children of Indian population are under the age of 15 years.
  - 30% of school-going children are suffering from malnutrition.
  - Rural areas have insufficient infant and child health services.
  - Under-5 mortality rate in India is very high. It is about 1/4 of the total under five year deaths in the world.
- **Causes of under-5 mortality by age group in India:**
  - Neonatal death from birth up to 28 days due to premature birth
  - Birth asphyxia
  - Difficult delivery and instrumental deliveries causing birth injuries
  - Hypothermia, starvation
  - Respiratory distress syndrome (RDS), ARI, neonatal tetanus, diarrhea, sepsis, etc.
- **Infant death from 1 to 12 months of age:**
  - Infections, diarrheal diseases, measles, whooping cough, ARI and malnutrition.
- **1 year to 5 years:**
  - Malnutrition, accidents, injuries, diarrhea, respiratory tract, infections, measles.

Objectives

- To reduce the infant and child mortality rate.
- To educate mothers and family members to give proper care to their children.
- To provide nutritious diet to the children.
- To establish the overall growth of the children by proper care and nourishment.
- Special efforts to preserve and promote the health of children below 5 years of age.
- Every child is immunized and protected from diseases.
- Early detection of ailments and defects, and appropriate treatment to prevent them from getting worse.
- To increase the health level of children through school health services and other programs.

Responsibility of Community Health Nurses toward Child Healthcare

- **Child health services are included in family health services.** It is the responsibility of the community health nurse to provide good environment and appropriate facilities for children. By guiding the family and community, and providing assistance and education on child care, the child health can be attained to optimum level. Prenatal, antenatal, intranatal, postnatal care are already discussed under maternal care. The major responsibility of community health nurses regarding immediate care of the newborn are:

- Clear airway.
- Establishing respiration.
- Maintenance of temperature by keeping baby warm by wrapping in the blanket.
- Prevention from infections by using aseptic technique while clamping and cutting the cord, no dressing has to be applied on the cord.
- Vernix caseosa is a protective covering, so should not be removed. Only change the baby sheet if it gets wet.
- Cleaning the baby's eyes with sterile saline.
- Watching for congenital anomalies, record weight, height and head circumference of the baby.
- Calling the physician if required in case of emergency.
- Early initiation of breastfeeding. As soon as the mother recovers from the stress and strain of labor, she should be encouraged and helped to feed the baby.

- **Care of the nutritional status:** Exclusive breastfeed should be encouraged for 6 months. A normal newborn baby requires 170 mL/kg body weight of milk with nutritious value of 120 kcal/kg body weight till 6 months of age. An average Indian mother can secrete 450–600 mL of milk per day which is sufficient for 6 months for baby. After that supplementary foods are started and then, gradually baby is weaned off from breast milk.
- **Immunization:** Community health nurse is responsible for immunization of children according to the National Immunization Program. This will protect the child from tetanus, diphtheria, whooping cough, tuberculosis, measles and poliomyelitis.
- **Assessment of growth and development:** Community health nurse should have the knowledge of growth and development of the child, weight, height and milestone should be measured according to the standard.
- **Prevention and treatment of common childhood accidents:** Once the children start crawling and walking, they are very prone to accidents like putting their finger in exposed electric sockets, opening the covers of the medicine bottles and drinking them. Any poisonous medicine or kerosene oil, etc. if kept within their reach, they are liable to drink. Parents should be educated to keep such things away from the reach of children. They may fall from staircase or sometimes from roof, they can go near the fire. All such things, hot milk, tea, water, and burning stoves should be kept out of reach of the children.
- **Educational functions:** Community health nurses should provide education to the parents regarding:
  - Education of mother about the benefits of breastfeeding, supplementary foods and weaning
  - About immunization of children
  - About personal and environmental hygiene
  - Encouraging them to attend under five clinics for children's health checkup and to know the growth and development of children
  - Educating them from prevention of infectious diseases and accidents
  - Making them aware of legal rights of children
  - Helping in the research work related to causes and treatment of child delinquency

- **Other functions of community health nurse toward child care:**
  - Providing remedies to check diarrhea, vomiting and dehydration.
  - **Conducting clinics:** Under five clinics, child guidance clinics and well-baby clinics.
  - Contacting various health organizations regarding child health, getting training about child health to update her knowledge and take their help to implement the latest child health plans.
  - Arranging rehabilitation services for disabled children.
  - Making the community aware of the prevention of child labor.
  - Helping in health checkups of children in orphanages and crèches.
  - Participating in school health programs such as, integrated management of neonatal and childhood illness (IMNCI), home based newborn care (HBNC) and Child Health Clinic Program.

Integrated Management of Neonatal and Childhood Illness (IMNCI)

Integrated Management of Childhood Illness (IMCI) was developed by WHO in collaboration with United Nations Children's Fund (UNICEF) and many other agencies working in the field of child care. IMCI aims to prevent and manage five major childhood diseases, i.e., ARI, diarrhea, measles, malaria and malnutrition. The main focus of the IMCI is on preventive, promotive and curative aspects. IMCI strategy is implemented in >100 countries in the world.

The IMNCI is the Indian version of IMCI. To introduce IMCI in India a core group was constituted. This group developed the Indian version of IMCI guideline and renamed as IMNCI.

The IMCI includes case management charts from 1 week to 2 months, from 2 months to 5 years of age. But in IMNCI, it includes 0–7 days' care of newborn neonates along with childhood illness.

Concept and Needs

Every year >10 million children die in developing countries before the age of 5 years. Most of the deaths are due to ARI, diarrhea, measles, malaria and malnutrition. So, an integrated approach was required to manage the sick children and to reduce the child mortality rate. So, WHO responded to the challenge and developed a strategy like IMCI and in India called, IMNCI. The major reason for developing IMNCI was curative care but it also covers nutrition, immunization and other important aspects of disease prevention and health promotion.

Objectives

- To reduce the mortality rate in children.
- To bring down the frequency of illness.
- To reduce the severity of illness and disability.
- To contribute to improvement of growth and development of children.

Components

The main components of the strategy are as follows:
- To strengthen the skills of the healthcare workers.
- To strengthen the healthcare infrastructure.
- To involve the community.

Principles of IMNCI Guidelines

- All sick young infants up to 2 months of age must be assessed for possible bacterial infection or jaundice. They must be assessed for major symptoms of diarrhea.
- All sick children from the age of 2 months to 5 years must be examined for dangerous signs that indicate immediate referral or admission to hospital. They must be routinely assessed for cough, difficult breathing, diarrhea, fever or ear problems.
- All sick young infants and children from age of 2 months to 5 years must be routinely assessed for nutritional and immunization status, feeding and other potential problems.
- Only a limited number of carefully selected signs are used based on evidence of their sensitivity and specificity to detect disease.
- The diagnosed children are classified for the specific action as:
  - They should be urgently referred to a higher level of care
  - They require specific treatment such as antibiotic or antimalarial
  - May be safely managed at home
  - The classifications are color-coded:
    Pink   — indicates urgent referral or hospital admission
    Yellow — indicates initiation of specific treatment
    Green — calls for home management
- IMNCI guideline does not describe the management of trauma or other acute emergencies due to accidental injuries.
- IMNCI management uses a limited number of procedures and encourages active participation of caretaker.
- An essential component of IMNCI guidelines in the counseling of caretakers about home care, feeding, fluids and when to return to a health facility.

Elements of Case Management

The case management of a sick child brought to the first-level health facility includes the following steps:

1. **Outpatient health facility (OPD cases)**
   - Assessment
   - Classification and identification of treatment
   - Referral, treatment or counseling of child's caretaker
   - Follow-up care
2. **Referral health facility**
   - Emergency triage assessment and treatment
   - Diagnosis, treatment and monitoring the patient's progress
3. **Appropriate home management:** Teaching mothers how to give oral drugs or treat local infections at home. Counsel mothers and other caretakers regarding feeding, fluids and when to return to the health facility.
4. **Child clinics:** Under five clinics and child guidance clinics are discussed in unit 6.

Family Welfare Services

Family welfare services include not only family planning services but the total package of health services to the family. Family welfare services are aimed at providing services to control and plan family size as well as complete healthcare of the family keeping in view the limited resources of the country and extensive population. The family welfare is given at the top most priority. The quality of health of the people and goal of Health for All is to be achieved through family welfare services.

Family welfare services are integrated package of services provided to the family to promote and maintain the health of the families. These services include:

- Maternal and child health services
- Family planning
- Family life education of parents
- Nutrition of the family
- Immunization services
- Healthful environment in the home
- Care of the sick, aged and handicapped in home
- Prevention and control of communicable diseases

Maternal and child health services are already discussed in this chapter.

Family Planning Services

For family welfare services, family planning is the most important component. Family planning is the voluntary planning regarding childbirth by a couple, i.e., childbirth should be according to their choice and not by chance or in other words, "planning for responsible parenthood" is called family planning. By controlling birth through family planning, the size of the family can be limited and population growth can be controlled. The objectives of family welfare can be achieved through family planning.

Family planning is defined as to limiting the size of the family and having spacing between the children and children according to the desire of the couple by adopting the methods of family planning. Family planning also includes the treatment of couples who do not have children so that they can also have children by treating the cause of infertility.

Infertility

Infertility is the inability of a couple to produce a child. It may be due to abnormality in male or female or both.

Causes of infertility:

- Abnormality of the reproductive system
- Immature sex organs
- Hormonal imbalance
- Psychological problems
- Malnutrition
- Excessive use of alcohol or tobacco

Management of infertility:

- Provide psychological support to the couple
- Identify the cause
- Investigation of the cause
- Appropriate treatment intervention, i.e., treatment of associated medical and surgical condition
- Proper referral system

Importance of Family Planning

Family planning is considered one of the basic human rights for a better quality of life. It is the woman who undergoes stressed life of pregnancy, labor and bearing the child. The small family norms and spacing help the woman gain greater freedom and equality. For the development of any nation, women's empowerment is essential. To empower women, women's education and employment are required to fight against poverty and solving economic problems. If both parents are working, they can have better social status and can give better education to one or two children rather than having more children. So, law and order, political system and economic development can be ensured only through family planning and by spacing childbirth, limiting the size of the family, women can contribute toward employment and raise the social and economic status of the country.

Objectives of Family Planning

- To plan pregnancy according to the choice.
- To avoid unwanted births.
- To limit the size of the family.
- To keep spacing between the pregnancies.

Goals of Family Planning

There are two main goals of family planning:
1. **Operational goals:**
   - To promote the voluntary acceptance of small family norms.
   - To motivate people to adopt the use of spacing methods to control the interval between pregnancies.
   - To ensure easy availability of contraceptives to all eligible couples.
   - To arrange the medical and surgical services to achieve demographic targets.

   Some other programs are also included in the family planning programs, like:
   - Child survival.
   - Status of women.
   - Employment.
   - Female literacy and education.
   - Poverty eradication.
   - Socioeconomic growth program.
   - Reproductive and child healthcare program.
2. **Demographic goals**: These are part of national population policy and continue to change with a change in the policy.

Scope of Family Planning

According to the expert committee of WHO, family planning includes the following subjects:
- Proper spacing between children
- Limited the number of births
- Premarital counseling
- Pregnancy test

- Providing services to unmarried mothers
- Preparing for the first birth
- Educating about nutrition and finances
- Sex education
- Genetic counseling
- Education about parenthood
- Marital guidance
- Adoption services

Aspects of Family Planning

Many aspects of life are affected by family planning. It affects the health services and controls the population. Some of the aspects of family planning are as follows:

Health aspects:

- **Health of women:** Pregnancy affects the health status of women. Anemia, pregnancy-induced hypertension, eclampsia, antepartum hemorrhage (APH), postpartum hemorrhage (PPH) and other abnormal conditions of pregnancy are dangerous to mothers. Maternal mortality and morbidity can be reduced to great extent by the use of family planning services. Mothers can be protected from many health problems by reducing the number of pregnancies and by spacing between the pregnancies and children can be protected from many congenital disabilities.
- **Health of children:** Planned pregnancy is important for better growth and development of the child. The health of the child is looked after right from intrauterine life. Children get better nourishment in small families resulting in better physical and mental development. Possibility of childhood diseases and communicable diseases is also reduced.

Economic aspects

The philosophy of a small family, a happy family explains the economic attitude of this program. Parents can look after and provide better education to one or two children. So the growth of individuals, community and economy of the nation can be achieved through the success of family planning.

Social aspects

Better economy of the country results in better social status, i.e., good education, good standards of living and proper nutrition are the bases of a good society and a strong nation. The social discrepancies are also narrowed down and personality of the individuals develops due to growing awareness. Marital relations become stronger and mental health improves.

Political aspects

Family planning affects the density of population. Success in family planning may bring improvement in the resources and qualitative change in the political system thus bringing transformation in the social, cultural, educational, economic and political perspective of individuals as well as countries.

Methods of Family Planning

- **Temporary methods** used for keeping spacing between the children include:
  - Barrier methods
    - Physical
    - Chemical
    - Combined

- Intrauterine devices (IUDs)
- Hormonal methods
- Postcoital *contraceptive* methods
- Miscellaneous
- **Terminal methods:** These are surgical methods and are employed only after the completion of the family. These are as follows:
  - Male sterilization, i.e., vasectomy
  - Female sterilization, i.e., tubectomy

Temporary methods

Barrier methods

- **Physical methods:**
  - **Condom:** It is an effective and most widely used device by the male without any side effects. In addition to preventing pregnancy, condom protects both males and females from sexually transmitted diseases (STDs). Failure rate 2–3%.

    Advantages of condom:
    - Easily available
    - Inexpensive and safe
    - Easy to use
    - No side effects
    - Protects not only against pregnancy but also against sexually transmitted diseases (STDs)
    - Light, compact and disposable.

    Disadvantage of condom: May slip off or tear during coitus due to incorrect use.

    - **Female condom:** It is a pouch made up of polyurethane with an internal ring which covers the cervix and an external ring which remains outside the vagina. It is prelubricated with silicone and spermicidal is not required. It is an effective barrier to STD infection. Due to high cost and failure rate of 5%, it is not used.
    - **Diaphragm:** It is a shallow cup made of synthetic rubber or plastic material in 5–10 cm of diameter. It has got flexible rim made of spring or metal. It is given to the woman according to the size. It is held in position partly by the spring tension and partly by vaginal muscle tone.

      A spermicidal jelly is used along with it. It is inserted into the vagina before sexual intercourse and remains in place for 6 hours after intercourse. Its side effects are nil but failure rate is 6–12%.
    - **Vaginal sponge:** It is a small polyurethane foam sponge measuring 5 × 2.5 cm saturated with spermicidal nonoxynol-9. It is less effective than diaphragm and failure rate is also high.

- **Chemical methods:** These are the chemical contraceptives which are placed in the vagina. The chemicals present in the devices destroy sperms. There are four categories of chemical devices:
  - i. Foam tablets and foam aerosols
  - ii. Creams, jellies and pastes
  - iii. Suppositories—inserted manually
  - iv. Soluble films

  Advantages: These were used before intrauterine devices (IUDS) and oral pills were invented. Nowadays, their use is only recommended with condoms for the sake of extra protection.

Disadvantages:

- Produce irritation and burning in the vagina
- Failure rate is high
- These are to be highly placed in the vagina.

- **Combined methods:**
    - **Combined devices:** Using chemical contraceptives along with condoms are known as combined devices. It provides double protection against pregnancy.
- **Intrauterine devices:** Intrauterine devices are devices which is when placed in the uterus provides protection against pregnancy. It is available in two groups:
  1. Nonmedicated, i.e., Lippes loop (Fig. 5.2)
  2. Medicated, i.e., Copper T (Fig. 5.3)
     - **Lippes loop:** It is made up of polyethylene and has the shape of a double S. It has a nylon thread attached to it which lies in the vagina and helps in pulling out the loop. It is available in four sizes A, B, C and D. It is nontoxic, reliable and stable. It may cause perforation of the uterus. It contains some amount of barium due to which it can be spotted on X-rays. Nowadays, it is not used.
     - **Copper T:** Copper reduces the fertility of a woman. Many types of copper T are made available with different amounts of copper in each type. It is available in the following types:

Copper T-200	ML Cu-250
TCu-380 A	ML Cu-375 and 250
TCu-220 C	
Nova T	

- **Insertion of IUCD:** Copper T should be inserted within 10 days of beginning of menstruation or 6–8 weeks after delivery.

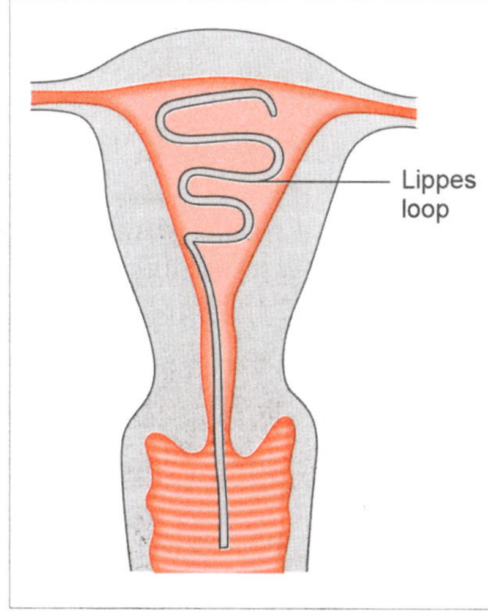

Fig. 5.2: Lippes loop

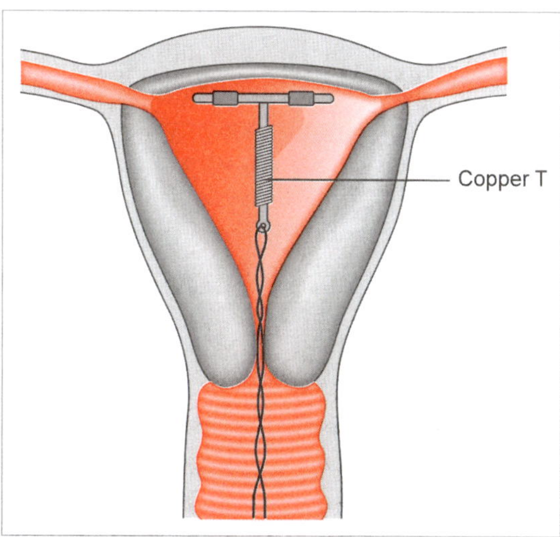

Fig. 5.3: Copper T

Advantages:
- An effective contraceptive
- Fertility can be restored after removal of copper T
- Inexpensive and easy to use
- Does not require continuous supervision
- Can be used up to 10 years
- Free from any harmful effects

Disadvantages:
- Pain and bleeding
- Ectopic pregnancy
- Spontaneous expulsion may take place
- Infection of pelvis
- Perforation of uterus.

- **Multiload 375 (Fig. 5.4):** This is a new Cu-T device used to prevent pregnancy.

Hormonal Methods

These are effective means of maintaining intervals between births. These are available in various combinations.

- **Mixed pills:**
  - Mala N, i.e., norethisterone acetate + ethinyl estradiol
  - Mala D, i.e., D-norgestrel + ethinyl estradiol.
- **Minipill:** This contains only progesterone. It should be taken throughout the menstrual cycle. It is not much popular because of high failure rate.
- **Mixed pills** are taken orally from the 5th day of menstrual cycle to the 21st day continuously, after that there is a break of 7 days during which the cycle begins again. It should be taken regularly. The day bleeding starts, is considered the 1st day of menstruation cycle. In case of no bleeding the day after 7th day should be considered the first day and course of pills should start again. Generally, menstrual cycle begins at the end of second course.

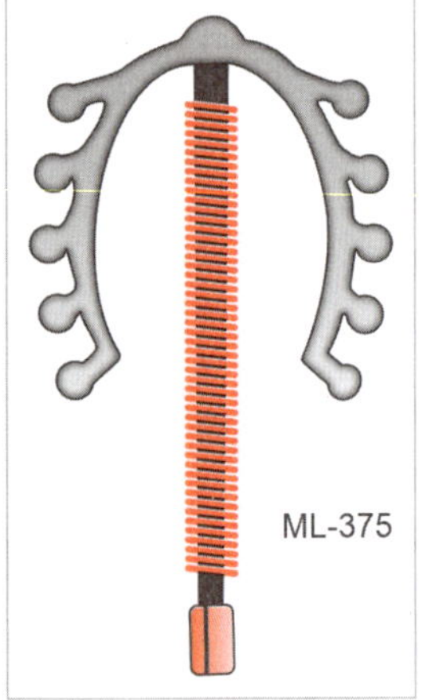

Fig. 5.4: Multiload

- **Postcoitus contraceptive pills:** These should be taken within 48 hours of unsafe coitus. Two mixed pills are advised to be taken immediately after unsafe coitus. These have less harmful effects than estrogen pills.
- **Male pills:** Safe male contraceptive pills have not yet been invented.
- **Nonsteroidal weekly oral *contraceptive* pill:** This pill is famous by the brand name "Saheli". It is free from side effects of nausea, vomiting, weight gain, dizziness, etc. The pill named "centchroman" and is to be taken once in a week.
- **Long acting/once-in-a-month pill:** In this, long-acting estrogen and short-acting progesterone are mixed. It is to be taken once-in–a-month. Its failure rate is high and has harmful effects. It is not used nowadays.
- **Emergency contraceptive pill (ECP) or E-pill:** It is used to prevent pregnancy in case of unprotected sexual intercourse. The pack consists of 2 pills. One is to be taken before 72 hours after unprotected sexual intercourse and the second one is taken 12 hours after the

first pill. The minor side effects include headache, nausea, vomiting and fatigue. It should not be taken as a regular contraceptive.

Advantages:

- Easy to use
- Inexpensive and easily available
- High rate of safety
- Regularity in menstrual cycle and reduction in breast disease.

Disadvantages:

- Cannot be used in case of heart disease.
- Metabolic effects may result into weight gain, high blood pressure, clotting of blood and heart failure, etc.
- Not suitable for women above 40 years of age.
- May result in tenderness in breast, uneasiness, pain, headaches and irregularity of bleeding.
- Other problems like liver disease, reduced lactation and ectopic pregnancy may arise.

- **Postcoital contraceptive methods**
  - **Menstrual regulation:** In this method, suction and evacuation of the uterine content is done within 6–14 days of stopping the cycle.
  - **Medical termination of pregnancy (MTP):** MTP is performed before the fetus is viable. According to the Termination of Pregnancy Act 1971, with the objective of reducing maternal mortality rate.

- **Miscellaneous methods:** This includes the following ways:
  - Abstinence
  - Coitus interruptus
  - Breastfeeding
  - Birth control vaccines
  - Safe period

Terminal Methods/Permanent Methods

- **Vasectomy:** It is the technique of male sterilization. A simple operation is performed under local anesthesia. In this method, both the vas deferens are cut 1 cm each and clamped and their heads are tied in a manner that they cannot unite again (Fig. 5.5).

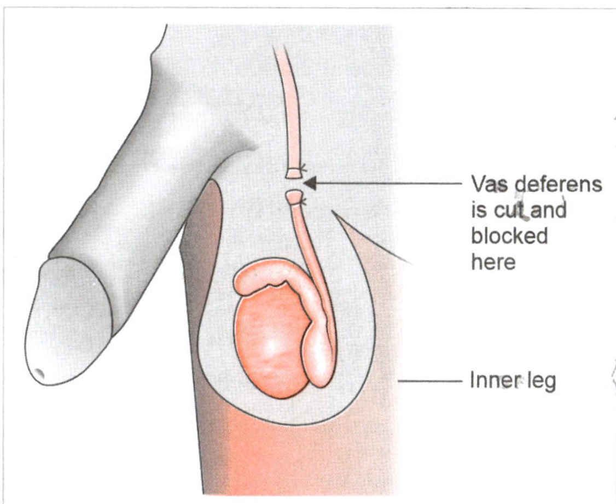

Fig. 5.5: Vasectomy

- **No scalpel vasectomy (NSV):** It is the latest and most popular technique of male sterilization.
  Advantages:
  - No side effects of hormones.
  - Cheaper and simpler than tubectomy.
  - No hospitalization is required as it is an outpatient department (OPD) procedure.
  - Recanalization is possible.
  - Permanent, safe and inexpensive technique.
  - Does not interfere with sexual pleasure.

  Disadvantages:
  - Local infection
  - Hematoma in the scrotum
  - Pain
  - Impotency, headache, uneasiness if a person is not properly convinced.

- **Tubectomy:** It is a permanent method of female sterilization. There are three types of tubectomy (Fig. 5.6):
  1. **Abdominal tubectomy:** Done under general anesthesia (GA) or spinal anesthesia. A lower abdominal incision is made, a part of fallopian tube is cut and clamped again, and abdomen is closed in layers. It works as blocking the path of ovum.
  2. **Minilap:** Minor form of abdominal tubectomy in which 2.5–3 cm incision is made on the abdomen under local anesthesia. A part of fallopian tube is cut and clamped. Safe technique and minimum complications. A good technique for postpartum sterilization.
  3. **Laparoscopy:** Using a laparoscope through abdomen, fallopian tubes are located and blocked by falope ring or rubber ring so that ovum cannot reach the uterus. Before inserting laparoscope, abdomen is expanded by using air or carbon dioxide. Incision is very small and few hours stay is required in hospital. It is done after 6 weeks of delivery. Lady should not have diabetes, respiratory disease or anemia.

     Advantages:
     - Minimum complication
     - Less expensive
     - 100% safe against pregnancy
     - Whole process completed in one attempt.

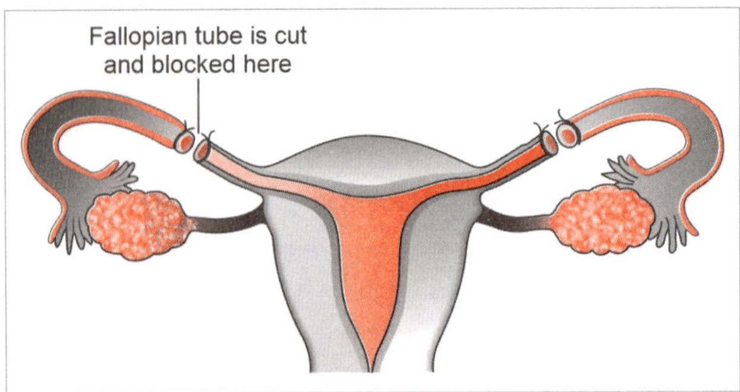

Fig. 5.6: Tubectomy

ROLE OF COMMUNITY HEALTH NURSE IN FAMILY HEALTH SERVICES

The role of a community health nurse in family health services is vast and varied (Fig. 5.7). She plays different roles in different settings of family health services. Some of her roles are described as under:

Survey work:

- Collect demographic facts.
- Make a list of the number of houses and find out their location.
- Collect information about pregnant mothers, eligible couples, contraceptive users, children and infants below the school-going age.
- Classify couples into low, medium and high priority groups. Review couples not using and using contraceptive to plan further action.

Health educator:

- Educates the individuals family and community regarding the prevention of communicable diseases.
- Teaches about nutrition and a balanced diet.

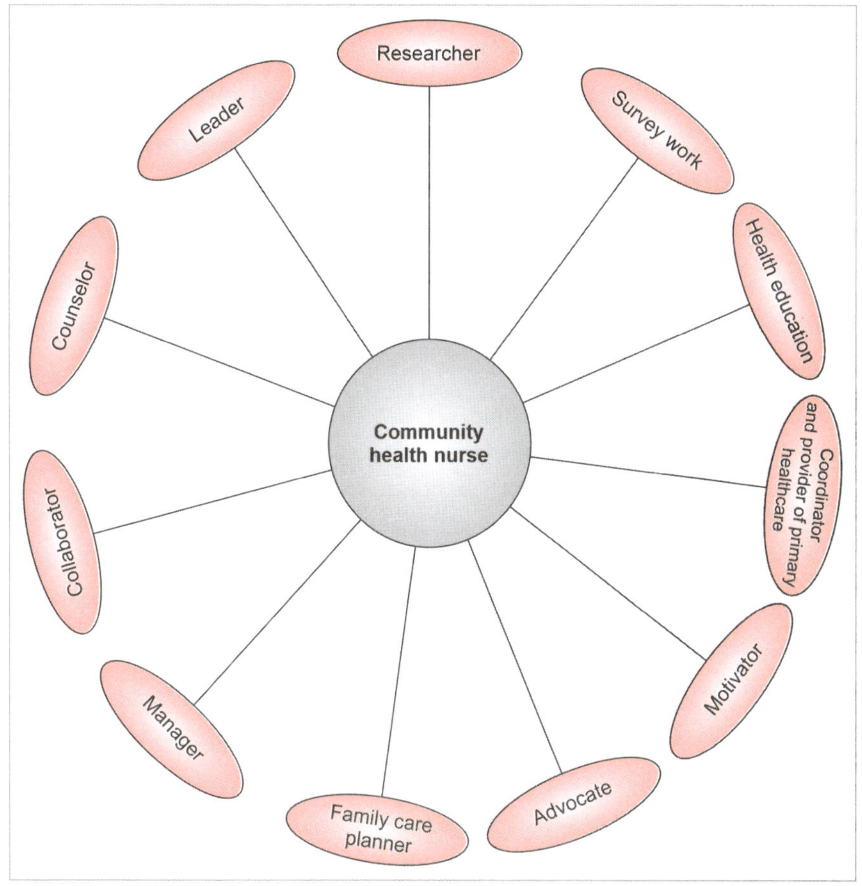

Fig. 5.7: Role of community health nurse in family health services

- Teaches the families about personal and environmental hygiene.
- Teaches mother about importance of breastfeeding and immunization of the child.
- Teaches families about first aid care and emergency management in case of snake bite, dog bite, etc.

Coordinator and provider of primary healthcare services:
- Provides direct care to the families within the legal and professional limits as per the standing orders of the state government and state's rules and regulations.
- Updates knowledge through conferences, seminars and attending short courses.
- Coordinates the services of physician, surgeon, dentist, nutritionist, social worker, Ayurveda, Yoga, Naturopathy, Unani, Siddha and Homoeopathy, abbreviated (AYUSH) and other specialists to meet family needs.

Motivator:
- Motivate the eligible couples about the use of contraceptive and adopting small family norms.
- Explain the importance and necessity of family planning.
- Identifying women needing MTP and referring them to the doctor.

Advocate for the family:
- Pleads and leads for the installation of facilities of healthcare in situ and required places.
- Encourages the implementation of laws and policies of environmental protection.
- Participates in the district government meeting and talks to administration in favor of folks for solution to the healthcare, social and financial problems available in her constituency.

Family care planner:
Nurse prepares the plan for health team as an integrated team approach is needed for better health of the family. She also plays a role in planning care in family health management.

Managerial:
- **Conducting clinics:**
  - Deciding the date and place of clinics
  - Arranging equipment and supplies and other resource of clinics
  - Supervising and guiding multipurpose health workers at clinics
  - Arranging and distributing contraceptives, and insertion and removal of IUDS
  - Assisting medical officers in conducting clinics
  - Organizing family planning camps and assisting the doctors in cases of operations, i.e., male and female sterilization operations
  - Following the aseptic technique during operation
  - Providing follow-up services for those couples who have accepted family planning methods.
  - Plans, conducts and evaluates health education programs.

Consultant:
Being a coordinator and direct care provider in family health services, advice is taken from her before starting any healthcare program in the community.

Collaborator:

- Community health nurse works in collaboration with other health teachers of government or nongovernmental organizations (NGOs) in community.
- She works with doctors, dispensers, vaccinators, TBA, midwives and lady health visitors (LHVs) in the community.

Counselor:

The community health nurse conducts the counseling of individuals, families and communities on various health and social problems.

Leadership and evaluator:

- The community health nurse after implementation of any project on health program, evaluates the success or outcome of the project.
- She evaluates the effectiveness of any program, drug, teaching, or vaccination in the community.

Researcher:

- Community health nurse finds the social and economic problems in the community that hinder care and cure.
- She searches for the causes of illness.
- She works hard for searching new methods of care and application of new principles of community health nursing.

FAMILY HEALTH RECORDS

Family health records are the written documents which provide information relevant to the health status of the members of the family. These are the important tools for the total healthcare of the family. Family health records are the important administrative and family guidance tool if written correctly and comprehensively contribute to the total care of the family. These records communicate specific information about the family's healthcare so that all interventions are directed toward the same goal. From the family records, the health workers can make out about family risk factors, illness or health behavior of the family members, an account of the services provided and guidance for future planning. Records should be written in scientific, informative and legally protective in nature.

Purposes of Family Health Records

- To make plan for family health services by providing baseline data.
- To improve the family healthcare services by providing facts about the rendered care.
- To provide data about the existing and potential health problems of the family.
- To document the services provided to the family.
- To provide data for nursing and other research work.
- To serve as a tool of communication between the health team members and other healthcare agencies.
- To provide facts about the assessment of the health status of family members and to evaluate family healthcare services.

Types of Family Health Records

The types of family health records are:
- Family folder
- Individual health cards
- Cumulative records or continuous records
- Process recording
- Registers

Family Folder

Family folder is used to maintain health records of all family members. It provides complete health history of the family. The information included in the family folder is as follows:

- **Identification:** Data of the family, age, education, occupation, gender, relation with each other and head of the family are included.
- **Structural deficit:** Information about widow/widower, old aged members and handicapped or mentally retarded child.
- **Nutrition status:** Nutrition status of the family along with information regarding nutritional deficiency and disorder.
- **Immunization:** Immunization status of children.
- Socioeconomic and cultural aspects of the family.
- Past medical history.
- Present health problems, need and immediate care.
- Details about contraceptives and family planning operation.
- **Environmental factors** such as surrounding environment.
- **Housing conditions:** Type, number of rooms, kitchen, storage, facilities.
- **Sanitation water:** Tap water or hand pump.
- **Health history** of each individual.

Individual Health Card

Individual health card is used to maintain the health of an individual. It provides complete health history of the individual. It provides information about age, education, sex, occupation, health status of the individual, past medical history, present health problems which need immediate care, immunization status, etc.

- **Types of individual cards:**
  - **Child health card:** The growth, development health history, immunization and general health status of under five children in the family and care given is noted.
  - **Maternity card:** It includes obstetric history, antenatal, natal or postnatal care given to the mother is recorded.
  - **Eligible couple card:** It is made for all married women of reproductive age to write menstrual history, use of contraceptives and records of guidance for infertile couple.

- **Medical card:** For any sick person in the family regarding the disease treatment started, follow up and termination of treatment, for example, tuberculosis patient.
- **Geriatric card:** This is used to record the health status and health problems, and care provided to the elderly members in the family.

Cumulative Records

The records which are maintained and continued for a longer period are called cumulative records. These are more useful, economical and time saving for the longer care of the family members. For example, the cumulative records of pregnant women begin from conception and cover antenatal, natal and postnatal care. Similarly, child health records are started from birth of the child to preschool period. Other examples, are HIV-infected family member records, old aged person records, diabetes, mellitus, tuberculosis patient's records. Cumulative records can be kept in family folder or a family diary, booklet or individual record of the family members. These are:

- Economical
- Time saving
- Used for longer period

Process Recording

Process recording is an event writing and is the written account of a situation. It includes nurse's family contact; for example:

- What was done by the nurse?
- What was said by the family during conversation?
- Reactions of the present family members.
- Any special situation that happened during contact.

It is helpful in evaluation of progress of family. It provides clues about better family healthcare. Video or tape recording may be used for the process of recording.

Registers

Registers are maintained to record the total volume of services provided to families and not for continuity of services. A comprehensive healthcare services register is maintained to keep a record of all families living in the area in a particular health center. Baseline data is recorded about families at the time of the survey and changes brought about in the family's health status over a month, quarter and year are all noted. Progress in the health services provided can be evaluated by analyzing family data from registers. For example, the number of children immunized at the end of the month can be compared with the number of children immunized at the beginning of the services.

Summary

- Family is a unit of healthcare. Family is a group of two or more members related by birth, marriage, adoption and residing together in a household.
- Family health nursing is the service provided by the community nursing personnel to prevent disease, to promote health, to ensure optimum health status of family members.
- Family healthcare services are provided to assess and coordinate the needs of family member. The services provided are antenatal, intranatal, postnatal, child health and family planning, reproductive health nutritional services, elderly care, care of physically and mentally handicapped, first aid and services related to environment health of family.
- Family health nursing care is provided by the community health nurse during home visits. She plans care according to the needs of the members of family according to the goals, policies, and objectives of the healthcare agency.
- Family healthcare nursing process is a systematic approach to assess, plan, implement and evaluate the care provided. The purpose of family health nursing care process is to prevent and promote the health of family members.
- The family health nursing or care process includes assessment, planning, implementation and evaluation. Maternal and child health services provide antenatal, intranatal, postnatal and neonatal care, growth and development care of children under 5 years of age and care for children having health problems.
- The family welfare services provide family planning services. Family planning services include methods such as mechanical methods, chemical methods, hormonal methods, emergency contraceptive methods and surgical methods.
- Other services of family welfare services include clinical services, domiciliary services, community services, setting up targets, family records, family welfare program, etc.
- The roles and functions of community health nurses in family welfare services include administration, supervision, direct care, education and roles in research and evaluation.

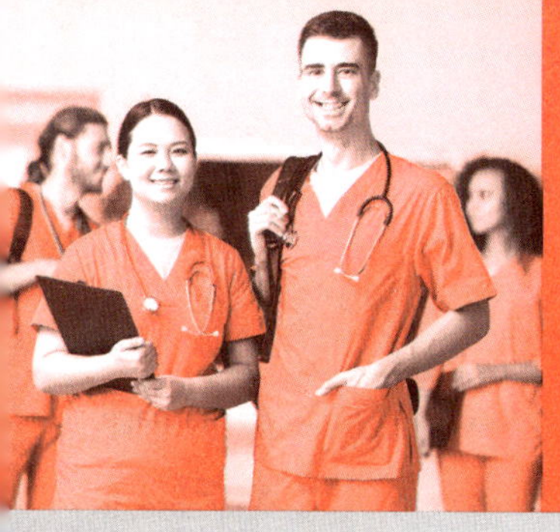

STUDENT ASSIGNMENT

LONG ANSWER TYPE QUESTIONS

1. Define family health and describe the family health nursing services provided to the family.
2. Define family health nursing process. Explain the phases of the family healthcare nursing process.
3. Describe the role and functions of community health nurse in family health nursing care.

SHORT ANSWER TYPE QUESTIONS

1. List the purposes of family health nursing care process.
2. Write short note about the family as a unit of health.
3. Enumerate the principles of working with families.

MULTIPLE CHOICE QUESTIONS

1. **The basic unit of health is:**
   - a. An Individual
   - b. The family
   - c. The community
   - d. Both b and c

2. **The concept of family health is:**
   - a. Physical and mental health
   - b. Spiritual and emotional health
   - c. Social and emotional health
   - d. All of these

3. **The planning phase includes:**
   - a. Setting goals and objectives
   - b. Establishing priorities
   - c. Planning appropriate intervention and formulating family health nursing care plan
   - d. All of the above

4. **The maternal health services include:**
   - a. Antenatal care
   - b. Intranatal care
   - c. Postnatal care
   - d. All of these

5. **The best method for spacing is:**
   - a. Tubectomy
   - b. IUCD
   - c. Condom
   - d. Pessary

ANSWER KEY

1. b	**2.** d	**3.** d	**4.** d	**5.** c

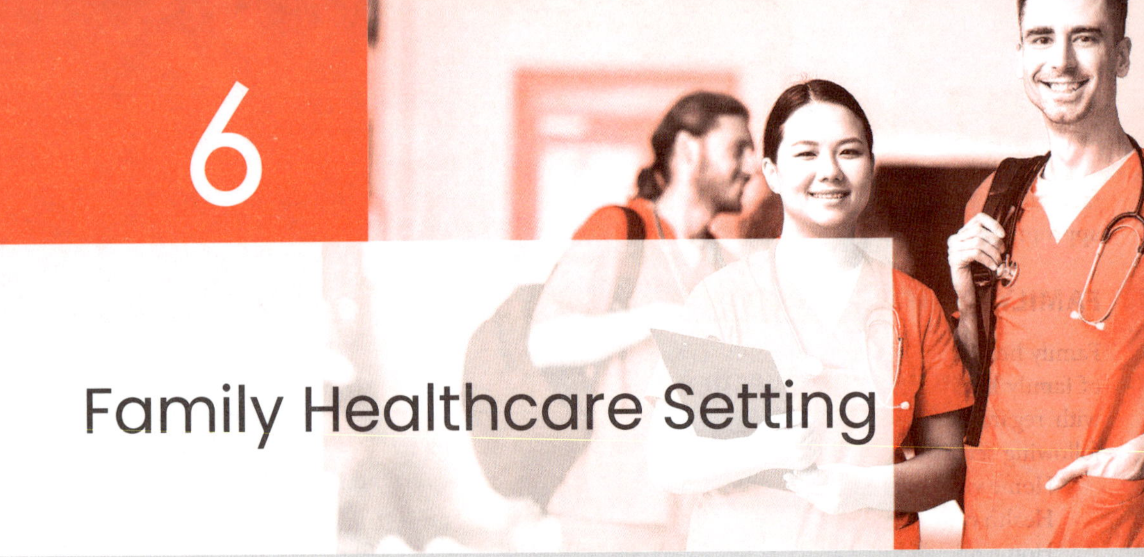

6

Family Healthcare Setting

LEARNING OBJECTIVES

After the completion of the unit, the readers will be able to:

- Describe the principles and techniques of family healthcare services at home and in clinics.
- Describe bag technique.
- State the purposes and functions of clinics.
- Appreciate the role of health personnel in clinics.

UNIT OUTLINE

- Introduction
- Family Healthcare Setting
- Bag Technique
- Clinics

KEY TERMS

Bag technique: The technique of opening and using the equipment placed in the bag for specific procedure or purpose.

Clinic: A small private or public health facility.

Healthcare settings: Institutions where healthcare is provided.

Home visit: A planned visit to families at their residence for the purpose of providing healthcare services.

INTRODUCTION

Family is the basic unit of providing healthcare to the community. In fact, family healthcare service is the nucleus of community healthcare services. If nation has to achieve optimum health, it has to be started from family healthcare services. In a family, the health of one member affects the health of other member of the family as the members of the family are interdependent on each other. They provide care and support to each other during sickness. Each family has different beliefs, customs, culture, lifestyle, education and socioeconomic status. The health workers engaged in providing healthcare services to the family need to know the background of the family, the community resources available and the goals and objectives of the healthcare agencies. Community health nurse plays crucial role as a direct care provider, coordinator, facilitator, teacher and an advocator in helping families to identify their need and receive appropriate care in family healthcare setting.

FAMILY HEALTHCARE SETTING

Family healthcare can be provided in a variety of settings but no single setting fulfils the objectives of family healthcare. All the settings have their advantages and disadvantages, so they are utilized with regards to specific problems in providing family healthcare to achieve the objectives. The following settings are utilized to provide family healthcare:

- Home visit
- Health centers
- Home nursing
- Clinics
- Factories and other work places

Home Visit

In India, the most needy and vulnerable group of population, live in rural and urban slums where the health facilities are hardly available. Secondly, the illiteracy and ignorance are the barriers to avail the existing facilities of health services, so majority of the population remains confined to home due to illness. Home visit is appropriate setting of family healthcare where all the family members are contacted at one time to inculcate health-seeking behavior in them. Home visit is the backbone of community health nursing services.

Purposes of Home Visit

The overall aim of home visit is to provide comprehensive healthcare to the family by delivering need-based quantum of healthcare with the participation of the family members in the home environment, so the purposes of home visits are:

- To identify the health problems of the family and investigate the associate causes of the problems.
- To provide best possible care in the home environment without disturbing family routine.
- To know the family and establish working relation with the family members so that they can actively participate as recipient of healthcare.
- To improve the health standards of the family.
- To plan and implement care with the family.
- To assess the health status, immunization, nutrition and environmental hazards of a family.
- To identify the sources of communicable diseases and educating families about the means of prevention.
- To follow-up treatment, care given and evaluate the healthcare.
- To reduce maternal and infant mortality rate.
- To provide health education during home visit while giving nursing care at home.
- To supervise and guide health workers in giving family healthcare.

Frequency of Home Visit

Frequency of home visit depends upon the extent of health problems of the family, need felt by the family and ability of the families to deal with their health needs. Families for visits are selected on the basis of priorities, health agency's policies, objectives and facilities available.

Priorities are established on the following guidelines:

- In case of acute and serious illness, frequent visits are required.
- During last trimester of pregnancy, approaching expected date of delivery.
- During labor.
- To visit premature infant.
- For information, education, counseling and guidance.

Principles of Home Visit

- Healthcare personnel visiting the families should have thorough knowledge of health policies and objectives of healthcare agencies.
- Visit should be planned according to the prioritized health needs.
- Regular visits are essential in selected units for continuity of the care.
- Establish rapport with kind approach, having concern with family members' health needs to gain their confidence, collection of data about family, home and environment, should be taken carefully.
- Scientific and up-to-date technique should be used while performing nursing procedures.
- Always respect the persons' feelings and needs and value, their culture and customs.
- Emphasis should be on quality of care rather than quantity.
- The family members should be motivated to accept the health aspects voluntarily instead of forcing one's concept on them.
- Visit can be made flexible due to prevailing circumstances at home, the aim of visit has to be changed or postponed.
- Health education should be an integral part of home visit. Family should be educated about personal hygiene, nutrition, immunization, family planning and about health problems in the community.
- Record of the work performed during each visit should be made. Evaluation of visit is essential to improve health facilities, so all the information has to be properly filled in family folder, daily diary, family card and result evaluated using health indicators.
- Never accept any gift from the family.

Advantages of Home Visit

- Family members get healthcare in relaxed home environment so their time to go to the clinics is saved.
- It helps the nurse/healthcare workers to observe family atmosphere.
- Health education becomes more realistic as the socioeconomic background becomes clearer.
- Care given to the patient by the family members can be observed closely.
- During home visits, the other members of the family can be educated who can take care of the patient at home.
- New health problems can be detected during home visit.

Disadvantages of Home Visit

- Home visits are more time consuming and more expensive in terms of trained manpower.
- Lack of up-to-date equipment, resources and inadequate skill, limit the efficiency of care through home visit.

- Lack of interest of the family due to low socioeconomic status and lack of education, make home visit ineffective.
- Dispute among the family members can create uncongenial environment for counseling of health education.

Planning and Evaluation for Home Visit

Planning: Home visit should be planned with definite aim, objectives and health resources, available at healthcare agency. It should be planned according to the needs of the family. There are three main steps in planning:

1. **Preliminary planning and preparation:**
   - Map of the area to be visited should be prepared after its survey. This will give the idea of community resources, like soft water supply, number of schools, health centers, environmental sanitation, roads, bus services, market and religious places like Temple, Church, Masjid, Gurudwara, etc.
   - Family folder, individual cards and health education material should be collected.
   - Preparation of the community bag. Home visiting bag has to be prepared which should contain medicine for treating minor ailments, sterile dressing material, delivery kit, urine testing articles, blood pressure (BP) instrument, stethoscope, fetoscope and other required instruments.
   - Newspaper and paper bags to receive soiled material.

2. **Procedure:**
   - Take permission to enter the house after knocking at the door or pressing the bell.
   - Introduce yourself by name and the health agency that you are representing.
   - Greet all the family members with pleasant smile.
   - Explain the purpose of your visit.
   - Develop good relations by talking to them in wise and friendly manner to gain their confidence.
   - Place the community bag at safe place beyond the reach of the children.
   - Interview the family members and motivate them to share their problems.
   - Provide care to the family, if required, like dressing, urine testing, checking BP and temperature and giving medicines as per their needs.
   - Maintain privacy and secrecy and the personal questions must be asked in privacy.
   - Note the following points are to be kept in mind during conversation with the family:
     - Type of family
     - Physical and ecological environment of home
     - Size of the family and per capita income
     - Education and employment of family members
     - Conveyance available in the family
     - Nutritional status, signs of malnutrition, if any
     - Health status of pregnant mothers
     - Health status of children under five years of age and signs of malnutrition, if any
     - Immunization schedule of children
     - Acceptance to the small family norms

3. **Document:** Record all the information gathered in family folder.
   - List the assessed healthcare needs in the folder and arrange to provide care accordingly. Specify the area in which the family can be helped to promote health. Plan for the next visit and record in the folder and diary.
   - Inform family about the next visit, terminate visit with the brief review of important points.
   - Write the attitude of the family toward prevention of disease.
   - Record visits in family folder.
4. **Evaluation:** Evaluation is a continuous process. A community health nurse should evaluate the home visits from the records made in family folder and assess the area for intervention of health services. She should enter the place, date and time of home visit in the register at the health center. The purpose of home visit is to note down the health problems of the family, provide guidance, do counseling and impart health education to the family during visit. The following information are gathered from the visit:
   - Immediate problems of the family
   - Origin of problems
   - Action taken to solve the problem
   - Reaction of the family members and their interest

BAG TECHNIQUE

Community bag is a vehicle to carry the tools required during home visit. It is made up of strong but light material like canvas, leather, plastic or light metal. It can be carried in hand or on the shoulder.

Articles of Nursing Bag

A nursing bag should have the following articles:
- Soap in soap dish, nail brush and towel   1 Each
- Apparatus for giving enema, i.e. enema can, tubing—one set, clamp, enema catheter, enema soap, strainer, vessel to dissolve soap in hot water or ready-made enema in disposable set is available and used commonly nowadays
- Urinary catheter, rubber or disposable Foley's catheter   1
- Clinical thermometer and two blood sliders wrapped in paper   1
- Rectal thermometer   1
- Pair of scissors   1
- Pair of artery forceps   2
- Pair of dissecting forceps   2
- Small gallipot 4″ and bowl 6″   1 Each
- Kidney trays   2
- Bag of sterile dressing   1
- Measuring tape
- Fetoscope   1
- BP instrument   1
- Stethoscope   1

- Bag of sterile swab sticks   1
- Spring balance   1
- Disposable gloves   1 Pair
- Large cotton bag to carry home equipment that cannot be disinfected in patient's house   1
- Disposable syringes and pricking needles   2
- Spirit and cotton swabs   1 Bottle
- Mucus sucker   1
- Cord ligatures   1 Set
- Eye antiseptics   Bottle
- Urine testing kit   1
- Glucometer   1
- Sterile delivery kit   1 Set
- Plastic apron   1
- Rubber sheet or plastic sheet   1
- Paper bag and newspaper
- Antiseptic lotions, e.g., betadine Savlon normal saline for dressing   1 Bottle Each
- Bandage and tape
- Baby feeding tube (Disposable)   1
- Prescribed medicine and injection
- Small diary, pencil/pen to be kept in outer pocket of outer shelf of bag

Articles of CHN in UNICEF Bag

The following articles are carried in UNICEF Bag:

UNICEF bags are light aluminum boxes containing following items of delivery kit.

- Plastic bag containing plastic apron and sheet, soap in soap dish, nail brush and towel in waterproof bag.
- Kidney dish   2
- Lotion bowls   2
- Small bowl for eye swabs   1
- Pair of artery forceps   2
- Pair of dissecting forceps toothed and nontoothed   1 Each
- Pair of scissors   2
- Bowl lifting forceps   1
- Gloves   2 Pairs
- Instrument box containing syringes and needles   1
- Complete set of enema can with connections   1
- Tubing, catheter and clamp   1
- Urethral catheter (Rubber)   1
- Mucus extractor   1
- Spring balance   1
- Clinical thermometer   1
- Rectal thermometer   1
- Stock of cotton for making pads and boiled swabs   Sufficient

- Cord ligatures   2 Set
- Sterile gauze pieces for cord dressing   Sufficient
- Prepacked sterile catgut with suturing needles   2 Packet
- Bottle of antiseptics—Dettol, Betadine, spirit   1 Each
- Bottle of antiseptic eye drops for baby's eyes (to be used when advised)   1
- Prescribed drugs or medicine in different containers
- Fetoscope   1
- Stethoscope   1
- BP instrument   1
- Measuring tape   1
- Note book, pen/pencil
  (Not to be kept inside box)
  Note: Nowadays prepacked sterile suturing materials with needles, cord ligatures, enema, disposable syringes and catheter are used.

Aftercare of Articles and Bag

Aftercare of articles and bag can be done in the following manners:
1. After coming back to health center, the used articles are cleaned and autoclaved.
2. The disposable articles and material are disposed of safely by burning.
3. Bag is emptied, cleaned with antiseptic from inside and outside, dried in sun. Articles are checked, rearranged and kept ready for next use.

Structure of Bag and Equipment to be Carried

Structure of bag and equipment to be carried in it for home visit include: Bag should have three main compartment and two pockets on both outer aspects of the outer compartments.
- The pockets on the first outer compartment contain soap, towel and nail brush for hand washing in one pocket and other pocket contains diary and family folder.
- First compartment, should contain medicine containers with medicine, like Tab. Paracetamol (PCM), antibiotic, multivitamin, analgesic and anti-inflammatory drugs, contraceptive pills, injection and disposable syringes.
- Middle sterile compartment contains sterile covered dressing tray with gauge pieces, cotton pads, sterile bowls, artery forceps, dissecting forceps, catheter sterile, delivery kit, sterile towel, autoclaved newspapers, sterile gloves, Gamjee pad, sterile stitching material.
- Second outer compartment contains android BP instrument, stethoscope, fetoscope, tape measure, thermometer, cotton swabs, spring balance and urine-testing kit, plastic sheet and plastic apron.
- One of the side pockets of the second outer compartment contains Savlon, Betadine, Spirit/Benedict's solution, and in the other pocket paper bags and newspaper.

Principles of Bag Technique

- Always check the contents of the bag before leaving for home visit.
- Bag and its contents must be kept clean and ready for use at all times.

- Hands must be washed with soap and water each time before touching the bag.
- Bag should be placed in a clean and safe area without danger of getting contaminated because of domestic animals, if any.
- All the articles used should be cleaned with soap and water, boiled and replaced for the next use.
- Things like pen, pencil, handkerchief, cell phone should not be kept inside bag.

Techniques of Using Bag During Home Visit

- Select the safe and clean area and spread newspaper and keep the bag on it.
- Open the side pocket and take out hand washing articles and wash hands.
- Remove apron from the bag and put it on.
- Prepare new paper waste bag to receive used swabs or contaminated material.
- Remove the required articles as per the requirement of the procedure and close the bag.
- Give nursing care to the patient based on the plan.
- When the procedure is over, make patient comfortable, wash hands with soap and water.
- Clean the articles with soap and water, boil and replace. Close the bag.
- Fold used newspapers with used side inside and dispose it.
- Dispose used paper bags with contaminated material by burning.
- Wash hands with soap and water.
- Record the observation, the procedure performed and care given to the patient.
- Plan for the next visit and inform the family about it.

CLINICS

Clinic is a type of healthcare setting to provide healthcare services to the people. It is a special place either in the hospital or in the healthcare centers where the specialist doctors along with the trained nurses and paramedical staff, diagnose, treat and provide follow-up care to the outdoor patients. Clinics are more convenient to the patients. They can get the consultation and treatment as outdoor patient according to the feasibility of their work schedule.

Purposes of Clinics

- Patients can directly approach to the specialist doctors with formal registration as an outdoor patient.
- Hospitalization is not required unless it is an acute emergency.
- Consultation, investigation, diagnosis and treatment is done as an ambulatory outdoor patient. The patient is spared of unnecessary expenditure of hospitalization.
- Patient can carry out treatment at his home environment with all home comforts and with emotional support of family members.
- Patient's routine job work is not disturbed much.
- Hospital is spared of overcrowding of the indoor patients.
- Requirement of trained staff also reduces.
- Referral system is very quick as the treating physician can refer directly to another specialist if need arises.

Features of Clinics

- Clinic should be set up at such a place where transport facilities are available.
- Clinic should be located near the emergency unit, laboratory and radiological department as the basic investigation may be required before starting treatment.
- There should be sufficient waiting area and chairs in front of the clinic and near the registration office where the patients can relax and wait for their turn.
- Facilities for drinking water and toilet are the basic requirements of every clinic.
- Small portable canteen should be available near the clinic where the patient can have some refreshment who come from far-off places or some patients come fasting for their investigations.
- Time for clinic should be fixed and working hours of the clinic are usually kept more than routine timings of the hospital.
- The physician and members of his team should be specialized and skilled in their work and sufficient in number.
- All equipment in the clinic should be up-to-date and in working conditions as patients are aware of latest technology of medicines through social media.
- Sufficient stationary should be available and records should be maintained accurately in register.
- Inside the clinic, hand-washing facilities, screen for privacy, arrangement for sufficient light should be there.
- Female attendant should be available while examining female patient.
- Staff working in clinic should be kind, sympathetic and tactful in answering the queries of the patient.
- There should be arrangement for effective health education.

Types and Functions of Clinics

The clinics are generally classified in following main groups:
1. General clinics
2. Maternal and child health clinics
3. Specialty clinics

Functions of General Clinics

The functions depend upon the aims and objectives and types of clinics. They are usually managed by general physician. The functions of the clinic are:
- To provide emergency care.
- To treat minor ailments.
- To examine routine laboratory investigation.
- For immunization through immunization clinic.

Functions of X-ray Clinics

X-ray clinic: X-ray clinic is managed by radiologist.
Its functions are:
- To provide radiological diagnosis.
- To provide radiotherapy to the cancer patients.

Functions of Dental Clinics

The dental clinics are run by dentist either bachelor of dental science (BDS) or master of dental science (MDS) in specific field.

Its functions are:

- Maintain oral health.
- Prevent and treat dental caries.
- Provide treatment for gingivitis, periodontitis, mouth ulcers.
- Warn patient about the use of oral tobacco.

Maternal and Child Health Clinic

The aims of maternal and child health clinic is to reduce the maternal and infant mortality rate and promote the health of the mothers and children. These clinics are in subcenters, primary health centers, community health centers, government hospital and in private hospitals. After 1980, a sizeable improvement has been noticed in the health of mothers and children due to implementation of primary healthcare.

The mother and child health (MCH) clinics are categorized as under:

- Antenatal clinic
- Postnatal clinic
- Under-five clinics
- Family planning clinic
- Child guidance clinic
- Reproductive and child health clinic

Functions of maternal and child health clinics: The functions of maternal and child health clinics depend on the category of the clinic.

- **Antenatal clinic:**
  - **Aim:** The aim of antenatal clinic is to take care of the health of pregnant women and their babies.

    Functions:
    - To promote and protect the health of mothers.
    - To prevent and treat malnutrition as nutritional anemia is very common in pregnant women.
    - To screen high risk cases and appropriate management of such cases.
    - To treat infections and teaching about personal hygiene.
    - To immunize the mother against tetanus.
    - Warning mothers against drugs, smoking and alcohol.
    - To assess the growth and development of the fetus during pregnancy.
    - Mothers are explained about frequency of visits to clinic.
    - To maintain the antenatal records like, weight, height, hemoglobin estimation, urine testing for sugar and albumen during each visit.
    - Preparing mother for mother craft.
    - Preparing for labor.
    - Sensitivity about the need of family planning.
    - Counseling of the family members about her care after delivery and to provide psychological support.
- **Postnatal clinic:** In postnatal clinic, care is provided to the mother and child after delivery, up to 6 weeks.

- **Aim:** The aim of postnatal clinic is to maintain optimum health of mother and child.
  Functions:
  - To help the mother to recover from stress and strain of labor.
  - To promote breast feeding to the infant.
  - To prevent infections.
  - To prevent complications.
  - To teach mother about care of newborn baby.
  - To provide family planning services.
- **Family planning clinics:** The National Population Policy of 2000 considered very essential to stabilize population for promoting equitable development of the country.
  Functions of family planning clinics are:
  - To provide guidance and counseling to legible couples.
  - To treat infertility.
  - To advise spacing between children.
  - To motivate couples to have small family.
  - To provide contraceptive devices to the couples.
  - To maintain records of mothers who adopt small family norms.
  - Records of tubectomy and vasectomy operations are maintained.
  - To provide health education on prevention of reproductive tract diseases.
  - Provide genetic counseling.
  - Sex education.
  - Education on nutrition.
  - Provide marital guidance.
  - Making available the contraceptive devices free of cost at all health centers.
- **Child guidance clinic:** Some children suffer from psychological disorders. These must be recognized by the parents and should seek medical help to resolve such problems. Some of the disorders are:
  - Bed wetting
  - Sensitive to normal situation
  - Cruel behavior toward children or animals
  - Stealing objects
  - No interaction with children of their age
  - Hating family members
  - Refusing to go to school
  - Child feels neglected
  - Not behaving as per the age
    Functions:
    Usually, the clinic is run by the psychologist, psychiatrist, pediatrician and community health nurse.
    - Detailed history of child is collected from the parents and diagnosis is made based on history.
    - Child is counseled about the problems.
    - Proper entertainment and sports facilities are provided to make child mentally healthy.

- Child is provided with number of options to solve his problem.
- Counseling is conducted frequently till problems are resolved.

- **Reproductive and child health clinics:** The aim of this clinic is to reduce maternal and child morbidity and mortality rate and promote optimum health of mother and child.

Functions:

- **For maternal health intervention:**
  - Provide essential obstetric care which includes antenatal care, institutional delivery and postnatal care.
  - Emergency obstetric care.
  - 24 hours delivery services at primary health centers (PHCs) and community health centers (CHCs).
  - Referral transport facility.
  - Medical termination of pregnancy on medical or social grounds.
  - Prevention, treatment and control if there is reproductive tract infection.
- **For child health intervention:**
  - Immunization on all vaccine preventable diseases
  - Essential newborn care
  - Oral rehydration therapy for diarrhea
  - Control and treatment of acute respiratory tract infection
  - Prevention and control of vitamin A deficiency

Specialty Clinics

These clinics are run by the specialist doctors in order to provide better medical and counseling services. It includes:

- **Diabetic clinic:** Diabetes mellitus is one of the major health problems and its incidence is increasing. Clinic is run by specialist with trained staff in this field. The functions of diabetic clinic are:

Functions:

- To screen high risk cases that are prone to get the disease. This group includes:
  - Obese patients above 40 years of age
  - Family history of diabetes
  - Premature atherosclerosis
  - Patients complaining of excessive appetite and frequency of urine
- To diagnose and treat such patients.
- Prevention of diabetes by healthy lifestyle.
- To provide modification of diet.
- To prevent and treat complications.
- Teach patients about self-care regarding:
  - Take regular meals
  - Take medicine as advised
  - Recognize signs of hypoglycemia and treat them
  - To keep sweets and chocolates in case, if signs of hypoglycemia are evident
- Teach patients about care of skin and feet.
- Avoid injury.

- Prevent infection
- Regular exercise and diet control
- Come for periodic medical checkup, always carry a diabetic card with phone number and address in it

- **Cardiac clinic:** Cardiac clinic is run by the cardiologist and his team. Due to sedentary lifestyle and consumption of alcohol, and cigarette smoking, heart disease is becoming a major health problem.

  Functions:
  - To diagnose and treat all problems related to heart.
  - Provide health education on prevention and care.
  - Counseling the heart patients about treatment and changing lifestyle.
  - Provide follow-up care.
  - To maintain records and reports.
  - To contribute for research work.

- **Tuberculosis clinic:** Tuberculosis (TB) is one of the communicable diseases. It is not only a problem for the patient suffering but also affects the family members and community if not treated and controlled.

  The TB clinic is run by the chest physician and health team specially trained in it to provide health education to the patient and family to prevent the spread of it.

  Functions:
  - To make diagnosis of any patient coming with cough more than two months and weight loss and sweating at night.
  - To provide antituberculosis drugs
  - To pay special attention on diet as TB is a wasting disease. To give health education on taking rest, diet with high protein and extra calories and vitamins
  - To teach the patient about the prevention of disease
  - If patient is not regular in taking medicine, he can be referred to directly observed treatment shortcourse (DOTS) clinic
  - To make records of all patients
  - To notify all the cases
  - To contribute to research

- **Sex clinic:** Sex health clinic is managed by the sex specialist and his/her team trained and specialized in the treatment and prevention of sex problems.

  Functions:
  - To diagnose the sexually transmitted diseases like chlamydia, gonorrhea, syphilis and acquired immunodeficiency syndrome (AIDS).
  - To provide treatment of such cases and follow-up care.
  - To provide sex education.
  - To advise the use of condom to prevent the spread of infection to another partner.
  - To educate about sex hygiene.
  - To testing urine for pregnancy.
  - To maintain records of all cases.
  - To notify the cases.

- **Nutrition clinic:** Nutrition clinic has become an essential component in every healthcare unit. Therapeutic diet in cases of diabetes mellitus, hypertension, cardiac, renal and tuberculosis cases, during pregnancy and lactation, diet requirement in growing children and nutritional deficiencies diseases call for the consultation of the dietician. Clinic is run by the dietician and his team trained in nutritional aspects. The models and health-conscious people routinely visit nutrition clinic.

Functions:

- To provide nutritional assessment, intervention and education to patients and family.
- To ensure nutritional needs are met by the meals and snacks planned in menu.
- To participate with healthcare team to provide dietary requirement of patients and growing children.
- To provide evidence-based medical nutrition therapy.
- To ensure standards of food are met through quality assurance.
- To provide knowledge and awareness of current nutritional information.
- To provide education on the healthy eating principles.
- To teach nursing and dietician interns about the nutrition aspects and therapeutic diets.
- To maintain records.
- To contribute to research work.

Functions of Health Personnel in Clinic

- To maintain good environment, cleanliness and sanitation of the clinic.
- To arrange for the drinking water.
- To arrange sufficient chairs in the waiting area.
- To have sufficient supplies, equipment like syringes, medicine, injections as per the requirement of particular clinic.
- To keep all equipment and devices used in the clinic in proper functioning condition.
- Arrangement for sufficient light in the clinic.
- To maintain good interpersonal relations among the health team and the patients.
- They should have positive attitude and good team spirit toward their work performance.
- It is the responsibility of the health personnel to have sufficient stock of health education material and pamphlets according to the type of clinic.
- To provide information and education on the concerned subject as per the clinic.
- To assist the doctors/specialists.
- To provide knowledge and demonstrations on certain procedure to the patient and family, which may be required to perform at home, like insulin injections, use of syringe and calculation of dose, etc. and checking temperature, blood pressure or use of nebulization at home.
- Assessing the health status and noting improvement following treatments and counseling.
- To inform patients about the next visit.
- To make accurate records.

Summary

- Family healthcare settings are the institutions where healthcare services are provided.
- The settings utilized to provide family healthcare are home visit, health centers, home nursing, clinics, factories, and other work places.
- Home visiting is the backbone of community health nursing. Before planning home visit, the base line survey of the community to be visited, should be done.
- The purpose of home visit is to observe the family composition role, responsibilities, to find out health problems, plan and implement care as per the need of the family.
- Nurse should use technical skill, kind and courteous approach. Home visit is the best setting to provide healthcare but it is expensive in terms of time and manpower.
- Clinic is a small government or private healthcare setting which is devoted to provide care to outdoor patients. Clinic settings are run legally to provide medical care.
- There are various types of clinics, i.e., general outdoor patient clinic, specialist clinic and polyclinic.
- Functions of health personnel in clinic to maintain cleanliness and good environment and maintain equipment and supplies; help the specialists; to provide information and education to the clients on the concerned subject; provide knowledge and demonstration on certain procedure to the patients and families and maintain accurate regards.

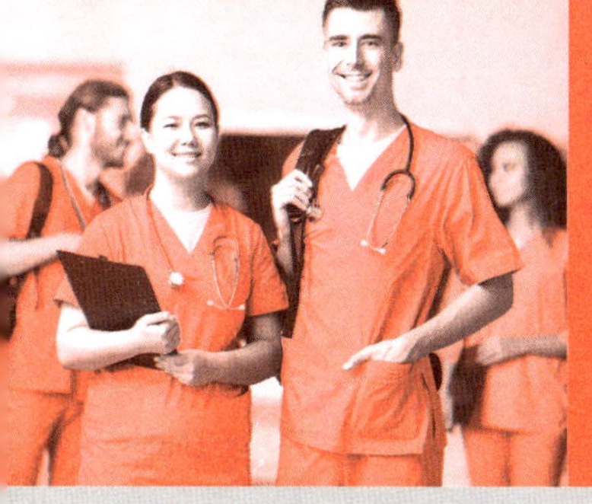

LONG ANSWER TYPE QUESTIONS

1. Describe the phases of home visiting.
2. Discuss the techniques of home visiting.
3. Explain the purpose and types of clinics.
4. Enumerate the principles of home visit.
5. Discuss in general the duties of health personnel at clinics.

SHORT ANSWER TYPE QUESTIONS

1. Define home visiting.
2. Enlist the purposes of home visit.
3. Write the features of good clinic.

MULTIPLE CHOICE QUESTIONS

1. **Which of the following is not correct in bag technique:**
   a. Survey area and prepare a map.
   b. Identify families who need home visiting.
   c. Keep all needed articles in bag for providing care.
   d. Visit communicable cases first and clean cases later on.

2. **The job of receptionist at the clinic is:**
   a. To welcome the patient
   b. To register the patient
   c. To guide the patient
   d. All of these

3. **The type of patients to be weighed in clinic:**
   a. Patients suffering from TB
   b. Pregnant women
   c. Children under the age of 5 years
   d. All of these

4. **The functions of nurse at clinic:**
   a. Taking vital signs
   b. Giving injections and dressing of wounds
   c. Providing family planning services
   d. All of these

5. **Which of the following is not the disadvantage of home visit:**
   a. It consumes lots of time and energy.
   b. Sometimes nurse has to face unforeseen events.
   c. Nonacceptance by family members.
   d. It is convenient for family members as they do not have to travel to visit health centers.

ANSWER KEY

1. d   2. d   3. d   4. d   5. d

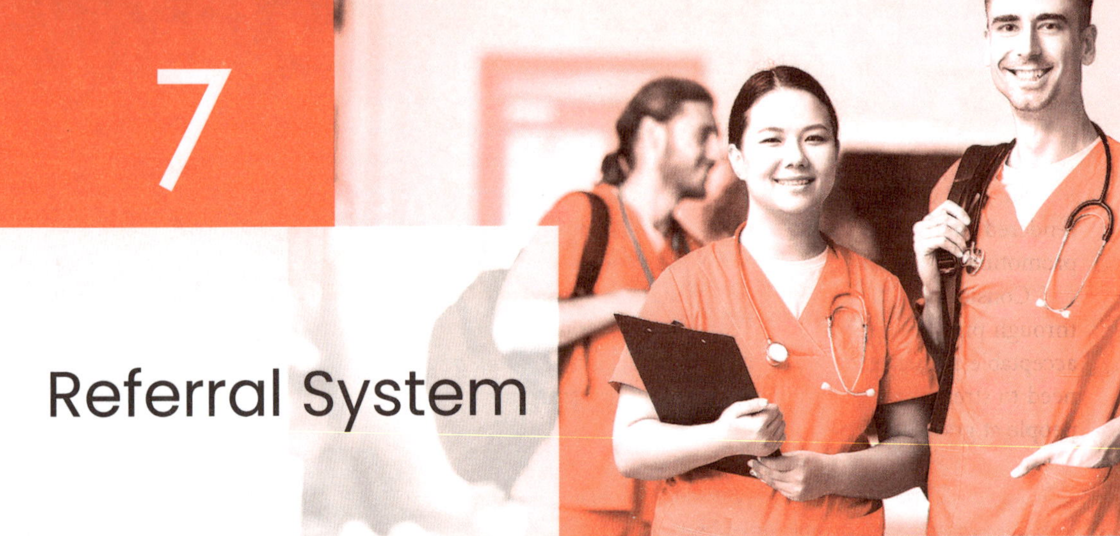

7

Referral System

LEARNING OBJECTIVES

After the completion of the unit, the readers will be able to:

- Define referral system.
- Describe the levels of healthcare.
- Explain the steps in referral system.
- Enlist the duties and responsibilities of nursing personnel at various levels of referring unit.
- State the staffing patterns at various levels of healthcare.
- Understand the importance of referral services.

UNIT OUTLINE

- Introduction
- Healthcare
- Healthcare Settings
- National Health Programs

KEY TERMS

Fatal condition: In this condition, a life cannot be saved even with treatment.

Referral: Sending the patient from one place to another.

Serious condition: In this condition, life can be saved but only with immediate treatment.

INTRODUCTION

A referral system in healthcare is a process that helps patients get access to specialized care when needed, while also making efficient use of resources. It's a key part of the health system, and it connects different levels of care.

HEALTHCARE

The dictionary meaning of healthcare is to protect health, to be concerned about health or to take care of health. World Health Organization (WHO) definition of health states, "Health is a state of complete physical, mental, and social well-being and not merely an absence of disease or infirmity".

So, in the light of the above definition, health can be understood as the "multiple services rendered to the individuals, families, and community by the health agency for the purpose of promoting, preventing, maintaining, monitoring and restoring the health".

Considering it, Government of India is committed to achieve the goal of "Health for All" through primary healthcare approach, the national health policy was reviewed in 2001 to achieve acceptable standard of health by strengthening the existing infrastructure and emphasizing the need to strengthen primary healthcare infrastructure making basic health services available to the people at grassroots level.

Characteristics of Healthcare

- Should be accessible to all within a specified geographical area taking care of their social and cultural values.
- Should be appropriate and adequate to satisfy the needs of the people.
- Comprehensive in nature.
- Within the capacity of available resources, like money, material and manpower.
- According to the priorities of the needs and policies of the government.

Purposes of Healthcare

- To reduce the morbidity and mortality rate.
- To improve basic environmental sanitation.
- To improve nutritional status.
- To increase the life expectancy of individuals.
- To investigate the new emerging health problems and take appropriate steps to deal with.
- To develop manpower and other resources.
- To explore the potentials of the people toward "Progressive India".

Levels of Healthcare

Healthcare in India is based on 3-tier system of services provided at three levels of care. These are Primary Level, Secondary Level and Tertiary Level.

Primary Level of Healthcare

It is the first level of contact between the community and healthcare providers at the grassroots level. At this stage many health problems are solved by the people themselves with some guidance, education and assistance provided by the health team (Fig. 7.1). The health agencies that provide primary healthcare are subcenters, primary health centers. These services are comprehensive in nature and provide basic healthcare by the team of health professionals. Health professionals include medical officer, health supervisors, multipurpose health workers male and female, sanitarian and extension health educator. At village level, the Anganwadi worker, trained dais and accredited social health activists (ASHA) and other leaders are active in contributing their services at primary level of healthcare.

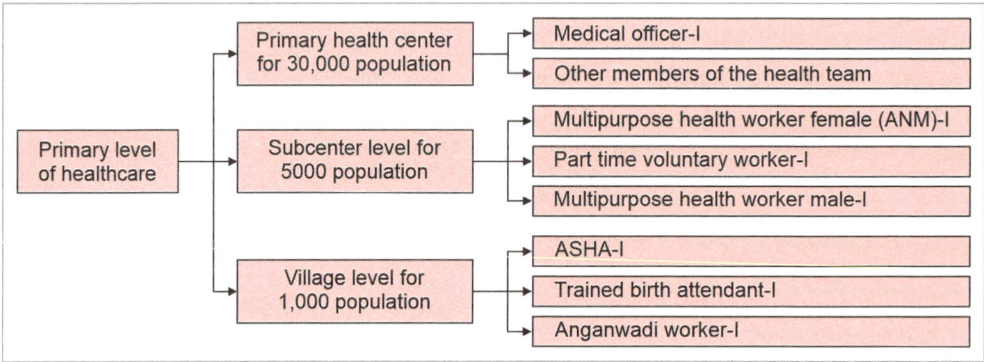

Fig. 7.1: Model of primary level of healthcare

Secondary Level of Healthcare

As per the policies of primary healthcare, the primary levels of healthcare settings are not equipped with the facilities and manpower to deal with all complex problems. So, the cases which require secondary level of preventive services, i.e., diagnostic, curative services and specialists' consultations are referred to as secondary level care (Fig. 7.2). The secondary level services are provided at community health center, district hospital, and district health center.

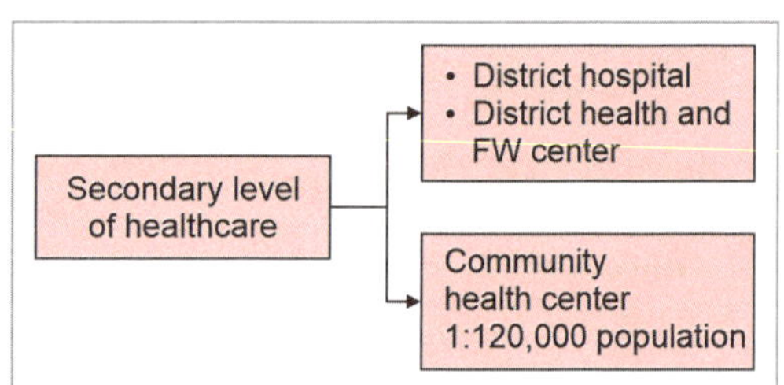

Fig. 7.2: Model of secondary level of healthcare

Tertiary Level of Healthcare

The health problems which cannot be treated at secondary level care setting are transferred to tertiary level care setting. The tertiary level care is provided at state level, regional level or central level. Institutions include specialist hospitals, medical college hospital and super specialiality hospital. These institutions serve as referral units for primary and secondary levels of care. In these institutions, the latest technology, facilities and super specialists, are available.

These institutions, in addition to provide tertiary level care, also serve as teaching institutions. The training and medical education is provided to the various categories of health workers. The planning, management and research work is also executed at this level.

HEALTHCARE SETTINGS

In the past, the health services were the privilege of the urban and allied community. The hospitals and dispensaries were available in the cities. In India 75% of the population belong to rural area where the facilities were very few and unevenly placed. People of rural area could not avail the health facilities due to poverty, illiteracy and ignorance; it resulted in high morbidity and mortality among the rural population.

The current commitment of all the countries to remove the inequalities in the distribution of healthcare services and resources and attainment of "Health for All" (HFA) by 2000 AD. That means minimum healthcare must be accessible and affordable to each individual of the society so as to maintain optimum level of health. To meet the global commitment of "HFA" the healthcare settings are restructured through primary healthcare approach to provide universal comprehensive healthcare to the people who can accept and afford it.

Factors Affecting Healthcare Settings

The following factors affect the healthcare settings:
- **Funds:** Funds are generated by the government through general taxes. It is up to the government how much funds are made available for healthcare services. Funds are also generated through private agencies and volunteers, and contribution from people.
- **Technical manpower:** It is the most expensive factor. How much trained manpower is employed by the government, depends upon government policies and decisions.
- **Consumers of healthcare:** These are the people to whom healthcare services are to be provided. The extent and nature of services depend upon the size, demographic characteristics, health status of the people, their health attitude, behavior, lifestyle, education, standard of living, sociocultural practices, physical surroundings of the people and health demands of the geographical area.
- **Other factors:** Constitutional obligation, political system, health policies, agenda and judiciary obligations.

Classes of Healthcare Settings

Keeping in view the abovementioned factors the health settings are classified as:
- Public sector
- Private sectors
- Voluntary health agencies
- National health programs
- Indigenous system of medicine

Public Sector

Public sector is a government-sponsored system. It is financed by public funds generated through taxes. Services are provided to rural and urban area by three-tier system at block level, district level and state level.

Health Services at Rural Areas

Health services in the rural area are provided through infrastructure, developed right form village to the block level.

Block Level

Organizational structure at block level is developed as under:
- Village level
- Subcenter level

- Primary health center level
- Community health center level

Village Level

To provide basic health facilities at village level, there are four categories of workers who provide healthcare to 1,000 population after getting training at subcenter and primary health center under the supervision of auxiliary nurse and midwife (ANM) and male health worker. They are:

- Traditional birth attendants (TBA)/trained DAIS
- Anganwadi worker
- Accredited social health activist (ASHA)

Trained dais

They are also known as traditional birth attendants. The national objective is to have one trained *dai* in each village. These *dais* have vital role in providing domiciliary midwifery services in rural areas. They are given training for 30 working days at primary health center and subcenter 2 days in a week and remaining four days, they accompany the auxiliary nursing and midwife (ANM) to the village. *Dais* are required to conduct two deliveries under the guidance and supervision of female health worker. Each dai is paid ₹300/- during the training. After completion of training, each dai is provided with a delivery kit and certificate. She is entitled to receive ₹150/- per delivery, provided the case is registered with subcenter or primary health center.

Functions:
- Contact every pregnant woman and get her registered.
- Attend every prenatal clinic.
- Ensure immunization of pregnant woman and newborn babies.
- Motivate eligible couples.
- Report about birth and death in the area to the authorities.
- Provide essential newborn care.
- Postnatal care to the delivery cases.

Anganwadi Workers

Under the Integrated Child Development Services (ICDS) scheme, one Anganwadi worker is appointed for 1,000 population. She is selected from the local community and undergoes training for 4 months. After training, she is paid an honorarium of ₹8000/- per month and if varies, with each state. She is a part-time worker.

Duties of Anganwadi worker include:
- Providing health checkups
- Providing supplementary food
- Taking care of immunization
- Providing informal education
- Taking care of lactating mother, adolescent girls, women of reproductive age (15–40 years) and children under 6 years.

Accredited Social Health Activist (ASHA)

The post of ASHA was created under national rural health service (NRHS) also known as National Rural Health Mission (NRHM). There is one ASHA for 1000 population. She is selected from the same community.

- **Selection of ASHA:** She should be married/divorcee or widow between age group of 25 and 45 years. Minimum education should be up to 10th standard. She should have good knowledge and art of communication and leadership qualities. She is a volunteer worker. The salary of ASHA is incentive based and provided by the state government according to the task performed. The Central Government pays ₹3000/- per month under the Rural Health Mission Scheme. ASHA also is provided travelling allowance for taking patients to health centers.
- **Incentive in ASHA**

  The student can see the Unit 2 of Textbook of Community Health Nursing-II to refer the list of ASHA incentives.
- **Duties of ASHAs:**
  - To create awareness and provide instruction to the community about health, nutrition, personal hygiene and sanitation.
  - To counsel the women on safe pregnancy, delivery, breastfeeding and complementary feeds.
  - To motivate people for adopting small family norms.
  - To work as depot holder for essential medicines, like ORS, iron, folic acid, tablets, chloroquine, oral pills, and disposable delivery kit.
  - To mobilize the community in accessing health services at subcenter and primary health centers.
  - To escort pregnant women requiring treatment.
  - To provide primary medical care for minor ailments.
  - To inform about births and deaths in the village and outbreak of unusual health problems to subcenter and primary health center.
  - To promote constructions of household toilets.

  So, three volunteer workers provide basic healthcare and referral services, at the village level.

Subcenter Level

It is the first peripheral health unit between the community and health services in rural area. It covers a population of 5,000 in plains and 3,000 in hilly area, tribal and backward area. Subcenter is managed by one multipurpose female health worker (ANM) and one multipurpose health worker male and one voluntary worker part time paid ₹100/- per month

Functions:
- Field visits
- Mother and child health (MCH) care and family welfare services
- Immunization of pregnant women and children under 1 year
- Training and supervision of Dais
- IUD insertion
- Simple laboratory investigations
- Health education
- Birth and death registration
- Record maintenance
- School health services

- Information, education and communication activities
- Attending review meetings and submission of reports to PHC medical officer
- Involvement in National Health Program
- Joined health activities with Anganwadi and Balwadi workers
- Coordinating with other agencies and sectors

Primary Health Center Level

Primary Health Center (PHC) is the first contact point between the village community and medical officer. It is the first structural and functional unit of public health services for rendering primary health services and healthcare in peripheral area. PHCs are established and maintained by the state government under the minimum need program. A PHC acts as a referral unit for 6 subcenters and covers a population of 30,000 in plains and 20,000 in hilly, tribal and backward area.

Staffing pattern:
- Medical Officer – 1
- Nurse midwife – 1
- Health worker female ANM – 1
- Pharmacist – 1
- Health educator – 1
- Health assistant male/health supervisor – 1
- Health assistant female/LHV – 1
- Upper division clerk/store keeper – 1
- Lower division clerk, Junior assistant – 1
- Laboratory technician – 1
- Driver (if vehicle is available) – 1
- Class IV workers – 4
  Total – 15
  There are 4–6 beds in some of the primary health centers.

Functions:
- Medical care
- Mother and child healthcare (MCH) and family planning services
- Prevention and control of communicable diseases
- Basic laboratory services
- Training of health workers, local dais and health assistants
- School health services
- Collection and reporting of vital statistics
- Safe water supply and basic sanitation
- Health education
- Referral services
- Prevention of food adulteration practices

Community Health Centers (CHC) Level

Community health centers are maintained by the state government under the Minimum Need Program (MNP). Each CHC has 30 sanctioned beds. It covers a population of 1,20,000 in plain and 80,000 in hilly, tribal and backward area. It acts as a referral unit for four primary health centers.

From community health centers patients are referred to district hospital/health centers if required for consultation and treatment. The specialist services provided at CHC are:

- Surgery
- Medicine
- Obstetrics and gynecology
- Pediatrics
- Dental and ENT

Staffing pattern:
- Medical Officer – 4
- Nurse Midwives – 7
- Dresser   – 1
- Pharmacist   – 1
- Lab technician   – 1
- Radiographer   – 1
- Ward boys   – 2
- Sweepers   – 3
- Aya   – 1
- Peon   – 1
- Dhobi   – 1
- Mali   – 1
- Chowkidar   – 1

　　　　　Total = 25

Functions:
- Routine and emergency surgery
- Routine and emergency medical care
- 24-hours delivery services including surgical intervention, like cesarean section
- Essential and emergency obstetric care
- Newborn care
- Routine and emergency care of sick children
- Blood storage facilities
- Essential laboratory services
- Safe abortion center
- Full range of family planning services including laparoscopic services
- All national health programs
- Other emergency measures, like tracheostomy foreign body removal and nasal packing, etc.
- Referral services

District hospitals, state level hospitals and medical college hospitals: The services to the urban community are provided through these hospitals. These hospitals are also referral units for the rural communities.

Central government hospitals: They provide general as well as referral services.

Defense hospital: These hospitals are financed by central government and provide services only to the defense employees and their families. Defense hospitals have their own medical college, nursing college and nursing schools.

Railway hospital: Railway hospitals are managed by central government and provide services to the railway employees and their families.

Autonomous institutes: Under this category, some institutions receive aid from central government but except few important matters, all other decisions are made by the institutions itself. All India Institute of Medical Sciences (AIIMS) New Delhi, National Institute of Mental Health and Neurosciences (NIMHANS), Bengaluru and Postgraduate Institute (PGI) Chandigarh are the hospitals which provide referral services to the rural and urban communities.

MUST KNOW

Various schemes introduced by government

Employees State Insurance Scheme (ESI): It was introduced in India on the principles of contribution by the employer and employee. It was started under the Parliament Act in 1948 to provide medical benefits in kind and cash during sickness, employment injury, maternity and pension for dependents on the death of worker because of injury. The Act covers employees drawing wages not exceeding ₹21,000/- per month.

Central Government Health Scheme (CGHS): It was introduced in 1954 to start at New Delhi to provide comprehensive healthcare to the central government employees. Later on, it was extended to other cities not only to the employees but also to their family members. It was implemented to the autonomous organization employees, members of the parliament, retired central government servants, widows receiving family pensions governors and retired judges. The scheme is based on the principle of cooperative effort by the employee and employer for the mutual advantages.

The facilities at CGHS are:
- Outpatient care
- Supply of necessary drugs
- Lab and X-ray investigation
- Domiciliary visits
- Hospitalization at government as well as private hospitals
- Referral services
- Pediatric services
- Obstetric services
- Family welfare services
- Emergency treatment
- Supply of optical and dental aids

Private Sectors

In private sectors, there are specialty hospitals, super specialist hospitals, medical colleges hospitals, dispensaries and health clinics. The people who can afford heavy expenses are taking the facilities of healthcare. But these hospitals provide only curative services. Poor and weaker section cannot avail the facilities of private sector clinics.

Mission/religious hospitals: This type of institutions is charitable and run by trust or mission. They provide medical services either free of cost or at minimum rate. They are present in urban areas but provide care to rural area also through camps.

Voluntary Health Agencies

These agencies are nongovernment and nonprofit making. They are initiated, established and administered by private citizens. They are financed by voluntary contributions and donations. These agencies are complementary to the government health agencies. The members of the agencies hold meetings, collect funds for its functioning from the private sources.

Functions

- **Supplementing the work of government agencies:** Government cannot provide complete health services because of financial and statutory restrictions.
- **Education:** Government alone cannot cope with the health education in India unless supplemented by voluntary efforts.
- **Pioneering:** Voluntary health agencies are in a position to find out ways and means of solving problems and getting the solutions of doing things in a fruitful way. Family planning program in India is an example of pioneering by the voluntary agencies.
- **Demonstrations:** By putting up experimental projects, the voluntary health agencies succeeded in its contributions toward healthcare services.
- **Guarding the work of government agencies:** Through their experimental approach, voluntary health agencies are capable of guarding and criticizing the work of government agencies.
- **Advancing health legislation:** It can mobilize public opinions and advance legislation on health matters for the future benefit of the community and country.

Types of Voluntary Health Agencies

Indian Red Cross Society

It was established in 1920 and has 400 branches all over India. It has been executing programs for promotion of health, prevention of disease and mitigation of suffering among the people. It performs the following functions:

- **Relief work:** The Red Cross Society mobilizes its resources immediately to rescue the people during natural calamities, like earthquake, floods, epidemics and drought.
- **Milk and medicine supplies:** Many orphanage homes, schools, maternal and child welfare centers, dispensaries and hospitals, etc. receive milk powder, medicines, vitamins and other supplies.
- **Armed forces:** Care of the sick and wounded in armed forces is the primary obligation of Red Cross. It has got the red cross home in Bangalore for permanently disabled ex-servicemen.
- **Maternal and Child Welfare Services:** There is a bureau of maternity and child welfare which provides technical advice and financial aid to its branches and other interested in improving maternity and child welfare scheme.
- **Family planning:** Several states in India are running family planning clinics under the auspices of Indian Red Cross.
- **Blood bank and first aid:** Some of the branches started blood banks, St. John Ambulance Association of India which is a part of Red Cross, trained lacs of men and women in first aid, home nursing and allied subjects.

Hind Kusht Nivaran Sangh

It was established in 1950 with its headquarter in New Delhi. It provides financial assistance to various leprosy homes and clinics. It also provides health education through publication and posters. Training to the medical workers and physiotherapists is also imparted by this agency. It conducts research and field investigations on leprosy. It has got branches all over India and works in close association with government and other agencies.

Indian Council for Child Welfare

It was started in 1952 and affiliated with international union for child welfare. It has branches in all states and districts all over India. The services are devoted to secure Indian children. These opportunities and facilities by law and other means, "helps enabling the children to develop physically, mentally, socially and spiritually in a healthy and normal manner and in conditions of freedom and dignity".

Tuberculosis Association of India

It was established in 1939. It has got branches in all the states of India. Its activities are organizing TB Seal Campaign every year to raise funds, training of doctors, health visitors and social workers in antituberculosis work, promotion of consultations and conferences. The institutions under the management of Association are: The New Delhi Tuberculosis Center, The Lady Linlithgow Sanatorium at Kasauli, The King Edward VII Sanatorium at Dharampur and the Tuberculosis Hospital at Mehrauli.

Bharat Sevak Samaj

The Bharat Sevak Samaj was formed in 1952. It is nonpolitical and nonofficial organization. It helps people to achieve health by their own action and efforts. Its branches are in all states and districts. Its important activity is to improve sanitation in villages.

Central Social Welfare Board

It was set up by the Government of India in 1953. It is an autonomous organization under the general administrative control of Ministry of Education.

Functions:
- Surveying the needs and requirements of voluntary welfare organization in the country
- Promoting and setting up of social welfare organizations on a voluntary basis
- Rendering of financial assistance to deserving existing organization and institutions

Kasturba Memorial Fund

This fund was created in 1944 after the death of Kasturba Gandhi. The main objective of this fund is to raise the standard of women, especially in the villages through *gram sevikas*. The trust is actively engaged in the various projects in the country.

Family Planning Association of India

It was started in 1949 with its headquarter at Mumbai. Association has branches all over the country and clinics with grants-in-aid from the government. Hundreds of doctors, health visitors and social workers have been trained on the aspects of family planning. Association has done commendable work in propagating family planning in India. Headquarter is answerable to enquiries on family planning.

All India Women's Conference

It was originated in 1926 and runs branches all over the country. It is the only women's voluntary welfare organization in India. Most of the branches are running MCH clinics, medical centers, adult education centers, milk centers and family planning clinics.

The All India Blind Relief Society

It was formed in 1946 with a view to coordinate different institutions working for the blind. It organizes eye relief camps and other means for the relief of the blind.

Professional Bodies

The Indian Medical Association, All India Licentiates Association, All India Dental Association and Trained Nurses Association of India are the voluntary agencies of men and women who are qualified in their respective fields of specialties and possess registrable qualification. These professional bodies conduct annual conferences, publish journals and arrange specific scientific sessions and exhibition, poster, research and set up standards of professional education. They also organize relief camps during periods of natural calamities.

International Agencies

There are international health agencies which provide technical and material assistance in planning and implementation of various health programs. These agencies include WHO, UNICEF, World Bank, United Nations Fund for Population Activities (UNPFA), United States Agency for International Development (USAID), Cooperative for Assistance and Relief Everywhere (CARE).

NATIONAL HEALTH PROGRAMS

In addition to various levels of healthcare settings, the Government of India has put up lots of efforts to deal with various health problems at national level. These problems include communicable and noncommunicable diseases, environmental sanitation, nutrition problems, population problems, etc.

Indigenous System of Medicine

During the last few years constructive efforts have been made to strengthen the indigenous system of medicine in the public sector of healthcare in both rural and urban areas. The services of indigenous system are provided through outdoor patient departments, dispensaries and hospital. The system includes—Ayurveda, Siddha, Unani, Homeopathy, Naturopathy and Yoga (AYUSH).

Referral Services

In India, health services are provided at three levels considering the three levels of prevention (Fig. 7.3). At each level, the facilities for health services are organized as per the planning to cater to the specific type of health needs of the client. No one level is equipped to meet all the health needs of the client and it is not possible to make each level functioning efficiently for providing comprehensive healthcare, WHO has identified the provision of referral system as one of the major supportive activities for primary healthcare, so the referral system has been established in such a way that cases can be referred from primary level of care to the secondary level of care to the tertiary level of care according to the clients health needs. This type of link between the healthcare settings is known as referral chain.

Primary health center is the first medical reference point in the health system chain. Each system performs its function for which it is established.

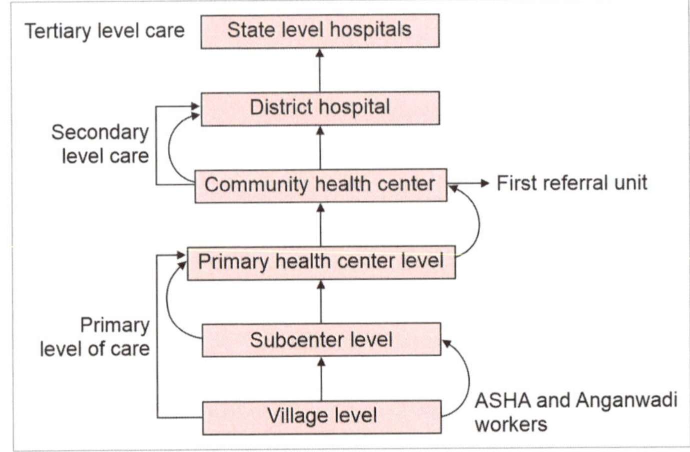

Fig. 7.3: Referral system

Purposes

- Helps in early diagnosis and treatment of the case under the specialist care
- Cost effective system
- Reduces the duration of stay of the patient in hospital
- Limits the progress of the disease
- Prevents complications by starting appropriate timely care
- Teaches the nursing personnel for reviewing of patients sent for referral

In the referral system chain, the patients can be referred from the village level by ASHA, trained dais and Anganwadi worker to the subcenter level. From subcenter, they are referred by health worker to the primary health centers, which is the first medical reference point. From primary health center, the doctor refers the cases which require specialist care to the community health center. The community health center is the first referral unit. Any unit which has got round the clock (24 × 7) services for emergency obstetric and newborn care in addition to all routine emergency care and blood storage facility for 24 hours is called first referral unit (FRU).

Functions of First Referral Unit

- Surgical function
- Medical treatment function
- Blood transfusion function
- Manual functioning
- Anesthetic function
- Obstetric and neonatal care function.

Steps in Referral

The steps to be taken are as follows:

1. Selection of Cases

It depends upon the condition of the patient and the facilities available in the health center. Patients to be referred are categorized under three groups.

i. **First group or fatal cases:** When it is known that prognosis of the case is poor and patient cannot survive in spite of best treatment made available to him/her. Referring such cases is simply wastage of time and money. Such patients are treated at the health center where they are admitted with the available resources. The relatives of the patients are made to understand about the condition of the patient and the reason for not referring.

ii. **Second group or serious patients:** This type of cases where the condition of the patient is serious but immediate treatment can save the lives of the patients. Such patients are immediately referred and shifted after giving emergency life-saving support.

iii. **Third group or common patients:** In this type of cases, the disease of the patient is serious but the condition of the patient is normal. Such patients are referred to as routine cases for diagnosis and treatment and consultation of the specialist.

2. Types of Cases to be Referred Urgently

- Any life-threatening conditions, like severe hemorrhage, shock, cyanosis, head injury, multiple fractures
- Severe chest pain
- Coma due to any cause
- Acute abdomen, intestinal obstruction hemoptysis, hematemesis, black-colored stool
- Convulsions more than one attack
- Severe pain in any part of the body that is continuous for >3 days
- Hyperpyrexia not responding to the treatment.
- Frequent vomiting, absence of bowel sound, severe diarrhea and dehydration, not responding to the treatment.
- Obstructed labor, complicated deliveries
- Suspected cases of tetanus
- Severe burns
- Poisonous cases
- Any other fatal or life-threatening condition

3. Preparation of the Case to be Referred

The patient and his/her family members are explained about the condition of the patient and need for referring to the next unit. Once the doctor has written the orders for referring, the referring form is filled and signed by the referring doctor. Patient's valuable and other belongings are handed over to the relatives. No dues are cleared by the patient. All medical documents, investigation reports, X-ray, ECG, etc., are kept ready to send along with the patient.

4. Shifting of Cases to the Next Referral Unit

After getting all the documents ready, the next referral unit is informed telephonically briefing about the condition of the patient, reason for referring so that before the patient could reach, bed is made ready with all the emergency equipment and drugs made available at the bedside and the concerned specialist to be informed about the time of arrival of the patient.

The referral unit will arrange an ambulance. The nursing staff collects all the patient's documents, the referral documents, the referral form and other emergency drugs or oxygen, IV drip, etc. required on the way according to the condition of the patient and doctor's advice in cases required, to be collected. If not used should be brought back and handed over to the head nurse. Staff nurse accompanying the patient should hand over the patient to the concerned staff in the referring unit with his/her vital parameters, treatment chart and case file with referral form and take the signature of the person.

5. Referral Form

All the units have printed referral forms which is filled by the referring doctors with patients' particular brief history of case treatment given and reasons for referring. A sample of Referral Form is as under:

Referral Form

Name of the health center/hospital:

Referral Registration No.: .... Date: ....

Name of the patient: .... Date and time of Admission: ....

Father's/Husband's/Guardian's Name: ....

Age: .... Sex: .... Religion: .... Occupation: ....

Permanent Address: ....

Telephone of next of kin: ....

Present diagnosis: ....

Case history in brief: ....

Description of treatment: ....

Reason for referring: ....

Enclosure and papers like:
- Case File
- X-ray, ECG
- Investigation reports, etc.

Sign of the Referring Doctor

(Name in Capital Letter)

Designation

Seal of the Health Center

6. Feedback

Referral system is usually two-way process and the retention of the patient in referral unit should be as brief as possible. As soon as the required investigations are over, the proper diagnosis made on the basis of clinical findings and the specialists' consultation, the line of treatment is decided which can be carried out at the parent health center. Patients should be returned to the parent center once the patient is responding to the new line of treatment. In this way, other serious patients will also get their chance for the consultation.

Role of Nurse in Referral Service

- Inform the referring unit telephonically before shifting about the condition of the case and treatment so that bed is readily available with all emergency equipment at bed side and specialist is available to see the case.

- Nurse should explain the patient and family for reasons of referring to secondary and tertiary level of healthcare.
- Nurse should check the condition of the patient whether he/she is fit to be shifted immediately or some emergency treatment is required till the condition is stable. In such cases, inform the doctor about the condition of the patient.
- Collect all the documents of the patient, like case file, investigation reports, X-rays, ECG treatment chart, vital chart, intake output chart, etc., which are to be sent along with patient.
- Check the referral form whether filled completely and signed by the referring doctor with brief history of the case.
- Patient's belonging and valuable to be handed over to his/her relatives.
- If the patient is to be shifted with life support treatment, like oxygen, IV life line drip, nurse should accompany the patient along with another attendant to the referring unit.
- Nurse should take clear instructions in writing from the treating physicians about the treatment to be given on the way if need arises in cases of emergency.
- Nurse should hand over the patient, his document and take signature of the person who has taken over the patient in the presence of some witness.
- All nursing personnel working in subcenters primary health center, community health center and district hospital should have knowledge of referrals system.

Interdisciplinary Referral System

Sometimes patients cannot be treated or diagnosed properly with the system of medicine and may not get satisfied with one type of therapy. They can be referred to another therapy. This type of referral system is called interdisciplinary referral system. In India, patients are shifted from allopathy to AYUSH. Government of India has made provision in some of the centers to avail such facilities. There is a plan to have all therapies under one roof.

Summary

- In public system of healthcare, the healthcare services are provided at three levels.
- Primary level of healthcare is the setting of healthcare which provides first level of contact between the community and healthcare provider at the grassroots level. At this level, most of the health problems are solved with some guidance, education and assistance and treatment by the team of health professionals.
- Primary healthcare is provided at subcenter and primary health center, secondary level of healthcare is provided at community health center and district hospitals, where the specialist services are available and tertiary level of care is provided at state level, regional level and central level institutions.
- Referral system is the system in which the patients are transferred from primary level healthcare to the secondary level of healthcare from secondary level to the tertiary level of healthcare.
- No one level is equipped to meet all the health needs of the client. The cases which cannot be managed at primary level of care are referred to secondary level and cases which cannot be managed at secondary level are referred to tertiary level of care. At each level, nurses should know the need of referral and type of cases to be referred.
- All documents should be collected and completed before sending the patient to referral unit. A feedback should also be taken about the patient from the referral unit.

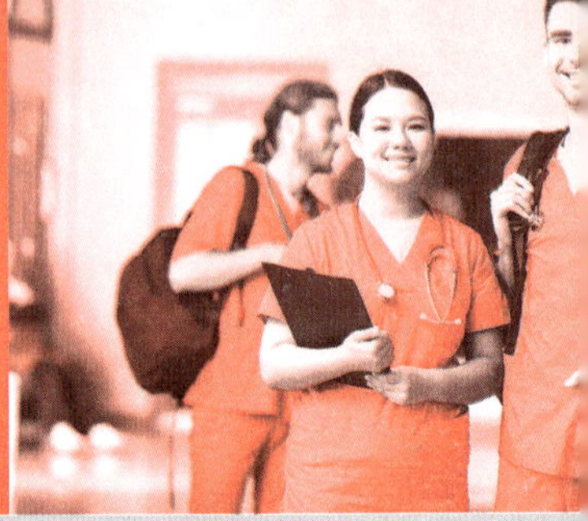

STUDENT ASSIGNMENT

LONG ANSWER TYPE QUESTIONS

1. Define referral system and explain the purposes of referring the client from one unit to another.
2. Describe the levels of healthcare.
3. Enlist the staffing pattern at each level of healthcare.
4. Explain the type of services provided at secondary level of healthcare.

SHORT ANSWER TYPE QUESTIONS

1. Write short notes on:
   a. Need for urgent referral
   b. Role of nurse in referral system
2. What do you understand by referral system?

MULTIPLE CHOICE QUESTIONS

1. **A patient at subcenter can be referred to:**
   a. Primary health center
   b. Community health canter
   c. District hospital
   d. Any of these

2. **The criteria for referring a patient:**
   a. Condition of the patient
   b. Availability of resources in referring unit
   c. Availability of specialist's services and advanced technology
   d. All of the above

3. **The functions of Indian Red Cross Society:**
   a. Blood bank and first aid
   b. Milk and medicine supply
   c. Maternal and child welfare series
   d. All of these

4. **The referral chain is:**
   a. Village → subcenter → PHC → CHC → state level
   b. CHC → subcenter → Village → PHC → state level
   c. Subcenter → PHC → village → CHC → state level
   d. PHC → CHC → subcenter → state level → village

ANSWER KEY

1. a   2. d   3. d   4. a

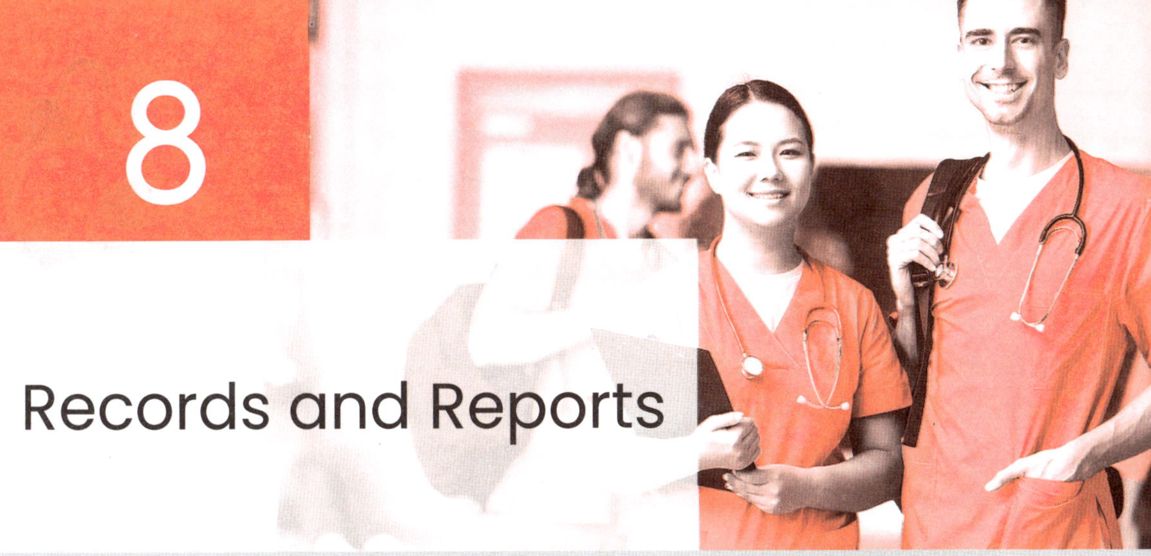

8

Records and Reports

LEARNING OBJECTIVES

After the completion of the unit, the readers will be able to:
* Differentiate between records and reports.
* Enlist the types of records maintained in hospitals, clinics and community area.
* Discuss the records and reports along with their principles.
* Explain the role and responsibilities of nursing personnel in maintaining records and reports.

UNIT OUTLINE

* Introduction
* Records
* Reports
* Essential Requirements of Records and Reports
* Preparation and Maintenance of Records and Reports

KEY TERMS

Records: The presentation of facts, figures, date and other information in writing are maintained in records.
Reports: Giving information about something to someone is done through reports which may be written or verbal.

INTRODUCTION

Records and reports are excellent tools of communication in any organization to function efficiently. Information is transmitted from downward to upward and from upward to downward. Effective communication is vital to the client care among health professionals. Nurses as a member of the healthcare team communicate information about the client's condition through records and reports among the healthcare providers. Clients depend on nurses to communicate their health problems to the doctors and others concerned with the doctors for best quality of care. It is essential for all the members of healthcare team to have accurate practice of maintaining records and reports.

RECORDS

Records are the presentation of facts, figures, date and other information in writing. A record is a permanent written presentation of information.

In healthcare setting, a record is a clinical, scientific, administrative and legal document relating to the nursing care given to the individual, family and community. Records are practical and indispensable tools of doctors, nurses and other paramedical staff to plan and deliver the best possible care to the client.

Principles of Writing Records

- Records should be written immediately, after an event has occurred.
- Records should be genuine based on facts, observation, conversation and action.
- Only accepted abbreviations should be used.
- Short and clear sentences should be used.
- Records should be appropriate, accurate and legible.
- Records are valuable legal documents; so, they should be kept confidential.
- Records should be written with blue ball point ink.
- Uniformity in writing records should be maintained.

Uses of Records

For Staff Nurses/Community Health Nurses

- Help to plan and implement care for the client.
- Help to evaluate the care and teaching given to the client.
- Prevent duplication of work.
- Help to assess the quality and quantity of care given.
- Provide protection in case of legal issues.
- Serve as a guide to the professional growth.
- Help in auditing the nursing care.

For Doctors

- Guide for diagnosis, treatment and follow-up care.
- Help in evaluating the services provided.
- Indicate the progress of the patient and continuity of care.
- Useful for doctors in making research and in medical practice.

For Health Agency

- Records are the proof of services provided by each worker.
- Help in auditing the care provided to clients.
- Help the administration in assessing the performance of their own institution.
- Used as an evaluation tool during conferences and meeting.
- Provide justification for expenditure of funds.
- Assist in finding out health problems of community unit.
- Legal document for community health activities.
- Assist in determining the need of resources like medicine, equipment and manpower.
- Means of communication between health workers, family and community.

For Individuals

- Help to make them aware of their health needs.
- Serve as a guide for future treatment and care.

Types of Records

Records are broadly divided into four categories:

1. **Periodical records:** These are of two types:
   i. **Temporary records:** These are casual or daily records.
   ii. **Permanent records:** These are cumulative or continuing records. These are the student's health records, once made and carried out to the next standard about health information of students like immunization, weight, height and other health check-up every year on the same card. It is possible to review the total history of the child/individual and evaluate the progress over a long period.

      Similarly, cumulative records of nursing students regarding their learning experience are added on the same record as and when they learn.

2. **Unit based records:** These include:
   - Individual records include individual health card
   - Family record of family folder
   - Community records—records of health problems of the community
   - National Health Program Records

3. **Subject based records:** These include:
   - Medical and nursing records pertaining to the treatment and medicine records
   - Economic records—financial structure of family and village
   - Social records—records of social structure
   - Political records

4. **Collection place-based record:** These include:
   - Collected at institutions, i.e., records of hospitals and health centers
   - Records to be kept with individuals, e.g., immunization card, disease card

Designing of Cards/Records

There are three designs of cards on which records are maintained:

1. **Folder type:** It is a broad card which can be folded into many parts, say 8 or 10. Some pages are kept blank for future entries.

2. **File type:** A file is maintained for each patient. The outer part of the file is usually printed for summarizing information. Periodical data is entered in separate papers and inserted into the file. The file type records are usually maintained in the hospital for patients.

3. **Envelope type:** It is a file type that is closed on three sides and kept open on one side. The data is entered on separate papers, tagged together and inserted into envelope.

Records Maintained at Hospitals, Health Centers, Nursing Education Institutes and Miscellaneous Sites

Records Maintained at Hospitals

It is the duty of the head nurse for keeping administrative and educational records. Some of the important records required to be maintained are:

- Admission and discharge register of patients
- Treatment register
- Laboratory investigation register
- Staff attendance and leave register
- Patients' day and night report register
- Equipment stock register
- Linen register, Dhobi book and laundry register
- Drug indent and maintenance register
- Medical officer on call duty register
- Condemnation register
- Census register
- Diet register
- Complaint register
- Birth and death register
- Accounts register
- Inventory registers
- Bed side charts, vital register (TPR and BP)
- Operation register
- Conferences/Meeting register
- Suggestion register

Records Maintained at Primary Health Centers

- **General information records:** These include records of individuals, families, village and map of community, facts, pictures and health information.
- **Outdoor patients records.**
- **Treatment and referral records:** These include records related to treatment of health problems and records of the referred patients to the other health unit.
- **Family welfare records:** These include medical termination of pregnancy (MTP) records, eligible couple record, family planning records.
- **Vital event records:** Register of birth and death.
- Stock register for equipment and drugs.
- Medicine distribution register.
- **Mother and child health records:** These include antenatal, postnatal and immunization records
- Infant and preschool children record.
- **Family folder:** This includes family structure and individual records.
- **Other records:** These include attendance register, medicine stock register, meeting records, monthly and yearly report register, stationery stock register, patients' registration records, depot holder record, daily diary cumulative records, training register.

Records Maintained at Subcenter Level

- Mother care register
- Child care register
- Program register
- Daily dairy
- Review register
- Stock register
- Monthly report register
- Family welfare register
- Referral register
- School health register
- General information register
- Eligible couple register

Records Maintained at Village Level

- Birth and death register
- Mother care record register
- Child care record register, growth chart
- Immunization register
- Eligible couple register

Records Maintained at Nursing Education Institutes

Student Records

- Admission application forms
- Health records
- Attendance register
- Leave records
- Progress reports
- Internal assessment
- Clinical experience record
- Daily diary
- Cumulative records
- Anecdotal records
- Course plan
- Unit plan
- Clinical rotation plan
- Student Nurses' Association (SNA) meeting register

Teaching Faculty and Other Staff Records

- Job description
- Education qualification, experience records
- Progress record
- Leave record
- Attendance record
- Staff development register
- Staff meeting register

General Records

- Inventory register
- Records of meeting of university
- Council/university inspection register
- Dispatch register
- Indent register
- Philosophy, purpose and curriculum of college
- Budget of the college
- Sports and extracurricular activities
- Copy of the school/college brochure
- Various files related to administration

Records to be Kept with Patients

- Health records of school going child
- Infant health records including immunization
- Records of antenatal and postnatal mother
- Records of tuberculosis patients
- Individual health cards

Though the cards are prepared and kept at health center, some records should be with the individuals. If a family migrates to some other place, information regarding their health is available.

> **MUST KNOW**
>
> **Relation between Records and Reports**
> Records and reports are interdependent. Reports are written based on records. Reports can also be presented as record. Records are always in written form, whereas report can be written as well as verbal. Records can be preserved, whereas verbal reports can be forgotten. In spite of being different, both seem synonymous and are interdependent. Both are important tools of communication and management in hospitals and community health centers and nursing.

REPORTS

Reports are the verbal or written information shared between health workers. They summarize the activities and services of nurses and healthcare workers.

Types of Reports

Reports are of two types:

1. *Verbal Reports*

Verbal reports are more convenient when the information is meant for immediate use. Sometimes in emergency, verbal reports are followed by written reports later on, e.g., nurse in charge of patient care reports about the condition of patient to the treating physician telephonically and takes instructions about patient care. Later on, she puts these instructions in writing. Similarly, while changing shifts, nurses handover with verbal reports along with written reports. Verbal reports are also made about certain complaints for immediate rectification, e.g., about emergency equipment, etc. or in case of occurrence of some unusual incident which should be immediately reported to the concerned authorities, verbally and later on in writing.

Types of Verbal Reports

- Report between head nurse and staff nurse during round of head nurse
- Report between the members of health team
- Reports on accident, mistakes and complaints while changing the shift
- Report between student nurses and clinical instructor

Advantages of Verbal Reports

- Help to deal with emergency when time is premium
- Help in implementing proper care of patients on verbal instructions
- Provide feedback
- Save time, build up confidence and maintain good interpersonal relations (IPR) among the health professionals
- Serve as a primary source of information

Disadvantages of Verbal Reports

- Possibility of mistakes due to wrong interpretation
- No proof, personnel can deny what was told.
- No permanent record is present.
- Can result in legal problems.
- Not useful in legal matters.

2. *Written Reports*

Reports are written when the information has to be used by several persons which is of permanent value. Examples of written reports are:

- Day and night reports
- Census
- Interdepartmental reports
- Weekly reports
- Monthly reports
- Special reports on unusual incidents
- Accident reports
- Evaluation reports
- Transfer reports
- Legal reports

Uses of Reports

Uses of reports are as follows:

- Reports give information about the condition of the patients and day-to-day progress of patients' health.
- They are used as an aid in planning patient care
- In community, they help in studying the health problems of an area so that an appropriate action can be taken to solve them.
- They are used in health planning.
- They show the kind and number of services rendered in a community.
- They help in future budget planning.
- They serve as a legal document.

ESSENTIAL REQUIREMENTS OF RECORDS AND REPORTS

Essential requirements of records and reports are as follows:

- These are valuable documents and should be filled carefully.
- They should be complete with complete details.
- Good filling system should be developed for records and reports.
- They should be easily available on time.
- Confidential records and reports should be shown to the authorized person only.

- They should be written in such a way that minimum clerical work is involved.
- Confidentiality should be maintained as they get legal importance.
- They should be placed at a definite and safe place.

PREPARATION AND MAINTENANCE OF RECORDS AND REPORTS

Preparation of records: Records should be filled properly in a systematic way to save time and energy. Filling of records further depends upon the objectives and methods adopted by the health center or hospital. Some of the methods commonly used are:

- Alphabetically
- Numerically
- Geographically

Some of the organizations use general and specific methods. They may combine the abovementioned methods/techniques.

Preparation of Reports

A report refers to a written document that includes the outcome of an investigation, project or initiative. It is supposed to be an in-depth analysis of a particular issue. It is prepared to inform, educate and present options and recommendations for further action.

Nursing Considerations

Guidelines while Preparing Records
- Records should be clear, appropriate with legible handwriting.
- Records should be based on facts and reality.
- Short and clear sentences should be used.
- Only acceptable abbreviations and short forms should be used in records.
- Special attention should be paid to numbers and statistics.
- Should be filled with royal blue ink as blank ink fades away with time.
- Person who is filling the records should sign in capital letters.

Guidelines while Preparing Reports
- Reports should be written in such a way that all essential information can be easily retrieved.
- Important information should be highlighted.
- Presentation should be attractive and important points should be stressed.
- The style of report writing should be made easy to understand.
- Vocabulary used in report writing should be simple.
- Reports should be written based on information and supervision.
- Reports should be presented correctly to avoid mistakes.
- Actual facts should be presented and reports should not contain personal feelings.
- All information and material should be collected before writing report.
- General method or outline of writing the report should be prepared before actually writing the report.
- Printed forms should be used as far as possible to save time.

Maintenance of Records and Reports

- Since the records and reports have legal implications, it is the duty of the nurse in charge of maintaining the records and reports and keeping them under safe custody.

- There should be no room left for leakage of information contained in the records and reports.
- Nurse should maintain records and reports immediately after the incident.
- Written records and reports should be preserved in a chronological order so that they are easily available whenever required.
- Records and reports should be handled carefully to avoid destruction.
- Records and reports should be protected from mice, termites, insects, etc.
- Records related to medicolegal cases, dying declaration, will, etc., should be handled carefully for giving witness wherever required.
- People get facilities and legal protection based on records. In such cases, the Xerox copy of the records can be given and entered in the register only with the written permission of authorized person.
- Records should be made accurate and there should be no mistake.
- Records and reports of medicolegal cases should be kept under lock and key.
- Legally accepted method should be used for destructing absolute records.

Summary

- Records and reports are necessary to collect useful information for assessing the health problems and health needs of the individuals, families and community.
- The records kept at subcenter levels are vital event records, eligible couple record, family folder, MCH care record, family welfare records.
- The records should be written promptly after providing services.
- Records should be clear, legible, accurate, complete and written with blue ball point ink.
- Reports are summarized services either in written or verbal form.
- Records have legal value; so, they should be kept under lock and key.
- No unauthorized person should have access to the records and reports.
- Nurses are responsible for maintaining records and reports in hospitals as well as in community settings.

STUDENT ASSIGNMENT

LONG ANSWER TYPE QUESTIONS

1. Describe the need to keep records and make reports.
2. Explain the various types of records maintained at hospitals, primary health centers and nursing education institutes.

SHORT ANSWER TYPE QUESTIONS

1. Write about the principles of record writing and importance of records.
2. Define reports.
3. Name different types of reports.
4. Write a short note on:
   a. Legal implications in record maintenance
   b. Elements of reports
   c. How to write records and reports
   d. Daily diary
   e. Monthly report

MULTIPLE CHOICE QUESTIONS

1. **Which of the following is not true about writing records and reports?**
   a. Write legibly
   b. Accurate and complete in all respects
   c. Consult the supervisor in case of difficulty in writing
   d. It is a formality and can be written at any time.

2. **The advantage(s) of patient related health records is (are):**
   a. Saves time in finding the card at the clinic
   b. It is of great value when patient moves to another place
   c. Useful for health workers visiting the home and an aid in health education
   d. All of the above

3. **Which of the following record is not maintained at subcenter?**
   a. Village records, family folders, individual health record
   b. Eligible couple register, contraceptive records
   c. Criminal and antisocial element record
   d. Daily diary, stock register for receipt, issue and balance of drugs, stationery, etc.

4. The element of report which presents facts not personal feeling to give true picture is called:
   a. Objectivity
   b. Correctness
   c. Clarity
   d. Brevity

5. **Which of the following is not true regarding records?**
   a. Recorded facts have value and scientific accuracy
   b. Records are a means of communication between the health worker and family
   c. Records help the nurse to organize work and save time
   d. Records can bring out certain hidden facts about a person which can be evidence against that person

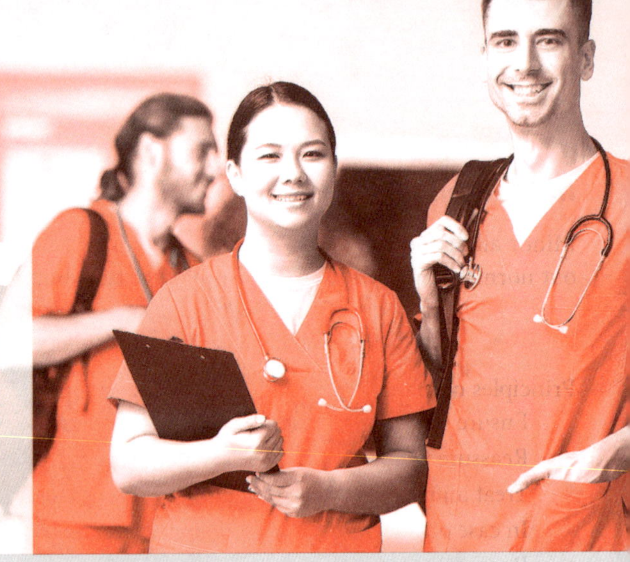

9

Minor Ailments

INTRODUCTION

Minor ailments include slight illness as well as emergencies of smaller nature. Minor ailment/illness may be acute which requires immediate treatment or it may be chronic which needs treatment for a longer period and continuous supervision, but associated complications require the help of a nurse. Since community health nurse is responsible to provide primary healthcare, she has to provide treatment of minor illness and manage the emergencies of smaller nature. Nurse should be capable of examining the signs and symptoms of the ailments and treating within her capabilities and following the limitation as per the standing orders prepared by the medical officer. People suffer from minor illnesses which are not necessarily long lasting and may not require doctor's attention but cause discomfort. Such ailments can be managed by community health nurse by following the guidelines of standing orders.

MINOR AILMENT/ILLNESS

Minor ailment/illness is defined as "any illness which does not prevent the patient from carrying out normal functions for a short period of time but is associated with some discomfort".

Principles of Managing Minor Ailments

Principles of managing minor ailments are as follows:

- Ensure safe and comfortable environment for the patient.
- Reassure the patient and family members.
- Treat injured/ill person properly to prevent any possible complication.
- In case of communicable diseases, isolate the patient to prevent the spread of infection.
- Record vital signs and keep continuous watch over patient's general condition.
- Help the patient to rehabilitate as early as possible.
- Provide health education to the patient and family during the treatment.
- Always follow the physician's instructions mentioned in standing orders and stick to the limitations in providing treatment.
- Help the family members in coping with the situations and prepare them for taking care of patient at home.
- Respect the belief of the patient if he has taken some other therapy for his treatment.
- In case of serious condition or whenever there is a doubt about the diagnosis, refer the patient to the hospital/or next referring unit immediately.

Classification of Minor Ailments

Minor ailments are classified (Fig. 9.1) into the following:
- General minor ailments
- Systemic minor ailments

General Minor Ailments

General minor ailments include common accidents, injuries, falls, fractures, burns, dog bite, high fever, heat stroke, diarrhea and fainting requiring immediate first aid treatment.

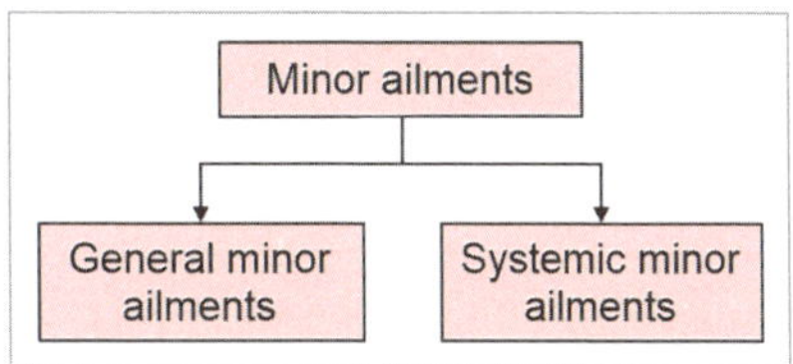

Fig. 9.1: Types of minor ailments

Systemic Minor Ailments

Systemic minor ailments include ailments of various systems of the body. Some of the common systemic minor ailments are the following:

- **Eye:** Accidental injury, foreign bodies, infections, poor eye sight, dry eyes and night blindness.
- **Ear:** Earache, foreign bodies in the ear, otitis media, itching, discharge from the ear, temporary deafness.
- **Respiratory tract:** Allergic rhinitis, common cold, sinusitis, sore throat, cough, dyspnea, asthmatic attack.

- **Cardiovascular system:** Hypertension, anemia, rheumatic heart disease, etc.
- **Digestive system:** Toothache, stomatitis, soreness in mouth, constipation, diarrhea, indigestion, vomiting, abdominal pain, distension of abdomen, hemorrhoid, etc.
- **Urinary system:** Burning micturition, urinary tract infections, renal stones, retention of urine
- **Neuromuscular system:** Headache, backache, convulsion, epileptic fits.
- **Reproductive system:** Dysmenorrhea, heavy bleeding, sores and discharge from genitals, breast lump, etc.

Apart from the abovementioned minor ailments, there may be behavioral problems, maladjustment or emotional disturbances which are also included in minor ailments but these require diagnosis and appropriate treatment.

Management of Minor Ailments

While providing treatment and first aid care in case of minor ailments, nurses must observe the following points:

- Assessment of the case by:
    - Taking history from the patient or relatives
    - Quick physical examination
- Finding the cause, making diagnosis and planning care as per the standing orders of the specific case.
- Providing the treatment and nursing care.
- Evaluating the outcome of the treatment, care given and condition of the patient.
- If there is improvement in the patient's condition, plan for follow-up care.
- If no improvement in patients' condition is seen and the condition is becoming serious, immediately refer to the hospital for necessary action.

STANDING ORDERS

Standing orders are the directions and guidelines about the management of ailments of specific nature made available in health units. On the basis of these, the nurses and health workers can follow the standing orders to treat emergencies at home, at hospitals or health institutions and in the community in the absence of doctor. These standing orders are issued by a team of doctors in which a nurse is also represented.

Objectives

Objectives of standing orders are as follows:

- To resuscitate the patient in case of emergency.
- To protect the life of the patient.
- To maintain the continuity of treatment of the patient.
- To ensure accountability of patient care being a member of the health team.
- To promote health services in the community.

Uses

Uses of standing orders are as follows:

- To provide first aid and emergency treatment in rural area in the absence of doctor.
- To minimize the complications of ailments.
- To strengthen the activities of health facilities in the community.
- To decentralize the health responsibilities.
- To build up the confidence of general public in community health service.
- To protect the general public from quacks.
- To enhance the primary healthcare services in the community.
- To create a sense of responsibility and confidence among the nurses and other members of the health team.

Types

Standing orders are divided into three categories (Fig. 9.2):

1. Specific Standing Orders

Specific standing orders are prepared for trained medical personnel, mainly for nurses. Technical knowledge and special skill are required to implement these orders. For example, giving injection, administering oxygen, home nursing, etc.

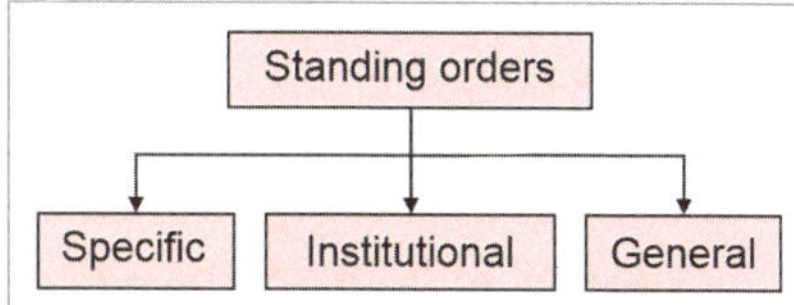

Fig. 9.2: Types of standing orders

These specific standing orders compensate for the need of a doctor. Most of the treatment-related decisions are to be made by the community health nurse or institutional nurse. Specific standing orders strengthen the healthcare services.

2. Institutional Standing Orders

Institutional standing orders are prepared considering the available resources, staff position and objectives of medical units. Standing orders for primary health centers are different than that for district hospitals. Similarly, standing orders for government medical institutions are different than that for private hospitals or clinics.

3. General Standing Orders

General standing orders are used for a large population and geographical area where there is a shortage of health resources to propagate the health messages. Examples of such standing orders include drinking ORS in case of severe dehydration and diarrhea, taking chloroquine tablets in case of fever with chills and rigor, giving hydrotherapy and plenty of oral fluids in case of high fever, creating awareness about protection from dengue fever, AIDS, etc.

STANDING ORDERS FOR THE TREATMENT/MANAGEMENT OF MINOR AILMENTS

Many times, nurses in the hospital, primary health centers, subcenters or in community health centers face the situations that patient require treatment when the doctor is not available or is likely to come late. In such condition, standing orders safeguard nurses to provide treatment to the patients. Standing orders for treating/managing various ailments are given in the subsequent sections.

Standing Orders for Management of Fever

Standing orders for management of fever are as follows:

- Make the patient comfortable and reassure him/her.
- Take history of fever, its onset, duration whether accompanied by shivering, headache, nausea, vomiting, running nose, allergy, skin infections, jaundice, cough, burning micturition, etc.
- Check temperature, pulse, respiration and blood pressure.
- Prepare blood slides to examine malaria parasite.
- Keep patient in well-ventilated room.
- Give plenty of oral fluids like fruit juice, soup, tea, coffee, coconut water, rice, water.
- Give antipyretics like Tab. Paracetamol after calculating the doze.
- Provide light meals like Khichri, Dalia, Suji, bread, etc.
- If fever is >39°C (102.7°F), give hydrotherapy.
- Monitor the pattern of fever for 2 days. If fever is accompanied with rashes over the body, keep the patient in isolation, and if necessary, inform the physician.
- If hyperpyrexia is accompanied with delirium, convulsion or unconsciousness, refer to the hospital for management.

Standing Orders for Management of Heat Stroke

Heat stroke occurs due to exposure of skin to hot weather for a prolonged period. It is characterized by high fever, headache, rapid pulse and dehydration.

Standing orders for management of heat stroke are as follows:

- Keep the patient in shade or in well-ventilated room. Open all the doors and windows and put on fans.
- Record temperature, pulse, respiration and blood pressure.
- Watch out for signs of dehydration.
- Remove all the clothes and wrap the patient in wet sheet, give cold sponge till the temperature falls below 100°F.
- If conscious, give plenty of cold fluids like lime juice with salt, coconut water, rice water, lassi.
- Reassure the patient and family members.
- Record temperature every 15 minutes till it falls below 100°F.
- As soon as there is improvement in patients' condition, refer to the doctor.

Standing Orders for Management of Burns

Standing orders for management of burns are as follows:
- Take quick history of burns.
- The immediate treatment for all kinds of burns is to pour cold water over the burnt area (except on acid burns where alkaline solution is poured). Cold water prevents further damage to tissue from heat.
- Do not try to remove the stuck clothes from the burnt area, it will cause more damage to the tissues.
- Pouring cold water separates the stuck clothes from the burnt area and reduces pain.
- Do not touch or break the blisters but bangles, rings and belt should be removed.
- Assess the percentage of burnt area. Check the condition of the patient and record vital signs.
- Keep the burnt area covered with clean clothes to prevent from dust and flies.
- If the patient is in shock, give him/her primary treatment of shock.
- If the patient is conscious and not vomiting, give ORS, fruit juice with plenty of salt to replace fluid and electrolyte.
- Superficial burns are more painful, give analgesic, if required.
- Record urinary output.
- Reassure the patient and family member.
- Refer the patient to hospital for further management.

Standing Orders for Management of Diarrhea

Diarrhea is passing of frequent loose stools due to intestinal infection (six or more loose stool in 24 hours). Standing orders for management of diarrhea are as follows:
- Watch out for the signs and symptoms of dehydration, i.e., dry skin, sunken eyes, coated dry tongue, rapid pulse, low BP and oliguria.
- If patient is having severe dehydration and is in a state of shock, immediately refer to the hospital.
- If there is no vomiting and patient is conscious, give ORS, lime juice, coconut water, weak tea, banana, khichri in small quantities at frequent intervals.
- If there is an epidemic of diarrhea and vomiting, stool should be sent for routine examination.
- If there is an outbreak of cholera, people should be vaccinated against it. Health officer should be informed.
- Educate people about control of flies, cleanliness of water, food and proper disposal of excreta.
- Provide medication as per the requirement.

Standing Orders for Management of Drowning

Standing orders for management of drowning are as follows:
- Loosen the clothes from the chest
- Make the casualty lie on his/her abdomen on a pitcher (*Matka*) with his head downward.
- Give gentle tapping over the upper back so that water will come out of the lungs.
- Resuscitate the patient and immediately refer to the hospital for further management.

Standing Orders for Management of Dog Bite

Dog bite is quite common especially in case of children while playing with dogs. Standing orders for management of dog bite are as follows:

- Reassure the patient and make him/her comfortable.
- Wash the wound with soap and water under running water.
- Check bleeding and depth of the wound.
- Clean with betadine solution.
- Stitches, if required, should be applied after 24 hours.
- Give injection TT 0.5 mL intramuscular.
- Do not kill the dog; observe the dog for 10 days.
- Refer the patient to hospital for Anti Rabies Vaccines.
- Always vaccinate the pet dogs.
- Never leave small children with pet as the temperament of the pet is never known.

Standing Orders for Management of Snake Bite

Snake bite is an acute emergency; and prompt management of the case is required to save the life of the patient in case of poisonous snake bite.

Snake bite may be from poisonous snake or nonpoisonous snake. But all snake bites should be treated as poisonous as many times patient may not be able to note the color and kind of snake. Standing orders for management of snake bite are as follows:

- Make the patient lie down and reassure him/her.
- Do not let the patient move.
- Immediately apply tourniquet just above the bite and make a cut of 1 cm in length and 1/2 cm in depth and allow to bleed and suck the bleeding with vacuum syringe.
- Release tourniquet every half hourly.
- Clean the place of bite with plain water or saline water.
- Ice can also be applied.
- Take history about the time of bite and color and kind of snake. Provide psychological support to the patient as well as family members.
- Give tea or coffee to drink.
- Refer the patient to hospital as early as possible for anti-snake venom (ASV) therapy.

Standing Orders for Management of Scorpion Bite

Standing orders for management of scorpion bite are as follows:

- Make the patient comfortable and reassure him/her.
- Apply tourniquet above the place of bite.
- Clean the place of bite thoroughly with soap and water.
- Remove the sting.
- Clean with betadine solution.
- Release the tourniquet after half an hour.
- Apply ice pack above the bite as it helps to reduce pain.

- Give injection TT 0.5 mL intramuscular.
- Give analgesics, if required.
- Give sweetened milk to drink.
- If the patient is in shock, refer him/her to the hospital immediately for management.

Standing Orders for Management of Fainting

Fainting is a state of temporary unconsciousness, which may be due to shock. Standing orders for management of fainting are as follows:
- Make the patient lie down in fresh air.
- Raise the foot end of the bed so that more blood reaches the vital organs.
- Remove the crowd.
- Check the vital signs.
- Give first aid if bleeding or fracture is there.
- As soon as the patient gains consciousness, ask him/her to take deep breath.
- Give some stimulating drinks like coffee, tea, fruit, juice, etc.
- If the person still remains unconscious, refer him/her to the hospital for management.

Standing Orders for Management of Injuries and Fractures

Standing orders for management of injuries and fractures are as follows:
- Keep the patient in comfortable position and reassure him/her.
- Clean the wound with antiseptic lotion, apply betadine solution and bandage with sterile pad.
- If fracture is present, immobilize the fractured part using splint.
- Check the vital signs.
- Monitor the condition of the patient with fractured bone.
- If signs and symptoms of shock are present, treat the shock.
- Give analgesics for pain.
- Give injection TT 0.5 mL intramuscular.
- Refer the patient to the hospital for further management.

Standing Orders for Management of Wound

Wound is a break in the continuity of the skin. Cuts and injuries cause wound. Wound may be incised, lacerated, punctured or clean wound. Standing orders for management of wound are as follows:
- Wash the wound with clean boiled water and antiseptic solution.
- Clean with betadine.
- Remove all foreign bodies like glass, pieces of wood, stone or dirt, etc. Clean and apply betadine lotion after removing foreign bodies.
- Apply sterile pad and bandage over the wound.
- Check the bleeding from wound.
- Give injection TT 0.5 mL intramuscular.
- Give analgesics and antibiotic as per the standing order.
- If the wound is deep, large and needs suturing or is caused by bullet injury or any other weapon, refer the patient to the hospital at the earliest for management.

Standing Orders for Management of Hemorrhage

Standing orders for management of hemorrhage are as follows:
- Make the patient lie down on his/her back with foot end raised.
- Reassure the patient.
- Apply pad on the bleeding point and press it till bleeding stops.
- Record temperature, pulse, respiration and blood pressure.
- Once the bleeding stops, apply pressure bandage.
- Give plenty of fluids to drink.
- Keep the patient warm.
- Take history and find out the cause of bleeding.
- If signs and symptoms of shock are present and bleeding is out of control, refer the patient immediately to the hospital for management.

Standing Orders for Management of Unconsciousness

Standing orders for management of unconsciousness are as follows:
- Make the person lie down in well-ventilated place in such a position that respiratory system functions properly.
- Open door and window to let the fresh air enter.
- Loosen the clothes from neck, chest and waist.
- Remove the dentures, if present.
- Clean the secretions from the mouth with gauze piece or by suctioning.
- Maintain clear airway.
- Check the vital signs.
- Give artificial respiration in case of blocked breathing.
- Find out the cause of unconsciousness from the relatives and refer the patient to the hospital as early as possible for treatment.

Standing Orders for Management of Poisoning

Standing orders for management of poisoning are as follows:
- Take history of taking poison from the relatives or friends.
- Make the patient lie down.
- Check the level of consciousness.
- Record vital signs.
- Keep the bottle of remaining fluid/poison, label or prescription brought by the relatives carefully to know the antidote if required or for medicolegal purposes.
- If the person is conscious within half an hour of taking poison, give one glass of cold water with one teaspoon of salt to drink to induce vomiting.
- If patient is conscious for more than half an hour, give one glass of warm milk to drink.
- If unconscious, refer the patient immediately to the hospital for management.

Standing Orders for Management of Epistaxis

Standing orders for management of epistaxis are as follows:
- Reassure the patient.
- Make the patient sit up with head erect and bent forward.
- Loosen the clothes around the neck.
- Clench the patient's nose at the junction of hard and soft part.
- Apply cold compress over the nose.
- Record blood pressure.
- Do not let the patient blow the nose.
- If bleeding is not controlled, refer the patient to hospital for management.

Standing Orders for Maternal and Child Healthcare

For Mother

- If vomiting and nausea is present in early pregnancy, give antiemetic to control morning sickness.
- In case of pregnancy-induced hypertension, advise to take salt-restricted diet and complete rest.
- If edema is present, refer her to the hospital.
- In case of high-risk pregnancy, APH or PPH, refer to the hospital.
- If fever is there after delivery, find out the cause like foul smelling scanty lochia, wound infection, engorged breast, give antipyretic and refer to the hospital.
- In case of stillbirth, provide psychological support. Provide comfort, treat breast engorgement and refer to the hospital for further investigation and management.

For Newborn Baby

- While taking care of newborn baby, maintain body temperature, respiration and clear airway.
- Watch out for the congenital anomalies like cleft lip, cleft palate, patency of rectum, clubbed feet, spina bifida, etc. and refer to the hospital if any abnormality is present.
- Record weight, length, head circumference and chest circumference of the baby
- Initiate breastfeeding as early as possible

For Convulsions in Children

- Make the child lie down on the bed.
- Take history of the child from the parents.
- Loosen the clothes from the chest and let the fresh air come.
- Keep the airway clear by suctioning or clearing secretions from the mouth with gauze piece so that respiratory tract functions properly.
- Record vital signs such as temperature, pulse, respiration, etc.
- In case of high fever, give cold sponge.
- Try to find out the possible cause of convulsion and refer the child to hospital for further management.

Nursing Considerations

Role of Community Health Nurse While Implementing Standing Orders
- Take general health history, special history about the onset of disease, symptoms and history of illness in the family.
- Find out any action taken and complication, if any.
- Record vital signs (temperature, pulse, respiration and blood pressure) and noting the condition of the patient.
- Identify the problems and personal needs.
- Provide first aid treatment and care as per the guidelines of the standing orders.
- Provide psychological support to the patient and family members.
- Implement the referral system as per the requirement of the case.
- Disclose the cause of illness, complication and follow-up treatment.
- Assess the work done.
- Regularly review the standing order manual and health book and keep up-to-date professional knowledge by periodically attending the health seminars, etc.
- Notify the communicable disease immediately to the health officer.
- Always keep the medicine kit ready for emergency.
- If there is any doubt about the standing orders, collect the correct and complete information from the concerned authorities at the earliest.
- Represent the nurses' view point while reviewing the standing orders.
- Be careful about one's limits and maintain the faith of doctors and health administration.
- Ensure safe and comfortable environment for the patient; ensuring patient's well-being is foremost important.

Summary

- Minor ailment indicates slight illness but does not prevent the patient from carrying out normal functions. The aim of management of minor ailment is to treat immediately to prevent any possible complication.
- Minor ailments are classified into general minor ailments and systemic minor ailments.
- General minor ailments include common accidents, burns, fractures, dog bite, fever, heat stroke and diarrhea requiring immediate treatment. Systemic minor ailments include ailments of various systems of the body.
- Standing orders are the directions and guidelines about the management of ailments of specific nature made available at health units. Based on these standing orders, the nurses and other health workers can treat emergencies at home and health institutions.
- The community nurse is responsible for updating the standing orders and reviewing them, thus ensuring up-to-date professional knowledge.
- Standing orders should be signed by the health authorities before implementing them.

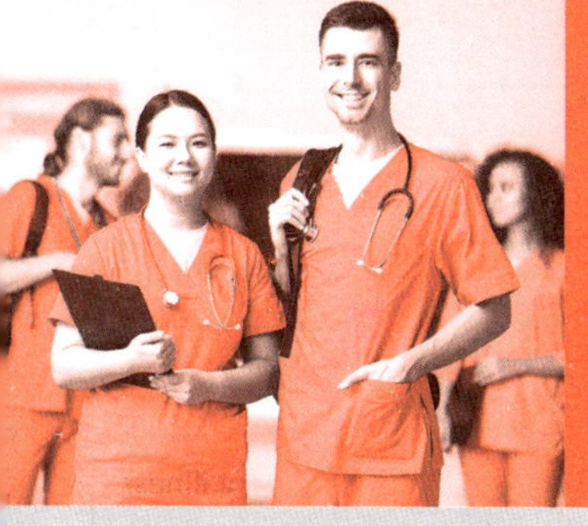

STUDENT ASSIGNMENT

LONG ANSWER TYPE QUESTIONS

1. Explain the classification of minor ailments and explain the management of minor ailments.
2. Discuss standing orders and discuss the types of standing orders.
3. Describe the responsibilities and limitations of community health nurse while carrying out the standing orders.

SHORT ANSWER TYPE QUESTIONS

1. Define minor ailments. Enlist the principles of managing minor ailments.
2. Enlist the objectives and uses of standing orders.

MULTIPLE CHOICE QUESTIONS

1. **The objectives of standing orders are:**
   a. To maintain the continuity of treatment of the patient
   b. To resuscitate the patient
   c. To create a feeling of responsibility in the members of health team
   d. All of the above

2. **Which of the following is not the responsibility of the community health nurses?**
   a. Proper recording and assessment
   b. Reassuring the client and family
   c. Provide treatment in emergency or in the absence of doctor
   d. Once she is trained, she need not consult the doctor

3. **Which of the following is not a minor ailment?**
   a. Heat stroke and fainting
   b. Diarrhea
   c. Severe chest pain in a heart disease
   d. Injuries, falls and burn

4. **The correct sequence of management of minor ailment is:**
   a. Assessment → diagnosis → evaluation → treatment
   b. Assessment → diagnosis → treatment → evaluation
   c. Diagnosis → evaluation → assessment → treatment
   d. Evaluation → diagnosis → treatment → evaluation

5. **All of the following are the principles of managing minor ailment; except:**
    a. Provide safe environment
    b. Record vital signs and keep continuous watch over the patient
    c. Manage the risk to prevent any possible complications
    d. Provide treatment as there is no need to consult the doctor

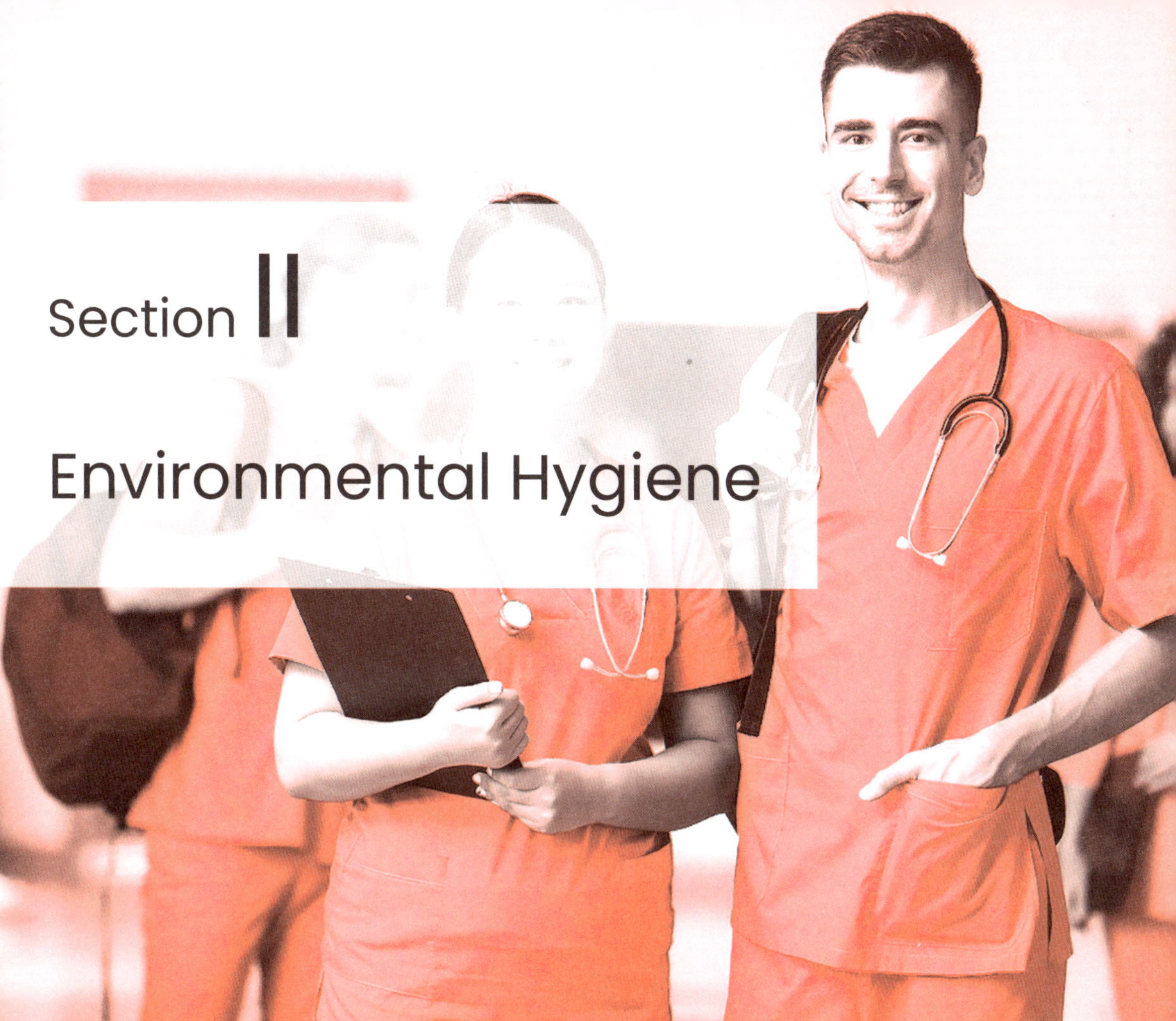

SECTION OUTLINE

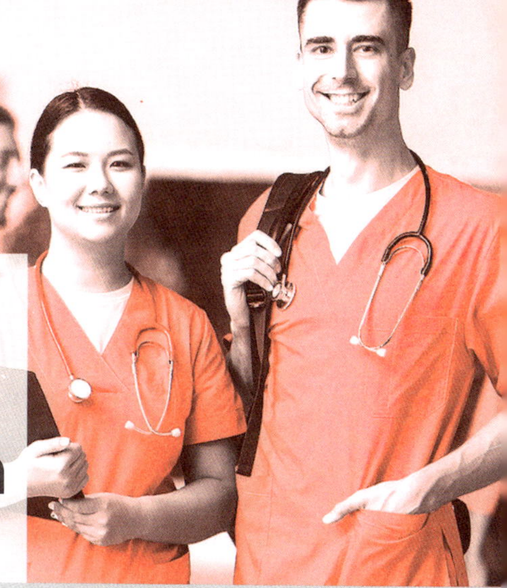

10

Environment and Environmental Health

LEARNING OBJECTIVES

After the completion of the unit, the readers will be able to:
- Discuss the area and components of environment.
- Explain the importance of healthy environment and its relation to health and disease.
- Discuss environment problems and enlist the factors affecting environmental health.

UNIT OUTLINE

- Introduction
- Definitions of Environment
- Sanitation
- Environmental Health
- Environment
- Importance of Healthy Environment
- Environmental Problems in India

KEY TERMS

Deforestation: The intentional removal of trees and forests from a place.
Environment: Factors affecting a person's life.
Green revolution: Increasing crop yields by using fertilizers.
Sanitation: A system that disposes of human waste efficiently, protecting health.
Urbanization: The development of rural areas like cities.

INTRODUCTION

In earlier days, the environmental sanitation was used to determine the relation between environment and health. The word sanitation means the science of safeguarding health; a way of living cleanly in all aspects of life, on the basis of which one can protect himself against disease and improve health. Cleanliness and hygienic conditions essential for good health are related to healthy environment. The health and environment have deep interrelation. Actually, the term sanitation covers the whole field of controlling the environment with a view to prevent disease and promote health. Man has already controlled some factors in his environment, e.g., water, housing, food, clothing and sanitation. These controllable factors are included in the standards of living. The control of these factors that are responsible for improvement in human health in the past century, in developed countries. Since the old problems are solved, new problems are emerging due to deleterious changes in the environment as a result of rapid development, industrialization and urbanization and demographic growth, hence, man himself is responsible for the pollution of his environment. Every change in environment affects the health. Clean and safe environment can be the basis of good health. There is a widespread concern among the general public health engineers, environmentalist, scientist, health administrators, epidemiologist, health professional and politicians, etc. Environmental degradation is of growing concern for international agencies like United Nations and World Health Organization. In 1972, UN conference on human environment focused the attention of whole world on the environmental hazards that threaten human being, since then World Environmental Day is celebrated on 5th of June every year to act as a reminder on the persisting environmental problems.

DEFINITIONS OF ENVIRONMENT

Environment is defined as "all that is external to an individual with which one is in constant interaction". It includes all external surroundings such as housing, air, water, food, soil, plants, animals, insects, microbes, etc. It also includes meteorological factors such as, temperature, humidity, sunlight, rainfall, etc.

"Environment is the sum total of all conditions, effects and system, which affect all creatures, their racial development, life and death".   **—Universal Encyclopedia**

"Environment refers to the sum total of all conditions which surround man at a given point in space and time".   **—Chris Park**

"Environment indicates all of the internal and external conditions, circumstances and influences surrounding or affecting the development and behavior of persons and groups".

—Roy (Nursing Theorist)

"Environment is the sum of all external conditions and influences on the development cycle of biotic elements over the earth's surface".   **—Herskovits**

SANITATION

The literal meaning of sanitation is "the science of safeguarding health". Sanitation is considered a way of life by National Sanitation Foundation of USA. It defines sanitation "as the quality of living which is expressed in the clean home, the clean farm, the clean business, the clean neighborhood and the clean community, it is nourished by knowledge and grows as an obligation and an ideal human relation."

Being a way of life, it must come from within the people. In the past, sanitation was focused on the sanitary disposal of human excreta. Even today also many people think, that sanitation means the construction of latrines. Actually, the term sanitation includes the whole field of controlling the environment.

Environmental Sanitation

Environmental sanitation is defined by WHO as "The control of all those factors in man's physical environment which exercise or may exercise a deleterious effect on his, physical development, health and survival".

Sanitation or environmental sanitation is not only concerned with sanitary disposal of human excreta, but also covers the whole field of controlling this environment, in order to prevent and control diseases and promote health. It includes prevention of pollution from industrial wastes, automobiles, nuclear technology, pesticides, etc. Therefore, the term environmental sanitation is replaced by environmental health.

ENVIRONMENTAL HEALTH

Environmental health can be defined as, "an art and science of promoting positive environmental factors and prevention and control of all the potential hazards including physical, chemical, biological and social factors which have deleterious effect on health of people".

Historical View

The relationship of the environment to health has been recognized by nurses since the time of Miss Florence Nightingale. She was the first nurse to recognize the importance of environmental factor in relation to health. Her concept of nursing care focused strongly on modifying the physical environment and included the "five essential points", i.e.,

1. Pure air
2. Pure water
3. Effective drainage
4. Cleanliness
5. Light

Thousands of years before the Christian era (3000–1500 BC), the Indus Valley Civilization showed the presence of planned cities with sophisticated drainage and water supply systems, well-developed houses, and public baths suggesting the practice of environmental sanitation. During the same period, environmental sanitation measures were taken by Egyptians and Romans. In India, sanitary conditions deteriorated during the Mughal Empire. The outbreak of leprosy and bubonic plague during 13th and 14th centuries in European countries was associated with poor environmental sanitation. The movement of true healthful living started in the middle of the 19th century in European countries and in America.

The impact of the environment on health was first documented by Edwin Chadwick, in 1842, in a report on the sanitary condition of laboring populations of Great Britain. In 1850, John Snow documented the spread of disease due to contaminated water in London, for the first time even before the discovery of microorganisms.

Later on because of the discovery of bacteria by Louis Pasteur and Robert Koch, the role of bacteria and environment in disease causation was understood, since then lot of efforts have been put in and measures have been taken by the Government at all levels in European countries and in America to assess, prevent and correct environmental hazards to promote health and prevent disease.

In India in 1859, Miss Florence Nightingale was involved by the British Parliament to investigate the heavy morbidity and mortality of British soldiers. Poor environmental sanitation was found to be associated with prevailing sickness among military and civil populations, since then the emphasis was put on improving sanitary conditions through public health department, local municipalities and health education departments. In India, after independence, various specific programs for improvement of environmental sanitation have been implemented through community development programs in rural and urban areas. The National Water Supply and Sanitation Program was started in 1954.

A drinking water board was set up in 1963, and some acts were enacted and promulgated, including the following:

- Comprehensive Water (Prevention and Control of Pollution) Act in 1974
- Air (Prevention and Control of Pollution) Act, 1981.
- Environmental Protection Act in 1986
- Prevention of Food Adulteration Act, 1975

In spite of all these efforts, the environment is getting polluted because of manmade pollutants like toxic gases, chemicals, radiation, nuclear wastes, domestic and industrial wastes are continued to be released in water, air and soil.

Purpose of Environmental Health

The purpose of environmental health is to create and maintain ecological conditions that will promote health and prevent diseases.

- Members of environmental team are:
  - Public health engineer
  - Epidemiologist
  - Physician trained in public health
  - Sociologist
  - Economist
  - Public health nurse or community health nurse
  - Health inspector
  - Town planner
  - Auxiliary staff

Factors Affecting Environmental Health

The environment in which we live is constantly deteriorating due to various factors, i.e., man-made and natural. Some of the natural factors are transient and seasonal, e.g., floods and draughts, etc. There are a number of man-made and natural factors which are making the environment unhealthy by affecting our ecosystem and environmental health. These factors are:

- **Population explosion:** This is the biggest problem. The population of India is increasing very rapidly and creating problems due to overcrowding, development of man-made resources by urbanization and industrialization and green revolution.
- **Urbanization:** People are migrating to urban areas for education, employment opportunities due to industrialization in the cities, they get jobs, as in the villages facilities for education and employment are lacking. People are poor in the villages and they migrate to cities for their livelihood resulting in overcrowding and development of slums, mostly on unauthorized land.
- **Automobiles:** The increasing number of motor vehicles and other automobiles results not only in overcrowding of the roads, but also the exhaust they release contains a number of harmful gases and other particles which tell upon human health. The exhaust of automobile released contains carbon monoxide, nitrogen oxide, lead and other unburnt hydrocarbons, which pollute the air we breathe and causes various respiratory diseases. Though the automobiles save time and energy, their hazards are dangerous to health.

- **Industrialization:** After independence, the industrialization has increased tremendously. There are small scale as well as large scale industries in towns. The industrial waste contains harmful waste products, such as gases, solid material, effluents, thermal waste, fumes of acids from acid factories and various chemicals are released into the atmosphere. These industrial wastes other than releasing into the air, it is also thrown into the rivers and streams, drains and on the land. It not only pollutes air, but also water and land too, thus deteriorate our environment causing harmful effects to the human health as well as to the animals and plants.

- **Deforestation:** Deforestation is another big threat to the environment pollution. The trees release oxygen and take up carbon dioxide from the atmosphere thereby purifying air. They also transfer water from ground to the air, thus maintaining temperature and also prevent soil erosion. But forests are being removed for need of wood for housing, building, industries and expansion of land due to increased population, modernization, urbanization, colonization and industrialization. This phenomenon is causing changes in the climate and has adverse effects on environmental health.

- **Green revolution:** The use of excessive fertilizers for increasing the yield of crops demands excessive water and as a result, the underground water is diminishing. It is causing a threat to water requirements for human beings and animals. The farmers are using excessive insecticide to destroy the pests and microorganisms, which have lasting effects on the agricultural products through the food chain. These products are passed onto various animals and human beings and cause various diseases, e.g., cancer is one of the diseases which is found in areas where excessive chemicals, fertilizer and insecticides are used.

- **Radioactive substances:** In power plants and hospital laboratories, where the radioactive substances are used, if human beings, working in such places do not take proper precautions and are exposed to radioactive elements like radium, and uranium, which emit radiation. This radiation causes cancer of various organs. The radioactive wastes from the power plants, if not disposed of safely with special disposal methods, pollute air and water and cause harmful effects on all living things, including humans, plants and animals.

- **Natural calamities:** These are not man-made, include floods, droughts, earthquakes, cyclones, volcanoes, landslides, tidal waves and tsunamis in the sea. All have harmful effects directly or indirectly on human beings, plants and animals.

ENVIRONMENT

The environment today has become a multidisciplinary subject. In earlier days, it was studied as a branch of natural science, but nowadays it is related to social sciences, history and literature. According to the system theory of environment, it refers to internal and external environment. The internal environment includes biological, physical, psychological, sociological and spiritual systems. The external environment consists of all external factors, living and nonliving, that surround the human beings and affect them, such as air they breathe, water they drink, the food they consume, housing, climate, heat, radiation, humidity geography, waste, microbial agent, insects, animals, rodent, plants and noise, automobiles, etc. The key to the good health largely depends upon the healthy environment. The most of the health problems are due to adverse environmental factors, such as water pollution, air pollution, poor housing conditions, presence of animal reservoirs and insects, vectors of diseases, which pose a constant threat to human health. The environment is getting deteriorated very fast because of population explosion, growing industrialization, increasing urbanization, deforestation, soil erosion, continuous nuclear technology and green revolution, etc.

Areas of Environment

The nature of environment is ever-changing. The areas that can be included in the study of the environment are as under:

- Ecological system
- Spatial system and analysis
- Study of biosphere
- Study of natural disasters
- The development of scientific forecasts of anthropogenic changes in the environment.

Although, the current concept of health and environment are more complex but nursing continues to be concerned with human beings' interaction with the environment in care and research. Providing an optimum environment for the maintenance of wellness is the responsibility of nursing personnel.

Components of Environment

There are three main components of environment, which are closely related to one another. These are as follows:

1. **Physical environment:** The physical environment is concerned with nonliving things and a variety of physical forces and factors, which directly or indirectly regulate the body mechanism and affect the health of the people. It includes housing, water, air, soil, lighting, friction, radiation, heat, sound, gravity, humidity, wind velocity, climate, geography and electromagnetic field, etc. A variety of pollutants are found to pollute air, water, soil, food and result into various acute and chronic diseases, e.g., gastrointestinal, respiratory and skin diseases.

2. **Biological environment:** The biological environment comprises all living things around human. It includes animals, plants, birds, insects, rodents, bacteria, virus, fungi, protozoa and other microorganisms. There are some diseases which are produced by arthropods, insects, microorganism, domestic and wild animals. Most of the time, there is harmonious coexistence, but sometimes, this is disturbed and results into ill health.

3. **Social environment:** The social environment includes customs, culture, belief, moral and ethical values. Income, education, social rules and regulation, religious practices, habits and occupation and living standards of the people. A favorable social environment helps individuals in their social development and maintenance of social health. The individual develops certain practices, which will have positive and negative social impact. Some of the negative social practices which have negative effects on health are *purdah* system, early marriage, dowry system, low status of women, caste system and segregation, etc. Some of the social conditions which also have negative impacts on health are broken families, single parent family, overpopulation, large families, poverty, illiteracy, unemployment, etc.

All these components of environment are related to each other. Every component of environment can help people to develop their potentialities to maximum and to attain optimum health.

IMPORTANCE OF HEALTHY ENVIRONMENT

Healthy environment is important for:

- Improving the health status of the individuals and community.
- Protecting the population against diseases.
- Controlling the environmental pollution.
- Protecting the people from environmental hazards.
- Reducing the morbidity and mortality.
- Protecting against communicable and noncommunicable diseases.
- Encouraging environmental education.
- Protecting the health of individuals and communities.
- Improving social status of the people.
- For the development and progress of the country and nation.

ENVIRONMENTAL PROBLEMS IN INDIA

- Air and water pollutions
- Reduction in forest area
- Soil erosion
- Sound pollution
- Poor housing and slum development
- Excessive use of chemicals, fertilizers in agriculture leading to soil pollution
- Industrialization and urbanization
- Unhygienic disposal of human excreta and refuse
- Insects and rodents
- Increasing pressure of traffic
- Depletion of natural resources
- Threat to biodiversity
- Radiation hazards
- Population explosion

Summary

- Environment refers to all that is external to an individual with which he is in constant interaction. It includes all the surroundings such as air, water, housing, food, soil, plants and animals. Sanitation is the science of safeguarding health.
- Environmental health is an art and science of promoting positive environmental factors and prevention and control of all potential hazards, including physical, chemical biological and social factors, which have deleterious effects on health.
- The components of environment include physical environment, biological environment and social environment.
- A healthy environment is important to attain optimum level of health.
- The environmental problems are increasing due to population explosion, deforestation, increasing urbanization and industrialization and also due to natural calamities. All these conditions have adverse effects on human health and there is strong need to improve the environment.

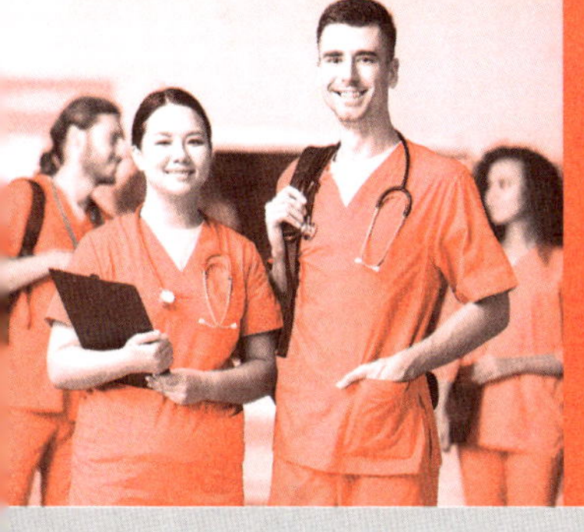

LONG ANSWER TYPE QUESTIONS

1. Describe the factors affecting environmental health.
2. Explain the environmental problems affecting human health.

SHORT ANSWER TYPE QUESTIONS

1. Define environment.
2. Enlist the components of environment.

MULTIPLE CHOICE QUESTIONS

1. **Which one of the following is not the component of physical environment?**
   a. Air
   b. Water
   c. Soil
   d. Microorganisms

2. **Which of the following is not the main component of our environment?**
   a. Physical
   b. Biological
   c. Spiritual
   d. Social

ANSWER KEY

1. d   2. c

11

Environmental Factors Contributing to Health

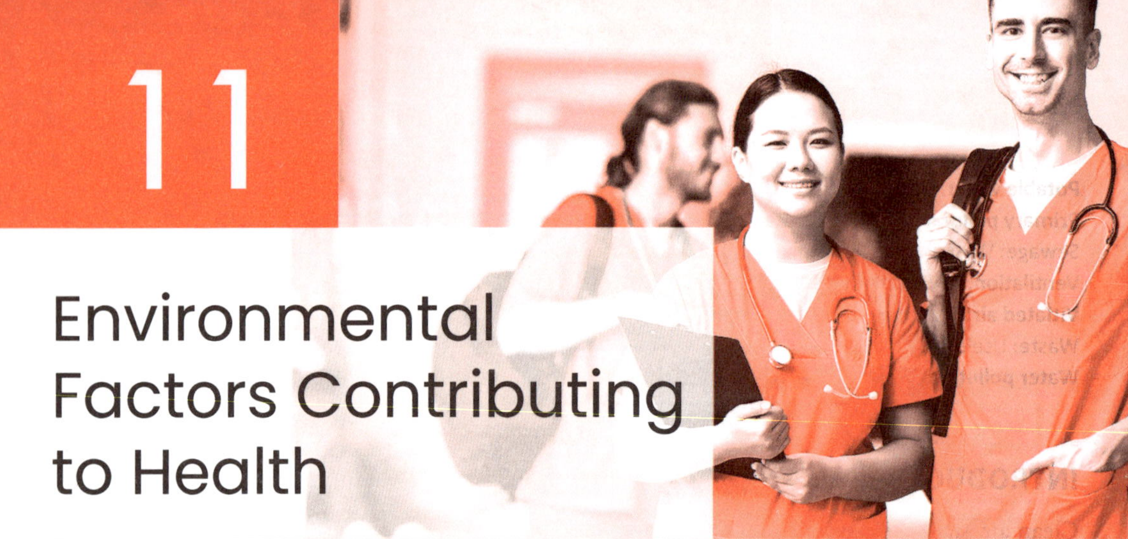

LEARNING OBJECTIVES

After the completion of the unit, the readers will be able to:

- State the meaning of wholesome water.
- Classify the different sources of water and enlist the uses of water.
- Describe the process of water purification on a small and large scale.
- Discuss air pollution and enlist the preventive measures of air pollution.
- Explain the causes and sources of solid waste.
- Describe the housing standards of India.
- State the minimum standards for living and enlist the effects of ventilation on health.
- Describe noise pollution and its control.
- List the diseases transmitted by arthropods of medical importance.
- Describe the environmental factors contributing to health and illness.

UNIT OUTLINE

- Introduction
- Water
- Water Pollution: Natural and Acquired Impurities
- Waterborne Diseases
- Water Purification
- Air
- Air Pollution
- Waste
- Excreta
- Sewage
- Health Hazards of Waste on Human Health
- Housing
- Noise
- Arthropods
- Rodents
- Insecticides
- Pest Control

KEY TERMS

Air pollution: Presence of undesirable substances in the atmosphere.

Chlorination: Addition of chlorine in water.

Garbage: Waste food, leftovers and peelings of food and fruits, leaves, etc.

Hardness of water: The presence of carbonates of calcium magnesium, chlorides and sulfates.

Housing: Physical structure which provides protection against storms, rain, lightning, snowfall, etc.

Impounding reservoir: Solid storage reservoirs across streams or rivers for the purpose of holding stream flow so that the stored water may be used when supply is insufficient.

Incineration: Disposal by burning.

Potable water: Water without impurities and is consumable.
Primary pollutants: Pollutants directly emitted from a source to the atmosphere.
Sewage: Wastewater containing organic, inorganic solids and liquids.
Ventilation: Removal of vitiated air and supply of fresh air.
Vitiated air: Physical and chemical changes in air especially reduced oxygen content.
Waste: Useless and unwanted material.
Water pollution: The presence of organic and inorganic salts, biological pollutants in water.

INTRODUCTION

Clean air, stable climate, adequate water, sanitation and hygiene, safe use of chemicals, protection from radiation, healthy and safe workplaces, sound agricultural practices, health-supportive cities and built environments, and a preserved nature are all prerequisites for good health.

WATER

Water is vital to all forms of life. Many health problems in developing countries are due to lack of safe drinking water. In India 50% of ill health could be reduced by providing safe drinking water.

Sources of Water

- Rainwater
- Surface water includes the following:
    - High level surface water, i.e., dams and artificial lakes
    - Low level surface water, i.e., tanks and ponds
    - Rivers and streams
- Groundwater
    - Springs
    - Wells
    - Tube wells

Characteristics of Safe and Wholesome Water

- It is clear, colorless and odorless.
- It is free from pathogenic organisms.
- It is free from harmful chemicals.
- It is pleasant in taste.
- It is fit for drinking.
- It should have an appropriate temperature.

Uses of Water

Water is the largest component of the body. The living things cannot survive without water. The uses and importance of water are explained as follows:

Physiological Importance

- Human body constitutes 60–70% of water
- Water regulates body temperature
- Water maintains circulation
- Water excretes waste material from the body
- Water maintains fluid and electrolyte balance
- Water is a major component of blood, tissues and bones.

Domestic Uses

- Drinking and kitchen work
- Personal health and cleanliness
- Cleaning house and washing clothes

Public Importance

- Swimming pools
- Public water supply
- Care of gardens
- Fire brigade
- Washing of drains
- Cleaning the roads

Agricultural Uses

- Rain water is a major source of irrigation
- Production of agricultural products can be achieved by adequate water supply.

Power Production

Water is used for power production in hydropower and steam power plants.

Occupational Importance

Water is used for establishment of industries, hotels, dairy, factories, tourism, laundry, and hospitals.

Water Harvesting

Recharging of groundwater by rainfall water is called water harvesting.

Rainwater Harvesting

Rainwater harvesting is a very important method of water conservation. By this method, we can preserve and build up underground water reserves in urban and semi-urban areas, where considerable water is drawn out by tube wells for domestic consumption. A vast quantity of water is discharged into drains. The rainwater can be added to the underground reserve by diversion of rainwater from rooftops and courtyards into soaking pits and trenches, instead of drains. This water can be cleaned, filtered and diverted into existing tube wells and wells (Fig. 11.1).

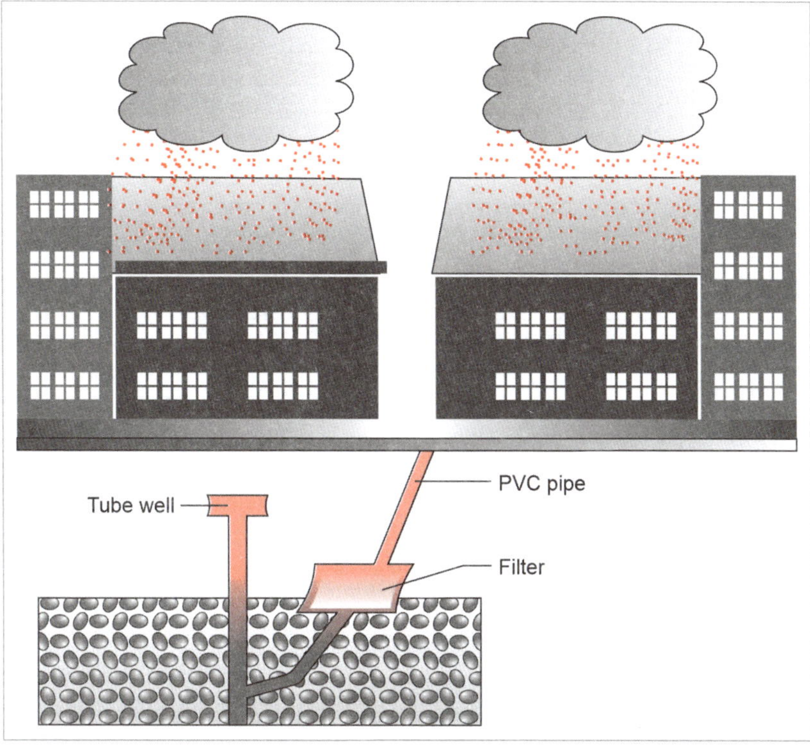

Fig. 11.1: Rainwater harvesting

WATER POLLUTION: NATURAL AND ACQUIRED IMPURITIES

Water pollution refers to the presence of any substance that changes the natural qualities of water and causes harmful effects on humans, animals and plants. Water being a good solvent can dissolve many substances in it. This property of water is responsible for the pollution of water. Water pollution means contamination of water due to any impurities. The main water pollutants include pathogens, toxic, chemical substances, industrial wastes, sewage, animal, and human wastes, nuclear wastes, insecticides, pesticides, chemical fertilizers, dyes soap and detergents, sediments and heavy metals like mercury, radioactive substances, brass, cadmium, and arsenic, etc. Contaminated water kills more people than all forms of violence, including war. According to UN report 2010, 90% of wastewater discharged in developing countries is untreated, contributing to the death of 2.2 million people a year from diarrheal diseases caused by unsafe drinking water and poor hygiene. At least 1.8 million children younger than 5, die every year due to water-related diseases. In India, the holy river Ganga and Yamuna are polluted due to adding of wastewater, untreated sewage, flowing of dead bodies of animals and human beings.

Sources of Water Pollution

The main sources of water pollution include waste matter from living habitants, industrial wastes, agricultural wastes and dead bodies of animals, etc. The sources of water pollution and impurities can be divided into two categories: (1) Natural and (2) Acquired (Flowchart 11.1).

Flowchart 11.1: Sources of water pollution

Sources of water polution

Natural impurities
• Dust and soluble gases
• Dissolved minerals
• Vegetable impurities
• Pathogenic agents
• Inorganic impurities

Acquired impurities
• Sewage
• Industrial waste
• Agriculture pollutant
• Physical pollutants
• Inappropriate social traditions

Natural Impurities

- **Dust and soluble gases:** Carbon dioxide, hydrogen sulfide, nitrogen, ammonia, etc.
- **Dissolved minerals:** Calcium, magnesium, sodium, salts of iron, lead, and manganese, etc.
- **Vegetable impurities:** Microplants, algae, and dry leaves, etc.
- **Pathogenic agents:** Bacteria, virus, ova, worms, cysts, etc.
- **Inorganic impurities:** Sand, soil, sludge, particles of sediments, etc.

Acquired Impurities

Acquired impurities are due to human activities. Due to increasing industrialization and urbanization, the acquired impurities are increasing. The main acquired impurities of water include:

- **Sewage:** Most of the rivers are polluted by the sewage. The sewage contains organic substances which absorb oxygen, kill the fishes and produce a foul smell in the water. The pathogenic organisms and other substances present in the sewage are the main causes of waterborne diseases.
- **Industrial refuse or waste:** The industrial waste of the industries like paper, cloth, alcohol, jute, sugar, steel, tanneries, oil refineries, paints and fertilizers completely pollutes the water when released in it. The properties and potability of water are destroyed and the toxic substances present in these wastes become a serious threat to the health. Water of rivers near factories is not fit for drinking due to industrial wastes thrown in it. (Mainly in Ganga and Yamuna rivers).
- **Agriculture pollutant:** Excessive and indiscriminate use of chemical fertilizers and insecticides to increase the agricultural production has not only damaged soil fertility but also polluted the water, as these substances flow into water and get dissolved in it. Similarly, disposing of weeds and other agricultural waste material into water also pollutes it.
- **Physical pollutants:** Physical pollutants such as radioactive substances, acid rain and thermal pollutants are also responsible for water pollution.
- **Inappropriate social traditions:** Water pollution also increases by disposing of the dead bodies and carcasses of animals and immersing the used items of worship in water.

MUST KNOW

Water-related Disasters
The water-related disasters include floods, drought, water epidemics, famine, landslides and the other water-related issues such as water pollution, salinization, tsunamis, land degradation, waterborne diseases, etc. These affect the ecosystem and life cycle.

Effects of Water Pollution on Health

There are many adverse effects on the health of people, animals and plants due to water pollution. There are various health disorders due to water pollution. The extent and nature of health disorders depend upon the type and quality of pollutants in water. Some of the disorders are listed here:

- **Gastrointestinal disorders:** These are due to the presence of pathogenic organisms such as bacteria, virus, protozoa and helminths. These disorders include diarrheal diseases dysentery, typhoid, paratyphoid fever, amebiasis, giardiasis, worm infestations, hepatitis A and E.
- **Neuromuscular disorders:** The disorders of nervous and muscular system are caused by metals like mercury, cadmium. Organic lead compounds in water cause headache, drowsiness, delirium, convulsions, coma and chronic constipation, loss of appetite and anemia.
- **Respiratory disorders:** These are due to the presence of free chlorine and hydrogen sulfide in water. These gases irritate the mucus membranes of the respiratory tract and cause acute bronchitis and lung disease.
- **Bone and teeth disorders:** These are due to presence of high concentrations of fluorides and cadmium in water.
- **Other factors:** Include cancer and disorders of liver, kidney and thyroid due to various chemical compounds present in water. Skin diseases like dryness of skin, ringworm infestation and eczema are caused by bathing in polluted water. Liver diseases like cirrhosis are also caused by the presence of algae in water.
- **Effects on animals and plants:** The presence of organic substances in water deoxygenates water, which is harmful for aquatic life and water plants. Oil spread on the surface of water sticks to the feathers of birds and due to this they cannot fly and finally, they die. Oil and chemicals in water destroy fish and other aquatic life. Black water is harmful for plants and vegetation.

WATERBORNE DISEASES

Waterborne diseases are classified into two groups:

1. **Waterborne diseases due to biological agents:**
   Those caused by infective agents present in water are listed in Table 11.1.

TABLE 11.1: Infective agents that cause waterborne diseases

Infective agents	Diseases caused
Viruses	Viral hepatitis, poliomyelitis, rotavirus, diarrhea in infants.
Bacteria	Cholera, typhoid, paratyphoid, bacillary dysentery, *E. coli* diarrhea
Protozoa	Amoebiasis, giardiasis
Helminths	Roundworm, threadworm, hydatid cysts
Leptospirosis	Weil's disease

Aquatic hosts	Diseases caused
Snail	Schistosomiasis
Cyclops	Guinea worm, fish tapeworm

2. **Waterborne diseases due to chemical wastage:** Mixing of chemicals, fertilizers, insecticides, industrial wastes containing chemicals and sewage changes the chemical composition of water, which causes ill effects on health. These are called waterborne chemical hazards. These include:
   - **Diseases caused by toxicity of water:** Excess of nitrates and fluorides cause fluorosis, while excess lead, arsenic and other toxic substances are responsible for many other diseases.
   - **Mixing of sewage with water:** Mixing of sewage with water may cause diseases of digestive system. It may cause spreading of communicable diseases through contaminated water supply. Besides this, the deficiency of fluoride may cause dental caries. Polluted water imbalances aquatic life and if used in irrigation, the agricultural products (vegetables and fruits) may become sources of diseases.

Prevention of Waterborne Diseases

- **Drinking water supply system:** Must be properly maintained and should follow all the hygienic standards during storage, filtration and distribution of the water supply.
- **Sanitation facilities:** The sewerage system must be properly maintained. The water supply should not clash with sanitation system.
- **Drink safe and potable water:**
  - Drink only thoroughly filtered water
  - Potable water should be stored in a hygienic place
  - Storage containers of drinking water must be thoroughly washed every day
  - If proper water purification system is absent, drinking water must be thoroughly boiled and then cooled in a hygienic container.
- Fresh cooked food should be consumed. Avoid such restaurants which are unhygienic.
- Keep finger nails short and clean at all times. Cut them every 3 days.
- Wash hands before and after every meal, after using toilet or washroom.
- Good hygienic behavior should be practiced by all family members.
- Always wash the vegetables, thoroughly with water containing salt before cutting.
- Fruits should be washed before eating.
- Do not store cut fruits in refrigerator. They should be consumed then and there.

WATER PURIFICATION

Water should be purified before supplying it for domestic use to the people and made free from pathogenic agents, impurities and contaminated agents. Water can be purified at large and small scale.

Purification at Large Scale

Water for the public supply is purified at a large scale. It is carried on by three processes:
1. **Storage:** Water is stored at natural or artificial constructed places. This process of water storage is a method of natural purification which is carried out in three steps:
   i. **Physical purification:** When the stored water is allowed to stand for 24 hours, most of the suspended and floating impurities settle down due to the influence of sunlight and gravity. Water is purified to a large extent and its properties also change.

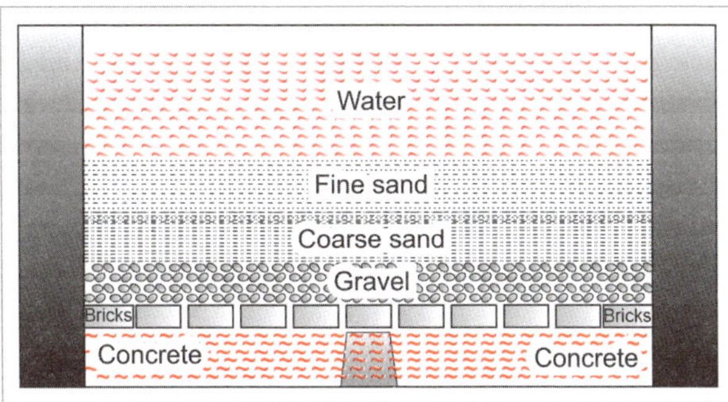

Fig. 11.2: Slow sand filtration

ii. **Chemical purification:** The aerobic bacteria present in the stored water oxidize the organic substances in the presence of dissolved oxygen in water. The process decreases the content of ammonia and increases nitrates. A change in the composition of water is initiated by chemical changes in the stored water by the bacteria.

iii. **Biological purification:** About 90% of the pathogenic bacteria die within 5–7 days in the stored water. However, if the water is allowed to stand for a longer period, the algae and foul smell may develop in it.

2. **Filtration:** By filtration, about 99% of the impurities can be removed. Filtration is of two types, slow sand filtration and rapid sand filtration.

   i. **Slow sand filtration (Fig. 11.2):** It is a standard practice of purification. Stored water is brought to the filtration plant for purification. This method works on the following basis:

   ◆ **Supernatant water:** The stored raw water is filled in the filter box up to a height of 1.5 m and this level is kept stable. It has got two advantages. One is that it ensures the flow of water through bed of sand and the second is that it provides a waiting period of 3–12 hours, depending upon filtration velocity. The water standing over the bed gets partially purified by the sedimentation and oxidation. The level of supernatant water is kept always constant.

   ◆ **Sand bed:** Sand is spread at the bottom of filter box at a depth of 1.2 m. Sand should be clean and sand grains should be 15–35 mm in diameter. Below the fine sand, there is a layer of coarse sand and then a layer of gravel below coarse layer of sand. The combination of fine sand, coarse sand and gravel is called filter bed. This is the most important part of the filter.

   ◆ **Under drainage system:** Below the filter bed lies the drainage system of water. The drainage system consists of perforated pipes that allow for an outlet of the filtered water and support the filter contained in the filter box. The filter box is a box of rectangular shape which is 2.5–4 m in depth.

   ◆ **Filter control system:** The pipes of filter are fitted with some valves and a system to regulate the continuity and speed of filtration. This maintains and measures the loss of head and the bed resistance.

Filter box is a rectangular construction which is 2.5–4 m deep. Its walls are made up of bricks, stones or cement. From top to bottom, the following order is maintained:

➡ **Raw water:** 1–1.5 m
➡ **Sand bed:** 1.2 m
➡ **Coarse sand and gravel bed:** Up to 0.3 m
➡ **Filter bed:** 0.16 m

The filter box can be cleaned as needed.

Advantages:

➡ Simple construction, easy working and low cost
➡ Easy monitoring
➡ Removes 99.2% bacteria
➡ Filtered water is of good quality.

Disadvantages:

➡ As the filter plant is uncovered, there is a possibility of contamination.
➡ Sedimentation is necessary before the beginning of filtration.

ii. **Rapid sand filtration (Fig. 11.3):** The rapid sand filters were installed in 1885 in the USA. Rapid sand filters are of two types:

1. Gravity type (Paterson's filter)
2. Pressure type (Candy's filter)

Steps involved in rapid sand filtration: The steps involved in rapid sand filtration include:

i. **Coagulation:** The raw water is treated with alum or aluminum sulfate to remove the turbidity of water. The amount of alum required is 5–40 mg/L, depending upon the turbidity, color, temperature and pH of the water.

ii. **Rapid mixing:** The treated water is subjected to violent agitation in a mixing chamber for a few minutes. This allows thorough mixing of alum in it.

iii. **Flocculation:** This involves the flow and gentle stirring of the treated water in a flocculation chamber for about 30 minutes. It results in the formation of a thick, copious white flocculent precipitate of aluminum hydroxide.

iv. **Sedimentation:** Coagulated water is passed into a sedimentation tank. It is kept for 2–6 hours in the sedimentation tank. In this tank, precipitates of aluminum hydroxide and other impurities settle down due to the process of sedimentation. This partially purified water and then passed into a rapid sand filter.

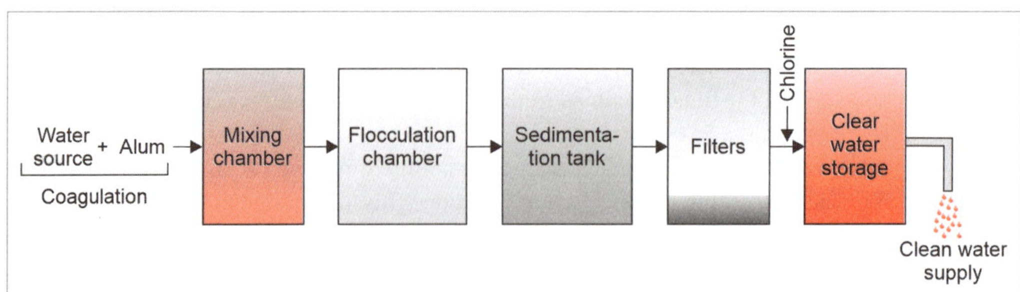

Fig. 11.3: Flow of water in rapid sand filtration

v. **Filtration:** After the above steps, the partially purified water is subjected to rapid sand filtration. Here, also sand is used for filtration. Thickness of the sand is about 1 m. Below the sand, there is a 30–40 cm thick layer of coarse and fine gravel. Sand is covered with a height of 1–1.5 m of water. Water is collected in under-drainage pipes after passing through sand and gravel. A slimy layer is formed on the sand bed with the filtration of water, similar to the biological layer formed in the slow sand filter. Process of filtration is stopped in rapid sand filtration when the loss of head rises above 7–8 feet and the filter is cleaned by backwashing.

vi. **Backwashing:** Rapid filters must be cleaned frequently daily or weekly. Washing is done by reversing the flow of water through the sand bed. The whole process takes 15 minutes.

Advantages:
- Storage of water is not required. Raw water is directly put under process of filtration.
- Filter occupies less space
- Filtration is 40–50 times more rapid than slow sand filtration
- More flexibility in operation of filter
- Washing is easy
- Every day 20 crore gallons of water per acre can be purified.

3. **Disinfection (Chlorination):** This is an important step in water purification and is necessary to kill all the remaining pathogenic organisms. This is done by chlorination of water. It makes the water safe for drinking. When chlorine is added to water, it reacts with water and forms hydrochloric acid and hypochlorous acid.

- Hydrochloric acid is neutralized by the alkalinity of water. The hypochlorous acid ionizes to form hydrogen ions and hypochlorite ions.

$$H_2O + Cl_2 \longrightarrow HCl + HOCl$$
Water + Chlorine   Hydrochloric acid + hypochlorous acid

$$HOCl \longrightarrow H^+ + OCl^-$$
Hypochlorous acid   Hydrogen ion + Hypochlorite ions

The disinfecting action of this reaction is mainly due to hypochlorous acid and partly due to hypochlorite ions.

- **Procedure of chlorination:** The equipment used for chlorination is called chlorination equipment (Paterson's chloronome), which is the most commonly used and available at all water supply centers. The amount of chlorine required for the specified quantity of water supply is added and all functions to control are performed by this equipment. Chlorination is always done by skilled and expert person or under their supervision. Other substances used for disinfection of water are chloramines, bleaching powder and prochloron, but chlorine is the most effective and safe chemical.

- **Chlorine demand of water:** This is the amount of chlorine required to destroy bacteria and oxidize the organic substances present in water. To estimate this, a fixed amount of chlorine is added to water having a fixed pH and at a fixed temperature, then the amount of residual chlorine is measured after an hour. It means the point at which the chlorine demand of water is fulfilled is called "Breaking point". Chlorine added after this point appears as free chlorine in water.

- **Amount of free residual chlorine:** This is needed to check the bacterial infection of water during storage and supply of purified water. To find out, the residual amount of chlorine in water "orthotolidine arsenite test" is used. After an hour of chlorination 0.5 mg/L of free residual chlorine is kept in the drinking water.

  The total quantity of chlorine is calculated by the formula: The total quantity of chlorine demand and free residual chlorine at the rate of 0.5 mg/L is required for certain quantity of water.

- **Control period:** Chlorine should remain in contact with water for at least one hour to ensure proper chlorination

- **Advantages of chlorination:**
  - It destroys pathogenic bacteria but has no effect on spores and viruses.
  - It makes the water safe and clean.
  - It helps in coagulation.
  - It influences the odor and taste of water.
  - It controls the algae and other impurities generating bacteria.
  - It oxidizes iron, manganese and hydrogen sulfide.

Purification at Small Scale

Water can be purified on a small scale by the following three methods for household purposes:

1. **Boiling:** This is the simplest method and is used for domestic purposes. Before boiling, it should be seen that water is not turbid or has suspended impurities. Suspended impurities should be removed by sedimentation or filtration. Water should be boiled in a storage vessel for 10–20 minutes. Water must be brought to a "rolling boil". It kills all bacteria, spores, cysts and ova. Boiling removes temporary hardness by driving off carbon dioxide and precipitating the calcium carbonate. The taste of water is altered but harmless. It is an excellent method of purifying water but offers no residual protection against subsequent microbial contamination, so it should be boiled in the same container in which it is to be stored.

2. **Chemical disinfection:**
   - **By using bleaching powder:** The freshly prepared bleaching powder contains 33% available chlorine. It is an unstable compound. On exposure to air, light and moisture, it decomposes and loses its chlorine content, but when mixed with an excess of lime, it becomes stabilized bleach. 5 g of bleaching powder is needed to purify 1000 L of water.
   - **Chlorine solution or tablets:** Tablets of chlorine are available of strength 0.5 mg each tablet. One tablet of 0.5 mg is used for 20 L of water to disinfect it. Chlorine solution is prepared from bleaching powder and 5% of chlorine solution is used.
   - **Alum:** Small quantity of alum is used to remove suspended impurities. Its excessive use causes diarrhea.
   - **Iodine:** It is used only in emergencies. Two drops of 2% ethanol solution of iodine are used for 1 L of water and it takes 20–30 minutes to disinfect water. It is expensive, changes the taste and odor of water and may increase thyroid activity.
   - **Potassium permanganate:** It can destroy only vibrio cholera and no other organisms, so it is not effective and is not used anymore.

3. **Filtration:** This method is used for the purification of water at the domestic level. The following filters are used for this purpose:
    - **Cloth filter:** A fine cloth or fine plastic sieve is used to remove impurities of water. A clean cloth or fine plastic sieve is placed over the mouth of pitcher and water is passed through it to remove the physical impurities. The cloth or sieve used for this purpose is cleaned every time before filtration.
    - **Ceramic filters (Fig. 11.4):** The Berkefeld filter is a type of ceramic filter. A long pipe-like structure is fixed in its center, which has innumerable holes in it, this pipe is called filter candle. 'Filter candles are made of porcelain or kieselguhr, a kind of clay. Water filters through these candles. The impurities, including bacteria and eggs of parasites, get removed by these candles and clear water gets collected in the chamber underneath.

        The candle filters get blocked after repeated usage and algae may also grow on the surface, so they should be cleaned with a soft brush and soap and washed thoroughly under running water. The candles should be boiled once a month and dried. This filter removes bacteria and impurities but not viruses.
    - **Ultraviolet filter:** It is most commonly used for domestic purposes. It works in four stages:

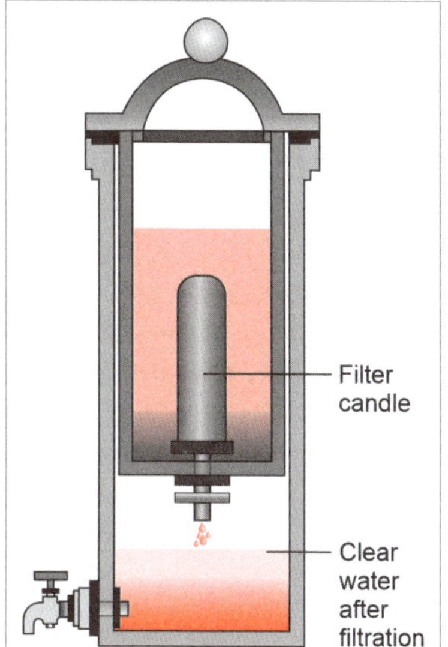

Fig. 11.4: Berkefeld filter

1. **Prefilter:** It removes dust, dirt and turbidity from water.
2. **Activated carbon:** It removes color, odor and biological impurities from water.
3. **Ultraviolet chamber:** Here, water is made free from pathogenic bacteria and viruses.
4. **Electronic monitoring system:** This controls the process of water purification. One liter of water is purified per minute. This is the best available technique used in houses. But due to its high-cost common people cannot afford it.

- **Disinfection of wells:** The main source of water supply in rural areas is the wells that need to be disinfected periodically. To ensure a safe drinking water supply and more frequently during the epidemics of cholera and gastroenteritis. The cheapest and effective method of disinfection of wells is by using bleaching powder.
    - **Steps in well disinfection:**
        i. Find the volume of water in well.
        ii. Measure the depth of water column = (h) meter
        iii. Measure the diameter of the well = (d) meter

$$\text{Volume of water} = \frac{\pi\, d^2 h \times 1000}{4}$$

The value of $\pi = 3.14$

$$\text{So, volume} = \frac{3.14 \times d^2 \times h}{4} \times 1000$$

One cubic meter is 1000 L of water

iv. Calculate the amount of bleaching powder required for disinfection. Roughly 2.5 g of bleaching powder is required to disinfect 1000 L of water.

v. Dissolve the bleaching powder in water and allow it to sediment for 5–10 minutes. When the lime settles down, the supernatant solution is chlorine solution. It is transferred to another vessel and the lime is discarded.

vi. **Delivery of chlorine solution into the well:** The chlorine solution is lowered below the surface of water and the well water is agitated by moving the bucket violently several times, so that chlorine mixes with the water inside the well.

vi. **Contact period:** For 1-hour water should not be used or drawn from the well to allow the disinfection of water.

- **Checking the free residual chlorine:**
  - **Orthotolidine test:** At the end of 1 hour, water is tested for free residual chlorine in water. If it is <0.5 mg/L, the chlorination procedure is repeated, before any water is drawn.
- **Apparatus to calculate the quantity of bleaching powder**
  - **Horrock's apparatus:** This apparatus is used to calculate the quantity of bleaching powder required for disinfection of water. The apparatus consists of the following:
    - Six white cups of 200 mL capacity each
    - One black cup with a circular mark on the inner side
    - Two metal spoons each with a capacity of 2 g bleaching powder when filled up to the level with brim
    - Seven glasses stirring rods
    - One special pipette
    - Two droppers
    - Starch iodine indicator solution
    - Instruction folder
    - **Procedure**
      - Take 2 g of bleaching powder
      - One level spoon in the black cup and make a thin paste with little water. Add more water to the paste up to the circular mark with vigorous stirring. Allow it to settle. This is called stock solution.
      - All six white cups are filled with water to be tested about 1 cm below the brim.
      - The stock solution with a pipette is added: 1 drop to first cup, 2 drops to second, 3 drops to third, 4 drops to fourth, 5 drops to fifth and 6 drops to sixth cup.
      - Each cup is stirred with a separate glass rod.
      - Wait for half an hour for the chlorine to react.
      - Add 3 drops of starch iodide to each white cup and stir with a clean glass rod.
      - Note the color of solution in each cup. Note the cup in which blue color appears first. This cup indicates the presence of free residual chlorine. Note the cup which shows distinct blue color, suppose the 3rd cup shows blue color, then 3 level spoons, i.e., 6 g of bleaching powder would be required to disinfect 455 L of water (2 g per spoon).

> ### Nursing Considerations
>
> **Nurses' Role in Prevention and Control of Water Pollution**
> Educating and motivating community about the following:
> - Importance of safe drinking water and teaching about various waterborne diseases
> - Purification of water at house
> - Safe storage and use of water
> - Surveillance of waterborne diseases
> - Notification and timely treatment of waterborne diseases
> - Keeping the records of wells, and tube wells in the area
> - Finding the source of water to be recharged
> - Providing information to the families, leaders and people at a large scale to make observations on color, odor, taste and turbidity of water and report to the concerned authorities
> - Identifying pollution of water at the source of water supply
> - Providing health education and creating awareness among families, community and leaders about the water crisis
> - In hospitals, taking an active part in water management, controlling the misuse of water in daily activities and creating the innovative water-saving techniques.

AIR

Air is a mixture of gases that form the atmosphere.

Composition of Air

- Oxygen 20.93%
- Nitrogen 78.01%
- Carbon dioxide 0.03%
- Traces of other gasses like argon, helium, neon, xenon, etc., are also present in the air.
- Besides these gases, dust, water vapors, small particles of ammonia, viruses, bacteria, and traces of vegetable debris are also present in the air. The composition of air remains constant but may change due to external factors.

Functions of Air

- Air is vital for all living things. Life is impossible without air.
- It purifies the blood. Blood is cleaned by the exchange of gases in lungs, i.e., carbon dioxide is removed from the blood and oxygen is taken up by the blood.
- It keeps the human body cool.
- It controls body temperature.
- It is the main medium for communication services.
- It is a medium for spreading pollen and bacteria.
- Air-conducted stimuli help in the functioning of auditory and olfactory sense organs.

Airborne Diseases

- These are mainly related to the respiratory system. Continuous coughing for no apparent reason may result in acute bronchitis due to air pollution. If the pollution of air is intense, it may result in immediate death by suffocation.

- The polluted air with droplets of infectious agents causes acute bronchitis, pneumonia, tuberculosis, lung infection, and infection of the upper respiratory tract.
- The other pollutants in the air can cause asthma, emphysema, lung cancer, respiratory allergies, heart problems and neurological problems in children, the elderly, smokers and others with chronic respiratory problems.
- Increased levels of lead can cause neuropsychological development issues in children.
- Sulfur dioxide causes asthma, chronic obstructive pulmonary disease (COPD), respiratory tract infections, and even death in severe exposure.
- Air polluted with hydrocarbons causes lung cancer.

AIR POLLUTION

Air is the basis of life in all forms. Clean air is essential for good health. Changes in the composition of air generate danger for health. In developing countries, air pollution has become a health hazard. The Bhopal gas tragedy in 1984 in India and the smoke from forest fires in Malaysia and Indonesia (1977) were disasters, resulting from air pollution. WHO estimated that about 2 million people die prematurely every year as a result of air pollution (2009). Air pollution is responsible for the diseases of respiratory system, nervous system and heart. There were 8.1 million deaths due to air pollution globally in 2021 and 2.1 million deaths in India.

> **MUST KNOW**
>
> **Pollution**
> Pollution is the process of mixing of the elements of natural environment with those of external environment and becoming active in negative and destructive direction, leaving their natural course of action. In the perspective of this definition, air pollution is a condition in which dust, smoke, toxic gases, chemical vapors and scientific experiments affect the natural composition of air. In other words, when the air becomes harmful for man and his environment, due to excess of external elements the condition is called air pollution.

Sources of Air Pollution

The main sources of air pollution are:

- **Automobiles:** Motor vehicles are the major sources of air pollution throughout the urban area and small towns. They emit hydrocarbons, carbon monoxide, lead, nitrogen oxides and particulate matter. These hydrocarbons and oxides of nitrogen may be converted in the atmosphere into 'photochemical', pollutants of oxidizing nature. All types of vehicles that run on diesel emit black smoke and malodorous fumes and increase air pollution. Due to increased number of vehicles and heavy traffic, Delhi has become the 4th most polluted city in the world, where about 400 kg of lead is released in the air through various gases and badly affects the brain, kidneys, heart. About 60% of air pollution is due to traffic and transportation.
- **Industries:** Industries emit a large number of pollutants into the atmosphere. Combustion of fuel to generate heat and power produces smoke, sulfur dioxide, nitrogen oxides and fly ash. Petrochemical industries generate hydrogen fluoride, hydrochloric acid and organic halides. Many industries discharge carbon monoxide, carbon dioxide, ozone, hydrogen sulfide and sulfur dioxide. Industries discharge their waste from high chimneys at high temperatures and high speeds.
- **Domestic sources:** Wood, coal, gas, oil, etc., used as fuel in homes for cooking food and other works, produce smoke, dust, carbon and other gases. These gases produced by the fuel used for

cooking in homes influence the composition of air. Due to domestic coal burning in 1952 in London, led to a disaster of air pollution in which thousands of people died.

- **Tobacco smoke:** The most direct and important source of air pollution affecting the health of people is tobacco smoke. It affects the health of passive smoker as they inhale the smoke produced by others.
- **Scientific research:** Explosions and reactions performed for the research and development of nuclear technique, space journeys and atomic power pollute the environment. Destruction of space crafts, missiles, weapons, and radioactivity and imbalance in the temperature ultimately results in environmental pollution.
- **Miscellaneous sources:** This includes:
  - Spraying fertilizers and insecticides.
  - Burning waste (Plastic, tires, etc.)
  - Greenhouse effect and change in the ozone layer of the atmosphere.
  - Decreasing forest resources, cutting down trees for industries and buildings for urbanization.
  - Use of chemical gases in war
  - Spilling of petrol and oil in the sea and its burning.
- **Air pollutants:** The major air pollutants are carbon monoxide, carbon dioxide, sulfur dioxide, hydrogen sulfide, lead, cadmium, hydrocarbons, ozone, particulate matter, and polyaromatic hydrocarbons.

Effects of Air Pollution

Air pollution is a slow poison and is becoming a serious environmental problem. It affects not only the health of people but also of all other animals. It has adverse effects on plants, soil, monuments, buildings and climate. Some of the hazards of air pollution are:

- **Effects on human health:** It affects the respiratory system, brain, heart and kidneys. On the respiratory system, it causes colds, coughs, acute bronchitis, tuberculosis, asthma, lung cancer, emphysema and respiratory allergies. The presence of lead in the air affects the brain, heart and kidneys.
- **Effects on soil and plants:** Air pollution, especially sulfur dioxide, fog and ill effects of fluorine compounds, check the growth of plants. Contaminated vegetables consumed by man and animals make them ill. Air pollution abrades, and corrodes metals. These affect the fertility of soils. It causes the disappearance of chlorophyll; the green coloring matter responsible for photosynthesis, the breakdown of plant cells and premature leaf fall. Ozone affects field crops, fruits and fruit trees.
- **Effects on monuments and buildings:** The black soot released by the Mathura refinery is causing blackening of the Taj Mahal. Similarly, other buildings and monuments are getting affected by polluted air. Lots of cleaning and maintenance and repair of buildings increase, besides causing esthetic nuisance.
- **Socioeconomic effects:** Smoke mixed with fog is called smog. Smog can be injurious to health as it contains sulfur dioxide, carbon monoxide and nitrous oxide in sufficient quantity. It reduces visibility due to smoke and fog, causing rail and road accidents and disturbances in road traffic. Uneasiness due to unpleasant smell, etc., are some of the major social effects of air pollution. Air pollution also affects general vitality and reduces the capacity to work and thus affecting economic development.

Control of Air Pollution and Use of Safety Measures

Control of Air Pollution

Air pollution has become a major health disorder related to various systems. To solve the problem of air pollution, and to develop protective measures against it, various countries have launched unified program under WHO. Lack of awareness and resources to solve the problem is a major hindrance in India. It can be controlled by joint efforts. The following measures should be taken to control and prevent air pollution:

- **Containment method:** In this method, the pollutants and toxic substances are prevented from escaping into the surrounding air. This is done by various engineering methods; for example, exhaust fans, suction apparatus and air cleaning devices, etc., are used in factories to improve ventilation. Building enclosures and installing arresters for removal of contamination are other engineering methods of containment.
- **Replacement method:** In this method, those technological processes which produce pollution are replaced with nonpolluting technological processes; for example, the use of compressed natural gas (CNG) instead of diesel in automobiles, use of nonleaded petrol instead of leaded petrol, the use of solar cookers, natural gas/gobar gas instead of firewood, coal, etc., for cooking.
- **Dilution:** Extensive planting of trees and vegetation around industrial and residential areas helps in diluting the pollutants. This is known as establishing a green belt. Dilution can also be achieved by the use of long chimneys high up to the atmosphere, where gases and smoke gets dispersed and diluted.
- **Disinfection of air:** Mechanical ventilation used helps in reducing vitiated air and bacterial activity. Operation theaters and infectious disease wards are disinfected by ultraviolet radiation. Chemical mists, triethylene glycol vapors are effective against bacteria. Dust control is another method of reducing the bacterial content of air in hospitals, wherein the oil is applied to the floors.

Use of Safety Measures

- **Legislative methods:**
  - To set up and strengthen industrial pollution control boards at the state and central level.
  - Imposing environmental tax to prevent pollution.
  - Pollution under control certification should be made compulsory and Air Act (1981) should be implemented properly (prevention and control of pollution).
  - Private organizations should be forced to protect environment.
- **Management of transport and road traffic to reduce the release of pollutants:**
  - Reducing the number of private vehicles.
  - Proper facilities of the public transport system.
  - Discourage the use of motorcycles, cars, scooters, and motorbikes and encouraging the practice of pooling of vehicles by a number of people working at the same place.
  - Stopping overloading of vehicles.
  - Determining the age of vehicles.
  - Industries should be set up away from the residential areas.
  - Proper methods of waste disposal to be used.
- **Mass education:** Public participation is essential to control air pollution. People should be educated about the hazards of air pollution and its control and prevention. People should be

made aware of their rights and duties. The health department, engineering, forest and transportation department, should be jointly and equally responsible for it.

- **Other techniques:**
  - Plantations should be encouraged by the government and voluntary organizations.
  - Deforestation should be discouraged.
  - Proper methods of waste disposal should be used.
  - Industries should be set up away from the residential area.
  - Use of helmet, mask, and glasses, while driving.
  - Alternative fuels to be used instead of wood.

Nursing Considerations

Roles of Community Health Nurses in Control and Prevention of Air Pollution

Air pollution is a worldwide problem. Government alone cannot control it without public participation. Community health nurse is a member of environmental health and has a significant role in solving this problem. She can help solve this problem in the following ways:

- **By providing health education:** By educating individuals, families and community about the composition of air, the need for clean air and sources of air pollution.
  - Informing people about the sources of air pollution and methods of its control.
  - Advising people to avoid crowded places, fairs and large gatherings.
  - Encouraging them to give up smoking.
  - Motivating people for early morning walks.
  - Teaching school children about the sources of air pollution and its ill effects on health will go a long way in controlling air pollution.
- **Legal roles:** Ensuring active participation in implementing the health laws regarding pollution and cleanliness of air. Reporting the responsible authorities about the breaking or violation of these laws.
  - Seeking cooperation of local administration and local bodies (like municipal committees, municipal corporation, etc.)
- **Technical participation:** Consulting air scientists and public health engineers about latest techniques and motivating the community to take benefit from them. Gathering knowledge about low-cost techniques of constructing well-ventilated houses and a lot of sunlight and passing on this information to the community.
- **Roles related to treatment:** Predicting the possible outbreak of diseases caused by air pollution with their ill effects on health, diagnosing these diseases at the primary level and making arrangements for proper treatment and referral services.

WASTE

Waste or refuse is the unwanted leftover substance that has been discarded. Waste, litter, garbage, etc., are other names of refuse.

Types of Waste

Waste is divided into two categories:

1. **Solid waste/refuse:** This includes street and household waste, i.e., peels of vegetable, fruits, ash packing material, bits of paper, rags, glass pieces, empty tins, newspapers, metal parts, electrical goods, electronic items and plastic bags, dead animals, manures and demolition products.

2. **Wet refuse/waste:** Sewage, liquid waste materials, contaminated water are the examples of wet refuse. This includes:
    - Sewage and animal excreta
    - Dirty domestic water
    - Water overflowed or wasted while collecting it from water supply
    - Contaminated water of markets, fairs, streets, slaughter houses, etc.
    - Industrial wastewater, especially of chemical factories, small scale industries like dyeing, printing, etc.

Sources of Waste

- **Street refuse:** It is collected by street cleansing service. It consists of leaves, straw, papers, animal dropping and litters of all kinds.
- **Market refuse:** It is collected from market and consists of large proportions of putrid vegetables and animal matter.
- **Stable refuse:** It is collected from stables. It contains animal droppings and leftover animal feeds.
- **Domestic refuse:** It consists of ash, rubbish and garbage. Ash is the residue from firewood used for cooking and heating. Rubbish consists of paper, clothing, bits of wood, metal, glass dust and dirt. Garbage is waste matter arising from the preparation, cooking and consumption of food, such as waste food, vegetable peelings and other organic matter. Garbage needs quick removal and disposal because it ferments on storage.
- **Industrial refuse:** It consists of waste ranging from completely garbage inert material, such as calcium carbonate to highly toxic and explosive compounds.
- **Biomedical waste or hospital refuse:** Hospital waste like soiled dressings, used syringes needles, plastic items, clothes, IV sets, bottles of medicine, plastic wrappers, foul smelling clothes with blood and plaster cast are the major chunk of the solid waste of hospital.
- **E-waste:** Electronic waste has become a major source of solid refuse. It is increasing day by day due to new models and discoveries.
    - **Storage of waste:** Before disposing the waste, it has to be stored at one place. The refuse can be stored in dustbins which are made of zinc, plastic, cement or steel or drums with closed lids.
    - **Collection of waste:** The method of collection depends upon the availability of funds. House to house collection is the best method, but it is expensive. In India, the people dump the refuse in the nearest public bin. The refuse is then transported by refuse collection vehicle to the place of ultimate disposal.
    - **Transportation:** The refuse from the dustbins is collected at different places and is transported in final disposal by following methods:
        - **Push cart and trolleys:** These are used to transport refuse collected from residential areas, markets and streets to other large vehicles.
        - **Tractor trolleys:** These are uncovered and can pollute the environment. Covered trolleys may be helpful for transportation of refuse.
        - **Dumpers:** These are better to transport refuse but covered vehicles should be used.

Methods of Waste Disposal

The principal methods of waste disposal are:

Dumping

In dumping method, waste is dumped into low-lying areas so as the level of ground can be lifted and brought to the same level of surrounding areas. The refuse decomposes into manure due to bacterial action.

- **Advantage:** It levels the ground and can be used in agricultural land.
- **Disadvantages:**
  - The refuse is exposed to the flies and rodents.
  - Air pollution and foul smell spread to the surrounding area.
  - Loose refuse is dispersed by the action of wind.
  - Drainage from dumps contributes to pollution of surface and groundwater.

The WHO expert committee (1967) condemned dumping as "a most insanitary method that creates public health hazards, a nuisance and severe pollution of the environment", dumping should be replaced by sound procedures.

Controlled Tipping or Sanitary Land Filling

This method is the most satisfactory method of refuse disposal, but sufficient land should be available. There are three methods used for controlled tipping:

1. **The trench method:** Where level ground is available, long trenches are dug out 2–3 m deep and 4–12 m wide. Refuse is dumped into it and covered with soil. Dumpers and bulldozers accomplish this work with ease.
2. **The ramp method:** This method is useful where the terrain is moderately sloping. Some excavation is done to secure the covering material.
3. **The area method:** This method is used for filling land depressions, disused quarries and clay pits. The refuse is deposited, packed and consolidated in uniform layers up to 2–2.5 m deep. Each layer is sealed on its exposed surface with a mud cover of at least 30 cm thick. Such sealing prevents infestation by flies and rodents and suppresses the nuisance of smell and dust. Chemical, bacteriological and physical changes take place in buried refuse. The temperature rises over 60°C within 7 days and kills all pathogens. It hastens the process of decomposition. After 4–6 months, the refuse is converted into good quality of manure.
   - **Advantage:**
     - This method is free from air pollution from burning.
     - It avoids the visual unpleasantness.
     - It also keeps the surrounding environment safe.
   - **Disadvantages:**
     - Too much land is required.
     - Nearby water sources may get contaminated.
     - If machines are not available, covering the trench with soil becomes a laborious task.

Incineration

Incineration is the best method of waste disposal. Presently, under the environmental management hospitals are directed to use incinerator to dispose of the biomedical waste. Tin, glass, sand, etc., should be removed from refuse before burning it. An incinerator can burn 250–450 kg of refuse every day.

- **Advantages:**
  - Less space is required
  - Reduced transportation cost
  - Quantity of refuse reduced to 1/4th
  - Economical to use
  - Useful for burning industrial waste
- **Disadvantages:**
  - Risk of infection for labor.
  - Reduced height of chimney can increase air pollution
  - Sorting of refuse is laborious and time consuming

Composting

Composting technique can be used to dispose of both sewage and refuse. Heat produced during the process is >60°C, which destroys eggs, larvae of flies, weed seeds and pathogenic agents. The compost produced at the end of decomposition process is the good quality of manure. There are two methods of decomposing:

1. **Anaerobic or Bangalore method:** In this method, a trench 90 cm deep, 2.5 m round and 10 m long is dug. First layer of refuse that is 15 cm thick is laid at the bottom of trench. A 5 cm thick layer of excreta is laid on it. This order is repeated till trench remains 30 cm from the ground level. Then, the pit is completely filled with soil and after 6 months, it is dug open to procure manure.

    In this method, human excreta are mixed by human labor which is an undignified and unpleasant work. This can also lead to infection. It can be used only at the small scale.

2. **Aerobic or mechanical composting:** In this technique, all work is accomplished through machines. Pieces of glass, metal, bones and rags are taken out and remaining refuse is grinded. After this, machine mixes excreta with grinded refuse, and the process of manure formation is completed in 4–6 weeks. This method is used on a large scale refuse disposal in big cities.

Manure Pit

Manure pit method is used in rural areas. A pit is dug about 1–5 m broad and 2 m deep away from the house. All the domestic refuse, i.e. garbage, cattle dung, straw and leaves, is dumped into the pit and covered with soil each day. It is closed properly when it is full and another pit is dug. The first pit is opened after 4–6 months and the manure obtained is used for agricultural purposes.

Burial

Burial method is suitable for small camps. A burial trench of 1.5 m wide and 2 m deep is dug. Every day refuse is put into it and covered with 20–30 cm thick layer of soil. When the depth of the trench is reduced to only 40 cm from the ground level, then it is covered compactly. After 4–6 months, the contents of the first trench are removed and used in the fields as manure.

Health hazards of solid waste, if allowed to accumulate:

- It decomposes and favors fly breeding.
- It attracts rodent and vermin.
- The pathogens which may be present in the solid waste, may be conveyed back to man's food through flies and dust.
- There is a possibility of water and soil pollution.
- Heaps of refuse present around residential areas, create bad odors and pollute air.

EXCRETA

Human excreta are a source of infection. Controlling the source of infection and breaking the disease cycle is an essential aspect of environmental health. Every society has a responsibility for its safe removal and disposal so that it does not constitute a threat to public health.

Health Hazards of Improper Excreta Disposal

Health hazards of improper excreta disposal are:

- Soil pollution
- Water pollution
- Contamination of food
- Propagation of flies and rodents
- Air pollution due to foul smell.

The resulting diseases are typhoid and paratyphoid fever, dysentery, diarrhea, cholera and worm infestations. These diseases are not only a burden on community in terms of sickness, mortality and low expectations of life, but deteriorate the social and economic progress of the community and country at large. Proper disposal of human excreta, therefore is a fundamental environmental service without which there cannot be any improvement in the state of community health.

Transmission of Diseases Through Excreta

Diseases are transmitted from the excreta of a sick person or a carrier through the following channels (Fig. 11.5):

- Water
- Food
- Fingers
- Flies
- Soil

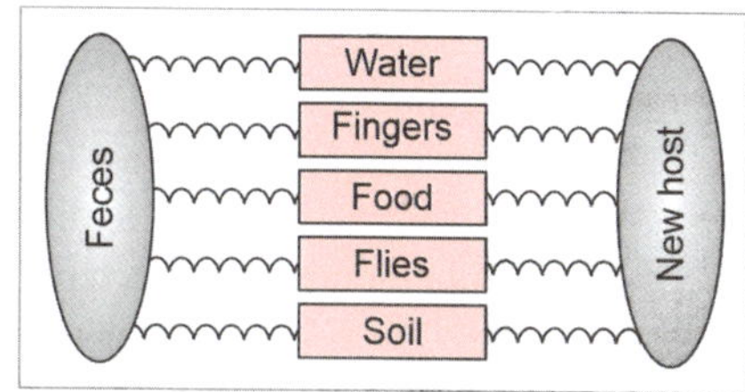

Fig. 11.5: Channels of transmission of diseases

Methods of Excreta Disposal

The methods of excreta disposal are divided into two groups:
1. Excreta disposal method for unsewered areas.
2. Excreta disposal method for sewered and urban areas.

Excreta Disposal in Unsewered Areas

- **Service latrine:** Night soil is collected from pails or buckets manually by human agency and later disposed by burning or composting. This type of latrines is against the dignity of man and responsible for infection, water and soil pollution. This type of latrines is not existing nowadays and is replaced by sanitary latrine.
- **Traveler's latrine:** This type of latrine is used in trains and ships. Latrines on trains spread the excreta in the center of tracks and produce foul smell and unpleasant view.
- **Sanitary latrine:** This type of latrine is also known as nonservice type. In this, the excreta is not disposed of by humans. A sanitary latrine is one which fulfills the following criteria:
  - Excreta should not pollute the soil.
  - Excreta should not pollute surface water.

- Excreta should not create a nuisance due to foul smell or unsightly appearance.
- Excreta should not be accessible to flies, rodents, animals and other vehicles for transmission of infection.
- **Types of sanitary latrines:**
    - **Borehole latrine (Fig. 11.6):** It was introduced by Rockefeller foundation during 1930's in campaigns of hookworm control. It consists of a circular hole of 40 cm diameter, 6 m in depth. A concrete slab with a hole and foot rest is placed on the hole.

        A suitable enclosure is built around it to provide privacy. Excreta falls in a deep hole below. This serves a family of 5–6 people in a year. When the contents of hole reach within 20 inches of the ground level. The squatting plate is removed, the hole is closed with earth and a new hole is dug similarly and used. This type of latrines is not used and is replaced by better innovations. Since the hole of this type of latrine is dug using a boring machine, this is called borehole latrine.

    - **Dug well latrine (Fig. 11.7):** This is similar to the borehole latrines, but to dig the pit, boring machine is not required. In this type, a hole of 3–3.5 m deep and 75 cm in diameter is dug. A concrete plate is placed over the hole to sit on. This was introduced in Singur, West Bengal in 1949–1950. A small family can use this type of latrine for 5 years. After that the pit is closed. The night soil undergoes **purification** by anaerobic digestion and is converted into a harmless mass.

    - **Water seal latrine (Fig. 11.8):** This is an improved version of sanitary latrine for small towns and rural areas. Here, excreta is "hand flushed by the users". The squatting plate is fitted with water seal; for this, a bent pipe is used that is called trap. Trap is always filled with water to a certain level. This trap prevents the escape of foul smell and excreta not exposed and also protects the flies. This latrine is of two types.
        1. **PRAI type:** The planning research and action institute, Lucknow has designed.
        2. **RCA type:** It has been designed under the sanitation project (Research cum Action) of

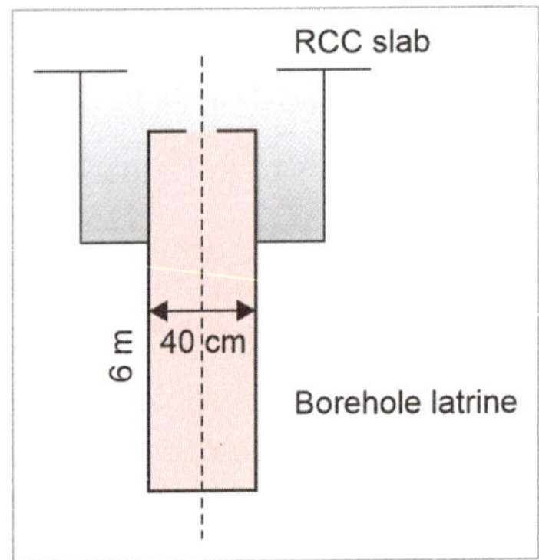

Fig. 11.6: Borehole latrine

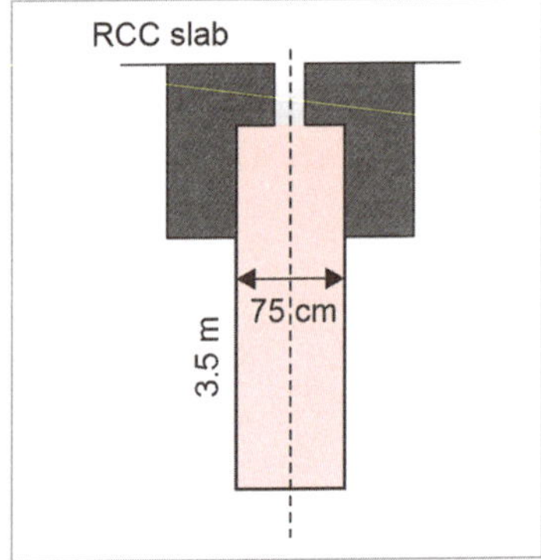

Fig. 11.7: Dug well latrine

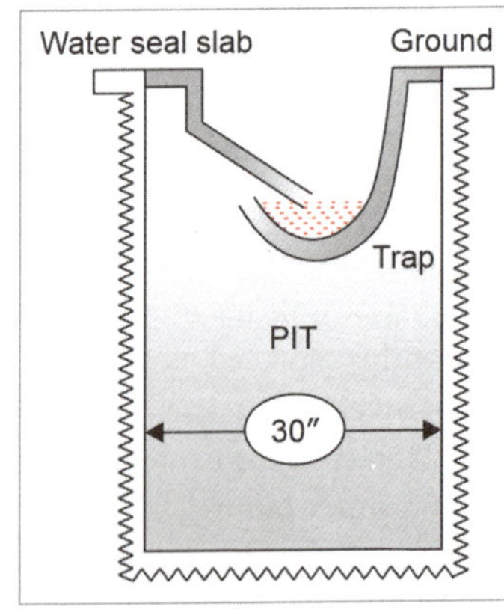

Fig. 11.8: Water seal latrine

the central government. RCA type of latrine is more used. Sulabh Shauchalaya latrine is also an example of a water seal latrine and its use and popularity is rising.

- **Sulabh Shauchalaya:** This model is the invention of Patna based firm. It is a low-cost pour-flush, water-seal type of latrine. It is an improved version of the standard hand flush latrine (RCA type). It consists of a specially designed pan and a water-seal trap. It is connected to a pit of 3 feet square and 3 feet deep. Excreta undergoes bacterial decomposition and is converted to manure. This method requires very little water.

- **Septic tanks:** These are used in residential and small organizations for excreta disposal. In absence of a public sewage system, sewage is disposed of by septic tanks. This is a tank made of bricks and cement having two chambers. The tank has an inlet through which excreta enters the tank and effluent is collected in a constructed pit through the outlet. The solids settle down in the tanks to form "sludge", while the lighter solids including grease and fat rise to the surface to form scum. The sludge is reduced in volume as a result of anaerobic digestion. Periodic removal of sludge from the tank is essential. The liquid escaping from the outlet is allowed to percolate into the subsoil, where it undergoes aerobic digestion by means of millions of bacteria present in the upper layer of soil (Fig. 11.9).

- **Aqua privy:** Its function is like a septic tank. Privy consists of a water tight chamber filled with water. A short length of a drop pipe from the latrine floor dips into water. The tank may be rectangular, circular in shape. The size depends upon the number of users. Night soil undergoes **purification** by anaerobic digestion. A vent pipe should be placed for the escape of gases into the atmosphere above the roof of the dwelling. The digested sludge is removed at intervals (Fig. 11.10).

- **Latrines suitable for camps and temporary use:**
  - **Shallow trench latrine:** A trench is dug about 30 cm (1 feet) wide and 90–150 cm deep (3–5 feet) the dugout soil is headed nearby. A foot rest is used to sit on the trench,

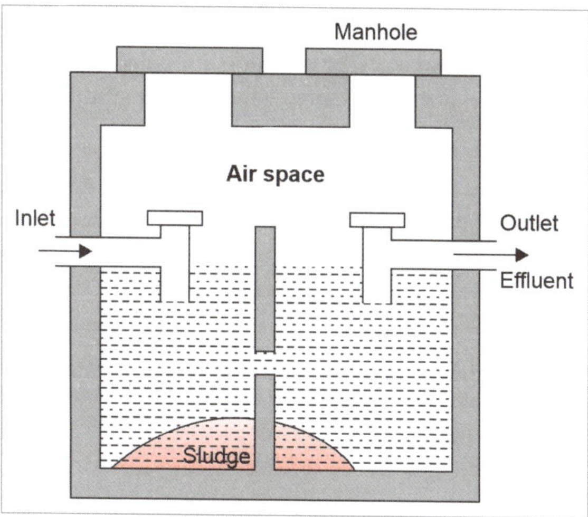

Fig. 11.9: Septic tank

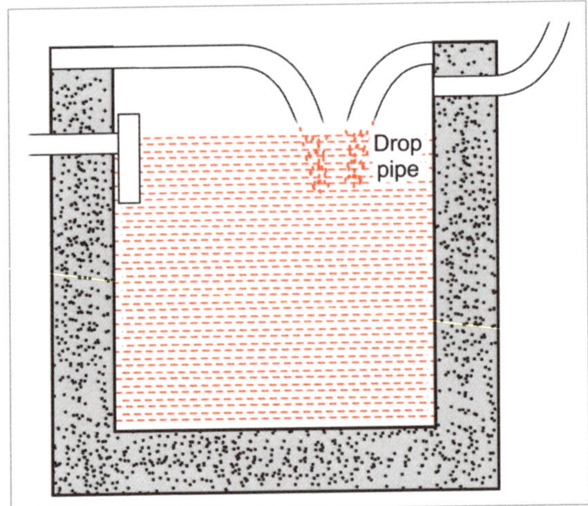

Fig. 11.10: Aqua privy

people are instructed to cover the excreta with soil. Separate trenches are dug for males and females. When the trench is 30 cm below ground level, it is covered with earth headed above ground level and compacted.

- **Deep trench latrines:** This type of latrines is used in long duration camps. The trench is dug about 2–2.5 m deep and 75–90 cm broad. The length is kept according to the number of users.
- **Pit latrine:** Also known as a long drop or dry latrine, is a basic type of toilet that collects human waste in a hole in the ground. They are a low-cost option for remote areas without a water supply.
- **Borehole latrine:** Description is already given.

Excreta Disposal in Sewered Areas

Sewage system is a good and healthy technique of disposing sewage and dirty water in cities or areas with systematic town planning. In this technique, sewage and dirty water are transported through underground pipes to the disposal area. The main methods of excreta disposal used in sewered areas are:

Water carriage system: In this method, the human excreta and wastewater from residential, commercial and industrial areas are transported via network of underground pipes called sewers to the ultimate disposal. From big cities, towns and high-density population areas, sewage is collected and transported to the area of disposal. Water carriage system is of two types:

1. **Combined sewer system:** In this type, the sewer carries sewage and surface water.
2. **Separate sewer system:** In this method, the surface water is not admitted into the sewers. The water carriage system consists of the following elements:
   - **Sewer appurtenance:** Manhole and traps, etc.
   - **Household sanitary fittings:** These are water closets, urinals, and washbasins. May be Indian squatting type or Western type of toilets. Water closets are provided with a 'flushing rim'. Human excreta are directly received in the water into the closet, without soiling the sides. The flushing removes all traces of excreta from the sides and keeps the closet clean.

The closet is connected to a small cistern by a pipe of 2.5–3.75 cm diameter. The flushing cistern holds about 15 L of water and works by siphonic action. The flushing cistern may be high-level or low-level.

- **House sewer/drain:** The house drain pipe is usually 15 cm below the ground level on a bed of cement concrete with a sufficient gradient toward the main drain. The house drain empties the sewage into the main sewer or public drain.
- **Street sewers or trunk sewers:** These are 22.5 cm (9 inches) in diameter. They are laid on a bed of cement concrete about 3 m (10 feet) below the ground level with a sufficient gradient to ensure self-cleansing velocity of 2–3 feet/second. The trunk sewers collect sewage from several houses and transport it to the main outfall or place for final disposal.
- **Sewer appurtenances:** These are manholes and traps installed into the sewerage system.
    - **Manholes:** Manholes are openings built into the sewerage system. These openings permit a person to enter the sewer for inspection, repair and cleaning. Workers entering manholes are liable to gas poisoning and asphyxiation, so due precautions should be taken for their safety.
    - **Traps:** Traps are devices designed to prevent foul gases from entering the houses and to remove sand, grit and grease from sewage. They are placed in three situations:
        1. Under the basis of water closet.
        2. Where the house drain joins the public drain
        3. Where surface wastewater enters the drain.

        The installation of a sewerage system involves specialized skill in planning, designing, construction, operation and maintenance.

SEWAGE

Sewage is the waste from residential, commercial and other organizations, containing solids and liquids excreta with an unpleasant smell. The dirty water collected from the joint sewage system is also known as sewage. The wastewater which does not contain human excreta, such as wastewater from kitchens and bathrooms is called "sullage".

Sewage contains 99.9% of water and 0.1% of solid matter in the form of excreta. The offensive smell of the sewage is due to the organic matter which it contains. The organic matter decomposes. During the process of decomposition, some foul-smelling gases like hydrogen sulfide, are liberated which gives an offensive odor. Home sewage contains 100–500 g/L of solid matter as human excreta. An adult expels 100 g of excreta per day. The quantity of sewage may be more according to the number of members in a family.

Objectives of Sewage Treatment

- To conserve the life of the aquatic animals, as the sewage can deplete the oxygen in water which may lead to the death of the plants and animals' life in water. So, to conserve this life sewage purification must be done.
- To participate in town planning.
- To aid the organic matter to liberate carbon dioxide, nitrate and water so as to treat the offensive odor due to hydrogen sulfide.
- To obtain pathogen effluent that can be disposed of without any problem.
- To prevent air pollution.

- To protect the water supply system, i.e., preventing the water supply from getting contaminated by improper sewage system.
- To prevent soil pollution.
- To protect from sewage borne diseases
- Water and sludge obtained after purification can be used safely for irrigation and other agricultural activities.

Methods of Sewage Treatment

The methods of sewage treatment are as follows:

Sewage Treatment Plant Method

This method is based on the biological principles, in which the treatment of sewage is done by the action of aerobic and anaerobic bacteria. This treatment is described under three headings:

1. **Primary treatment:** It has three stages:
   i. **Screening:** Sewage is passed through a metal screen, where pieces of wood, rags, garbage and dead animals, etc., are separated. This removal is done to prevent the clogging of the treatment plant. Screening can be movable or non-movable. Matter collected by screening is removed by hand or with the help of a machine and then disposed of either by burial or by burning.
   ii. **Grit chamber:** After screening, sewage is passed through a 20–30 m long grit chamber. Here, a steady flow of sewage is maintained due to which, heavy particles like sand and gravel settle down. These substances are removed periodically and disposed of by dumping or trenching.
   iii. **Primary sedimentation:** After passing through the grit chambers, the sewage reaches the primary sedimentation tank. This tank is rectangular in shape. Sewage is allowed to pass very slowly at a velocity of 1–2 feet/minute and kept in this tank for 6–8 hours, 50–70% of the organic solid matter settles down under the influence of gravity in the form of sedimentation. The settled organic matter is called sludge. The sludge is removed by mechanically operated devices without disturbing the operation in the tank and pumped into the digester. Very small bacteria present in the tank attack the solid substances and break them into simpler soluble elements and ammonia. A certain amount of fat and grease rises to the surface to form scum, which is removed from time to time and disposed of. The effluent from the primary sedimentation is greatly cleaned.

2. **Secondary treatment:** The effluent coming out of primary sedimentation tank still contains organic matter and bacteria. It has got great affinity for oxygen and can cause pollution of soil and water. This is subjected to secondary treatment by aerobic oxidation by any of the following methods:

MUST KNOW

Decomposition of Organic Matter

It takes place by aerobic and anaerobic process.

- **Aerobic process:** Aerobic decomposition of organic matter takes place in the presence of dissolved oxygen. The organic matter is broken down into simpler compounds by the process of oxidation. The compounds formed are carbon dioxide, water, ammonia, nitrates, nitrites and sulfites by the action of organism, i.e., bacteria, fungi and protozoa.
- **Anaerobic process:** Anaerobic decomposition of the organic matter takes place when the sewage is highly concentrated and contains plenty of solids. The end products of decomposition are methane, ammonia, carbon dioxide and hydrogen. In anaerobic decomposition, the reactions are slower and the mechanism of decomposition is extremely complex.

- **Trickling filter method:** This filter is a layer of gravel 1–2 m deep and 2–3 m in diameter. The size of the filter is determined according to the amount of collected sewage and the size of population. The effluent of primary sedimentation tank is sprinkled uniformly on the surface of filter by revolving device of perforated pipes. The process of purification begins with the action of aerobic bacteria; the bacteria form a slimy layer called zoogleal layer. This layer is responsible for the treatment of sewage. Oxidized sewage is sent to a secondary tank. This tank is also known as the manure tank. Sludge collected in the tank changes into a good quality of manure.

- **Activated sludge process:** The effluent from the primary sedimentation tank is passed through an aerated chamber. Here, it is mixed with activated sludge, which is rich in aerobic bacteria. Mixing is done by pumping compressed air in the chamber. The process continues for 6–8 hours, after which the aerobic bacteria oxidize organic matter in the sewage into carbon dioxide, water and nitrates. This method is suitable for big cities and is the modern method of purifying sewage.

3. **Disposal of remainders:** The sludge obtained after 2–3 hours of sedimentation is called activated sludge or aerated sludge. Some part of it is carried back to aeration chamber, while the remaining is sent back to the sludge digester. The sludge is disposed by following methods:

   - **Sludge digestion:** Sludge obtained from sedimentation tanks is pumped into sludge digestion tank. Here, sludge is incubated under favorable conditions of temperature and pH is treated with anaerobic bacteria. Here, it undergoes anaerobic autodigestion and the complex organic solids are broken down into carbon dioxide, methane, water and ammonia. The volume of sludge is greatly reduced. It takes 3–4 weeks or longer for complete digestion. The residue is inoffensive, sticky, and tarry mud which dries of readily to form good quality of manure.

   - **Disposal of effluent:** Disposal of effluent obtained from last sedimentation tank is chlorinated and used for irrigation or it can be mixed with river or streams. Effluents of Okhla sewage treatment plant, Delhi is used for irrigation.

     - **Sea outfall:** Here, sewage is directly discharged into sea which disappears in the vast and deep expanse of water. Solid part of the sewage gets oxidized but sewage should be released deep into the water far away from the coast. Nearly 2/3rd of the sewage of Mumbai is discharged into Arabian sea.

     - **Land treatment:** After primary treatment, sewage is released toward the land through pipes. This method of using effluents for irrigation is known as land treatment. Crops that do not come in contact with the sewage on land can be cultivated through this method, or trees which bear fruits high above the ground should be grown on this soil.

Oxidation Pond

This is very cost-effective method of sewage treatment for small population or commercial establishments. The oxidation pond is referred by different names, i.e., waste stabilization ponds, redox pond, sewage lagoons, etc. At present, 50 ponds are functioning in India. It works in the presence of sunlight, algae and certain types of bacteria.

- **Construction of oxidation pond:** The ponds are 1–1.5 m deep and have an inlet and an outlet. For the proper and efficient working of oxidation ponds, there should be proper sunlight, presence of algae in the pond, a specific type of bacteria which receive nutrition from decomposed organic matter. Ponds should be constructed in an open area and entry of children and animal should be banned in that area.

- **Working system:** The organic matter present in the sewage is oxidized by the bacteria into carbon dioxide, water and ammonia. Algae consume carbon dioxide and organic chemicals with the help of sunlight and release oxygen that is required for oxidation. Thus, algae and bacteria maintain biological balance for their mutual benefit. Algae release oxygen in the presence of sunlight. Sunlight is essential for oxidation ponds. Oxidation ponds work at full capacity during sunny days. Anaerobic bacteria play a major role in treatment of sewage, while aerobic bacteria have a minor role to play in this process.
  - **Advantages:** Effluent obtained from the outlet of these ponds may be used for growing vegetables, crops or sewage farming or can be released in river or a stream after purification.
  - **Disadvantages:** Oxidation ponds are the suitable methods of sewage treatment on a small scale but increase the chances of breeding mosquitoes in the surrounding area. To control the mosquito population, minimum vegetation should be allowed to grow on the banks of ponds. Foul smell emanating from oxidation pond is also a problem.

Other Methods of Sewage Treatment

Other recommended methods of sewage treatment are:
- Oxidation ditches
- Aerated lagoons

These are low-cost treatment methods for the purification of sewage.

HEALTH HAZARDS OF WASTE ON HUMAN HEALTH

Human health is related to his environment. Presence of refuse and excreta in the environment has an ill effect on the health. Waste management has become a major health problem. Refuse and waste can cause the following health problem:

- **Increasing the number of disease-carrying agents:** Refuse and waste are the sources of flies, insects, rats, dogs, pigs and other stray animals. The flies, insects and rodents can be the cause of cholera, plague, dysentery and other intestinal infections.
- **Air pollution and foul smell in the environment:** Foul smell of decomposed refuse and smoke due to burning of refuse cause respiratory problems.
- **Pollution of water resources:** Drinking water may get contaminated due to leakage of pipes, if the refuse is collected near the source of water or waste may be blown into the water. Refuse can contaminate rainwater. Consumption of contaminated water leads to waterborne diseases.
- **Destroying the esthetics:** Foul smell of refuse destroys the esthetic of the city and residential areas, and residents may suffer from hesitation, inhibition and depression due to unpleasant odors.
- **Contamination of food:** If refuse and waste are collected near the residential area, the flies and insects may contaminate food and cause gastrointestinal infections.
- **Pollution of soil:** If the refuse and waste are kept collected on soil, it causes soil pollution.

HOUSING

Housing is defined as the physical structure, that is required for a person including all necessary services, facilities, equipment and devices needed for the physical and mental health and the social well-being of the family and individuals. Housing is the most important component of man's total environment.

Housing provides shelter, protection, all basic needs, rest, sleep, cooking, bathing, family life and care. Housing provides physical, sociological and psychological support of family members to each other through thick and thin. Good housing is responsible for man's health and total well-being.

Location

The place selected for constructing house should be located in a healthy area. There should be an access to the community facilities, such as health services, schools, shopping areas, swimming pool, place of worship, parks and community hall.

Types of Housing

- **Pucca house:** This type of house is made of bricks, cement, waterproof ceiling with all electrical and drainage facilities. This kind of houses is built in cities, towns and also in developing rural areas of the country.
- **Kutcha house:** This type of house is made of clay, wood and bamboo. These kinds of houses are found in villages and in poor community.
- **Mixed type:** For example, pucca and kutcha houses. These houses are made of bricks, clay, wood, etc. and are found in villages in poor community.
- **Wooden house:** This type of house is made of wood and bamboo and is found in earthquake prone areas.
- **Tent houses:** The tents are made of thick canvas used for making temporary houses in fairs, festivals, etc.

Characteristics of Good Housing

An expert committee of WHO (1974) recommended the criteria for good housing:
- Healthful housing provides physical protection and shelter.
- It provides adequately for cooking, eating, washing and excretory functions.
- It is designed, constructed and maintained in such a way as to prevent the spread of communicable diseases.
- It provides protection from sound pollution and air pollution.
- It is free from harmful and toxic materials released due to construction work.
- It encourages personal and community developments, promotes social relationship and reflects a regard for ecological principles and hence promotes mental health.

Basic Amenities/Housing Standard

Housing standard varies according to social and economic status, family size, composition, living standard, lifestyle, stages in life cycle, education and cultural factors. It also varies from country to country and from region to region. The minimum standard recommended by (EHC) (1947) are as:

- **Site:**
  - Should be elevated from its surroundings, so that it is not subjected to flooding during rains.
  - Should have an independent access to streets and link roads of adequate width
  - Away from breeding places of mosquitoes and flies
  - Away from traffic, excessive noise, dust, smoke and smell
  - Should be safe and dry for foundation structure
  - Surrounding should be pleasant.
- **Set back:** For proper lighting and ventilation, there should be open space around the house. This is called "set back".
- **Walls:**
  - Walls should be reasonably strong
  - Should have low heat capacity, should not absorb heat and conduct the same
  - Weather resistant
  - Unsuitable for harborage of rats and vermin
  - Not easily damaged
  - Smooth

  These standards can be maintained by 9″ brick wall plastered smooth and colored cream or white.
- **Floor:** Floor should be pucca and satisfy the following criteria:
  - It should be impermeable, so that it should be easily washed and dried.
  - It should be smooth and free from cracks and crevices to prevent the breeding of insects and harborage of dust.
  - It should be damp proof.
  - The height of the plinth should be 2–3 feet.
- **Roof:** The height of roof should not be <10 feet in the absence of air conditioning for comfort. The roof should have low heat transmission coefficient.
- **Rooms:** The minimum number of living room should be at least two, one of which can be closed for security. The number and area of rooms should be increased according to the size of the family so that recommended floor space per person may be made available.
- **Windows:** Unless mechanical ventilation and artificial lighting are provided, every living rooms should have two windows and one of them should open directly to an open space.
  - The windows should be placed at height not >3 feet above the ground in living room
  - Window area should be 1/5th of the floor area. Doors and windows combined should have 2/5th of the floor area.
- **Floor area:** The floor area of a living room should be at least 120 sq ft for occupancy of >1 person and 100 sq ft for a single person is optimum, and minimum area per person is 50 sq ft.
- **Lighting:** There should be proper arrangement of lighting. The day light factor should exceed 1% over half the floor area.
- **Kitchen:** There should be separate kitchen for every dwelling house. Kitchen must be protected against dust, smoke, fly proof and insect and rodent proof. Lighting should be adequate with provision for storing food, grocery, crockery and cutlery and water supply provided with sink for washing utensils. Floor should be impervious fitted with arrangement for proper drainage.

- **Privy:** A sanitary privy is must in every home, belonging exclusively to it and readily accessible.
- **Garbage and refuse:** These should be removed from the dwelling daily and disposed of in a sanitary manner.
- **Bathing and washing:** Bathing and washing facilities belonging exclusively to the house and proper privacy should be there.
- **Water supply:** Safe and adequate water supply should be available at all times.

Town Planning

Before construction of houses, town planning is mandatory to provide basic amenities in the dwelling units. Wherever the towns or dwelling units are to be established, a suitable site is to be selected. Then, the architects and engineers plan proper housing with adequate and safe drainage system, water supply, lighting, streets and parks, shopping centers, place for worship, schools and play grounds for the children. So, the preparation and implementation of plans related to basic infrastructure of cities and towns is known as town planning.

Objectives

- Providing basic amenities to the citizens which include healthful housing, safe water supply, appropriate lighting and proper medical facilities.
- Good transport system is very important. It includes developing public transport system and transport facilities of the town according, to the traffic engineering and looking at the present and future population.
- Conservation of environment. It includes proper disposal system of waste and refuse, control of air pollution and sound pollution.
- Provision of citizen welfare facilities like parks, playgrounds, swimming pools, community centers, labor welfare center and orphanages, etc.
- Establishing the outlines and standards of plans, making arrangement for estimated cost, revenue collection and local institutional management.
- Increasing the participation of the citizens in development of towns, evaluating it according to the feedback.

Advantages

- Raising the living standards of the people by providing basic amenities like healthful housing, safe water supply, and adequate lighting and ventilation, helps in improving their living standards, which in turn increases their working capacity.
- Reduction in the number of accidents. Wide and clean roads ensure a smooth flow of traffic and help in reducing the number of accidents.
- **Conservation of environment:** Proper methods of waste disposal, appropriate sewerage system, plantation, and parks to keep the environment of the planned city clean. Similarly implementing preventive laws and control air and sound pollution, makes the environment conductive for good health. Citizens should be motivated to conserve the environment and contribute in maintaining the standard of cities.
- **Promotion of health:** Healthy housing, raised standard of living, comfortable transportation, protected environment and availability of health services protect the citizens against diseases

and improve their level of health. Facilities of entertainment centers, parks, swimming pools, community centers and gardens also improve the status of mental health of the citizens.

- **Improved esthetics:** Well-designed homes, crossing streets, roads and circles, markets, commercial complexes and parks of planned towns, add to the beauty of the town. It increases tourism and people feel proud of their cities. The Examples of good town planning are Chandigarh, Jaipur and Ahmedabad.
- **Other advantages:** Checking the stray animals, insect control, generating more revenue, night shelters (Rain Basera) and conducting other welfare programs are the other important aspects of town planning.

Central governments, the ministry of urban and town development, department of town planning, housing boards, public works department, water supply, electricity, medical and health and the department of transport play important role in town planning. At the local level, urban development authorities, local bodies, municipalities and other autonomous organizations bear the responsibilities of town planning.

Ventilation

Ventilation means the "exchange of air between outdoors and indoors", or the entry of fresh and pure air to replace the stagnant and vitiated air from the room.

The modern concept of ventilation implies not only the replacement of vitiated air by a supply of fresh outdoor air but also control of the quality of incoming air with regard to its temperature, humidity and purity with a view to provide a thermal environment that is comfortable and free from risk of infection.

Thus, we can say that "ventilation is the science of preserving or maintaining the environmental conditions to keep human body healthy and provide comfort to man".

Standards of Ventilation

Most of the standards of ventilation have been based on the efficiency of ventilation in removing bad odor. Some of the standards of ventilation are:

- According to some environmental scientists, 1000–2000 cubic feet of air supply per person per hour is required, while other recommend the limit between 300 and 3000 cubic feet per person per hour. This standard is not very popular in these days.
- Room air should be changed 2–3 times every hour and that of conference halls 4–6 times.
- In residential buildings, about 500 per cubic feet per person is desirable.
- According to the categories of hospitals and units, 1200–1800 cubic feet of space should be reserved for each patient.
- The optimum floor space area should be between 50 and 100 sq ft per person in the hospitals. For communicable diseases, this index should be 144 sq ft per patient.
- In the hospital, the minimum distance between the beds of the patients should be 3 feet.
- In residential buildings, the height of the roof should be 11–12 feet.
- There should be sufficient windows and doors in every house for proper ventilation.
- The continuously rotating air, moderate temperature and 50% humidity should be there in the room.
- Air in the premises should be free from dust, smoke and unpleasant smell.

Types of Ventilation

Ventilation is of two types:

1. **Natural ventilation:** This is the simplest system of ventilating small buildings, schools, offices and primary health center, buildings, etc.

   Types of natural ventilation are:

   - **Air movements or currents/wind:** Air moves through open doors and windows and impure air gets away with it. So, arrangement should be made for cross ventilation while constructing a building. Closed doors and windows increase the humidity of the room as there is no movement of air and no ventilation.

   - **Diffusion and expansion of gases:** Air passes through the smallest openings or spaces by diffusion and the exchange of air can take place. There is no significant contribution to ventilation, but it is important in crowded residential areas.

   - **Temperature:** Air flows from high density to low density. When the air in the room is warm, it spreads in the room and rises up, goes out through the ventilator build at a height. The outside air which is cooler and denser will enter the room through inlets placed low. In summer, this difference in the density and temperature of the air is affected; therefore, fans are used to maintain the movement of air.

   - **Entrance and exit way:** The ventilators and windows built at higher levels function as exit point, whereas the entrance doors and windows at lower levels are entry points of air.

   The natural ventilation can be maintained in a stable and healthy manner by architecture and engineering.

2. **Artificial or mechanical ventilation:** Artificial ventilation can be achieved by the following:

   - **Exhaust ventilation:** In this technique, exhaust fans are used to expel air, this process creates a vacuum in the room which gets filled by the fresh air coming through entrance way. This system is used to expel smoke from the kitchen and toxic gases from the factories.

   - **Plenum or propulsion system:** In this system, centrifugal fans are used into the room to blow fresh air as these fans create a positive pressure and displace the vitiated air. The plenum or propulsion system is used for supplying air to air-conditioned buildings and factories. Air is delivered through ducts at desired points.

   - **Balanced ventilation:** In this type of ventilation, air is forced into the room from one end using plenum system while it is expelled from the other end using exhaust system. A balance between these two systems is called balanced system. This system is used for large conference halls. The only drawback of this system is total blockage of natural ventilation.

MUST KNOW

Ventilation and Health

The poor ventilation in residential quarters or workplaces may have ill effects on human health and people may have the following complaints:

- Headache
- Insomnia
- Loss of appetite
- Loss of working capacity
- Fatigue and irritability
- Weakness of immune system
- Frequent attacks of cold, cough and respiratory diseases
- Hot flashes and complain of excessive sweating.

Air Conditioning System

This system helps in cleaning, cooling or heating the air at the same time. The technique of air conditioning uses filters, refrigerators cooling coils, humidifier wheels, eliminator plates and electric fans in a joint working system. Air conditioning is popular in large institutions, hospitals, industries and dwellings.

Ventilation can be achieved through natural or artificial system. It is best to use the natural system of ventilation. In residential buildings, healthy natural ventilation can be maintained with the help of sufficient a number of windows, doors, ventilators, arrangement of cross ventilation, hand or electric fans, use of mats or blinds made of khas roots and conservation of environment. Air coolers or air conditioning may also be used to maintain ventilation.

Lighting

Lighting is an essential component of the environment. In addition to pure air, water, food, housing, and ventilation, appropriate light is also very important.

Advantages of Good Lighting

- Protects the eye from fatigue, stress, and defects of vision.
- Enhances the working capacity.
- Protects from accidents as improper light is the major cause of many accidents in old age.
- Adequate light helps in proper functioning of hospitals, research laboratories, factories, multistory buildings, housing, offices, etc.
- Good light protects against headaches and psychological fear of darkness.
- Light is essential for plant life, conservation of environment, as photosynthesis takes place in the presence of light.

Requirement of Good Lighting

If lighting is not adequate, the visual apparatus is subjected to strain which may lead to general fatigue and loss of efficiency. Appropriate lighting is essential for good eyesight and vision. The following points should be considered while arranging adequate light:

- **Sufficiency:** The intensity of light must be sufficient while reading, writing or doing the desired work to avoid strain on the eyes.
- **Absence of glare:** Very bright light is not good as it generates uneasiness, harms the eyes and reduces the critical vision.
- **Shadow:** Shadow obstructs the light. There should not be any shadow on the book while reading.
- **Steadiness:** Light should be steady, flickering of light, color changes and movements of light in circles are not signs of an adequate light system.
- **Color and distribution of light:** Colored light is not good for reading. White light (tube light) helps in working. There should be an even distribution of light.
- **Distribution:** The distribution of light should be even, having the same intensity over the entire field of work. The contrast differences in light strain the eyes and affect the visual acuity.

Natural and Artificial Lighting

The source of light can be natural or artificial.

Natural Sources

The sun and its reflected light are the natural sources of light. The amount of natural light depends upon the day, time, weather cycle and clouds. Efficient utilization of natural light calls for careful design, architecture of the house, its entrance and exit, area of the room, number of doors and windows, glass, color and arrangement of curtains, etc., which determine the amount of natural light received. Whitewash or cream-colored distemper helps in reflecting light. A sufficient number of ventilators and windows also bring light in the room.

Artificial Sources

The natural light is superior to artificial light, but it may not be easily available in all places, such as floor areas for constructing homes, multistory buildings, streets of the city, dark godown and stores, and too many offices. Faulty maps and constructions obstruct the entry of natural light. Moreover, natural light is available only during the daytime. Artificial sources of light used are:

- **Electric source:** This source can be in the form of hydroelectricity, solar electricity, nuclear electricity, thermal electricity and wind electricity, etc., and we get light through bulbs or tube lights. Electricity is the most important and major source of light.
- **Petroleum source:** We receive artificial light through kerosene, LPG, candles, gas lanterns and generators running on diesel, similarly lamps using oil or ghee, and gas produced in "Biogas plants" can also be used for providing artificial light.
- **Filament and fluorescent lamps:** These are widely used. In filament lamps, electric current heats the tungsten filament and the light emitted depends upon the temperature. The hotter filaments produce the blue light. Accumulation of dust on the bulbs reduces illumination by 30–40%. The bulbs and shades should be cleaned regularly. Fluorescent lamps are economical in the use of electric current. They are cool and efficient. The light emitted simulates natural light. The lamps consist of a glass tube filled with mercury vaporous and an electrode fitted at each end. The inside of the tube is coated with fluorescent chemicals, which, when absorbed, practically all the ultraviolet radiation and remit the radiation in the visible range.
- **Compact fluorescent light (CFL):** A compact fluorescent tube is a gas discharge lamp that uses electricity to excite mercury vapor. CFL converts electrical power into useful light more efficiently than an incandescent lamp. CFL is also known as an energy saver. CFL uses less power and has a longer- rated life.
  - **Advantages:**
    - Energy saver
    - More visible light
    - Lower luminosity
    - Longer life in comparison to incandescent lamps.
  - **Demerits:**
    - Frequent switching shortens its life.
    - If broken, a very small amount of mercury can contaminate the surrounding environment.
    - The emission of ultraviolet light can cause a variety of health problems in sensitive persons.
    - Effects on watercolor paintings and many textiles.

NOISE

Noise is an unpleasant sound. It is another cause of environmental pollution and imposing a serious threat to human health. It is a serious hazard in all big cities such as Delhi, Kolkata, Mumbai, Chennai and Bengaluru. Noise threatens the health, not only of human beings but also all other living organisms. The undesirable sound makes the child cry and awakens the patient from sleep.

A sharp sound generates stress. But it is difficult to define noise as everyone has a different attitude toward sound. Sound forms the basis for speech, which is the main mode of communication in human beings. Three conditions are necessary for the production and hearing of sound, i.e., sound producing vibrating body, a medium for the sound waves to travel and an ear to detect the sound waves. Musical sounds are those sounds which have regular and periodic vibration. These are pleasant to the ears, stimulate brain activity, and cause relaxation. Noises are those sounds that are irregular and nonperiodic. They produce jarring and unpleasant sensations in the ear. It is of high- intensity sound that causes pollution and is harmful. The noise pollution or sound pollution is the high-intensity sound produced from various sources and can cause harmful effects on human beings and all living things.

Definition

Noise is a sound whose undesirability is determined by the time and place. It means noise is an undesirable sound at the wrong place and at the wrong time. Presently, the word noise is replaced by sound.

Sources of Sound Pollution

- **Domestic sources:** These include sounds of kitchen, i.e., mixers, grinders, sounds of radio, television, record player, coolers, air conditioners, generators, grass-cutting machines and noise produced by domestic quarrels, scolding, screaming and shouting.
- **Traffic sources:** These include the sound of vehicles running on the roads, their engines horns and their stereo systems. Aircrafts, trains also produce significant noise near airports, and railway stations, trains, buses and other automobile produce loud noise.
- **Industrial source:** The noise produced by machines like drilling and milling machines, rollers and cranes and publicity of products on loud speakers. These produce sound of very high intensity which is deafening and harmful to workers and people in the surrounding area.
- **Political source:** Sound pollution generated in dharna, demonstration of protest, slogan shouting, election campaigns, and rallies, etc.
- **Construction site:** Sound produced by bulldozers, concrete mixers, cutting and crushing machines, hammers strikes, etc. All these produce thundering and roaring sound which can cause noise pollution.
- **Source of sound pollution in hospitals:** Sound produced by the trolley, wheel chairs, equipment, oxygen cylinders and other machinery, sound of shoes, unrestricted conversation of workers, patients and relatives, commotion of emergency and noise produced by their shouts and shrieks and also the wailing of relatives at the death of patient.
- **Other sources:** These include the use of loudspeakers during religious and cultural functions till late night, use of crackers and fireworks during function is very disturbing for small children and elderly sick people.

Effects of Noise Pollution

World Health Organization (WHO) prescribed optimum noise level, 45 db during day and 35 db during night time and anything above 80 db is hazardous. The harmful effects produced by noise pollution are:

Auditory Effects

- **Auditory fatigue:** It occurs in places where sound intensity is above 90 db. It is characterized by whistling and buzzing of ears.
- **Deafness:** The noise can cause temporary and permanent hearing loss. Temporary loss occurs between 4000 Hz and 6000 Hz ranges; a noise of 90 db disappears after 24 hours, if the noise exposure is avoided. If the ears do not get chance to recover due to repeated continuous exposure to noise, permanent deafness occurs. A sound of 160 db can cause complete deafness either due to rupture of eardrum or damage to inner ear or both.

Nonauditory Effects

- Obstruction of conversation.
- **Changes in psychosocial behavior:** Continuous exposure to noise causes annoyance, tension, anxiety, and temper tantrums. It can also cause fatigue, insomnia, inefficiency of work and impaired concentration.
- **Physiological changes:** Exposure to noise affects the cardiovascular system, and increases heart rate and blood pressure. Decreases peripheral circulation.
  - Increasing intracranial tension.
  - Affecting the digestive system and causing peptic ulcer.
  - Can cause visual disturbances such as constriction of pupils, impaired color perception and reduced vision at night.

Prevention and Control of Noise Pollution

- Noise pollution can be reduced by using good quality of silencers in the vehicles.
- Railway yards, aerodrums, industries and factories should be installed away from the residential areas. Wherever this provision is not possible, green belts should be laid down around these installations.
- Noise producing activities should be limited to the specified hours of the day and night by air flights and construction work, social functions and parties, where loud speakers or DJ is played, it should be limited up to 10 pm.
- The use of pressure horns and loud speakers should be banned in residential areas.
- Earplugs and earmuffs and other barriers should be used in industrial setup.
- The workers should be exposed for limited hours to high intensity sound in industries. They should be changed frequently from high intensity zone to quiet zone.
- The use of soundproof or insulating materials in building house and health institutions.
- Proper maintenance of motors and machines should be done.
- Providing health education to people, regarding noise pollution and to promote voluntary organization.
- Enacting specific legislation control to noise pollution from various sources. In India, making loud noise is punishable by law with imprisonment up to five years and fine up to 1 lakh or both.

If it continues, an additional fine may be extended to ₹5000/day. If the above contravention continues beyond a period of one year after due date of conviction, imprisonment may be extended to 7 years.

Nursing Considerations

Nurses' Role in Prevention and Control of Noise Pollution
- Identifying and helping families and communities to identify the source of noise pollution in their houses, neighborhoods, and communities.
- Educating and motivating people regarding prevention and control of noise pollution in their household, neighborhood and community.
- Creating awareness among families, leaders and people at large regarding the harmful effects of noise on human health.

ARTHROPODS

Arthropods are invertebrates and belong to the phylum *Arthropoda*. These include mosquitoes, housefly, sand fly, human louse, rats, fleas, rodents, ticks, etc.

Medical entomology: The branch of preventive medicine that deals with the arthropods of medical importance is known as medical entomology.

Arthropods and transmission of diseases: Arthropods transmit diseases in the following ways:
- **Transmission through direct contact:** Arthropods transmit diseases from one person to another either through direct contact or due to proximity and spread diseases.
- **Mechanical transmission:** The diseases are transmitted from one place to other by carrier arthropods. The insects and parasites mechanically carrying infections with them when they sit at a place, spread infections, e.g., housefly transmits diarrhea, dysentery, typhoid, cholera, gastroenteritis.
- **Biological transmission:** Some diseases like malaria, filariasis and plague are transmitted through biological transmission. In this case, pathogens grow in the arthropod host or part of their life cycle is completed in the insect host and then disease is transmitted through the insects or arthropod host.

Mosquitoes

Mosquitoes are found all over the world, but in tropical countries, they are found in large numbers. The human blood-sucking mosquitoes are more dangerous. There are four important groups of mosquitoes in India which are related to the disease transmission:
1. Anopheles
2. Culex
3. Aedes
4. Mansonia

Body Structure

Body of mosquito has three parts:
1. **Head:** It is semicircular in shape, has a pair of large compound eyes, needle-like structures in front of head called proboscis with which mosquito bites, a pair of palpi on either side of proboscis and a pair of feelers, also known as antennae.

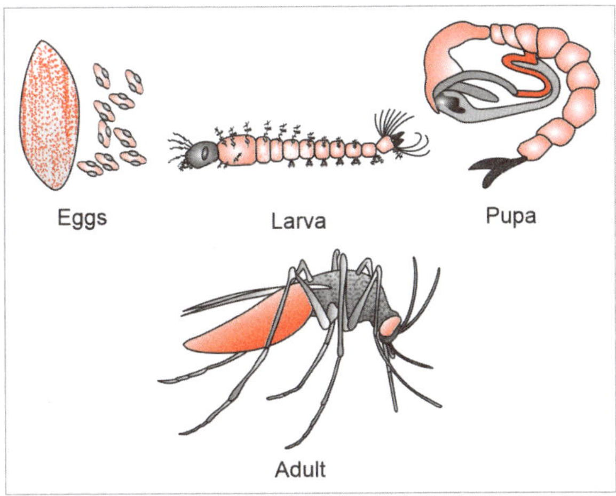

Fig. 11.11: Life cycle of mosquito

2. **Thorax:** It is large and round. It has a pair of wings located dorsally and three pairs of legs ventrally. When the mosquito is at rest wings are folded. The buzzing noise (Bhin Bhin) which the mosquito produces is due to beating of its wings.
3. **Abdomen:** It is long and narrow with ten segments. The last two of which are modified to form the external genitalia.

Life Cycle of Mosquito

There are four stages in the life cycle (Fig. 11.11) of mosquito:

1. **Eggs:** The female *Anopheles* mosquito lays 100–250 eggs at a time. The shape, size and nature of eggs may vary with the tribe of mosquito. Mosquito remains in egg stage for 1–2 days.
2. **Larva:** Larva is a free-swimming creature with an elongated body. It lives in dirty and stagnated water and floats freely. It feeds on bacteria and small plants like algae. This stage lasts for 4–14 days.
3. **Pupa:** Pupa is a comma-shaped with large round cephalothorax and narrow abdomen. At this stage, it does not eat anything and continues to float on the surface of the water. It goes underwater on sensing danger. This stage lasts for 1–4 days.
4. **Adult:** On completion of its development, the adult mosquito comes out by bursting the outer layer of pupa. Male has a shorter life compared to the female mosquito. Under normal circumstances, a mosquito lives for 2 weeks.

Habits of Mosquitoes

- Mosquitoes are found in dark places, corners, stagnated water, cooler, kitchen cabinets, bathrooms, toilets and more in rainy season.
- Only the female mosquito bites, as it requires blood to lay eggs. Male mosquitoes do not bite.
- After a blood meal, they rest on the surface of walls. The spray of DDT on the walls to kill mosquitoes is based on this habit.
- Mosquitoes may fly up to 3 miles. They are more abundant during rainy season. *Anopheles* breeds in clean water, *Culex* prefers dirty water and *Aedes* prefers artificial collection of water.

- There are 44 species of *Anopheles'* mosquito are found in India. Only six of these spread malaria. *Culicine* mosquitoes spread filarial and can fly for long distance.
- The *Aedes* mosquito bites during the day and is found in the flower pots, earthen pots, coconut shells and coolers.

Mosquito-borne Diseases

The mosquito-borne diseases are given in Table 11.2.

Control Measures of Mosquitoes

There are three methods to control mosquitoes:
1. **Protection against mosquito bites:**
   - Use of mosquito nets at night.
   - Fixing the wire mesh in doors and windows to prevent the entry of mosquitoes.
   - Wearing full-sleeve shirts and pajamas to cover the body.
   - Use of a fogging machine to repel mosquitoes.
   - **Use of mosquito repellents:** Mosquito repellents like odomos, indolon, diethyltoluamide, etc., are rubbed on the skin due to which mosquitoes do not sit on the skin.
   - Massaging mustard oil is also an effective measure.
   - **Smoke:** Smoke produced by burning neem leaves, mosquito repellent coils, tablets, or liquid chemicals in electrical devices or other substances repels mosquitoes.
2. **Eradication of mosquitoes:** The adult mosquitoes as well as larvae are attacked to eradicate mosquitoes.

   Larvae eradication measures include:
   - **Controlling the environment:** In this, the breeding places of mosquitoes are eliminated. Stagnated water, cesspools, drains, etc., are either filled or leveled. By doing so, the source of reduction, the breeding process and the resting place of mosquitoes are studied and accordingly, effective steps are taken.
     - Piles of waste materials and refuse should be removed and disposed of properly to prevent mosquito breeding.
   - **Use of larvicide:** The larvicidal oil, diesel, kerosene, petrol, crude oil, etc., are sprayed at the breeding places of mosquitoes. Due to reduced surface tension and toxic nature of oil, mosquitoes are eliminated at the larvae and pupae stages only. Use of oils makes the water unfit for consumption but it is an effective method of larvae eradication.

     Larvicides like, Paris green powder (copper acetoarsenite), fenthion, chlorpyrifos, abate, etc. are sprayed at the breeding grounds of mosquitoes. DDT and BHC are not used nowadays as the mosquitoes are becoming more and more resistant to them.

     Adult eradication measures include:
     - **Use of insecticides:** DDT, Malathion, Lindane, BMC, etc., are used as residual spray on walls. This remains affective for 3–12 months. Presently, due to extreme use of these

TABLE 11.2: Diseases spread by different types of mosquitoes

Types of mosquitoes	Diseases
Anopheles	Malaria, filariasis (not in India)
Culex	Bancroftian filariasis, Japanese encephalitis, West Nile fever, viral arthritis (epidemic poly arthritis)
Aedes	Yellow fever (not in India) Dengue, dengue hemorrhagic fever, chikungunya fever, filariasis (not in India)
Mansonia	Filariasis, chikungunya fever

substances, the mosquitoes have become resistant. Smoke of insecticides can repel mosquitoes for some time.

  ♦ **Genetic control:** This technique is very effective and less expensive. This includes methods such as male sterilization, chromosome, transference, sex distortion and genetic change as the malaria is a major health problem, so different techniques to be used to eradicate mosquitoes.

3. **Biological control:** Certain types of fish, (Gambusia fish) feed on mosquito larvae therefore, such fish are released in ponds, lakes and small lakes, etc.

Housefly

The presence of flies indicates insanitation. Housefly is another insect which is closer to man and found in large numbers in India throughout the year and more in spring season. Majority of the flies are nonbiting.

Body Structure

Musca domestica is the most common species of housefly. It is 1/4 inch in length and the body is divided into:

- **Head:** It bears a pair of antennae, a pair of large compound eyes and a retractile proboscis which is adapted in sucking liquid foods. The eyes of male are closer.
- **Thorax:** It has 2–4 dark longitudinal stripes, two wings and 3 pairs of legs. The legs and body are provided with numerous short and stiff hairs which secrete a sticky fluid that helps in transmission of disease.
- **Abdomen:** It is segmented and shows light and dark markings.

Life Cycle of Housefly

There are four stages of life cycle of housefly (Fig. 11.12):

1. **Eggs:** The female fly lays 120–150 eggs at a time on human excreta, manure heaps, garbage and vegetable refuse.
2. **Larvae:** Eggs hatch into larvae and remain under manure heaps. They crawl to reach their food. Larvae measures 1–2 mm in length. Its anterior end is narrow and posterior end is broad. This stage lasts for 2–9 days.
3. **Pupa:** Pupa is dark brown and barrel-shaped and measures about quarter of an inch. This is a resting stage and lasts for 3–6 days.
4. **Adult fly:** The life cycle from egg to adult takes 5–6 days in summer in India, but at other time it may take 8–20 days.

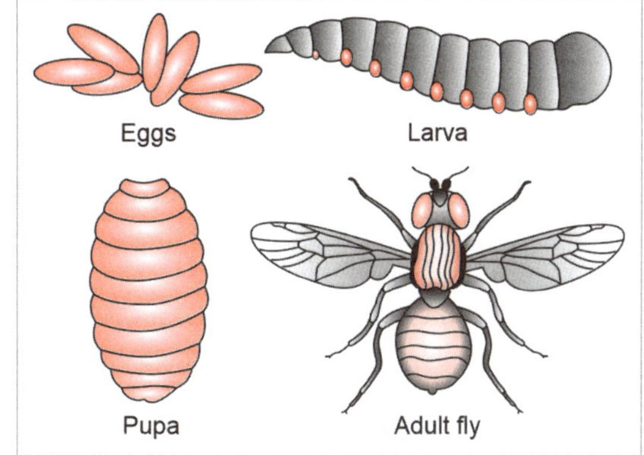

Fig. 11.12: Life cycle of house fly

Habits of Flies

- Flies grow on filth, heaps of refuse, manure garbage and animal excreta
- Sputum, pus and drained body fluids attract flies
- Flies cannot consume solid substances. They vomit on them and suck the food in the liquid state
- Flies fly in circles and can fly up to 6–7 km
- Flies usually remain close to the breeding places, always hovering around garbage and resting on hanging objects on vertical surfaces
- Flies do not bite; they are attracted to food by its smell
- Flies defecate constantly all day and deposit countless pathogens on exposed food
- Generally, they live for 15 days in summer and 25 days in winter.

Fly-borne Diseases

- Typhoid and paratyphoid fever
- Diarrhea and dysentery, gastroenteritis
- Cholera
- Amebiasis
- Helminthic infestations
- Poliomyelitis
- Conjunctivitis
- Trachoma
- Anthrax

Most diseases are spread through mechanical transmission.

Transmission of Diseases by Flies

- **Mechanical transmission:** Flies sit on the infected materials and carry the bacteria or other pathogenic organisms on their legs and feet and leave it on the uncovered edible food stuffs, there by transmitting diseases by mechanical transmission.
- **Food pipe transmission:** The disease producing organisms are stored in the food pipe of flies. They are harmless till excreted through vomit or defecation. Since, the flies have habit of vomiting on edible substances and thus spread diseases. Similarly, they defecate on food, milk and other food stuffs and transmit diseases.

Control Measures of Flies

The best methods to control flies are to destroy their breeding places and to improve environmental sanitation in the community. The objectives of the fly control program are:
- To control the breeding places of flies
- To destroy the flies
- To protect the edible substances from being infected by the flies
- To educate people about the maintenance of cleanliness through health education.

The methods used to achieve these objectives include the following methods:
- **Environmental control:**
  - Proper collection and disposal of garbage and refuse
  - Maintenance of proper cleanliness of the kitchen. Kitchen should be made fly proof by using wire mesh
  - Stopping open air defecation and using sanitary latrines

- Building sanitary latrines in campus and conferences
- Improving the level of personal hygiene and domestic and environmental cleanliness.
- **Destruction of flies:**
  - Flies can be destroyed by using insecticides as DDT, BHC, Lindane, etc.
  - Using fly paper to attract, trap and kill the flies. Similarly, fly swatter, tube light, etc., can also be used
  - Flies can be controlled by dusting some special powders on table, cloth, furniture, etc.
- **Preventive measures:**
  - Using wire mesh on the doors and windows of the houses, hospitals, hotels and restaurants
  - Food and other eatable substances should be kept covered
  - Cut fruits and vegetables should be kept covered till consumed
  - Glasses and cups used for consuming, tea, milk juices and liquids should be immediately cleaned and kept at proper places.
  - Toilets and urinals should always be closed
  - Washing of hands before handling the food.
  - Proper cleanliness of the kitchen, utensils and disposal of kitchen waste.
- **Health education:** Health education on frequent washing hands, keeping the kitchen and the house clean, making fly proof houses and kitchen. Keeping all eatables covered and proper drainage of the kitchen waste, helps in controlling the flies and thus preventing the diseases.

Sandfly

Sandfly is the second most harmful fly after housefly. It is a small insect, light or dark brown in color and smaller than mosquitoes. Their bodies and legs are full of hair. There are about 30 species have been found in India. The important ones are:

- *Phlebotomus papatasi*
- *Phlebotomus argentipes*
- *Phlebotomus sergenti*
- *Sergentomyia punjabensis*

Body Structure

Body of the sand fly is similar to the mosquito and consists of three parts: It cannot fly but can jump to a certain distance.

1. **Head:** It has a pair of long, slender and hairy antennae, palpi and proboscis. Only female bites.
2. **Thorax:** It bears a pair of wings and three pairs of legs. The wings are upright and extremely hairy.
3. **Abdomen:** It has 10 segments and covered with hair. In female, the tip of the abdomen is rounded whereas in males there are clusters attached to the last abdominal segment.

Characteristics Features

The characteristics features of sand fly which distinguishes it from mosquito are:

- It has long legs compared to the size of body.
- Wings are upright.
- Body is extremely hairy.
- It cannot fly but can jump to a certain distance.
- Being smaller than mosquito, it can pass through an ordinary mosquito net.

Life Cycle of Sandfly

The life cycle of sand fly is shown in Figure 11.13.
- **Egg:** The eggs are laid in damp dark places in the vicinity of cattle sheds and poultry. Eggs hatch within 7 days.
- **Larva:** The Larva is hairy with a distinct head, thorax and abdomen. It feeds on decaying organic matter and becomes pupa in 2 weeks.
- **Pupa:** This stage lasts for 1 week.
- **Adult:** The average life of sand fly is about 1 week.

Diseases Transmitted by Sandfly

Kala-azar, Sandfly fever.

Control Measures of Sandfly

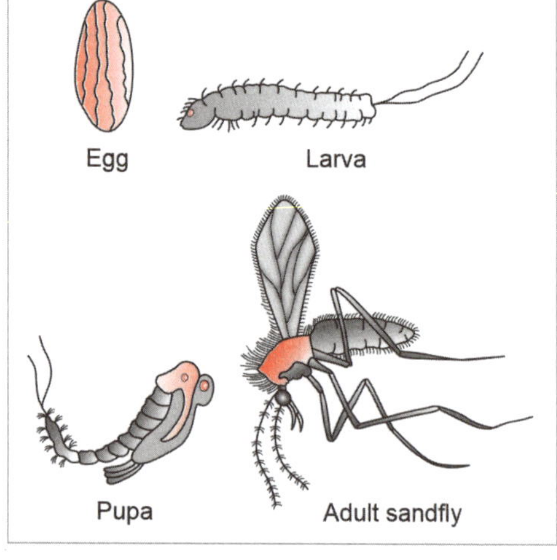

Fig. 11.13: Life cycle of sandfly

Sand fly can be easily controlled as it cannot move long distance.
- **Use of insecticide:** Spray of DDT 1–2 g/m^2 or lindane 0.2 g/m^2 area is useful in effective controlling.
- **Sanitation:** Paying attention to the cleanliness of animal sheds, homes, healthy eating habits within the premises. Removing shrubs and vegetation within 50 yards of human dwelling, filling up of cracks and crevices in wall and floors. Location of cattle sheds and poultry forms at a fair distance from human habitations.

Louse

Louse is a small wingless parasite which lives on the bodies of mammals and birds). Poor personal hygiene and sanitation are directly related to louse infestation. More women and small children are infected than men. There are three types of louse (Fig. 11.14).

1. Head louse (*pediculus humanus capitis*)

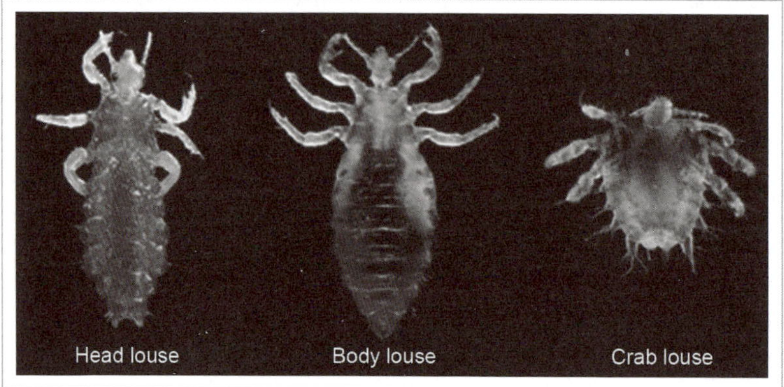

Fig. 11.14: Types of louse

2. Body louse (*pediculus humanus corporis*)
3. Pubic/crab louse (*pthirus pubis*)

Infestation by louse is called pediculosis. Head louse is found in head, body louse on body and crab louse in pubic region. It is difficult to remove them manually.

Body Structure

The body of the louse is flattened dorsoventrally and composed of three parts:

1. **Head:** Head is pointed in front and bears five jointed antennae. Mouthparts are adapted for sucking blood.
2. **Thorax:** Thorax is square-shaped. Three pairs of legs are attached ventrally to the thorax. Legs are strongly developed and provided with claws which help the louse to cling to the hair and clothing.
3. **Abdomen:** Abdomen is elongated and segmented. Last abdominal segment is pointed in case of male and bilobed in female.

Life Cycle of Louse

There are three stages in the life cycle of louse (Fig. 11.15):

1. **Egg:** Female lays 300 eggs at a rate of 4–9 eggs per day. These are firmly attached to the root of hairs. Their common name is 'nits'. This stage continues for 6–9 days.
2. **Larvae:** Larva is similar to an adult louse but smaller in size. It remains in this stage for 10–15 days.
3. **Adult:** Under favorable conditions, an adult louse lives for 30–50 days.

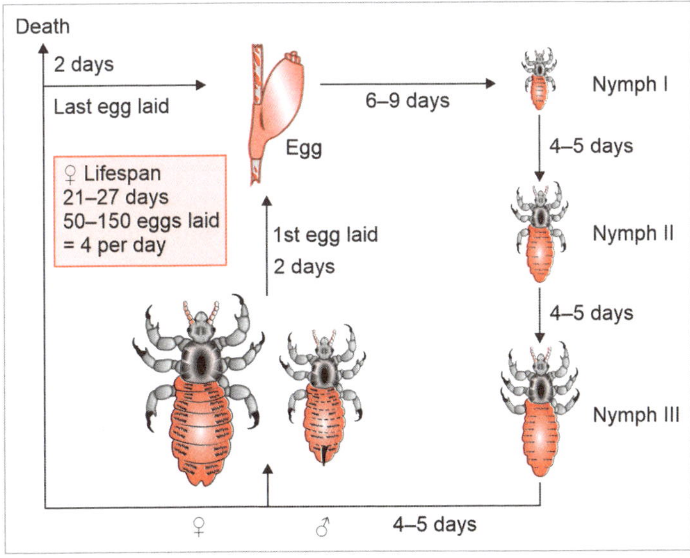

Fig. 11.15: Life cycle of louse

Diseases Transmitted by Louse

Louse transmits diseases through bites or infected excreta.

- Epidemic typhus
- Relapsing fever
- Trench fever
- Dermatitis and itching, etc. major diseases caused by louse.

Modes of Transmission

Direct contact:
- Sleeping with infected person
- Contacts in crowded places
- Children playing at school when their heads come in contact.

Indirect contact:
- By using combs, towels, clothes or beds of the infected person
- Infected items of hotels, dharmshalas, etc., and clothes and combs of saloons.

Control Measures of Louse

Protection against louse:
- Maintaining personal hygiene, frequent washing of hairs to remove dirt.
- Undergarments should be changed every day.
- Special care of female child and women's hair.
- Hot water can be used for washing clothes, clothes should be dried in sunlight and hot iron to be used.
- Combs should be kept clean, hair brushes, hair pins and clips should be separate.
- Every person should have separate towel.

Use of insecticide for killing the lice:
- Application of 10% DDT on hair and head; then covering head with cloth for 24 hours and thereafter washing the hair. This process should be repeated every week, till the nits and lice are destroyed.
- 1% malathion should be sprayed on the undergarments on the inner surface to destroy body lice.
- Mixture of coconut oil and kerosene also destroys lice.

Fleas

Fleas are small, wingless insects bilaterally compressed, having hard powerful chitinous exoskeleton and covered with backwardly directed bristles. They have powerful hind legs with which they jump. Their mouthparts are designed to suck blood.

Types of Fleas

There are more than a thousand species of fleas known. But in India, 37 species are known to occur. From public health point of view, the following types of fleas are:

- Rat flea (Fig. 11.16)
- Human fleas
- Dog and cat fleas
- Sand fleas

The rat fleas are the vectors of plague and typhus.

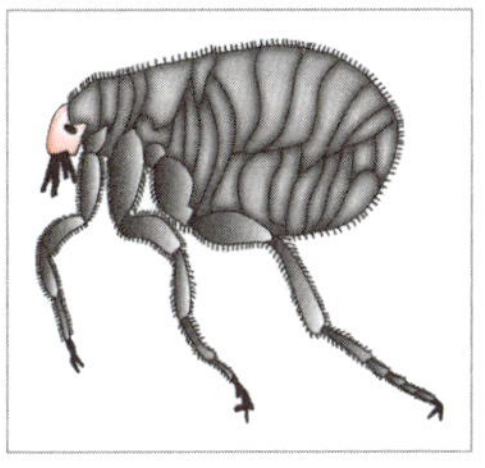

Fig. 11.16: Rat flea

Body Structure

The body of the rat flea is made up of three parts:

1. **Head:** It is conical in shape and attached to the thorax without neck. Head bears short piercing mouthparts.
2. **Thorax:** It composed of 3 segments: Prothorax, mesothorax, and metathorax. Three pairs of legs attached to thorax. Flea has no wings.
3. **Abdomen:** It consists of 10 segments. On the posterior part of abdomen, there is a coiled structure known as penis. In the female, there is a short stumpy structure on the posterior part of abdomen called spermatheca.

Life Cycle of Flea

There are four stages in the life cycle of flea (Fig. 11.17):

1. **Egg:** The eggs are deposited in the rat holes and on the hair of rat. The size is 0.5 mm and a female lay up to 300–400 eggs in lifetime, 2–6 at a time. The eggs hatch in 2–7 days.
2. **Larvae:** The larvae are small, legless caterpillars, whitish in color and have sparse long hair on its body. They are found in dust and debris and feed on the organic matter. Duration of larva stage is 2 weeks.
3. **Pupa:** Pupa develops inside the cocoon. Pupal stage lasts for 1–2 weeks.
4. **Adult:** The life cycle of flea may be completed within 3 weeks. Normally, the flea lives for one month. Infected flea may live one year.

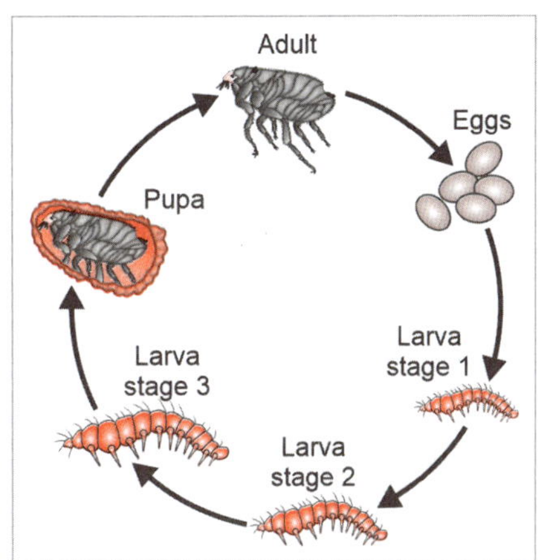

Fig. 11.17: Life cycle of flea

Habits of Fleas

Fleas cannot fly as they have no wings. They can make vertical jumps of 3–4 inches from the ground. Both sexes bite and suck blood. Fleas are transported from place to place, not by rats but by transport vehicles and in commodities like grains, cotton, gunny bags, etc., in this way plague is transmitted.

Diseases Transmitted by Flea

- Plague (Bubonic)
- Endemic or murine typhus
- Chiggerosis
- Hymenolepis diminuta, a cestode of rodents infrequently seen in humans.

Transmission of Disease

Fleas transmit disease by following ways:

- **Biting:** Some fleas which ingest plague bacilli become blocked or hungry due to multiplication of plague bacilli in their proventriculus or stomach. This blockage prevents the fleas to obtain further blood feeds. Because of hunger, flea begins to bite more ferociously making frantic efforts to obtain blood feed. During this process of sucking blood from host, it injects plague bacilli into the wound.
- **Mechanical transmission:** This takes place from the proboscis of the flea that has recently fed on the infected rodent. The flea deposits fecal matter, while sucking which may contain numerous bacilli. If the host scratches the flea-bitten area, there is direct inoculation of the infected agent at that spot.

Control of Fleas

- Rat eradication
- Spraying insecticides (10%, DDT, or 5% malathion) to be sprayed over the rat runs, area, i.e., carpets, gunny bags or other harborage areas or on the rat holes to kill the fleas.
- **Use of flea repellent:** Diethyltoluamide repels fleas for more than a week. Benzyl benzoate is also an excellent flea repellent.

RODENTS

Rats and mice are part of the human environment. They are in close association with humans and cause ill health and damage to buildings, and food materials. Rodents are reservoirs of some communicable diseases like plague and typhus fever; therefore, destruction of rats and elimination of their habitat are important measures to protect environmental health.

Types of Rodents

- **Domestic rodents:** They live in close association with man are:
  - Black rat (Rattus rattus)
  - Norway rat (Rattus norvegicus)
  - House mouse (Mus musculus)

  Black rats infest ships, shops, homes, etc. It climbs fast and lives in the roofs of buildings and also live in the burrows. Norway rat frequently occupies sewers, drains as well as house.
- **Wild rodents:** The common wild rodents in India are:
  - Tatera indica
  - Bandicota bengalensis varius
  - B. indica
  - Millardia meltada
  - Millardia gleadowi
  - Mus booduga

> **MUST KNOW**
>
> In India, *Tatera indica*, has been found to be the natural reservoir of plague.

Modes of Transmission of Diseases

- Directly biting the human body
- Contaminating food and water
- Through rat fleas

Diseases Transmitted by Rodents

- **Bacterial:** Plague, tularemia, salmonellosis.
- **Viral:** Lassa fever, hemorrhagic fever, encephalitis.
- **Rickettsia:** Scrub typhus, murine typhus.
- **Parasitic:** Hymenolepis diminuta, leishmaniasis, amebiasis, trichinosis, Chagas disease.
- **Others:** Rat bite fever, leptospirosis, histoplasmosis ringworms, etc.

Methods of Rodent Control

Rodents need food, water and shelter to grow. So, the proper control on these three can eradicate rodents. The important methods of rodent control are:

- **Maintaining the cleanliness:**
    - Construction of rat proof buildings, kitchens and shops, etc., so that rats cannot enter to get shelter.
    - Proper disposal of waste.
    - Filling the cracks and holes of walls and floors.
    - Roof should not become their shelter place.
    - Keeping the residential area clean
- **Trapping:** Rats can be trapped using rat traps and their number can be reduced.
- **Use of rodenticides or rat poisons:** Zinc phosphate (1-part zinc phosphate 10 parts of wheat flour), barium carbonate, warfarin, pindone, etc., are placed near the burrows of rats in the form of balls or powder as such rodents consume these and get killed due to their toxic effects. Poisonous wheat flour balls, and rice flour used to attract rats are called baits.
- **Other methods:** Cyano gas pumped into the shelter and the burrows of rats can kill the rats as well as fleas. This is a very effective technique.

Disease Transmitting Ectoparasites Born by Rodents

Ticks

Ticks are ectoparasites of vertebrate animals. Sometimes, they attack humans and transmit diseases. Their bodies are oval-shaped and not distinctly separated into head, thorax and abdomen. Ticks are of two types:

1. **Hard tick:** It bears a hard shield on its dorsum called the Scutum. It is absent in soft ticks. The body of the tick is oval-shaped. It has head on its anterior end. Adult has four pairs of legs. Sexes are separate, males are smaller than females. Both sexes bite and suck blood (Fig. 11.18A).
2. **Soft tick:** It is called a soft tick as it does not possess a hard shield on its back. The body does not show any division, head is present ventrally and not seen from above. This makes it easy to identify the soft tick from the hard tick (Fig. 11.18B).

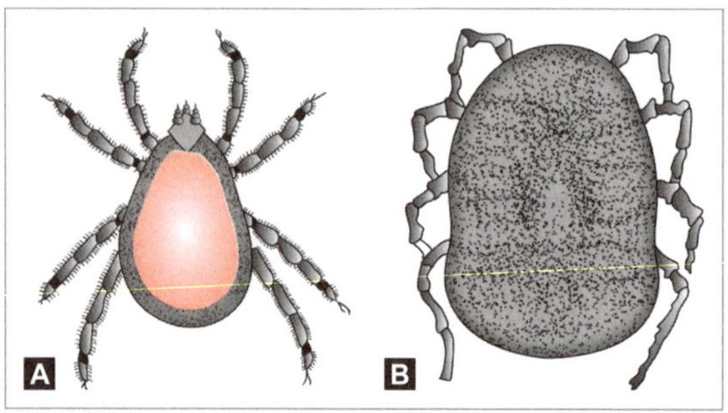

Figs 11.18A and B: **A.** Hard tick, **B.** Soft tick

Life Cycle of Ticks

There are four stages in the life cycle of both hard and soft ticks (Fig. 11.19):

1. Eggs
2. Larvae
3. Nymph
4. Adult

The entire life cycle from egg to adult takes 3 months in case of hard tick, and 9–10 months in case of soft tick. Ticks live for a year or more.

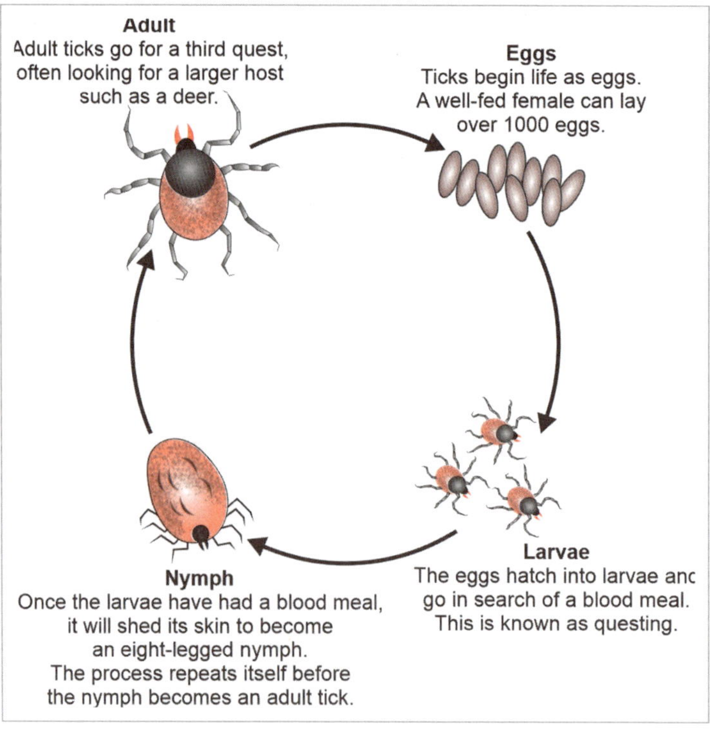

Fig. 11.19: Life cycle of tick

Diseases Transmitted by Hard Tick

- Tick typhus
- Viral encephalitis
- Viral fevers, e.g., Colorado tick fever
- Viral hemorrhagic fever, e.g., KFD in India
- Tularemia
- Tick paralysis
- Human babesiosis

Diseases Transmitted by Soft Tick

- Q fever
- Relapsing fever
- Kyasanur forest disease (KFD)

Control Measures of Ticks

- **Maintaining cleanliness:** Cracks and crevices in ground near buildings should be filled up.
- **By insecticides:** Spraying DDT or malathion 1–2 pounds per acre should be sprayed in tick infected area.
- **Protection of workers:** They should wear protective clothing impregnated with insect repellents. At the end of days' work, they should examine themselves for ticks and remove them immediately.

Mites

There are two varieties of mites. Out of these two, the itch mite infests the human habitat.

1. **Itch mite:** This is an extremely small round arthropod that lives as a parasite on human skin. It can be seen by naked eye and it measures 0.4 mm in size. It is an ectoparasite of man. It lives and breeds on human skin. It lays eggs just below the epidermis. When the eggs hatch, the larvae begin to crawl out of the skin causing itching and irritation. This itching results into scratch on the skin which leads to bacterial and fungal infection. At this stage, anyone coming in contact with infected person gets infections.

2. **Trombiculid mite:** The larval stage of trombiculid mites, also known as chiggers, are vectors for scrub typhus, a potentially fatal febrile disease in humans. Chiggers are also known to carry other pathogens and bacterial symbionts, and may play a role in transmitting viral diseases.

Life Cycle of Mite

There are four stages in the life cycle of mite (Fig. 11.20).

1. Egg
2. Larva
3. Nymph
4. Adult

Life cycle gets completed within 10–15 days. Mite lives for 1–2 months.

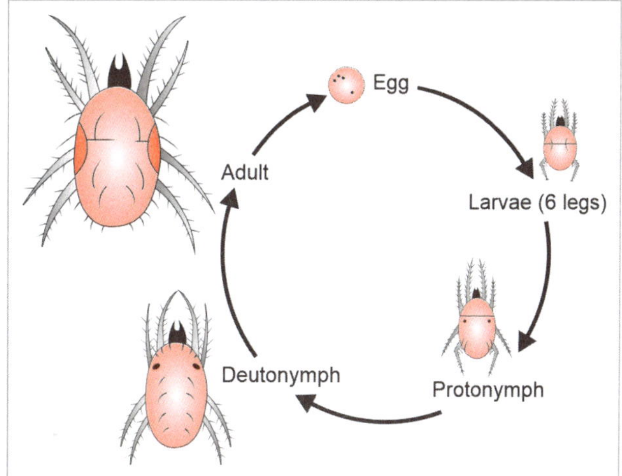

Fig. 11.20: Life cycle of mite

Mites and Scabies

Scabies is a disease that is caused by mites. Fingers and the places in between, wrist, underarm, hips, lower abdomen, feet and palm are the places where terrible itching is felt, especially in the night. In acute cases, papules, boils and lesions might be present.

Control Measures of Mites

- Using insecticides to destroy mites.
- **Environmental control:** Filling the cracks of the walls of houses and enhancing the level of cleanliness.
- Paying proper attention to personal hygiene.
- Using antimite formulations (repellent on skin).
- Treatment of scabies includes the application of 25% benzyl benzoate on the skin after having bath, a sulfur ointment, 10% thermosole and benzene hexachloride.
- For affective control, all members of the family should be treated together.

Bugs

The bug problem is of great interest in the field of community health, both in the rural and urban communities. They are found in homes, in furniture, beds, mattresses, boxes, books, on railway station, bus stops, Dharamshala and even unhygienic hotels, in walls and crevices. The bugs are found in areas of poor sanitation. They create a lot of discomfort and loss of sleep at night (Fig. 11.21).

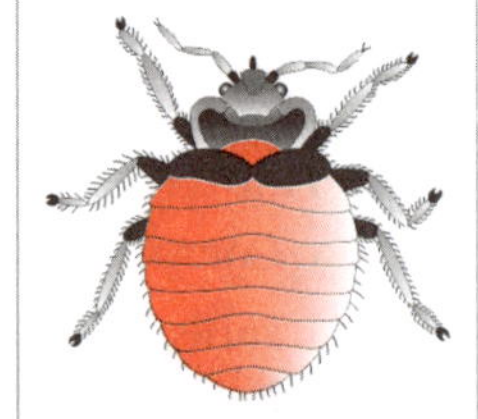

Fig. 11.21: Bed bug

Bugs feed on human blood and are also the vectors of many communicable diseases caused by blood parasites, protozoa, helminths, bacteria and virus. They are dark brown in color, flat and oval-shaped, having three pairs of legs, two eyes, two antennae and a short, broad head. They have proboscis-like structures below their head. Bugs use the structures to suck blood.

Control of Bugs

Cleaning the house, furniture, beds, etc., and environmental sanitation is of utmost importance. There should be entry of good sunlight in the house. If the bugs are present, they should be killed by spraying dieldrin at 1 g/m^2, a hexachlorocyclohexane (HCH) at 0.5 g/m^2. Houses should be whitewashed once a year and debugging compounds should be sprayed. The linen, mattresses and furniture should be exposed to sunlight for a couple of days.

Cyclops

Cyclops is a water flea found in freshwater. It is pear-shaped transparent structure having body, a tail and pair of feelers, five pairs of legs and an eye (Fig. 11.22). It swims in water. Average life of cyclops is 3 months.

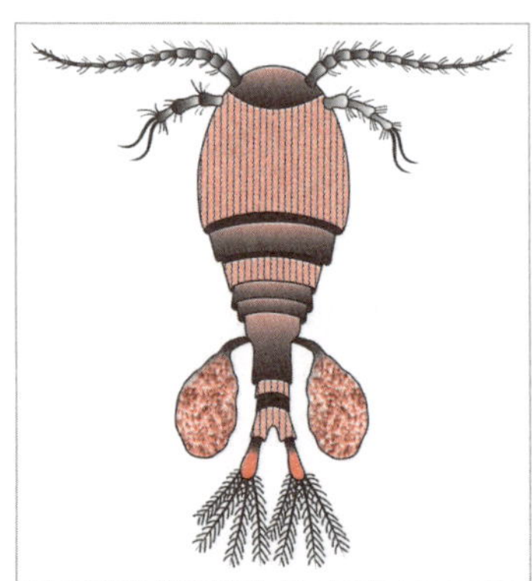

Fig. 11.22: Cyclops

Human beings contact guinea worm infection by drinking water which contains infected cyclops. The cyclops acts as an intermediary host for guinea-worm disease. Nearly 5 million people are living in, such endemic area in India. Cyclops is also an intermediate host of fish tapeworm infestations, but this disease is rare in India.

Control of Cyclops

Cyclops can be controlled by the following methods:

- **Physical method:** Cyclops is killed by heating water at 60°C. Filtering the water with a piece of fine cloth will remove cyclops.
- **Chemical:** By chlorination of water in strength of 5 ppm or adding 4 g of lime to one gallon of water will kill the cyclops.
- **Biological:** Certain kinds of fish, e.g., Barbel and Gambusia, have been found to feed on Cyclops. These fish have been successfully used to eradicate Cyclops in some parts of India, but the permanent method of controlling Cyclops is to provide purified piped water for drinking.

INSECTICIDES

The chemical substances used to kill or destroy insects are called insecticides. Insecticides used are liquids, powder, gases spray and painting with residual action.

Types of Insecticides

- **On the bases of mechanism of killing:**
  - **Contact insecticides:** Insects are killed when they come in contact with it, e.g., DDT, HCH, pyrethrum, dieldrin, etc.
  - **Stomach poisons:** These insecticides kill the insects on reaching its stomach, e.g., Paris green, sodium fluoride, etc.
- **On the bases of chemical nature:**
  - **Fumigants:** These insecticides either fumigate or produce smoke when burnt, which have destructive effects on insects and they either get killed or become inactive, e.g., sulfur dioxide. Insecticides can be organic and inorganic compounds, some commonly used insecticides are:
  - **Dichlorodiphenyltrichloroethane (DDT):** This is white powder, having strong smell and insoluble in water. It kills the insects by damaging their nervous system. It does not have repellent action on insects. Spray of 5% solution of DDT works like an insecticide, it is effective in controlling malaria.
  - **HCH/BHC hexachlorocyclohexane/benzene hexachloride:** This is a white or chocolate colored powder and smells like fungus. It is less effective as compared to DDT. It destroys the insects either through contact or by evaporation. Its 5% solution is used for spray.
  - **Paris green:** This is an emerald green fine crystal or powder that is soluble in water. It is used for killing larvae or malaria parasites.
  - **Pyrethrum:** This is an herbal insecticide; 0.1% solution is used for spray. It acts as contact poison.
  - **Malathion:** This is less toxic than DDT and used as a substitute for it. It is used for killing adult mosquito and is available in the powder form.
  - **Mineral oils:** Mineral oils like kerosene oil, crude oil, etc., used to kill larvae and pupa of mosquito.

Insecticide Resistance

Extensive use of insecticide develops resistance in insects against toxic insecticide substances. This is known as insecticide resistance. According to WHO, resistance is the capability developed in insects against toxic insecticide substances for that quantity of insecticides that is dangerous for that group of insects or the normal quantity of insecticide cannot destroy the insects because insects have developed resistance against it.

- **Reasons for insecticide resistance**
  - Wrong selection of insecticides
  - Improper use and concentration of insecticides
  - Extensive use of insecticides in agriculture
  - Effect of biochemical and genetic factors.
- **Disadvantages of insecticides**
  - All effects on the nervous system
  - Skin diseases
  - Make edible stuff toxic
  - Reduce nutrient value of plants and agricultural products
  - Improper use may cause death
  - Environmental pollution.

PEST CONTROL

Arthropods or insects are responsible for many diseases like malaria, filariasis, kala-azar, plague, diarrhea, dysentery, cholera, typhoid, etc. which have become a serious public health problem. Insects transmit disease through direct contact, mechanical transmission, biological transmission, etc; therefore, it is very essential to control them.

Techniques of Pest Control

Individual Protection

The person should protect himself or herself from the attack of mosquitoes, insects, flies and parasites by:
- Maintaining good personal health and hygiene
- Making mosquito and fly-proof houses by using mesh wires on doors and windows, etc.
- Using mosquito repellents, e.g., Odomos on the skin, fumigating substances to repel mosquitoes and insects
- Using mosquito nets.

Environmental Control

- Maintaining cleanliness inside and outside the house, maintaining proper sanitation
- Eliminating the breading places of pests
- Making provision for a safe water supply system
- Proper disposal of sewage and refuse

Use of Chemicals

- Making use of various insecticides, e.g., DDT, BHC, antilarval oil and fumigating substances, etc., to destroy pests.
- Protecting oneself from the ill effects of the chemicals as well as from the pests.

Biological Control

This is achieved through biotechnology. Gambusia fish is used to control mosquitoes and cyclops. However, this technique is not considered safe as it may disturb the biological balance.

Genetic Control

- Sterile technique for mosquito control
- Cytoplasmic incompatibility
- Chromosomal translocation

Nursing Considerations

Responsibilities of community health nurses in pest control:
- Community health nurses should educate the community about the diseases caused by insects and pests.
- They should explain to the community about the habitat and habits of pests and insects.
- They should teach the community methods of control of pests and insects.
- They should teach the community about individual protection, by using all measures to protect themselves from pests and insects.
- They should teach people about environmental cleanliness and sanitation to eradicate pests and insects.

Summary

- Potable water is free from impurities and used for drinking purposes.
- The sources of water are rain, rivers, streams, wells, springs, and impounding reservoirs.
- Water pollution is a main problem in India.
- Water gets polluted by agricultural waste, municipal and industrial waste. These wastes change the taste, and odor due to the presence of chemicals, organic nutrients and pathogens. Water is purified on a small scale as well as a large scale by various methods.
- Air pollution occurs due to industrialization and population explosion and gases emitted from factories, power stations exhaust and automobiles. Polluted air affects our health. Air pollution can be controlled and prevented by installing pollution control equipment.
- There are three types of wastes: (1) Solid, (2) Liquid and (3) Gas.
- Sources of solid waste are domestic sources, industrial, agricultural and commercial. The main causes of solid waste pollution are overpopulation, increased production and decreased consumption and advanced technology.
- Pollution due to solid waste causes diseases such as plague, salmonellosis, endemic, typhus, diarrhea, dysentery, dengue, tuberculosis, poisoning, GI disease, jaundice and hepatitis.
- Solid waste management includes collection, transportation and transfer to a suitable site by using environmentally compatible methods to dispose of solid waste.
- The methods used are dumping, controlled tipping, ramp method, area method, volume reduction method and compositing method.
- Disposal of sewage includes land treatment, dilution and artificial methods: primary and secondary and nonservice treatment.
- Human excreta are disposed of by installing sanitary latrines.
- Housing is the physical structure that provides protection against cold weather, summer, rainfall, and snowfall, etc.
- Housing protects against harmful effects of naturally occurring space and the spread of communicable diseases from exposure to pollution.
- Housing should be designed in such a way as to provide adequate ventilation and sunlight, fresh air, light water supply, rodent and insect-proof.
- Health problems due to poor housing are asthma, bronchitis, influenza, tuberculosis, arthritis, rhinitis cough and skin problems. These can be prevented by ensuring good ventilation, light, and exhaust system. There should be no leakage, floor crevices, cracks or slipperiness.
- Noise is undesirable sound that disturbs natural processes and causes harm to human health.
- The sources of noise are transport, agricultural machines, industries, loudspeakers, entertainment equipment and social functions, etc.
- Health hazards due to noise are headache, tachycardia, hypertension, muscular strains, tinnitus and nervous breakdown and auditory defects.
- Noise pollution can be controlled at source level, at receivers and by enacting legislative control.
- Arthropods are living things in the surroundings of man.
- The diseases transmitted through arthropods are malaria, filariasis, dengue, yellow fever, chikungunya fever, diarrhea, dysentery typhoid, paratyphoid, amebiasis, sleeping sickness, etc.
- Diseases are transmitted by direct contact, mechanical contact and biological ways.
- Arthropod diseases in humans can be controlled and prevented by adopting measures to kill mosquitoes or by protecting oneself from mosquitoes.
- The diseases caused by rodents are plague and typhus. These can be controlled by providing health education to humans to control rodents.

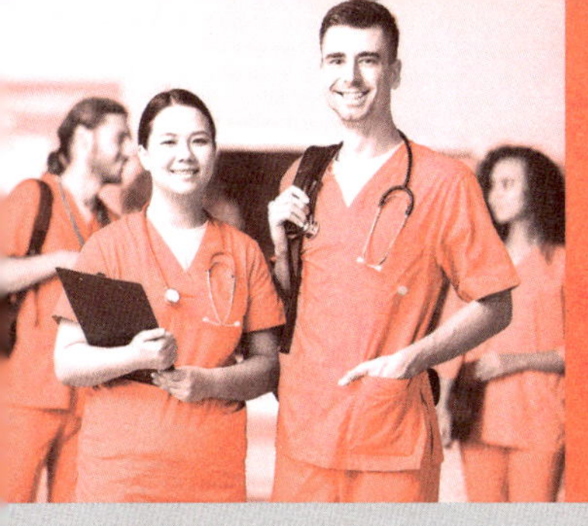

LONG ANSWER TYPE QUESTIONS

1. Explain the process of water purification on a large scale.
2. What are the principles of chlorination? Describe methods of chlorination.
3. What are the causes of air pollution? Discuss in detail the preventive measures of air pollution.
4. What are the ill effects of air pollution? Write the control measures of air pollution.
5. Describe controlled tipping. Write the advantages and disadvantages of controlled tipping.
6. What is a septic tank? Describe the treatment process that occurs in a septic tank.
7. Enlist the purposes of housing. Describe the health problems occurring due to poor housing.

SHORT ANSWER TYPE QUESTIONS

1. Write short notes on:
   a. Types of ventilation
   b. Natural ventilation
   c. Effects of poor ventilation on employees.
   d. Requirement of good lighting
   e. Improving day light illumination
   f. Noise pollution and its impact on health
   g. Suppression measure at source of noise.
2. Enlist the diseases transmitted by mosquito.

MULTIPLE CHOICE QUESTIONS

1. **Water that is good enough to drink is called:**
   a. Potable water
   b. Groundwater
   c. Surface water
   d. Artesian water

2. **Which one of the following does not cause hardness of water?**
   a. Calcium chloride
   b. Magnesium chloride
   c. Sodium chloride
   d. Magnesium carbonate

3. **Which of the following is the example of nonbiodegradable waste?**
   a. Food waste
   b. Cavan waste
   c. Paper waste
   d. Metal waste

4. **The cattle should be kept away from house:**
   a. 100 feet
   b. 75 feet
   c. 50 feet
   d. 25 feet

5. The height of the roof should not be less than:
   a. 10 feet
   b. 12 feet
   c. 14 feet
   d. 15 feet

6. The recommended floor area for a single person is:
   a. 100 sq ft
   b. 150 sq ft
   c. 200 sq ft
   d. 250 sq ft

7. The optimum floor space requirement per person is:
   a. 50–100 sq ft
   b. 100–150 sq ft
   c. 150–200 sq ft
   d. 200–250 sq ft

8. Which of the following transmits Q fever?
   a. Hard tick
   b. Soft tick
   c. Mite
   d. Fleas

9. Guinea worm disease is transmitted by:
   a. Fleas
   b. Mites
   c. Cyclops
   d. Flies

Community Organization to Promote Environmental Health

LEARNING OBJECTIVES

After the completion of the unit, the readers will be able to:

- Describe the community organization that promotes environmental health.
- Describe the levels and types of agencies involved to protect the environment.
- Enumerate the legislation and acts regulating the environment.
- State the major areas of activities for pollution control.

UNIT OUTLINE

- Introduction
- Environmental Health Risk
- Protection of Environment
- Environmental Protection and Laws in India
- Major Areas of Activities for Pollution Control
- The Air (Prevention and Control of Pollution) Act, 1981
- The Water (Prevention and Control of Pollution) Act, 1974
- Noise Pollution and Legislative Measures

KEY TERMS

BOD: Biomedical oxygen demand.
Emission: To release or discharge.
Penalty: It refers to the punishment decided by law for a criminal offence or illegal act.
Violation: Contrary to the rules.

INTRODUCTION

Environmental health is a global concern. Environmental health problems play important role in the health status of man, family and community. There is a growing awareness about these problems in the minds of people. Environmental factors such as lack of safe water supply, inadequate sanitation, indoor pollution resulting from the use of biomass fuels, air pollution and noise pollution are responsible for many diseases which can be prevented by controlling these environmental pollutant factors. The greater portion of environmental burden of ill health is born by the rural population in rural areas due to lack of facilities of safe water supply, proper disposal of refuse and waste and unavailability of commercial fuel. By improving environmental sanitation inside and outside the house such as safe water supply, sanitation, smokeless vehicles and clean cooking fuels can reduce mortality and morbidity rates. Premature death and illness due to major environmental health risks account for 20% of the total burden of the disease in India.

ENVIRONMENTAL HEALTH RISK

Environmental health risks fall into two categories:
1. **Traditional hazards:** These are related to poverty and lack of development such as lack of safe water, inadequate sanitation and waste disposal of indoor air pollution and vector-borne diseases.
2. **Modern hazards:** These are caused by development that lacks environmental safeguards such as urban air pollution and exposure to agro-industrial chemicals and waste.

PROTECTION OF ENVIRONMENT

Environmental pollution is protected at national, state and local levels. Voluntary and social agencies also participate to reduce the environmental pollution.

National Level Organizations

Ministry of Environment and Forest

As there is a strong need for the conservation of environment and forest. Due to the cutting of forests for housing constructions, setting up of industries and for the developments of urbanization and widening of the roads for the purpose of fuel, lacs of trees and forests are axed and new implantation of the trees is very less as compared to the destruction. As a result, not only the wild life is being distinguished but the environment is also getting polluted day by day so to conserve the environment and forests, central government has set up a separate Ministry of Environment and Forest in 1985, to conserve the environmental health and forests. The departments working under this ministry are environment, forest and wildlife.

Department of Environment

This department has central authority to plan, encourage and coordinate environmental programs. The success of environmental conservation depends on environmental programs to create awareness and make people conscious of environmental hazards. A national environmental awareness campaign has been launched to sensitize people to the environmental problems through audio-visual programs, seminars, symposia and training program, etc. *"Paryavaran Vahini"* has been constituted in 184 districts, involving the local people to play an active role in preventing *poaching*, deforestation and environmental pollution. An environmental information system network has been set up to disseminate information on environmental issues. India has a large network of NGOs which are involved in spreading message of sustainable development to the public.

Institutions involved in environyental activities are:
- **Environmental training institute:** It was established in 1994. Over the years, the institute has conducted 124 technical programs involving 1965 participants and 36 special environmental awareness programs have been conducted for NGOs, Government officials, professionals,

universities and educational institutions. The similar environmental training institutes have been established by the government in various states.

- **Tata Research Institute:** This has launched the "Growth with Resource Enhancement of Environment and Nature" (GREEN India 2047) project. The major cause of indoor pollution is that the weaker section of society is dependent on low-grade biomass energy sources. This emits harmful gases which pollute the atmosphere as well as the residents of the houses, especially the women, children and old population who stay at the house are exposed to the smoke. This causes various respiratory problems, heart diseases, pregnancy-related problems and eye diseases. These problems can be solved by making good quality of fuel available. Currently, efforts to produce methane gas or other gases from organic matter are emphasized so that they can lead to clean combustion for cooking purposes.

Central Pollution Control Board (CPCB)

It is an autonomous body affiliated with the Ministry of Environment and Forests. This was set up in September 1974 under water pollution prevention and control ordinance 1974. This is the highest national authority to control environmental pollution. Central pollution control board has responsibility to implement the laws, rules related to state pollution control board and societies. This board develops the rules, which describe the standard of pollution discharged in air and water and the degree of noise. It advises the central government on all issues related to prevention and control of air, water and noise pollution and it provides technical services to the ministry of environment and forest for the implementation of the environment (Conservation Act 1986).

Functions and Activities of CPCB

- Assessing and monitoring the quality of water and evaluating the quality of Ganga, Yamuna and Kaveri river water is included in this.
- Assessing and monitoring the quality of air.
- National Air Quality Monitoring Program.
- Assessing the quality of air in National Command Authority (NCA), Delhi.
- Assessing and monitoring the traffic pollution.
- Setting up authorized pollution checkup center.
- Assessment of carbon dioxide emanated from catalytic converter and noncatalytic converter vehicles and taking remedial steps for it.
- Discovering nontraditional sources of energy.
- Monitoring generation and disposal of solid waste.
- Providing technical advice, research publications, water testing kits, etc.
- Running public awareness programs.
- Providing help to nongovernmental organization, etc.

National Museum of Natural Science (New Delhi)

This museum was established to educate the public and make them aware of the environment-related issues.

Central Ganga Authority

It was set up in 1985 to make Ganga pollution free by implementing the Ganga work plan.

Ecological Department Board

This board encourages and creates awareness among students, youth and women for conservation of environment.

Indian National Human, Animal Kingdom and Environmental Research Society

This society encourages environment-related education and research. Central Public Health Engineering Research Institute is also working in these directions.

Environmental Protection Authority

This Authority looks after all the environment-related aspects of National Capital Region (NCR). It was established in 1998. Other than these many central government organizations and departments of family welfare, town planning, urban housing and transport departments are responsible for the health and conservation of the environment.

State Level Organizations

Forest and environment departments of state governments are conducting, coordinating and directing the programs related to conservation of the environment. State Pollution Control Board gives environment certificates to industries or factories. Departments of health, energy, mining, transport and housing, etc., also carry the responsibility of maintaining environmental health and its conservation. Formation of environmental corps or wings is also an important step.

Local Level Organizations

Panchayats, municipal corporations, town development authorities, urban improvement trust, municipal committees and other autonomous societies encourage the conservation of environment at the local level.

National Level Voluntary Organizations

- Bombay Natural History Society (BNHS)
- World Wide Fund (WWF) for Natural India
- Center for Science and Environment (CSE)
- Center for Environment Education (CEE)
- Bhartiya Vidhyapeeth Institute of Environmental Education and Research (BVIEER), Pune
- Wildlife Institute of India (WII), Dehradun
- Botanical Survey of India, Kolkata
- Uttarakhand Seva Nidhi, Almora
- Ranthambore Foundation—*Sawai Madhopur* (Rajasthan), etc.

ENVIRONMENTAL PROTECTION AND LAWS IN INDIA

The actual awareness about environmental protection was recognized at the global level at the UN Conference on Human Environment held in Stockholm (Sweden), in June 1972. The late prime minister Mrs Indira Gandhi took keen interest and initiative to take appropriate steps for protection and improvement of the human environment and formulate the Indian laws to control environmental pollution in India. These are:

- Indian Forest Act, 1972
- Wildlife Protection Act, 1972
- Water Act, 1974
- Forest (Conservation) Act, 1980
- Air (Protection and Control of Pollution) Act, 1981
- Environment Protection Act, 1986
- The National Environmental Tribunal Act, 1995
- Public Liability Insurance Act, 1991.

Legislation Related to Environment

The legislation related to environment is given in Table 12.1 and the legislations and acts regulating environmental hygiene are shown in Box 12.1.

TABLE 12.1: Legislation related to environment

Legislation Act	Provisions
Forest Act, 1972	This act stipulates that no forest land or any portion there may be used for non-forest purpose. It provides for the constitution of an advisory committee to advise the government on cutting the trees.
Forest (Conservation) Act, 1980	This act has been passed to control deforestation which causes ecological imbalance and results in environmental degradation. It has provision to put restrictions on the use of forest land for nonforest purpose.
Wildlife Protection Act, 1972	This act provides the constitution of a wildlife advisory board, regulations of hunting of wild animals and birds, laying down procedures for declaring the areas of sanctuaries and national parks and regulations of trade in wild animals.
Water (Protection and Control of Pollution) Act, 1974	This act provides for the establishment of central and state pollution control boards for the prevention and control of water pollution. The act seeks to control pollution primarily through standards to be laid down by the boards and the consent orders issued by them. Stiff penalties are imposed for violation. The boards are given ample powers for investigations and inspections and to take samples and establish laboratories for analyzing the samples.
Air (Protection and Control of Pollution) Act, 1981	Air pollution is to be controlled primarily through standards laid down (1981) by the boards and the consent orders issued by them. For contravening the standards laid down by the boards and for violating the provision relating to consent by the board, stiff penalties have been provided.
Environment Protection Act, 1986	This act provides for: • Covering some of the major areas of environmental hazards not covered by the existing laws. • Linkages in handling matters of industrial and environmental safety and control mechanism to guard slow insidious buildup of hazardous substances especially of new chemicals in the environment. • An authority not only to coordinate the activities of the various regulatory agencies but to assume the role of studying, planning and implementing long-term requirements of environmental safety.

Contd...

Legislation Act	Provisions
National Environmental Tribunal Act, (1995)	The tribunal shall consist of a judicial as well as a technical member with appropriate knowledge and experience of legal administration, scientific and technical aspects of the problem related to environment and wildlife. In addition, to provide compensation to the people for death, injury or damage to the property or to the environment.
Public Liability Insurance Act, (1991)	This act provides liability insurance for individuals injured by accidents with hazardous materials. The measure mandates that business owners operating with hazardous will take out insurance policies. An environmental relief fund was established and is maintained by industry operators.
Forest Conservation (Amendment) Act, 2023	This act amends the Forest Conservation Act of 1980 to clarify the act's applicability, exempt certain types of land, and allow for infrastructure to support national security.

BOX 12.1: Legislations and Acts regulating environmental hygiene

The environmental conservation and control of pollution is about 150 years old in India. Some of the Indian laws on the environment are:

- Shore Bombay Nuisance Act, 1853
- Indian Panel Code, which gave some provisions to control Nuisance (Pollution), 1860
- Indian Fisheries Act, 1897
- Indian Ports Act, 1907
- Bengal Smoke Nuisance Act, 1905
- Motor Vehicle Act, 1938
- Factory Act, 1948
- Maharashtra Prevention of Water Pollution Act, 1953
- Orissa River Pollution and Prevention Act, 1954
- Prevention of Food Adulteration Act, 1954
- River Boards Act, 1960
- Atomic Energy Act, (Radiation Protection Rules) 1962
- Gujarat Smoke Nuisance Act, 1963
- Insecticides Act, 1968
- The Environment (Protection) Act, 1986
- The National Green Tribunal Act, 2010

The government of India has taken the following steps to control environmental pollution:

- **Formation of Ministry of Environment and Forest:** The Central Department of Environment was established in November 1980 under the control of Ministry of Environment on the recommendation of ND Tiwari committee. It was renamed Ministry of Environment and Forest on 4th April, 1985. This ministry handles the affairs of environment, forests and wildlife. Central pollution control Boards have been formed for this purpose.
- **National Environment Awareness Campaign:** Under this campaign, the important programs started by the government of India to create awareness among the people are:
  - **Environmental education:** The Supreme Court of India has directed University Grants Commission (UGC) to prescribe a course on "Man and Environment". UGC has insured circulars to various universities to introduce the course on "Environmental Education". The main focus of environmental education is the following:
    - Overpopulation and ways to check its rapid growth
    - Afforestation as a preventive measure against soil erosion and water pollution
    - Afforestation to prevent air pollution
    - Insisting on smokeless cooking
    - Discipline in playing radio and TV and a ban on the use of loudspeakers

- ◆ Elementary knowledge of the scientific and philosophical basis of man and the environment
- ◆ Rules regarding the disposal of household wastes
- ◆ General principles of sanitation

■ **National Environmental Campaign:** This campaign was started in 1986 through the mass media of TV, various TV channels, National Geographic channels, Animal Planet, etc. Telecast of the regular programs on the environment, e.g., Ham Zameen, Earth file, wildlife, living on edge, etc.

■ **Paryavaran Vahini:** The Ministry of Environment and Forests started a scheme called *Paryavaran Vahini* or Environment Brigade in 1992 to create awareness among common people. The people's program extends over 168 districts of India with the objective of involvement of people through active participation. Each *Vahini* has 20 members like students, teachers, doctors, engineers NGOs, etc. belonging to different fields.

■ **Special drive for rural areas:** Special awareness programs regarding environmental sanitation and use of nonconventional energy resources have been launched in rural areas.

■ **Environmental Friendly Product Scheme (1991):** Under the environmentally friendly scheme, the environmentally unsafe (from a pollution point of view) products will be tested before marketing and will bear the Label 'ECOMARK' (with an earthen pot logo). A notification regarding this was issued on February 21, 1991 covering four articles of soaps, detergents, paper and paints.

■ **Celebration of important days:** By celebrating important days, awareness is created through media , seminars, lectures, public meetings, TV films, audio and video cassettes, puppet shows, etc.

MUST KNOW

The important days concerning the environment are:
- World Environment Day on 5th June was declared in 1972 in Stockholm conference (Sweden)
- Earth Day: 22nd April is celebrated as, 'Save Earth' from greenhouse gases (GHGs) and ozone depletion
- World Population Day: 11th July
- World Health Day: 7th April
- Anti-Tobacco Day: 31st May
- World Forest Day: 21st March
- World Nature Day: 3rd October
- National Science Day: 28th February
- World Food Day: 16th October
- United Nations Day: 24th October
- United Nations (UN) International Day for lessening natural disasters: 13th October
- Wildlife Week: 1–7th October
- National Environmental Awareness Month: 19th November to 18th December
- The first national environment awareness program was started in 1986 at environmental education center Ahmedabad on "Save Water".

● **Important national level awards:** Some national level awards for individuals and organizations with outstanding work in the field of environment protection have been instituted by the

Ministry of Environment and Forest. The main aim of these awards is to motivate people for active participation in environmental protection programs. Some of these awards are listed as under:

- Pitambar Pant National Environment Fellowship Award, 1978
- Indira Priyadarshini Vrikshamitra Award, 1986
- Indira Gandhi Paryavaran Puraskar, 1987
- Incentive on Hindi Books of Environment, 1987
- National Award for Prevention and Control of Pollution, 1991
- The "Sultan Qaboos" Prize for environmental preservation. This prize has been instituted by United Nations Educational, Scientific and Cultural Organization (UNESCO).
- Paryavaran Evam Van Mantralaya Vaigyanik Puraskar, 1992
- Mahavriksha Puraskar, 1993
- Rajiv Gandhi Wildlife Conservation Award, 1998

MAJOR AREAS OF ACTIVITIES FOR POLLUTION CONTROL

- **Air quality monitoring:** A national network of ambient air quality monitoring stations was initiated in 1984 and was set up in cities and towns in India. The parameters to be measured are sulfur dioxide, carbon monoxide and oxides of nitrogen. Suspended particulate matter (SPM), temperature humidity, wind speed and directions.

- **Assessment of water quality:** Under the national water quality monitoring program, the water quality of rivers is being monitored. The stations covering all major rivers of country monitor in respect of 19 parameters such as Total Dissolved Solids (TDS), Biomedical Oxygen Demand (BOD), metals and nitrates.

- **Assessment of coastal water quality:** The Central Pollution Control Board (CPCB) in collaboration with the department of ocean development has identified 173 monitoring stations all along the Indian coast to assess the water quality. Four State Pollution Control Boards (SPCBs) suspended particulate matter have also been involved. 25 parameters are being processed to formulate schemes to control and monitor pollution of the wasted water.

- **Preparation of environmental standards:** These are based on the standard prepared by CPCB and the Bureau of Indian Standard (BIS), effluent and emission standards for different kinds of industries, including thermal power plants have been notified under Environmental Protection Act, 1986.

- **Enforcement of standards:** This is very helpful to control pollution at source. Minimum National Standards (MINAS) have been evolved by CPCB for major categories of water and air polluting industries respectively. These standards refer to the minimum limit of effluents and emissions that an industry may discharge into any water body or the atmosphere. The SPCBs can stipulate the same or more stringent standards for effluent and emission of discharges.

- **Ganga Action Plan:** There are 27 stations along the river at Rishikesh, Kanpur, Allahabad, Varanasi, Patna and Rajmahal, Biochemical Oxygen Demand (BOD) values and other parameters have been recorded to assess the pollution.

- **The Environmental (Protection) Act 1986:** It was formulated in 1986 to provide protection and improvement of environment and matters connected herewith. The Act consists of 26 sections and extends to the whole of India and came into force on November 19, 1986.

Objectives of (Section 1)

- The environment quality has been declining since the 1960s. This has resulted in increasing pollution, loss of vegetal cover, excessive concentrations of harmful chemicals in atmosphere and threat to life support system. The concern over the state of the environment has grown.
- There are many laws existing that concern directly or indirectly for protection of environment, but it is necessary to have general legislation for environmental protection.
- There is an urgent need for enforcement and general legislation on environmental protection, speedy response in the event of accidents, threatening environment and deterrents punishment to those who endanger human environment, safety and health.

Definitions (Section 2):

- Environment includes water, air, land and the interrelationship which exists among and between water, air land and human beings, other living creatures, plants, microorganisms and property.
- Environment pollutant means any solid, liquid or gaseous substance present in such concentration as may be, injurious to environment.
- Environment pollution means the presence of any environment pollutant in the environment.
- Hazardous substance means any substance or preparation which, by reason of its chemical or physical properties is liable to cause harm to human life, plant life or property.

Powers and measures of the law:

- Central government has the power to take all necessary measures for the purpose of protecting and improving the quality of environment and preventing, controlling and abating environmental pollution.
- Central government shall have the power to take measures:
  - It must coordinate with the state government.
  - To execute nationwide programs.
  - To lay down standards for the quality of environment.
  - To lay standards for emission or discharge of environmental pollutants.
  - To restrict location of industry in certain area.
  - To lay down procedures and safeguards for the handling of hazardous substances.
  - To examine manufacturing processes as they are likely to cause environmental pollution.
  - To prepare manuals, codes or guidelines relating to the prevention and control of environmental pollution.
  - To establish environmental laboratories.
  - For collection and dissemination of information on environmental pollution.

Central government can issue directions and it can order:

- Closure of an industry
- Stoppage of the supply of water, electricity, or any other service

The rules of central government for the protection of environmental quality: The rules may provide:

- Standard of quality of air, water and soil
- Maximum permissible limit of concentrations of various environmental pollutants (including noise and dust)
- The procedure and safeguard for handling hazardous substances
- Restriction on the location of industry
- Procedures and safeguards for preventing accidents

Measures to control environmental pollution:
- The act prohibits every person carrying on any industry from discharging or emitting any environmental pollutant in excess of the prescribed standards.
- Hazardous substances shall be handled only in accordance with prescribed safeguards.
- The person in charge of premises (industry) from where excess emission occurs is bound to inform the board. He is also bound to render all assistance, if called upon.
- Any authorized officer of the board has the right to enter any place for performing his duty or to examine and test any equipment and industrial point or to determine whether rules are being followed or not.
- Any authorized person of the board can take samples.
- For the analysis of samples, government has set up environmental laboratories and appointed analysts.

Punishment or penalties:
- Any authorized person of the board can lodge a complaint in court.
- Any person can lodge a complaint in court after a notice of at least 60 days.
- The central government has power to make rules regarding various matters.
- If a person is found guilty, does offense again and again then additional fine of up to ₹5000/- and an imprisonment of 7 years can be extended in this case.

THE AIR (PREVENTION AND CONTROL OF POLLUTION) ACT, 1981

The Air Act was framed in the year 1981, but came into force on March 29, 1982 for the effective prevention control and abatement of air pollution in the country. The Air Act extends to the whole of India and is a welfare legislation dealing with the special evil of pollution. Therefore, it is considered a Modern Act or Special Act. Central and State Pollution Control Boards (Constituted under Water Act, 1974) shall exercise the power and perform functions for the Prevention and Control of Air pollution to improve the quality of air.

Amendment of the Air Prevention and Control of Pollution Act, 1987

Measures to Control Air Pollution

The Air Act was amended in 1987 to remove the difficulties encountered during implementation, to confer more powers on the implementing agencies and to impose more stringent penalties for violation of the provision of the Act. Definition of air pollutant was amended to include noise. Also, Section 19 was added (Air pollution control area can be declared).

The state government after consultation with the state board can:
- Declare any area within the state as a pollution control area. This power provides measures which are preventive in nature, particularly use of only approved appliances in the premises.
- Prohibit the use of any fuel other than the approved fuel in any air pollution control area.
- Prohibit the burning of any material (other than fuel) in any air pollution control area.
- The state government has to notify this declaration in the official gazette:
    - No person without the previous consent of the state board in writing can operate any industrial plant in air pollution control area.

- No person operating an industrial plant in any Air Pollution Control (APC) area shall discharge the emission of any air pollutant in excess of the standard laid down by the state board.
- Emission of air pollutant in excess of the standard laid down by the state board is an offence and punishable under section 37 of Air Act. In such cases, board can lodge an application to the court.
- On receipt of application, the court can order the person to check the emission of air pollutants or can authorize board to implement the directions. All expenses incurred by the board shall be recoverable from the person concerned
- Any person authorized by the board has the right to enter any place:
  - For the purpose of performing his duty.
  - For the purpose of determining whether the provisions and directions under this Act are being complied with.
  - For the purpose of examining or testing any control equipment, industrial plant, record register or any other document.
  - Any obstruction or willful delay is punishable offence.
  - State board has the power to obtain any information from a person carrying on any industry.
  - State board has the power to take samples of air emissions. The board has set a procedure to be followed in this connection.

Penalties

- Violation of act under any circumstance may lead to imprisonment from 1½ years to 6 years and a fine (no limit).
- Whosoever damages the property of board leads to imprisonment up to 3 months or a fine up to ₹10,000/- or both.
- Offence by a company or government department may lead to punishment to the director of company or head of the government department according to the offence.
- Court shall take cognizance of any offence if the complaint is made by:
  - Board or its authorized officer
  - Any person who has given notice of not <60 days.
- State government has the power to supersede state board, if the board persistently makes defaults in the performance of its functions.
- Central government has the power to make rules.

THE WATER (PREVENTION AND CONTROL OF POLLUTION) ACT, 1974

The Water Act was enacted on March 23, 1974 to implement the decision reached at the Stockholm conference under article 252 section-1 of The Indian Constitution. It is a social welfare legislation enacted for:

- Prevention and control of water pollution.
- Maintaining and restoring the wholesomeness of water.

- Establishing pollution control boards.
- Assigning powers and functions relating to water pollution to boards.

The Act has been adopted by states of Assam, Bihar, Gujarat, Haryana, Himachal Pradesh, J&K, Karnataka, Kerala, Madhya Pradesh, Rajasthan, Tripura and West Bengal and all union territories with effect from (WEF) March 23, 1974, the state of Uttar Pradesh adopted it on February 3, 1975.

Definition of Water Pollution

- Contamination of water or alteration of physical, chemical and biological properties of water.
- Discharge of sewage or trade effluent discharge of gaseous substances which may likely to (a) create nuisance (b) render the water harmful or injurious to public health, safety, domestic or commercial, industrial or agricultural uses or the life and health of animals or plants or aquatic life.

Legislation regarding prevention and control of water pollution are: State Pollution Control Board is powered to prevent and control water pollution.

The powers of the state board are:

- To make survey of any area of industry
- To take samples of water of any sewage or trade effluent for the purpose of analysis
- To enter any building to examine any plant or record
- To order closure of any industry or stoppage of supply of electricity and water

Punishment or Penalties

- Failure to comply with the directions of the board to give information results in imprisonment up to 3 months or a fine up to ₹10,000/-.
- If anybody destroys property of the board, will be fined ₹10,000/- or imprisonment or both.
- Anybody who pollutes water will be fined up to ₹5000/- and imprisonment from 1½ year to 6 years.
- Anybody who interferes with monitoring devices (Meter or gauze) will be awarded imprisonment up to 3 months or a fine of ₹10,000.
- If any offence is committed by company, the director or manager of the company will be punished.
- Court shall take cognizance of any offence under this act if the complaint is made by:
  - Board or any authorized officer
  - Any person who has given notice of not <60 days
- Parliament amended the water act in 1988 to make it more effective and also to deal with air pollution.

NOISE POLLUTION AND LEGISLATIVE MEASURES

Noise is defined as a loud, unpleasant or unwanted sound that disturbs unwilling ears. It adversely affects our physiological and mental health. Noise is measured in units called decibels (dB). A sound above 80 dB causes noise pollution (Table 12.2).

TABLE 12.2: **Permissible noise level in different areas**

	Daytime (6 am–9 pm)	Night time (9 pm – 6 am)
Industrial area	75 dB	65 dB
Commercial area	65 dB	55 dB
Residential area	55 dB	45 dB
Silence zone	50 dB	45 dB

Legislative Measures

- Excessive noise has been recognized as a crime under section 268 of the Indian panel code (Nuisance Act, 1860).
- Noise has been recognized as a pollutant under Sections 6 to 26 of Environment Protection Act, 1986. This Act was amended in 1989 to prescribe day and night limits of noise level. An area with 100 meters radius around a hospital or institution or court can be declared a 'silence zone'. The use of vehicular horns, loudspeakers and burning of crackers is banned in areas of a silence zone under this Act.
- Under section 133 of Indian Penal Court (IPC), the use of loudspeaker is a public nuisance.
- Making loud noise is punishable with imprisonment up to 5 years or a fine up to 1 Lakh or both. In case it continues, and additional fine may be extended to five thousand rupees per day. If the above contravention continued beyond a period of 1 year after the date of conviction, imprisonment may be extended to seven years.

Summary

- Environmental factors such as air pollution, water pollution, noise pollution, etc., are responsible for environmental health risks.
- The environmental pollution is protected at the national and state levels.
- The voluntary and social agencies also participate to reduce environmental pollution.
- A comprehensive approach to pollution control based on principles such as to prevent pollution at source, encourage, develop and apply the best available practicable, technical solutions has been undertaken.
- To prevent and control environmental pollution, *Paryavaran Vahinis* have been constituted.
- There are some institutions that are involved in controlling environmental activities such as Environmental Training Institute and Tata Research Center.
- To control environmental pollution, the government of India has formulated various laws and acts. Any violation of these laws results in penalties. These laws are:
  - Indian Forest Act, 1972
  - Wildlife Protection Act, 1972
  - Water Act, 1974
  - Forest (Conservation) Act, 1980
  - Air (Protection and Control of Pollution) Act, 1981
  - Environment Protection Act, 1986
  - National Environmental Tribunal Act, 1995
  - Public Liability Insurance Act, 1991
- The government of India has started programs to create awareness among the people to protect environment such as environmental education, national environmental campaign, *Paryavaran Vahini*, environmentally friendly product scheme and celebration of important days to create awareness about environment protection.

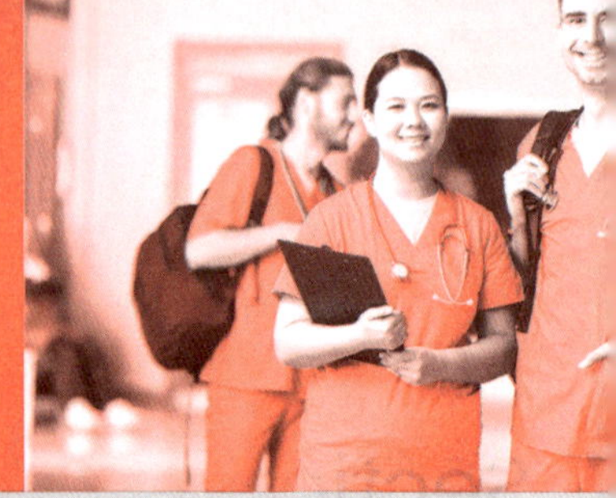

LONG ANSWER TYPE QUESTIONS

1. Explain the principles of pollution control.
2. Discuss the role of NGOs in pollution control.

SHORT ANSWER TYPE QUESTIONS

1. Write short notes of the following:
   a. *Paryavaran Vahini*
   b. Environmental agencies at the national level categories of environmental health risk
2. Enlist various acts to prevent environmental pollution and briefly describe each.

MULTIPLE CHOICE QUESTIONS

1. **Forest Conservation Act was enacted in:**
   a. 1984
   b. 1976
   c. 1972
   d. 1980

2. **The Prevention of Food Adulteration Act was enacted in:**
   a. 1953
   b. 1954
   c. 1950
   d. 1963

3. **The Insecticide Act was enacted in:**
   a. 1948
   b. 1978
   c. 1958
   d. 1968

4. **The Motor Vehicle Act was enacted in:**
   a. 1948
   b. 1953
   c. 1938
   d. 1928

5. **The Shore (Bombay) Nuisance Act was formed in:**
   a. 1963
   b. 1853
   c. 1933
   d. 1973

6. **Which of the following Act was made in 1972?**
   a. Water Act
   b. Indian Forest Act
   c. Wildlife Protection Act
   d. Both (b) and (c)

ANSWER KEY

1. a   **2.** b   **3.** b   **4.** c   **5.** b   **6.** d

Health Education and Communication Skills

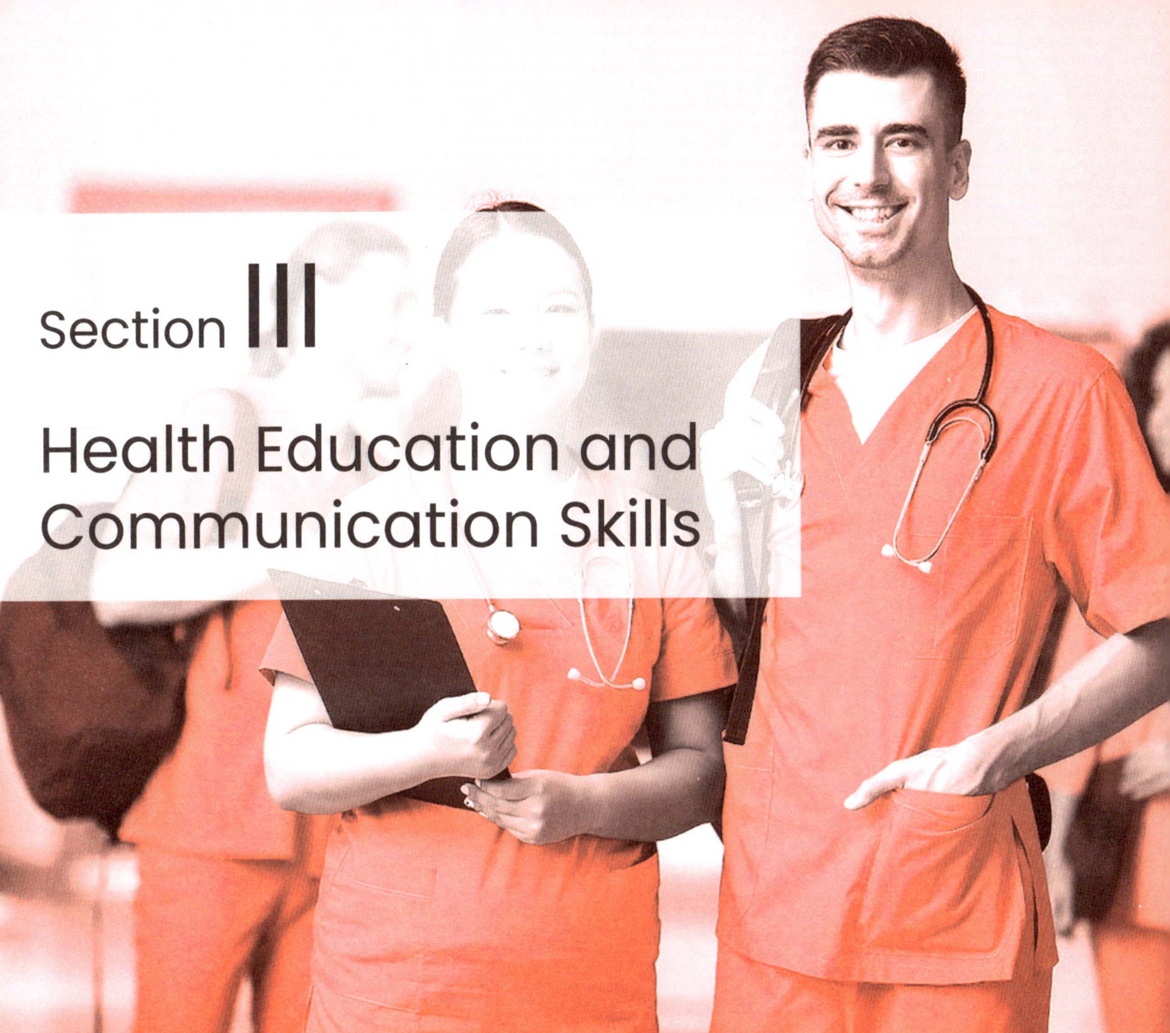

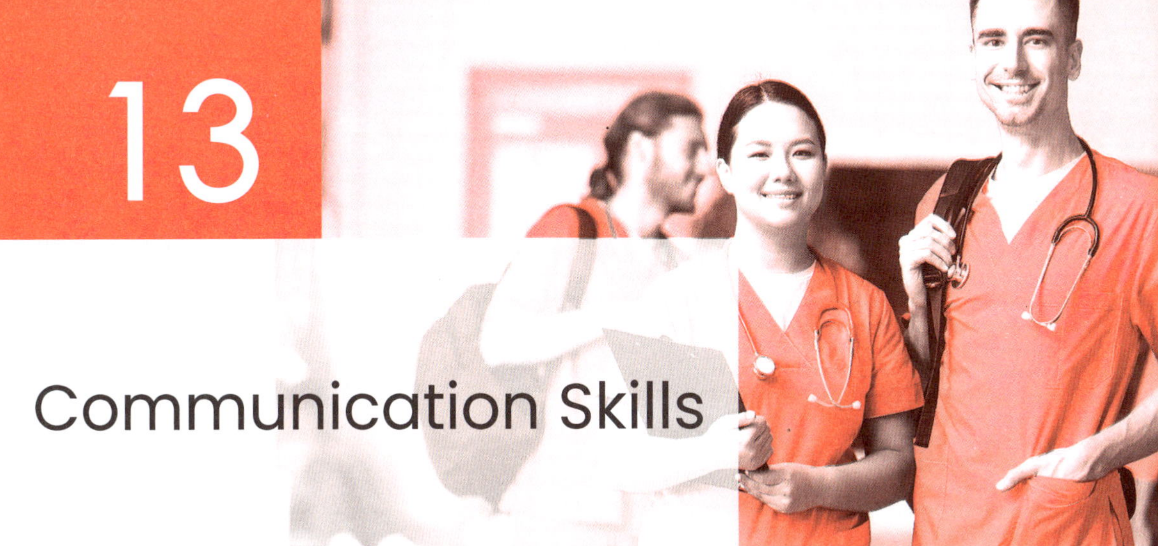

Communication Skills

LEARNING OBJECTIVES

After the completion of the unit, the readers will be able to:
- Describe the concepts and different aspects of communication.
- Understand the need and importance of communication in health.
- Describe the principles and process of communication.
- Acquire observing and listening skill of communication.

UNIT OUTLINE

- Introduction
- Communication
- Establishment of Successful Communication
- Observing and Listening Communication
- Communication Models
- Health Communication

KEY TERMS

Barrier: Interruptions in communication.

Channel: Medium by which information is transmitted.

Communication: Conveying information from a sender to receiver.

Downward communication: Flow of information from higher level to lower level.

Horizontal communication: Flow of information between the individuals of same status.

Interpersonal communication: Interaction between two or more people.

Message: Content or subject matter.

One-way communication: Communication from sender to receiver. No feedback from receiver.

Receiver: Audience or the person or the group for whom the communication is intended, or the person who receives the message.

Sender: Originator of message.

Two-way communication: Communication from sender to receiver, from both sides, i.e., feedback included.

Upward communication: Flow of information from lower level to higher level.

Verbal communication: Conveying information by speaking.

Written communication: Conveying information by writing.

INTRODUCTION

Communication is any means of exchanging or sharing ideas, information or feelings between two or more people. It is a basic component of human relationship including nursing. Broadly, it refers to the countless ways that humans have of keeping in touch with one another. On this basis, communication is the participation and exchange of thinking, experiences, views, opinion and facts between individuals and groups.

COMMUNICATION

Communication is more than exchange of information. It is a process necessary to give way for desired changes in human behavior and informed individuals and community participation to achieve predetermined goals. Communication has developed into an interdisciplinary science drawing richly from social science. With the development of newer methods of communication and information explosion, the mental development of the humans has expanded considerably for clearer thinking and better social intersectoral coordination. Since communication and education are interwoven, communication methods enhance learning and the ultimate aim of communication is to bring a change in the desired direction of the person who receives the communication. Communication is an important part of our normal relationship with other people. Our ability to impress other people depends on our communication skills. Good communication is important in imparting health education to the people. The term "Health Communication" is often used with health education. The developing countries are on the move to exploit the current "communication revolution" to put today's health information at the disposal of families, to help people to achieve health by their own actions and efforts.

Meaning

The word communication comes from Latin word, "Communicare" which means to share, to impart, to inform, to participate, etc. It means transmitting and sharing of ideas, opinions, facts and information between persons/groups in such a way that the meaning received is equal to those, that is perceived and understood by the sender.

Definitions

- Communication may be defined as the process of conveying information from a sender to a receiver with the use of a medium in which the information is understood in the same way by both the sender and the receiver.
- Communication can also be defined as social interaction, where at least two or more people interact and share ideas through common language.
- It may also be defined as a process of exchanging of information and ideas between two or more people.

Process

Communication which is the basis of human interaction is a complex process (Fig. 13.1). The main components of communication are:

- Sender or source
- Message

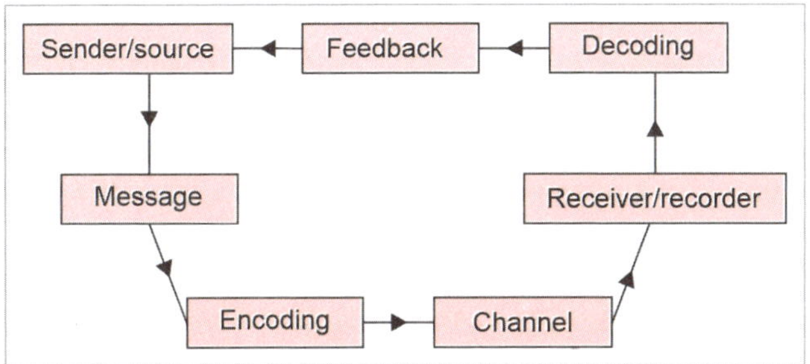

Fig. 13.1: Process of communication

- Encoding
- Channel
- Receiver or Recorder
- Decoding
- Feedback

As shown in the Figure 13.1, the communication process passes through the seven stages:

1. **Sender or source:** Sender or source is the originator of the message. He delivers information to others. For effective communication, the sender must know:
   - His objectives are clearly defined
   - The interests and needs of the audience
   - The message to be communicated
   - Channel of communication
   - His professional abilities and limitations

   The impact of the message will depend on his own social status, knowledge and prestige in the community.

2. **Message:** Message is the content or subject matter or ideas. The message is the information of communication which the communicator transmits to his audience to receive, understand, accept and act upon. It may be in the form of words, pictures and signs. Health education may fail in many cases if its message is not clear, adequate and accurate. A good message must be:
   - As per the objectives of the message
   - Based on the felt needs
   - Meaningful
   - Concise, clear and understandable
   - Specific and accurate
   - According to the audience
   - Interesting
   - Culturally and socially acceptable

   For successful communication, the right message to the right people at right time should be conveyed.

3. **Encoding:** To convert content, information and ideas into codes (words, actions, pictures, etc.) is known as encoding.

4. **Channel (medium):** Channel is the media of communication between the sender and the receiver. The whole communication is based on the following media systems:
   - **Interpersonal communication:** This is the most common channel. In this channel, there is face to face communication. It is more effective than any other channel. As there is personal and direct communication, it is more influential in persuasion about decision making of the undecided persons. Interpersonal communication channel is superior for the motivational effect and counseling.
   - **Mass media:** This channel utilizes TV, radio, printed matter, cell phones, internet, films, posters, videos, etc. to communicate to the large number of population in a town, district, state or nation within a short time than other means of communication. As it is a

one-way channel of communication, it can convey the messages to the people from center to periphery, but the feedback mechanism is poorly organized. It is not very effective in changing established modes of behavior.

- **Traditional or folk media:** This media is important in preserving the cultural heritage as every community has its own network of traditions, customs, folk dances, singing, dramas, etc. This media can be utilized in the rural population for health communication in the form of role play, dramas and folk dances, etc.

5. **Receiver (Audience):** It is the person for whom the message is sent. All communications must have recorder or audience. This may be a single person or a group of persons. Without audience, communication has no meaning other than mere noise. The audience may be of two types:
   i. **Controlled audience** is one in which people are held together by a common interest. It is a homogeneous group.
   ii. **Uncontrolled audience** is one in which people have gathered for the motive of curiosity. The more homogeneous audience, the greater chances of an effective communication.
6. **Decoding:** The opening of the code is called decoding. It provides meaning to the received content.
7. **Feedback:** Feedback is an answer from the receiver. Feedback is necessary to ensure whether the message has reached in the right form. If the message is not clear or not acceptable, the audience may reject it. The feedback provides an opportunity to the sender to modify his message and render it acceptable. In interpersonal communication, feedback is immediate whereas in mass communication it takes time to get feedback. Feedback is obtained through interviews, attitude surveys, polls, etc. It can rectify transmission errors.

Purposes

- Communication is essential for every organization for meeting its objectives.
- It provides cooperation, coordination, good interpersonal relationship and motivation among the workers.
- It ensures public participation in health education and other health programs.
- Good communication is very effective in teaching-learning activities.
- It helps in exchanging information, ideas and opinions regarding health.
- It provides publicity to the health policies, actions and activities and removes rumors.
- It maintains continuous public contact.
- It helps in maintenance of health records and in receiving correct information.
- It helps to obtain feedback from community or health workers.

Principles

The principles of communication which should be observed by the community health nurse and all health professionals in health education are:
- The message should be based on the client's health needs and priorities before planning for health teaching.
- The communicator must understand the values, interests, needs and sociocultural patterns of the community to promote acceptance, assimilation and practice.

- The message should be very specific, significant, adequate and accurate.
- The message must be properly designed and organized to attain intended health behavior.
- Principles of psychology of teaching and learning must be kept in mind, e.g., principles of known to unknown, simple to complex, etc.
- The information must be brief and in positive statement as far as possible. The message should be appropriate and in simple and correct language.
- There must be effective communication of message, i.e., the message communicated should be thoroughly and easily understood by the audience. The communicator should make proper use of medium, i.e., verbal and nonverbal language, examples, phrases, proverbs, anecdotes, reinforcing technique, etc.
- There should be both way communication to receive the feedback to ensure whether the message is properly understood, accepted, assimilated or not.
- Preferably there should be direct communication as direct communication is more effective and it provides immediate feedback which is taken care then and there.
- The environment must be conductive to communicate health education. The time and place should be convenient to the client and the communicator. There should be no disturbance, noise, etc. The audience should be able to pay attention, look and listen clearly.
- Communication should involve as many sense organs as possible when the message is given and received. By involving more than one senses, it becomes more effective.
- The communicator must pay attention to his/her image while presenting message. The presenter must be professionally dressed up. No untoward posture or gesture should be there. Voice should be audible, clear, well-modulated to have an impact on audience.
- Message should not exceed 45 minutes as audience will not be able to pay attention.
- Presentation should be concluded by highlighting key messages. This helps in retaining the messages.

Types

The types of communication are shown in Figure 13.2.

- **One-way communication (didactic method):** The flow of communication is "one-way", from the communicator to the audience. Examples of this method are lecture method in classroom and mass media communication. The drawbacks of didactic method are:
  - Knowledge is imposed.
  - Learning is authoritative.
  - Audience's participation is very little.
  - No feedback or very slow feedback.
  - Does not influence human behavior.
- **Two-way communication (Socratic method):** In this method, both the communicator and the audience take part. The feedback is fast. The audience may raise questions and add their own information, ideas and opinions to the subject. Hearing process is active and "democratic". It is more likely to influence the behavior of the audience in desirable direction.
- **Verbal communication:** In this, written or spoken words are used for communication. Verbal communication is of two types:
  - i. **Oral communication:** This is done through conversation, telephone, interviews, lectures, conference and other means but unclear words and absence of permanent records can lead to misunderstanding.

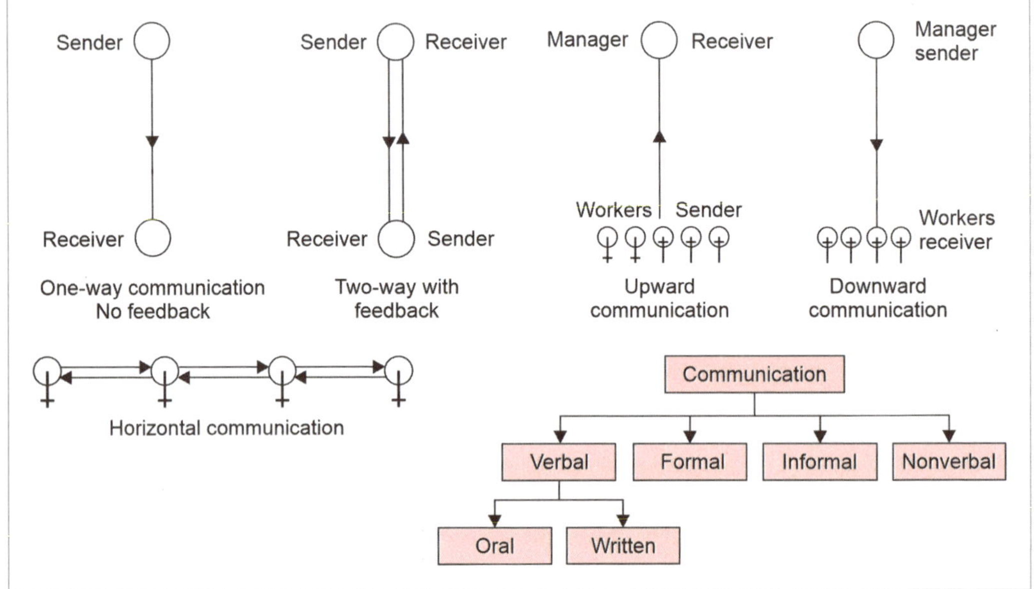

Fig. 13.2: Types of communication

ii. **Written communication:** Written communication can be done through newspapers, posters, handbook, booklets, letters, magazines, bulletins and notice board, etc. But the readers and viewers should be able to understand or read the language for effective communication.

- **Nonverbal communication:** In this type, communication is done without words. It includes whole range of body movements, postures, gestures, facial expressions, e.g., smile, raised eyebrows, frown, staring, gazing, etc. Silence is nonverbal communication. It can speak louder than words.

- **Formal and informal communication:** The formal communication occurs in the organization under the organization structure and follows the line of authority. Informal (grapevine) communication network exists in all organizations, e.g., gossip circles. The informal channel may be more active, if the formal channel does not cater to the information needs.

- **Downward communication:** This type of communication flows from top to bottom and the main objective is to convey orders, directives, instructions, standing orders and protocols, etc.

- **Upward communication:** This communication is from the subordinate staff to the superior, which flows in the form of reports, complaints and suggestions. Message runs from lower level to the higher level.

- **Horizontal communication:** In this type of communication, there is an exchange of information between individuals of the same status or designation, for example, communication between two health workers regarding a service.

- **Visual communication:** The visual form of communication is through charts, graphs, pictograms, tables, maps, posters, etc.

- **Telecommunication and internet:** Telecommunication is the process of communicating over distance using electromagnetic instruments designed for the purpose. Radio, TV and internet, etc., are the mass communication media, whereas telephone, telex or teletype and telegraph are known as point-to-point telecommunication system. The point-to-point telecommunication system is closer to interpersonal communication.

Importance

- Communication is one of the important invisible factors of production.
- Communication helps in the process of organization. It is important in directing and motivating employees in the management in getting things done by other personnel in the organization.
- Communication makes better understanding between labor and management in industry as prerequisite of conductive climate is necessary for overall advancement and productivity.
- Communication is the lifeline of any organization to bring an effective change to influence action.
- Communication serves as a lubricant fostering the smooth operation of the management process.
- Good communication is important in healthcare industry for smooth functioning of the hospitals and healthcare settings.
- Communication is the basis of decentralization and delegation. Every person must have clear understanding of their objectives and responsibilities and must be aware of how his/her job is related to the job of others.

MUST KNOW

Importance of Communication in Planning and Coordination

The success of planning depends on an efficient network of communication. If the system of communication is good, useful suggestions will flow from the subordinate to the superior and this will considerably help in formulation of plans.

- **Basis for democratic management:** Effective communication will go a long way in bringing about democratic management in organization.
- **Basis to good external communication:** Effective communication helps in creating good public image.
- **Helps to mold attitude:** Communication helps to mold attitude and imparts belief in order to persuade, convince and influence behavior.
- **Binds people together:** Force of effective communication binds the people of an organization together. It promotes group spirit.
- **Orient people to their environment:** Communication helps to orient people and their physical and social environment.
- **For avoiding misunderstanding and ignorance:** A good system of communication is also necessary to avoid misunderstanding and ignorance.
- **For higher productivity:** It has been proved that a definite relationship exists between communication and employee's productivity.

Barriers

Effective communication is necessary for the achievement of objectives of health education. The obstructed or faulty communication can lead to undesired results. The barriers of communication should be taken care while passing the message. The barriers of communication are:

- **Linguistic barriers:** These include incorrect message, faulty translation and use of technical language, etc.
- **Physiological barriers:** Difficulties in hearing or listening expressions
- **Psychological barriers:** Emotional disturbances, immaturity, haste, carelessness, jealousy, lack of interest, prejudices, poor retention power, fear, phobia, superstitions and opposite thinking, etc.
- **Organizational barriers:** Breakdown in communication sometimes may arise due to:
  - Several layers of management
  - Long lines of communication
  - Special distance of subordinates from top management
  - Lack of means of communication
  - Incorrect policies
  - Lack of instructions for passing information to the subordinates
  - Heavy pressure of work at certain levels of authority
- **Personal barriers:** Lack of interest in communication, false promises, lack of knowledge, confidence and time, fear of criticism, difference in formal education.
- **Environmental barriers:** Geographical distance, mechanical and electrical failure, sound pollution and physical obstacles can block communication.
- **Cultural barriers:** Customs, beliefs, religions, attitudes, economic and social class differences, language variations, cultural difficulties between foreigners and nationals and between urban education and rural education.
- **Barriers due to status or position:** The attitude exhibited by the superior sometimes causes disturbance in two-way communication.
- **Semantic barrier:** Semantic is the science of meaning. The words may not have same meaning to two persons. One cannot convey meaning only one can convey words. But the same words may be perceived differently by different persons.
- **Tendency to evaluate:** People may try to judge the statement of another person. Everyone tries to evaluate others from his point of experience. Communication requires an open mind and willingness to see things through the eyes of others.
- **Lack of ability to communicate:** All persons do not have the skill to communicate. Some people may have natural inborn skill whereas an average person may need some training and practice by interviewing and public speaking.
- **Inattention:** Failure in communication results when the person does not listen to the instructions properly or fail to read the messages, bulletins, notices, minutes and reports due to lack of attention and preoccupied by family problems, etc.
- **Heighted emotions:** Barriers may arise due to emotional reactions, physical conditions like noise, insufficient light, past experience, etc. It is easy to communicate to people with balanced emotions.
- **Resistance to change:** There is a general tendency of human being to maintain status and ego. When new ideas are communicated, the listening apparatus may act as a filter in rejecting new ideas. Thus, resistance to change is an important obstacle to effective communication.

MUST KNOW

Communication Gap
Causes of communication gap:

- Communication gap may occur when the message is conveyed through various channels.
- It may arise due to lack of coordination between the various departments which leads to conflicts and interdependent rivalries.
- Strict demarcation between various functions of organization that restrict the interaction resulting in tight compartments.
- Lack of flexibility to accommodate the changing conditions and emergencies

Remedies to overcome communication gap:
Communication gap can be overcome by:

- Encouraging feedback
- Encouraging suggestions
- Issue clear cut instructions
- Encouraging personal communication and avoiding impersonal communication
- Establishing rules and regulations for smooth functioning of the organization
- Organizing various functional areas to avoid compartmentation

Essentials

- Think before communicating
- Know your objectives well
- Know your audience
- Consult
- Determine your medium
- Help the receiver
- Proper tone and content
- Timing and timelines
- Check the result
- Look for tomorrow
- Listen
- Climate of trust and confidence
- Support with actions
- Continuous process
- Feedback

ESTABLISHMENT OF SUCCESSFUL COMMUNICATION

- Message should be simple, clear and the language in which the audience can understand.
- For the effective feedback, use the two-way communication.
- Health message should be useful.
- Proper use of audio-visual aids, gestures, words and pictures.
- Latest and reliable information
- Credibility and genuineness of communication.
- Topic for health education should be according to requirement, feelings, beliefs and experience of people.
- Correct medium and method for communication should be used.
- Appropriate attention to verbal as well as nonverbal message.
- Increase communication skills by observing the following qualities:
  - **Confidence:** Be confident in your ability to relate to people.
  - **Honest:** Always be honest with your feelings.
  - **Sensitive:** Be sensitive to the needs of others.

- **Consistent:** Be consistent and know yourself.
- **Anxiety:** Recognize symptoms of anxiety.
- Recognize differences.
- Use words carefully.
- Recognize and evaluate your own actions and responses.
- Be careful in your nonverbal communication, e.g., gestures, position, touch, physical appearance, facial expressions, distance, etc., are included.

OBSERVING AND LISTENING COMMUNICATION

Observation

- **According to dictionary:** Observation means to see the events on right perspectives and to record them for knowing the mutual relationship between the cause and effect.
- **According to CA Mojer:** The broad meaning of observation is to use the eyes more as compared to the ears and tongue. Observation and inspection are the collection of facts about realities and incidents.

Observation and inspection are qualities of a good manager, supervisor and health educator. Observation is completely a scientific process. In health education, during communication, the observation must be goal oriented. The medium and method of observation should be selected according to the level, i.e., personal, group or community. For effective communication in the healthcare industry, the following facts are to be observed:

- The health educator should adopt the method which is being received or welcomed by the individual or the group.
- Subject chosen should be relevant to the individual, group or the health problems of the community.
- The results of the efforts made to solve health problems.
- Determining the topic for future health education.
- Use of specific audio-visual aids by community health nurses/workers/health educators.
- The advantages or gains to the individuals or groups by health education.
- Observations should be close to reality and should be focused on the present or immediate problems, e.g., if a person is suffering from jaundice or anemia, the color of eyes, skin, nails and the dietary status should be observed.

Types of Observations

- Participatory observation
- Nonparticipatory observation
- Semiparticipatory observation
- Controlled observation
- Uncontrolled observation

Observation in Health Education

- Observation should be limited only to the reference subject.
- The objective of observation should be clear.
- The observer should be familiar with special technique and methods used for observation.
- The observer should have previous experience and knowledge of health education.
- The observer should have interest and expertness of communication skill.

Limitations of Observations

- Reaction of individual/group toward health education
- Bias or favoritism of the observer
- Limited area of study
- Inability to observe special events

Listening

Being a good speaker is easy but being a good listener is difficult. Most people try to impress by speaking or giving a speech but do not bother to hear anyone with patience. But in communication, it should be kept in mind that apart from speaking, one should have the art of listening.

Just listening by keeping mum is not a sign of good listener. The listener should hear others with attention and patience. The health problems should be well-listened, understood and evaluated, to make health education effective. The meaning of good listener is to be attentive and pay attention on the "total individuals". For effective communication, one should be a discreet listener, keeping concentration and patience.

Mnemonics

The methods used to become a good listener can be described as **LADDER** pattern.
 L : Look at others, keep good eye contact
 A : Ask appropriate questions only
 D : Do not interrupt
 D : Do not change the subject
 E : Express emotions with control
 R : Responsively listen.

Good art of listening enhances improvement in personality, saves time, decides the focus of the problems, fulfills objectives and facilitates feedback.

Good listening has two aspects:

1. **Physical:** One should attain a forward looking posture and should look at the person who is speaking. He should keep his ears toward speaker.
2. **Psychological:** It means that the listener should pay attention to the speaker and show interest in him by nodding, encouraging with suitable small responses such as "go on", etc. The facial expressions should show acceptance to the speaker, and should not show anger.

Nursing Considerations

Golden Rules of Communication
For successful communication, the following rules should be studied:
- Communication skill
- Behavior of the sender and receiver
- Social and cultural system
- Knowledge of the subject and the receiver
- Purpose of communication
- Feedback

COMMUNICATION MODELS

Model 1

Continuous loop model (Fig. 13.3): This is the earliest model of communication that has been presented and accepted by others who study the field. It is the simplest model. It includes all of the basic parts in the communication process. This model is based on the fact that language is a system or machine. In this machine, communication acts as the "gears" for the machine to work properly. Any breakdown or interference hurts efficiency.

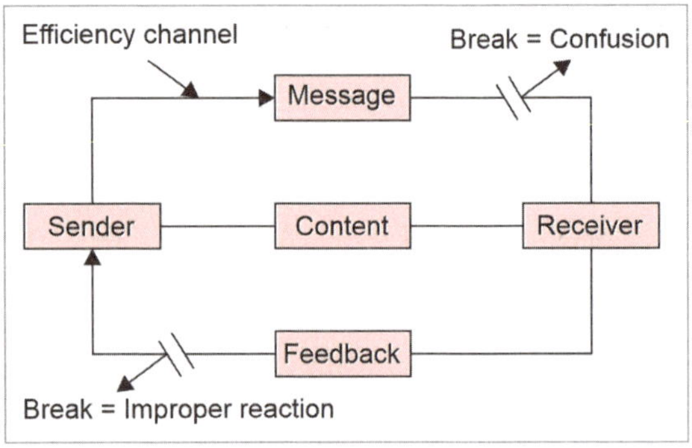

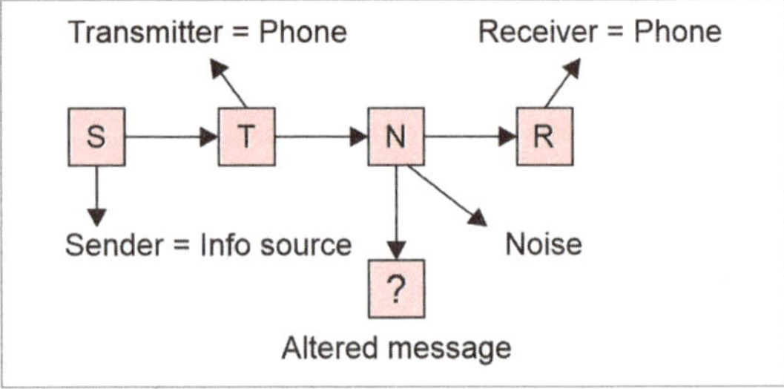

Fig. 13.3: Continuous loop model

Model 2

Shannon and Weaver created this model (Fig. 13.4) in 1949. This model was designed to be practical. Just as loop model was more academic, the Shannon and Weaver model is more down-to-earth. The basis for this model was a study of telephone conversation over a very lengthy time for a period of 2 years. The team studied only what they deemed to be important or significant calls of some length. The focus was on the mechanism of the message.

Fig. 13.4: Shannon and Weaver model

HEALTH COMMUNICATION

Health communication is an important area of communication. It links the domains of communication and health. Health communication includes the study and use of communication strategies to inform and influence individuals and community decisions that enhance health. Health communication can contribute to all aspects of disease prevention and health promotion. Its main functions are information, education, motivation, counseling, raising morals and making people agree to do something about health concern. Health communication is an important tool for health development and is the milestone of all health organizations.

- **For Individuals:**
  - Effective health communication can create health awareness, health risks and solution.
  - Can change attitude and result in health-seeking behavior.
  - Provides motivation and skill needed to reduce the health risk.
  - Helps individuals to find support from available resources.
  - Can motivate to protect and promote their health.

- **For the community:** Health communication can be used to:
  - Influence the public agenda
  - Advocate the policies and programs
  - Improve in delivering of public health and healthcare services
  - Promote positive changes in the socioeconomic and physical environment
  - Encourage social norms that benefit health and quality of life

Summary

- Communication is the process of conveying information from sender to receiver with the use of a medium in which the information is understood in the same way by both sender and receiver.
- The communication provides cooperation, coordination, good interpersonal relations and motivation among the workers.
- The components of communication process include sender, message, encoding, channel, receiver, decoding and feedback.
- Communication can be one-way, two-way, upward, downward, horizontal, verbal, nonverbal, formal and informal communication.
- The success of communication depends upon the clarity of thought, simple language, clear-cut instructions, well-defined objectives, correct medium and communication skill.
- Barriers of communication can be due to faulty use of technical language, difficulty in hearing or perceptions, emotional disturbances, carelessness, prejudice, poor retention power, organizational barriers, personal barrier, environmental barrier or lack of ability to communicate.
- Communication gap may result due to lack of coordination between the various departments, or it can also be due to lack of flexibility to accommodate changing conditions and emergencies.
- Communication gap can be overcome by encouraging feedback, encouraging suggestion, issue clearcut instructions and establishing rules and regulations for smooth functioning of an organization.
- Health communication is important to motivate and encourage people to inculcate health-seeking behavior and to solve many health problems.
- Health communication is an important tool for health department. It contributes to achieve Health for All.

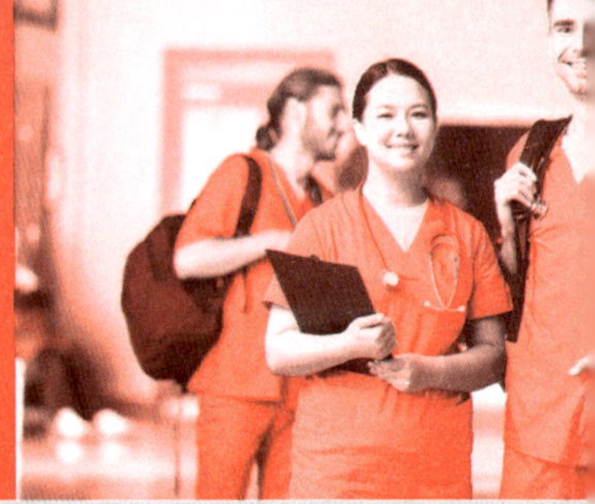

STUDENT ASSIGNMENT

LONG ANSWER TYPE QUESTIONS

1. Define communication. Explain the process of communication.
2. Enlist various types of communication.
3. What are the purposes of communication? Explain them.
4. Describe the barriers of communication.

SHORT ANSWER TYPE QUESTIONS

1. Write short notes on:
   a. Upward communication
   b. Horizontal communication
2. Differentiate between the following:
   a. Formal and informal communication
   b. Verbal and nonverbal communication
   c. One-way and two-way communication

MULTIPLE CHOICE QUESTIONS

1. **Barriers of communication include:**
   a. Information overload
   b. Exploring
   c. Focusing
   d. Summarizing

2. **Mental processing of the message and understanding the sender's message is:**
   a. Decode
   b. Encode
   c. Feedback
   d. Imagination

3. **A technique where by repeating the main message, the client has expressed:**
   a. Listening
   b. Restating
   c. Clarification
   d. Reflection

4. **Which of the following is an example of nonverbal communication?**
   a. Vernacular language
   b. Smile
   c. Jargon
   d. Slang

5. **A person is communicating with his friend on telephone is referred to as:**
   a. Intrapersonal communication
   b. Interpersonal communication
   c. Media communication
   d. Mass communication.

ANSWER KEY

1. a	2. a	3. c	4. b	5. b

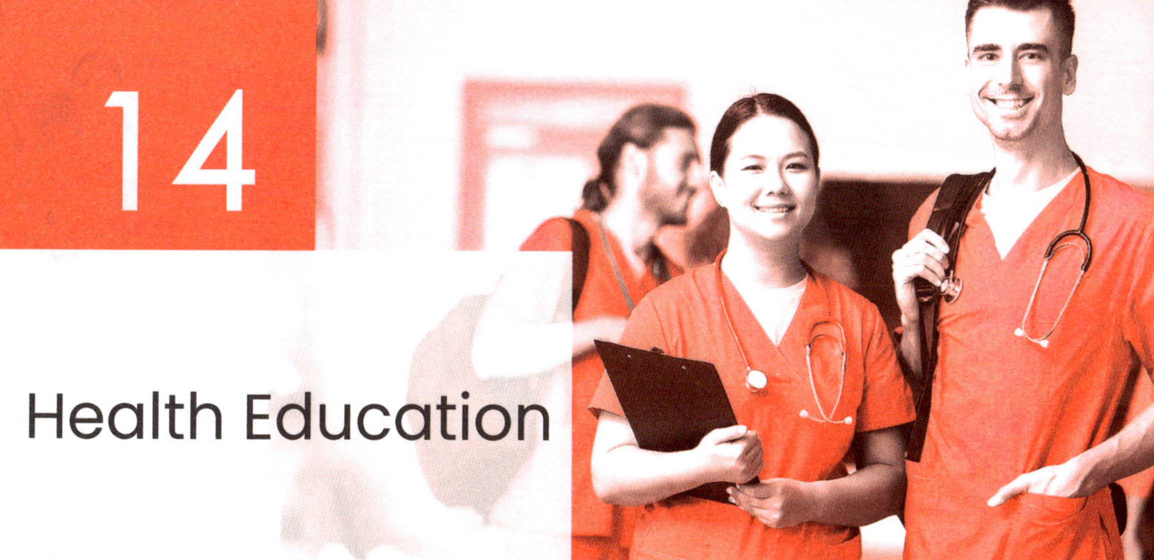

14

Health Education

LEARNING OBJECTIVES

After the completion of the unit, the readers will be able to:

- Describe the aims and objectives of health education.
- State the principles and scope of health education.
- Discuss the levels, approaches and process of health education.
- Enlist the methods of health education.
- Describe the role of nurses in health education.

UNIT OUTLINE

- Introduction
- Health Education
- Process of Change/Modification of Health Behavior
- Levels and Approaches of Health Education
- Methods of Health Education
- Scope of Health Education and Opportunities for Health Education in Hospital and Community
- Nurse's Role in Health Education

KEY TERMS

Adoption: To take over or accept; the act of taking something as your own.

Counseling: Giving advice which a therapist or other expert gives to someone about a particular problem.

Motivation: To create interest; an internal state that propels individuals to engage in goal-directed behavior.

Reinforcement: To make repetitions; the action of strengthening or encouraging something.

Simulation: To create functional condition with model; an imitative representation of a process or system that could exist in the real world.

INTRODUCTION

Health education is a way of educating people about health. It is concerned not only with the communication of information, but also motivating people and developing their skill and confidence to recognize their health needs and take appropriate action to meet those needs.

Health education includes not only physical health, but also environmental health, social health, emotional health, intellectual health and spiritual health.

HEALTH EDUCATION

Education helps to increase knowledge and is an important tool in bringing about a desirable change in personality building and in behavior modification. Similarly, health education provides knowledge about health and motivates individuals toward developing healthy habits to improve their health by practicing healthful ways of living. Health education is an instrument which is being utilized to bring about a positive change toward health attitude among the people to meet the goal of Health for All (HFA).

Definitions

- World Health Organization (WHO) defined health education as "comprising of consciously constructed opportunities for learning, involving some form of communication designed to improve health literacy, including improving knowledge and developing life skill which are conductive to individuals and community health".
- According to Alma Ata (1978), health education has been defined as "a process aimed at encouraging people about the need to be healthy, to know how to stay healthy, to do what they can do individually and collectively to maintain health and to seek help when needed".
- The Joint Committee on Health Education and Promotion Terminology of 2001 defined health education as "any combination of planned learning experiences based on sound theories that provide individuals, groups and communities, the opportunities to acquire information and the skill needed to make quality health decisions".
- According to Griffith (1972), "health education attempts to close the gap between what is known about optimum health practice and that which is actually practiced".
- According to Green (1980), "health education is any combination of learning experiences designed to facilitate voluntary adaptations of behavior conductive to health".

Purposes

- Health education improves the health status of individuals, families and communities.
- It helps to prevent the transmission of communicable diseases.
- It helps to control the noncommunicable diseases.
- It improves the quality of life of people.
- It reduces the morbidity and mortality rates.
- It reduces the premature deaths.

Aims and Objectives

- To provide knowledge to the people to adopt health promoting activities and practices.

- To encourage people to adopt healthy lifestyle.
- To improve skill and change attitude toward health-seeking behavior.
- To motivate people to become self-reliant regarding health.
- To create a feeling in them about the belief that "health is wealth".
- To change the behavior of people by changing attitude.
- To motivate people to make their own health-related decisions.
- To create a positive self-concept and increase self-awareness.
- To develop an understanding of appropriate factual information and concepts.
- To create an awareness that diseases are significant health problems.
- To increase and improve the knowledge and attitude of public about detection, treatment and control of diseases.
- To allow public to experience social relations that will encourage desirable behavior, leadership and cooperation with others.
- To make people aware of availing the available health facilities.

Principles

The principles of health education (Fig. 14.1) are based on the fundamental principles of general education and behavioral sciences. The main principles are listed as follows:

- **Interest:** Health education should be based on the need of the individuals so that they will show interest; and learning becomes easy and long lasting.
- **Motivation:** It arouses interest to learn. Health education becomes effective if the people are motivated.
- **Participation:** In health programs, people should be included so that psychologically they accept it willingly and recognize it. It is a two-way process in which the speaker and listener take part.
- **Learning by doing:** A person can learn better by doing things instead of listening or watching. A Chinese proverb emphasizes the importance of learning by doing:
  "If I hear, I forget; If I see, I remember; If I do, I know".
- **Known to unknown:** The rules of teaching should be applied in health education. Start from "known to unknown", from "simple to more complicated", from "particular to general" and from "concrete to abstract". We should start where the people are, what they understand and then proceed to new knowledge.
- **Comprehension:** We must know the level of understanding and literacy of the people to whom the teaching is to be given. The medium of teaching should be according to the community language.
- **Credibility:** It is the degree to which the message to be communicated is perceived trustworthy by the receiver. It should be based on fact which is consistent and compatible with scientific knowledge and local culture.
- **Reinforcement:** Some grasp new things quickly in a single period, whereas others may not accept the new facts in one attempt. So, repetition at intervals is necessary. If there is no reinforcement, people are likely to forget.
- **Good human relationship:** Good interpersonal relationship (IPR) is essential between the health educator and the audience to share information, to know the interest and to understand the feelings and ideas of people.

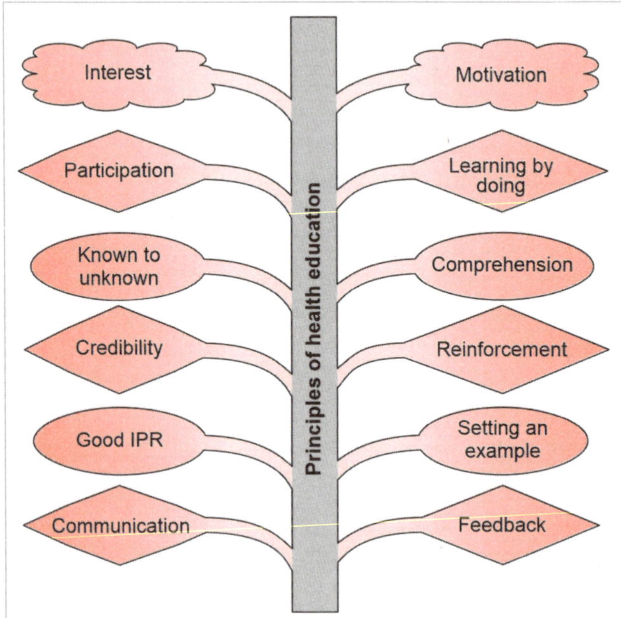

Fig. 14.1: Principles of health education

- **Setting an example:** The educator should be a role model in things which are taught to the people.
- **Communication:** Health education is a two-way process. Language should be simple and understandable by the people.
- **Feedback:** It is necessary to know the effectiveness of teaching.

PROCESS OF CHANGE/MODIFICATION OF HEALTH BEHAVIOR

To achieve positive impact of health education, health behavior of the people undergoes modification (Fig. 14.2). It takes place under the following stages:

- **Awareness/knowledge:** In this stage, the person has some knowledge or information about the new facts about health and its usefulness.
- **Interest:** At this stage, the person likes to know about the things in which he/she is interested. He/she seeks more information.
- **Self-assessment:** In this stage, the person evaluates advantages and disadvantages to the family and to him/her. This thinking will enable him to decide whether to accept the change or reject it.

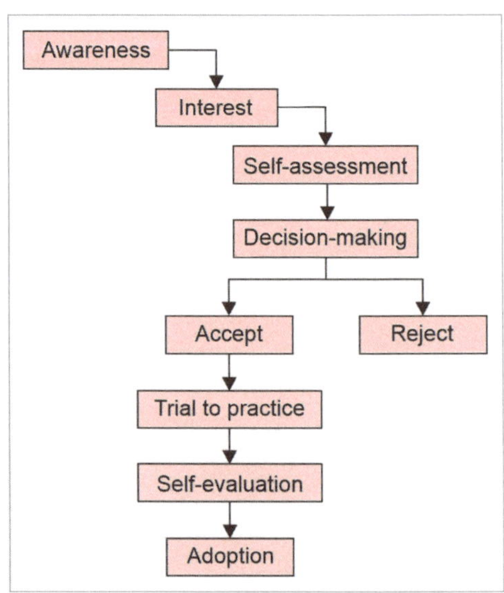

Fig. 14.2: Process of modification of health behavior

- **Decision-making:** During this stage, the person takes final decision.
- **Trial to practice:** In this stage, the person puts the decision into practice and seeks more information and needs help to overcome the problems.
- **Self-evaluation:** At this stage, the person decides that the new practice is helpful for himself/herself and for the family or not, whether it can be practiced in their daily life or not.
- **Adoption:** In this stage, people accept the new practice and continue it in their daily life. Acceptance of new thinking and habits is called adoption. But adoption is very slow in the beginning, and later it may increase.

LEVELS AND APPROACHES OF HEALTH EDUCATION

Levels

There are mainly three levels of health education:

1. **Individual or family level:** At this level, health education is imparted to a limited number of persons. The doctors, nurses and health workers have great role in imparting health education in the hospitals and in homes during home visits. Health education is more effective when it is provided at home visit as the individuals can exchange ideas and clear their doubts. It helps to motivate people to change their health behavior.
2. **Group level:** At this level, health education is aimed at a particular group of people as per their needs. For example, breastfeeding and immunization for postnatal mothers, sex education for adolescent youth and family planning for eligible couples and personal hygiene for school children.
3. **General public level or community level:** At this level, the health message is conveyed to a large population. The message chosen should be of common interest. For example, control of communicable diseases, personal hygiene, first aid treatment of fever and diarrhea.

Approaches

There are four main approaches of health education:

1. **Legal approach:** In this approach, there are some rules and laws framed by the authorities and passed by the government. The public should follow these rules strictly. The person who disobeys these laws is punished by fine or imprisonment or both. Compulsory vaccination of smallpox and polio has eradicated these diseases. Similarly, smoking in public area is banned to prevent air pollution and protect the environment health.
2. **Educational approach:** Health education is very effective means of changing people's attitude toward health. Though it is a slow process and reinforcement is required, but this is positive and democratic approach.
3. **Service approach:** Health services are made available to the people but people do not avail these facilities either due to lack of knowledge or ignorance, e.g., health and wellness centers at subcenter and primary health center (PHC) level are opened in rural areas for providing health services. Similarly, community health centers and district hospitals are opened in urban areas to provide health services.
4. **Primary healthcare approach:** The aim of this approach is to help the person to become self-dependent in their health matters. But this approach is successful only with people's active participation and involvement in the planning and delivery of healthcare services.

METHODS OF HEALTH EDUCATION

Based on the gathering or social groups, the following are the methods of health education:
- Methods used at individual and community level
- Methods used at group level
- Methods used at general public level

Methods Used at Individual and Community Level

At individual level, health education is imparted to individuals/patients in the hospital while performing treatment and care. At community level, health education is imparted to patients during home visit by health personnel while taking history and making assessment.

Counseling is also provided at individual level on matters of selection of family planning methods, child health problems and reproductive health problems which may not be discussed in the group during counseling. Privacy, confidentiality and trust should be maintained.

Methods Used at Group Level

- **Lecture method:** This is one-way method usually practiced not only in health education, but also in general education. The speaker plays the main role and participation of the group is almost nil. The following points should be considered in lecture method:
  - Lecture should be well organized with ideas developed in a logical sequence. Local experience should be used while illustrating general statement.
  - It should be complete with fundamental facts and information.
  - Lecture should relate to past, present and future material on the subject.
  - Lecture should not exceed >15–20 minutes.
  - To make the lecture more effective, maximum use of audio-visual aids should be made like charts, graphs, models, specimen, posters, films, etc.
  - It is an ideal method for presenting huge amount of information in a short period of time.
  - It is also called talk and chalk method as chalk may be used to write important words and headings on the board.
  - It is useful in introducing new subjects, in summarizing the literature in a field, in reviewing, in integrating different ideas and concepts into an orderly system of thought.
  - It is difficult to meet individual needs as there is little personal relationship between the educator and audience.
- **Group discussion (or two-way method or Socratic method):** This method is useful when there is a common topic of interest. Group members can exchange their thoughts and experience and clear their doubts. This method provides wider interaction among members than other methods of health education. The following facts are important in group discussion:
  - The group should have 6–12 members for effective discussion.
  - The role of group leader is influential in group discussion. Group leader initiates the discussion, extends the debate, controls the discussion, motivates members and presents conclusion in the end.
  - In group discussion, every member has equal opportunity to contribute the ideas, experience and knowledge on the problem. The individual learns to think independently.

- There should be maximum participation by all the members.
- The members should have the liberty to express themselves clearly without any fear. Discussion should be healthy, free from bitterness and undue interference.
- Discussion should be subject centered.
- The whole proceedings are recorded by the recorder. At the end, conclusions are written and they should be signed by all the group members.

- **Panel discussion:** In this discussion, there are 4–8 experts who discuss the given subject in front of the audience. One person from the experts group starts proceeding as a chairman.
  He/she introduces the experts and subject and its role in brief and invites the experts to express themselves. Its features are:
  - There is no special agenda or sequence of lectures.
  - The audience are invited to participate after the experts have expressed their views.
  - The discussion should be natural, self-inspired and easy going.
  - The success of panel discussion depends on the chairperson to a great extent. If well planned and conducted in correct manner, it proves to be very effective method of health education.

- **Workshop:** In this method, the participants are divided in small groups and each group is assigned some special task and solution of a particular problem. Each group has a leader and recorder. The special features of the group are:
  - Each group is allotted one topic only.
  - Each individual has an important role in it.
  - Education is carried out under the guidance of experts in an effective, friendly and democratic atmosphere.

  In this way, small groups combine to study the subject in totality and together find out the solution of the problem. In the report of workshop, conclusions are presented. This method has proved to be very good in the field of education.

- **Symposium:** In this method, 4–5 expert speakers are there with chairperson who introduces topic to audience. Symposium is a series of speeches on a selected topic. Experts present their views on different aspects of the topic in brief. There is no discussion among experts like panel discussion. In the end, the audience can contribute in the topic by asking questions. In the end, the chairperson summarizes the topic and closes the session.

- **Role play:** Expression by acting can be more impressive than words. Keeping this fact in mind, acting or social dramas are staged or played for health education. Its features are:
  - The audience can actively participate and express or demonstrate their own experience.
  - About 25 participants can participate in the group.
  - Useful for presenting real-life situations.
  - It is valuable in discussing problems of human relationship.
  - At community level, the health education imparted in this way is very effective in changing the attitude of the people.
  - It is very interesting to see the participants acting out real situations; and learning in this way becomes permanent and long lasting.

- **Demonstration:** It is a method of health education involving practical exhibition and explanation for performing a certain act or procedure. Practical demonstration is an important technique of health education for demonstrating baby bath, taking temperature, giving hair wash to a bedridden client, back care, changing position, etc. By this method, education takes place under realistic condition and the audience queries can be satisfied. The group should not have >20 participants. There are opportunities for return demonstration also. The method has got its limitations. The material required for demonstration may be expensive, limited or difficult to transport.

- **Simulation:** This is the method of experiencing real situation with the help of models designed to perform certain activities, for example, showing cardiopulmonary resuscitation (CPR) on a dummy or showing various stages of mechanism of labor on a simulator model. This is also very effective method of teaching.

Methods Used at General Public Level

The mass media methods are used in combination with other methods to make them more effective. The following methods are used:

- **Television:** It is an excellent method to change the people's attitude, views and behavior regarding health concern. It is one-way method; it has great potential to educate people.
- **Radio:** It is also very effective means for a large population. Health information is represented through dramas, plays, discussion programs; and people can get benefit at their household.
- **Newspaper:** It is the quickest method of disseminating information of all forms from news to entertainment, education, health problems, science and literature. It is very popular in urban community and literate people of rural areas.
- **Posters:** These are visual presentations and are used to convey health messages about implementation of health programs or any happening through pictures, words or symbols. They can be displayed at public places where people can see and realize the importance of the message being conveyed.
- **Health exhibitions and health museum:** Health knowledge about health problems can be presented through health exhibitions and health museum. These suggest their remedial and preventive measures. The models, charts, posters, objects, photos, diagrams, etc. are used to arrange health exhibitions and health museums. These exhibitions and museum attract more people.
- **Printed material:** It includes health magazines, pamphlets, booklets and handouts prepared by different institutions, organizations and government. Ministry of Health and Family Welfare is involved in circulation of printed material and caters to the needs of the people.
- **Folk media:** Folk dance, folk songs, puppet shows, *nukkad dramas, katha, keertan* are folk methods which are very popular in India. Health information presented through these methods is very interesting, effective and entertaining besides providing education.
- **Direct mailing:** Folders, newsletters and booklets on family planning, immunization, nutrition, etc., are printed and mailed from the health department. They reach the village leaders, literate persons and local bodies.
- **Internet:** This has revolutionized the communication system. It is the fastest means of communication and provides direct and instant communication across the world. One can communicate by means of email or an online chat on WhatsApp. Health-related information from Ministry of Health and Family Welfare, Government of India; and World Health Organization (WHO) is available online.

SCOPE OF HEALTH EDUCATION AND OPPORTUNITIES FOR HEALTH EDUCATION IN HOSPITAL AND COMMUNITY

Aspects of Health Education

The scope of health education is vast. The subject matter of health education includes every aspect related to health. The contents of health education are divided under the following topics:

- **Human biology:** A brief description of the anatomy and physiology of human biology forms the basis of other topics of health education. It is necessary to explain in short about structure and functions of human body, how to keep the body physically fit and the importance of exercise, rest and sleep. Ill effects of smoking, drugs and alcohol on the body result in a variety of diseases.
- **Nutrition:** Body needs fuel to provide energy for work. Balanced diet is important to prevent deficiency diseases. The nutritive values of different foods, methods of cooking for preservation of nutrients, food hygiene, storage and preservation of food are also important. Diet in pregnancy and lactation, diet for infants/toddlers and elderly people is also a vital part of nutrition.
- **Hygiene:** People should be educated about:
    - **Personal hygiene:** Taking bath, care of hair, nails, feet, importance of hand washing, care of mouth, eyes, ears, nose and maintaining cleanliness.
    - **Environmental hygiene:** Includes good housing, lighting, ventilation, fresh air, sunshine, safe water supply, control of insects, rodents, proper disposal of excreta and waste, use of latrine and collection of refuse.
    - **Food hygiene:** Hygiene of vegetables, fruits, milk, hygienic storage of food and prevention of diseases caused by unhygienic food.
- **Maternal and child health (MCH) and family planning:** Mothers are taught to improve their health and keep themselves healthy during pregnancy and lactation. They need to be taught about balanced diet, baby care, and infant feeding. They should be educated about small family norms and need for family planning.
- **Prevention of communicable and noncommunicable diseases:** Health education regarding prevention of communicable diseases and protection by immunization against vaccine-preventable diseases should be given. Health education to control noncommunicable diseases like hypertension, heart disease, dental caries, malnutrition, drug addiction, etc., should also be imparted.
- **Prevention of accidents:** Accidents may occur at home, at work place or on the road. People should be educated about safety measures against accidents.
- **Utilization of health services:** People should be educated about how to make use of available community health services. Many people in rural areas are ignorant about those facilities due to lack of awareness. People should be motivated to participate in the national health programs and make use of available health facilities.
- **Sex education:** Community should be educated about prevention of sexually transmitted diseases and acquired immunodeficiency syndrome (AIDS) especially in the adolescent group.
- **Mental health:** This area is of increasing importance. Drug dependence, smoking, alcoholism, juvenile delinquency, crime and violence are becoming major problems. People require proper health education for optimum mental health.

- **Health statistics:** To educate people regarding:
  - Importance of health surveys
  - Importance of birth and death reporting
  - Cooperation in activities like census collection

Scope of Health Education

The scope of health education refers to the breadth and depth of knowledge, skills, and strategies that are involved in promoting and improving health. Health education is a multidisciplinary field that encompasses various aspects of health and wellness, including physical, mental, social and emotional well-being. Overall, the scope of health education is vast and encompasses a range of disciplines and strategies that can be used to promote and improve health at the individual and community levels. The scope of health education includes:

- **Health promotion:** It aims to increase awareness and knowledge about healthy lifestyles and behaviors that can prevent the occurrence of illnesses and diseases.
- **Community health:** It is the study and practice of promoting health at the community level. It involves working with communities to identify and address health problems and to promote healthy behaviors.
- **Disease prevention:** It focuses on strategies and interventions that can help individuals avoid and manage chronic conditions, such as diabetes, heart disease and cancer.
- **Environmental health:** It focuses on the relationship between human health and the environment, including air, water and soil. It aims to prevent environmental hazards and promote healthy living environment.
- **Health communication:** It is the process of conveying health-related information to individuals and communities through various channels, such as mass media, social media and interpersonal communication.
- **Public health policy:** It refers to the development and implementation of policies and regulations that promote health and prevent diseases. It involves working with government agencies, health organizations and communities to promote public health and well-being.

Opportunities for Health Education in Hospital and Community

- **Health education in hospitals:** The nurses and other health workers get ample opportunities for health education in hospital. Planned health teaching requires preparation, whereas incidental health teaching continues as long as the health workers come in contact with patients while providing care to them.
- **Health education in outpatient department:** Patients spend a lot of time for health check-up, i.e., for registration, consultation, investigation, diagnosis, treatment and admission procedure. During the waiting period, health education can be provided by the following methods:
  - Displaying pictures, posters, charts and models in waiting area.
  - Distributing pamphlets.
  - Showing documentary film on important and common health problems.
  - By arranging group discussion.
  - Giving health education at personal level in consulting room.
  - Health education in family planning clinic, psychiatric clinic and nutrition clinic.
  - Arranging street plays, etc.

- **Health education in inpatient departments:** Nurses get opportunities to educate patients on health matters while providing nursing care by the following methods:
  - Motivating patients to adopt health-seeking behavior while performing certain procedures, e.g., bed making, during sponge bath, giving back care, hair care, feet care, etc.
  - By arranging demonstration on nutrition, baby care, teaching about taking insulin injection at home, on minor dressing and first aid treatment of fever, how to give hydrotherapy, how to prepare ORS at home in case of diarrhea.
  - Providing incidental teaching to patients and relatives about specific procedure, for example, care of bedridden patient at home.
  - Providing clinical and bedside teaching.
- **Education in the community:** The community health nurse can educate community in the following ways:
  - **During home visit:** In this, the community health nurse can impart health education to the individuals and families by counseling, group discussion or demonstrations.
    - Providing information related to their health problems.
    - Providing education on family planning, prenatal and postnatal care to the mothers
    - Providing education on personal hygiene, nutrition, immunization, prevention of communicable and noncommunicable diseases.
    - Providing information and creating awareness to utilize the available health services and referral services.
    - Providing education on environmental hygiene, housing, ventilation, lighting, use of latrines and disposal of waste.
  - **In the school:** While assessing the health status of the students, the school health nurse gets opportunities to provide health education to the students and parents. At the student level, the health messages have long lasting and permanent effect of health education. This enables the students to take care of their health from the childhood and prevent and solve their health problems. Health education has to be included in their curriculum so that they learn and practice healthful living and also coordinate, promote and evaluate the health programs.
  - **At college or university campus:** Health educators should be a part of team working to create an environment in which students make healthy choices and create caring community. Students should be educated on disease prevention, environmental health, emotional and sexual health, first aid, safety and disaster preparedness, substance abuse prevention, human growth and development and nutrition. Students may manage grants and conduct research.
  - **In companies:** The industrial nurse provides education about safety measures of workers. She helps and guides the employers to provide healthy environment for workers to protect their health. Routine medical checkup of the employees is conducted to screen industrial hazards. She guides the management to take special care of the workers who are at risk due to working conditions of the industries and provide adequate rest and safety to protect their health.
  - **In community organization:** The community health nurse helps the community to identify its needs, its problem-solving abilities and mobilize its resources to develop, promote, implement and evaluate strategies to improve its own health status.

NURSE'S ROLE IN HEALTH EDUCATION

Nurse plays a vital role in imparting health education to the patients, families and community by virtue of her duties. Nurse remains in contact with the patients for a longer time than doctors and other health professionals. Right from the time of admission till discharge of patients from hospital, she is with them, providing care and carrying out the doctor's instructions. Nurse builds good interpersonal relations with the patients. Nurse should consider the following points while providing health education:

- To win the confidence of the people.
- To arouse interest in people toward health-seeking behavior and motivate them to keep themselves healthy.
- To motivate people to inculcate healthy habits.
- To create awareness and encourage people to make use of available health services.
- To develop a sense of responsibility among people to maintain their own health and also the health of whole community.
- The subject for health education should be selected according to the priority and need of the people.
- There should be effective communication so that the people can clear their doubts.
- To enhance the effect of health education, appropriate audio-visuals aids should be used.
- Health education should be planned and continuous.
- Nurse should seek the cooperation of government and voluntary organizations on health education.
- The nurse should evaluate and do the expected corrections of health education program with the help of various tools and observation.
- Health education imparted should be practical and genuine.
- The nurse is a coordinator in providing care to the patient; so, she should make best use of her position in providing health education to the patients, families and community.

Summary

- Health education is a way of educating people about their health.
- The concept of health education seeks to increase knowledge and modify health behavior.
- The aim of health education is to achieve Health for All by educating them and making them solve their health problems themselves.
- The principles of health education are good communication, good interpersonal relations, reinforcement, motivation, interest and people's participation in health programs.
- The process of change of health behavior takes place by creating interest and by helping people for making self-assessment and taking decisions.
- There are three levels of providing health education—individual level, group level and general public level or community level. The approaches of health education are legal approach, educational approach, service approach and primary healthcare approach.
- The methods of health education are used according to the group level such as interview, counseling and home visit (at individual level); group discussion, panel discussion, workshop, symposium, role play, demonstration and simulation (at group level); television, radio, newspaper, posters, exhibitions, health museum, printed material, folk dance, internet, etc. (at general public level).
- The role of nurse is vital in health education by virtue of her duty as she spends more time with patients/clients and community.

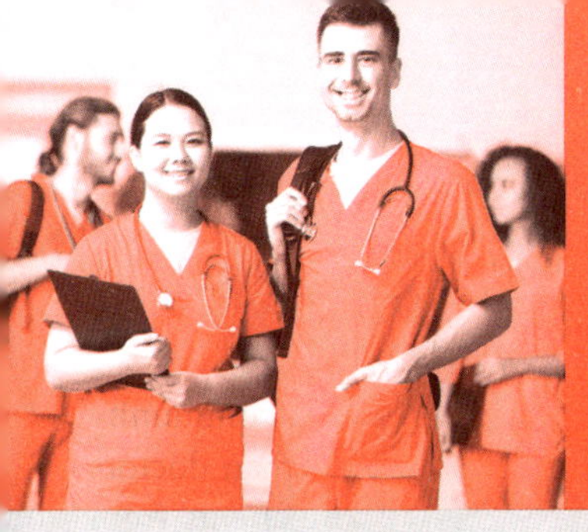

STUDENT ASSIGNMENT

LONG ANSWER TYPE QUESTIONS

1. Describe the principles of health education.
2. Explain the methods of health education.

SHORT ANSWER TYPE QUESTIONS

1. Define health education. Enlist the purposes of health education.
2. Write a short note on:
   a. Levels of health education.
   b. Approaches of health education.
   c. Process of change/modification of health behavior.
   d. Nurses' role in health education.

MULTIPLE CHOICE QUESTIONS

1. **Which of the following methods is used for health education?**
   a. Lecture and demonstration method
   b. Interpersonal discussion and panel discussion
   c. Seminar and symposium
   d. All of the above

2. **Health education can be provided by:**
   a. Receptionist
   b. Health personnel
   c. Microbiologist
   d. Radiologist

3. **Health education can be given in:**
   a. Only in the clinic
   b. Clinic and hospital
   c. Community setup
   d. All of these

ANSWER KEY

1. d   2. b   3. d

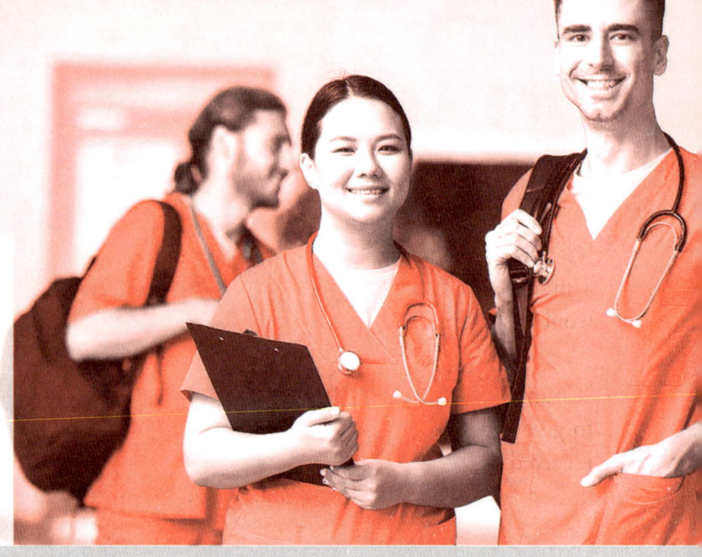

15

Counseling

LEARNING OBJECTIVES

After the completion of the unit, the readers will be able to:

- Define counseling and differentiate between health education and counseling.
- Enlist the principles and scope of counseling.
- Explain the qualities of good counselor.
- Describe the role of nurse in counseling.

UNIT OUTLINE

- Introduction
- Counseling Process: Steps/Phases
- Qualities of a Good Counselor
- Role of Nurse in Counseling

KEY TERMS

Adapt: To make adjustment to the new situation.

Counsel: To give professional advice and help to somebody with a problem.

Crisis: A condition of instability or danger, as in social, economic, political, or international affairs, leading to a decisive change; a dramatic, emotional or circumstantial upheaval in a person's life.

Exhort: To advise strongly.

INTRODUCTION

Counseling denotes "giving advice". It is a process that helps the client to recognize problems and manage stress by using problem-solving technique when the help is provided by the counselor. The counselor finds out the client's problems. He/she finds many solutions to solve problems and helps the client to choose the best possible solution to solve problem.

Definitions

- "Counseling is a dynamic and purposeful relationship between two people who approach a mutually defined problem with mutual consideration of each other to the extent that the troubled or less matured person is aided to a self-determined solution of his problem."
  Wren, 1962

- "Counseling is the helping relationship that includes someone seeking help, someone willing to give help, who is capable or trained to help, in a setting that permits help to be given and received". **Cormier and Hackney, 1987**

Purposes

- Helping individuals through temporary crisis
- Helping individuals to make wise choices
- Improving the understanding of self
- Providing the needed information and assistance
- Identifying the disturbed behavior at the earliest
- Facilitating adjustment
- Helping in adaptation to changes or new environment
- Making self-sufficient and independent
- Referring care needing special treatment
- Using capabilities and talent efficiently
- Promoting the optimal, personal, and professional development
- Balancing physical, psychological, emotional, social and spiritual growth
- Helping in overall development and creating conditions for living productive life

Principles

- Client's need to be placed first
- Maintain dignity of individual as individual is primary concern in counseling
- Avoid dictatorial attitude
- Maintain relationship of trust and confidence with the client
- Emphasize thinking with the client
- Make the client feel comfortable and free to talk about the problems
- Confidentiality is to be maintained
- Warmth, friendliness, openness and empathy are ingredients of successful counseling process
- Counselor has to concentrate on attentive listening, answering questions objectively and reinforcing important information
- Let the client make voluntarily informed decision
- Supremacy of client's values and culture

Scope

Every individual faces certain level of stress and strain in fast moving life, which gives rise to the need for counseling. Scope of counseling is as follows:

- Counseling helps to achieve positive mental health by overcoming stress.
- It maximizes individual's freedom to make right choice and act within conditions imposed by environment.
- It helps to resolve the problems of individuals.
- It helps the students in the selection of educational courses, profitable occupation and job placement.
- It helps the students in improvement of study skills and study habit formation.
- Counseling services can help in getting loans, scholarship and help from the voluntary organizations to complete their studies for students who are financially weak.
- It improves personal effectiveness. Vocational, health and living conditions, personal, social, moral and marital issues fall within the scope of counseling.

Types

Directive or Prescriptive Counseling

Directive counseling is counselor centered. Counselor plays a leading role. He/she directs the counselee to take steps in order to resolve conflicts. Directive counseling believes in the limited capacity of the client. The counselor tries to direct the thinking of the client by informing, explaining, interpreting and advising.

Tools Used

- Advice
- Warning
- Exhortation
- Praise
- Reassurance

Steps of Directive Counseling

The steps followed in directive counseling (Fig. 15.1) are:

- Collecting the relevant data
- Analyzing the problems
- Diagnosis, formulating conclusions regarding the nature and cause of the problem exhibited by the client
- Prognosis
- Prescribe remedial measures
- Follow-up

Nondirective Counseling

Nondirective counseling is client centered and the role of counselor is passive. The client makes the final decision. Counselor has to accept the capability of the

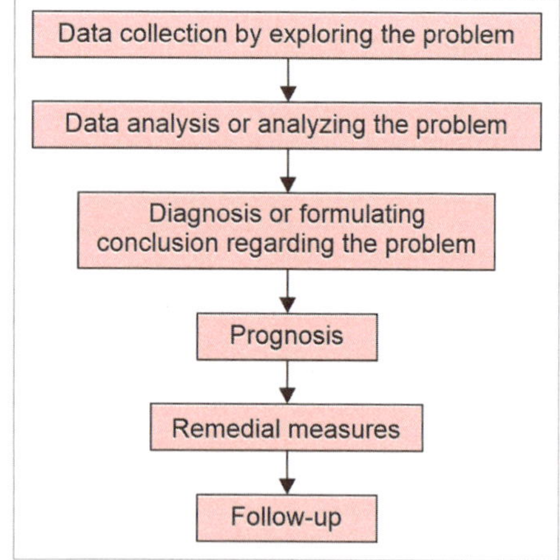

Fig. 15.1: Steps of directive counseling

client to make adjustment and adaptation. Counselor only creates an atmosphere in which the client works out his/her own understanding. The emotional aspects are emphasized more. It leads to voluntary choice of action. The principles of tolerance and acceptance are extremely important.

Steps of Nondirective Counseling

The steps followed in nondirective counseling (Fig. 15.2) are:

- Establishing rapport
- Exploration of problem
- Exploration of the cause of problem
- Find out alternative solution
- Termination of the session
- Follow-up

Elective Counseling

The counselor makes use of both directive and nondirective counseling which may be useful for the purposes of modifying client's ideas and attitudes. It puts check on the client's expression whenever it is in his/her interest.

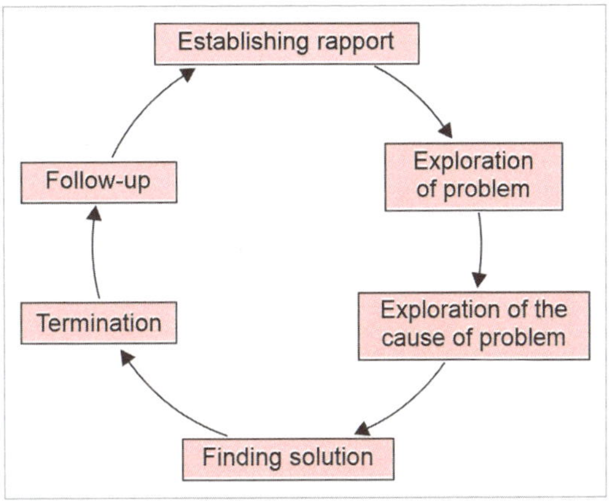

Fig. 15.2: Steps of nondirective counseling

The technique is effective because it has been derived from all sources of counseling, selecting the best and leaving out what is least required. The goal is independent with integration of the client rather than problem oriented. The counselor creates an atmosphere in which the client can work out his own understanding. It leads to a voluntary choice of action.

Steps of Elective Counseling

The objectives of elective counseling are as follows:

- Facilitate the development of self-insight component
- Release of tension
- Leading the client to a point of self-realization, self-actualization and self-help.

This method is useful in solving educational, vocational and marital problems.

Steps followed in elective counseling (Fig. 15.3) are:

1. Interview
2. Establishing rapport with client
3. Collecting relevant data
4. Analyzing the problem
5. Formulating conclusion regarding the nature of problems
6. Creating an atmosphere in which client works out to solve problems

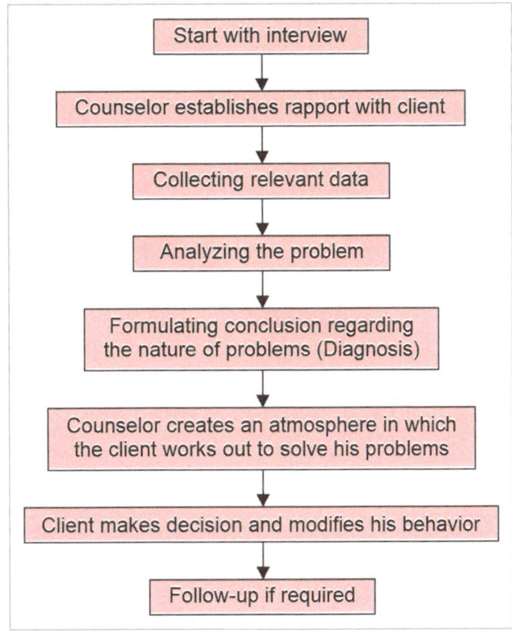

Fig. 15.3: Steps of elective counseling

7. Enabling client to make decision and modify behavior
8. Follow-up, if required

Group Counseling

Group counseling (Fig. 15.4) is useful when the client has not responded to individual counseling. This type of counseling is helpful for the adolescent group where peer group values are more important. The individual may gain an insight and understanding into his/her own problems. Ideas and values may become more understandable and acceptable by listening to others who discuss their difficulties. The counseling group encourages individuals to develop desired abilities through their relationship in an acceptable and meaningful social situation. The counselor should provide comfortable environment for group counseling. He/she should encourage team spirit, create a climate of harmony, cooperation, understanding and acceptance. For homogenous group of 6–8 or below 20 members, group counseling is advised. Counselor should have sound knowledge and sufficient skill.

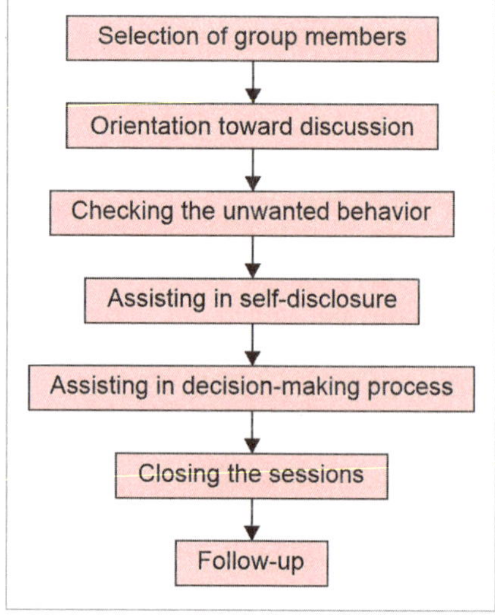

Fig. 15.4: Steps of group counseling

Short-term Counseling

- Short-term counseling is used in situational crisis
- It focuses on the concerns of client or family
- It can be relatively minor or major concern, but it needs immediate attention irrespective of the situation.
- Counselor will assist the client and guide problem solving in a systematic way or decision-making in a logical manner.

Long-term Counseling

- Long-term counseling extends over a long period of time and varies on daily, weekly or monthly basis.
- It is focused on the client who experiences development crisis.

Student Counseling

Students are not considered mentally ill, but may need help to solve their problems pertaining to the choice of educational institute, course, method of study, adjustment, vocational choice, etc. Student counseling deals with total personality of the individual. It connects directly to the needs of the individual.

Placement Counseling

The counselor will advise the client regarding jobs which are most suitable for him/her depending upon interest, abilities and attitude.

Psychotherapeutic Counseling

Psychologically trained individual (counselor) consciously attempts to assist the client to modify his/her maladaptive behavior. The counselor makes an attempt in making the client to speak out the repressed feelings and emotions. Various methods of psychotherapy are:

- Behavior counseling
- Encouragement
- Giving information and advice
- Hope

Marriage Counseling

- To advise and help in selecting the suitable spouse
- To identify the positive aspects of relationship as well as those cause conflict
- To solve marital problems
- To focus on the need for understanding the point of view and feelings of each other
- To help couples to talk constructively about problems in marital relationships

Vocational Counseling

- If any problem arises within a specific vocation, necessary steps are taken to solve those problems.
- It helps an individual in establishing greater control over his/her own frustration.
- Counselor will help the client/counselee to improve overall personality and will also help in training counselee to develop skills and gain mastery over the vocation so that counselee will be best among his/her co-employees in the profession.

Individual Counseling

Individual counseling involves mutual interchange of opinion to receive and impart information. The counselor will try to establish rapport; and structuring has to be done so that the client understands what to expect at counseling. Individual counseling involves gathering all available pertinent facts, and making diagnosis on the basis of available pertinent facts. This helps in formulating an appropriate plan of action. Counselor will help the client to assimilate the information. Client achieves an insight and a sense of emotional release which alters his/her perception and attitude toward himself/herself and his/her situation. During closing phase, client makes decision and plans, modifies behavior and solves problems.

Follow-up contact may be planned.

Motivational Counseling

Motivational counseling involves discussing feelings and incentives with the client. The counselor can encourage to establish helping relationship to avoid feeling of despair and work through the feelings of their motivation. For example, if the client shows unwillingness to participate in learning activities, counselor has to assess any factor from the past or present that might be negatively influencing motivation.

Health Counseling

The purpose of health counseling is helping the individual to learn more about health and healthy habits. Health counseling helps individuals to become more aware of the role of education, nutrition, rest and sleep. It also helps the client to seek referral services and guidance for social, mental and physical health.

Crisis Counseling

Crisis counseling helps the client to overcome the effect of crisis situation. Crisis may be due to family conflicts or loss of family member. These situations may affect the normal behavior of the individual who may develop feeling of anxiety or guilt. The counselor helps the individual to understand the situation and develop a new pattern of behavior.

Personal Counseling

Most of the students usually face certain problems about which they may be very anxious. They generally try to cope with the problems. Counselor helps the students to understand and solve these problems. Counselor helps students by providing advice on personal problems. He/she helps the students to develop interpersonal skills, improve study habits and accept themselves and others.

Educational Counseling

Educational counseling helps students to get maximum benefits out of education and solve their problems related to education. Students orient themselves to the new purpose or philosophy of education. They develop study habits and choose specialization according to their interest and need.

Orientation Service Counseling

Orientation service counseling helps students to become fully aware about themselves and the new environment of institution.

COUNSELING PROCESS: STEPS/PHASES

Counseling process takes place according to the nature of the problems of the client who needs help (Fig. 15.5). Counselor will use different approaches which are suitable to change the behavior and attitude of the counselee to adjust with new environment. There are five phases or steps of counseling process which are in progressive movements and collectively describe the counseling process. The phases may overlap with each other, for example, the assessment may begin, while the phase of establishing relationship is in process.

Phase-1: Establishing relationship:
- Phase 1 is a very important phase in the process of counseling as it affects the progress of the process. The relationship of the counselor and counselee is unique and it is influenced by factors

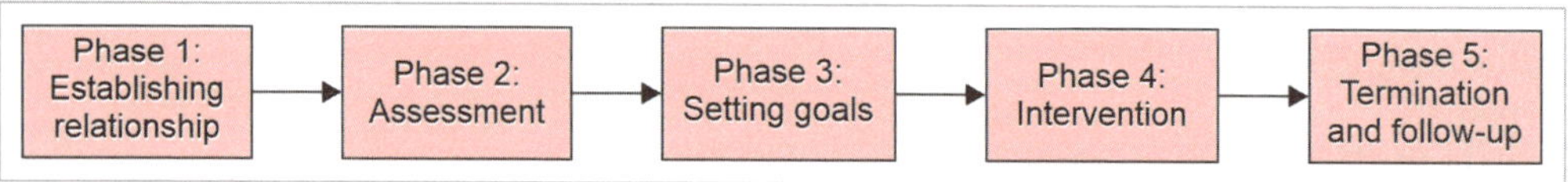

Fig. 15.5: Phases of counseling

such as respect, trust and a sense of psychological comfort. The skills of the counselor as required in establishing relationship are:

- Introduction of the counselor to the counselee
- Listening attentively to what the counselee says
- Addressing the counselee by name
- Ensuring physical comfort
- Encouraging open communication
- Not interrupting the counselee when he/she is talking
- Observe nonverbal communication
- Being patient as it may take several sessions to establish relationship

Phase-2: Assessment or data collection:

- In phase 2, the counselor encourages the clients to talk about their problems. The counselor uses his/her skills of asking questions, collecting information and making observation; and seeks views to help the individuals clearly state their problems (Fig. 15.6). The skills involved are:
  - Observation
  - Enquiry
  - Making association naming facts
  - Recording
  - Making educational guesses

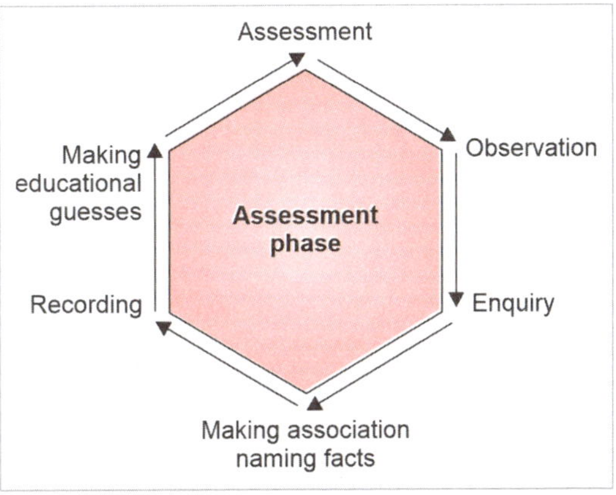

Fig. 15.6: Assessment phase

Phase-3: Setting goals:

- In phase 3, setting goals is cooperatively done by the individual and the counselor. Main purpose of this phase is to provide directions to the individual and the counselor. Goals are set based on the educated guesses made in assessment phase. Setting goals helps to know how well counseling is working, and when counseling may be conducted. The skills needed are:
  - Skill of drawing inference
  - Differentiation
  - Teaching individual to think realistically
  - Dynamism, i.e., goals are not fixed for all time to come as they may be changed whenever new information is received or new insight is developed.

Phase-4: Intervention:

- The intervention used will depend upon the approach used by the counselor, the problem and the individual. The choice of intervention is a process of adaptation. The counselor should be prepared to change the intervention, if the selected intervention is not working. The counseling skills needed are:
  - Skills in handling the intervention

- Knowledge of its effects
- Ability to read the client's reaction

Intervention is planned with the consultation of the counselee.

Phase-5: Termination and follow-up:

- The successful termination of counseling depends upon planned activities in each phase. It must be done without destroying the accomplishment gained and should be done with sensitivity and good intention. The individual may feel a sense of loss. Hence, termination should be planned over a few sessions. Follow-up appointments can be fixed.

QUALITIES OF A GOOD COUNSELOR

- **Intellectual competence:** Counselor should have deep knowledge of his/her field, theories as well as desire and ability to learn.
- **Interest:** Counselor should have keen interest in a wide range of activities.
- **Pleasing personality and voice:** Counselor's voice should be clear and he/she should have a balanced personality.
- **Energy:** Counseling is physically demanding and emotionally draining. Counselors must have the ability to remain active in entire session and sustain the activity when they see a number of clients in a row.
- **Flexibility:** Effective counselor is not tied to one specific set of responses. He/she adapts to meet the needs of client.
- **Support:** Counselor supports the clients in making their own decision.
- Sympathetic understanding
- Respect client's ability and need
- Friendly nature
- Emotionally matured behavior
- Well trained in counseling technique
- Should be authentic, sincere and honest
- Superior intellectual ability and judgment
- Should be fair, tactful and sincere
- Should maintain the confidentiality of the client
- Should possess high ethical values
- Should be open to change
- Must appreciate the values of culture
- Should have self-control and stability
- Professional dedication
- Good listener
- Makes good pleasing eye contact
- Should have sense of humor, be perceptive and be calm
- Approachable, genuine, objective, creative and imaginative

MUST KNOW

Differences between health education and counseling

Health education	Counseling
Health education is an organized service related to health which provides knowledge about health to individuals, families and community.	It is a specialized service offered to help individuals to solve their problems by themselves.
It is an educative service providing education, information and communication regarding health.	It is a therapeutic service provided to the individuals who need help to solve their problems.
Motivation is directed toward forming healthy habits.	Motivation is directed toward talking about the problems.
Aim is to control diseases.	Aim is to relieve stress and rehabilitate individuals.
It is a process which brings about changes in the health practices of the people.	It is a process that helps the client to recognize his/her problems and manage stress by problem-solving techniques.
Health education can be provided by health workers through health exhibitions, posters, and electronic media.	Counseling can be provided by only specialized person who is trained for counseling.
It is an instrument through which positive changes can be brought in the community's knowledge and behavior regarding health attitude and habits.	It is an interaction between two individuals; the one who provides help and the other who receives help.
It can be provided in any health care setting, i.e., hospital, health centers, clinics or even at home.	It can also be provided in clinic or at client's home.
The topics are planned according to the priority, need and interest of the individuals, families and community.	The topic starts with introduction, history taking, setting goals and lastly the intervention.

ROLE OF NURSE IN COUNSELING

The nurse as a counselor should ensure the following:

- The room is comfortable, not noisy and distracting.
- Distance between the counselor and counselee should be 30–35 inches so that the counselee feels comfortable.
- The chairs should be at 90° from one another so that the client can look either at counselor or straight.
- There should be no table during the session but small desk can be placed as physical and symbolic barrier against the development of close relationship.
- The auditory and visual privacy should be maintained by professional codes of ethics and assure client's maximum self-disclosure.
- The nonverbal behavior of the client should be observed clearly; client's facial expression, eye contact, sitting style and body gesture should be noted during counseling.

- Nurse should—help client to recognize and cope with stressful psychological or social problem to develop and improve interpersonal relationship and to promote personal growth.
    - Provide emotional, intellectual and psychological support
    - Focus on helping a client to develop new attitudes, feelings and behavior rather than promoting intellectual growth
    - Encourage the client to look at alternative behavior, recognize the choice and develop a sense of control
    - Help patients to make decisions that promote their overall well-being
    - Use interpersonal skills, warmth, friendliness, openness, empathy and caring
    - Listen carefully
    - Use therapeutic communication technique
    - Make referral, if needed
    - Work with patient and family to help them cope with illness and lifestyle changes, many may have to cope with permanent alternation. Examples are stress management and grief counseling.

Summary

- Counseling is giving advice to a client to help him/her recognize problems and find solutions.
- The purpose of counseling is to provide alternate solutions to the client so that he/she can select the best suitable options.
- The principles of counseling are to maintain confidentiality and maintain a relationship of trust with the client.
- The scope of counseling is to maintain positive mental health by overcoming stress.
- Counseling can be provided on health education, placement, marriage, motivational counseling, crisis counseling and orientation service counseling.
- The steps of counseling include establishing relationship, making assessment of clients' problems, setting goals, intervention, termination and follow-up.
- The counselor should have intellectual competency, and a lot of patience and tolerance. He/she should be sympathetic, supportive and flexible.
- The difference between counseling and health education is that in counseling the specialized services are offered to the client to resolve his/her problems by himself/herself, whereas health education is an organized service to provide knowledge regarding health to the individuals, family and community.
- Nurse should provide comfortable environment by arranging room for counseling without distortion and noise, provide emotional, intellectual and psychological support to the client, and provide referral services, if needed.

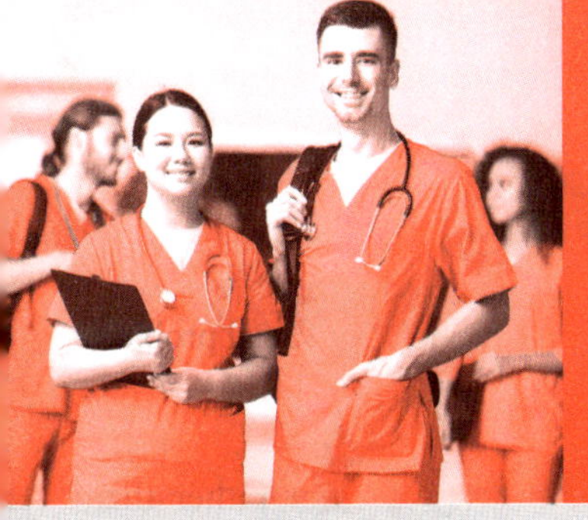

LONG ANSWER TYPE QUESTIONS

1. Describe the types of counseling.
2. What is the scope of counseling? Explain the process of counseling.
3. What is the difference between counseling and health education? Write the qualities of a good counselor.

SHORT ANSWER TYPE QUESTIONS

1. Define counseling. Enlist the purposes of counseling.
2. State the principles of counseling.

MULTIPLE CHOICE QUESTIONS

1. **The role of counselor in nondirective counseling is:**
   a. Active
   b. Passive
   c. Both active and passive
   d. None of these

2. **Listening in counseling is which process?**
   a. Passive process
   b. Dual process
   c. Active process
   d. None of these

3. **The final step of directive counseling is:**
   a. Prognosis
   b. Diagnosis
   c. Synthesis
   d. Follow-up

4. **Who plays a proactive role in counseling?**
   a. Counselee
   b. Counselor
   d. Administrator
   d. Referee

5. **Counseling is provided to:**
   a. Educate on health matter
   b. To relieve stress and rehabilitate
   c. To control disease
   d. To promote health

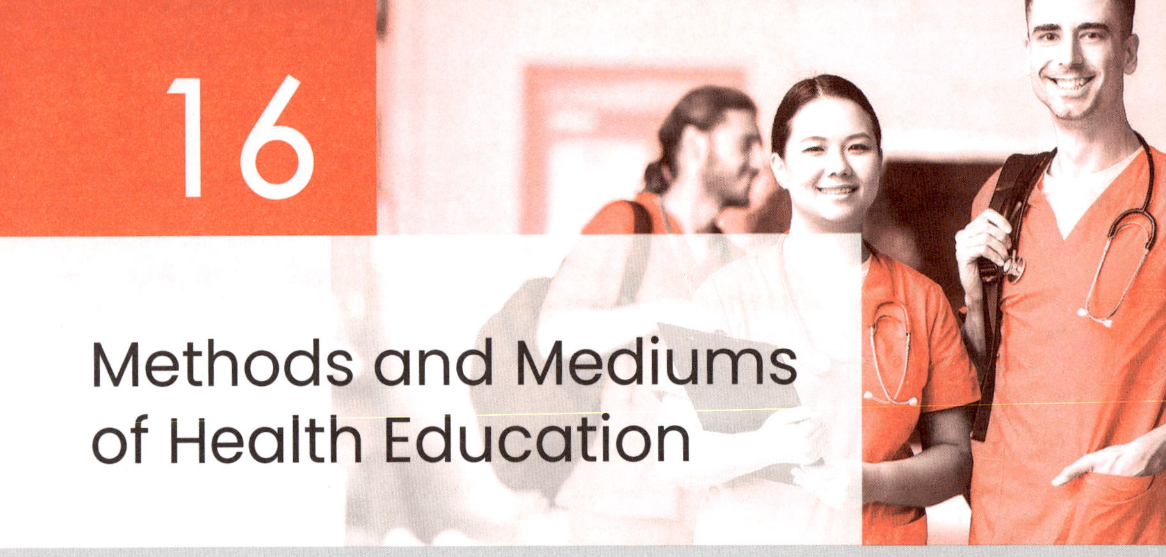

16

Methods and Mediums of Health Education

LEARNING OBJECTIVES

After the completion of the unit, the readers will be able to:

- Define audio-visual aids.
- Enlist the purpose of audio-visual aids.
- Describe the various types of audio-visual aids.
- Demonstrate skill in preparing and using different kinds of audio-visual aids.

UNIT OUTLINE

- Introduction
- Methods of Health Education
- Mediums of teaching Health Education
- Selection, Preparation and use of Audio-visual Aids
- Health Education Plan for a Group of Postnatal Mothers

KEY TERMS

Audio aids: Involve the sense of hearing; an instructional device in which the message can be heard but not seen.

Combined aids: Involve techniques and devices with both hearing and vision.

Visual aids: Involve the sense of vision; visual materials, such as pictures, charts, and diagrams, that help people understand and remember information shared in an oral presentation.

INTRODUCTION

Audio-visual (A-V) aids are the tools used to impart health education more effectively. It involves more senses of the learner. The A-V aids motivate curiosity in the learner by listening to them, by seeing to them, or by both to learn more. It creates interest to learn and the learning becomes permanent and long lasting.

METHODS OF HEALTH EDUCATION

Methods of health education are discussed in Unit 14.

MEDIUMS OF TEACHING HEALTH EDUCATION

Definitions

- Audio-visual aids are the devices that make learning easy and interesting.
- "A-V aids are those aids which help in completing the process of learning. They stimulate thinking, motivation and interest in learning". **—Carter V Good**
- "Audio-visual aids are any devices which are used to make learning more concrete, more realistic and more dynamic." **—Kinder S James**

Purposes

- To enhance learning
- To make the learner attentive toward the topic
- To impart health education with the help of A-V aids is of permanent nature
- To initiate thinking and reasoning in the learner
- To provide motivation for self-activities to make learning more effective
- To help keep continuity of thought and avoid drifting away from the subject

Types

The types of audio-visual aids are given in Figures 16.1 and 16.2.
- **First classification:** On the basis of communication (Fig. 16.1).
- **Second classification:** On the basis of technique used (Fig. 16.2).

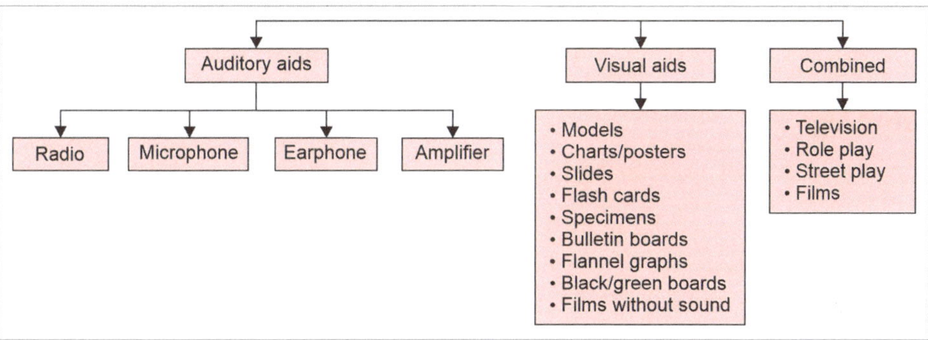

Fig. 16.1: First classification of audio-visual aids (medium) on the basis of communication

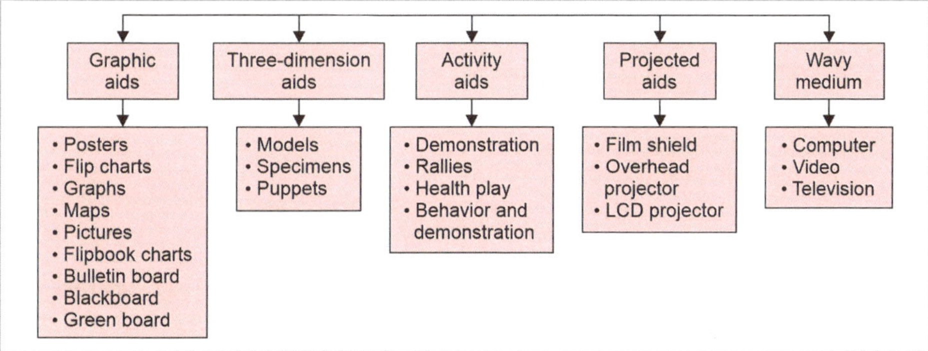

Fig. 16.2: Second classification of audio-visual aids (medium) on the basis of technique used

- **Third classification:** On the basis of operation (Fig. 16.3).

Projected aids	Nonprojected aids			
	Audio aids	Graphic aids	Display boards	Activity aids
• Film • Film strips • Opaque projector • Overhead projector (OHP) • Slides • Multimedia • Videotape	• Radio • Television • Recordings	• Charts • Cartoon • Diagrams • Flash cards • Graphs • Maps • Photographs • Pictures • Posters • Models	• Black board • Bulletin boards • Flannel boards • Magnetic board • Peg board	• Demonstrations • Experimentation • Field trips

Fig. 16.3: Third classification of audio-visual aids (medium) on the basis of operation

SELECTION, PREPARATION AND USE OF AUDIO-VISUAL AIDS

Based on the need, the audio-visual aids can be selected. Audio-visual aids can be of following types:

- Graphic aids
- Printed aids
- Three-dimensional aids
- Projected aids

Graphic Aids

The graphic aids include the following:

- Posters
- Flip charts
- Graphs, maps and pictures
- Charts
- Bulletin boards
- Blackboard/chalkboard/green board

Posters

The posters are visual presentation and are used to convey health messages, about the implementation of health programs or any happening through pictures, words or symbols.

Preparation

- Posters are prepared from large-size paper.
- Should be written in the local language.

MUST KNOW

Criteria for Selection of Audio-visual Aids

Audio-visual aids are very effective aids for imparting health education. They enhance learning and make the learning process interesting and easy. The selection of A-V aids depends upon the following:

- **Audience/learner:** Before the selection and preparation of A-V aids, the background of the audience, age group, level of knowledge, their needs for learning, their capacity to learn should be known. People with visual impairment, require audio and tactile aids, e.g., audiotapes and large printed material with bold letters. A person with auditory impairment requires visual aids.
- **Objectives:** A-V aids are prepared according to the learning objectives.
- **Place/settings:** A-V aids should be selected according to the setting whether it is to be used in clinics, hospitals, outdoor departments, or in the community setting.
- **Characteristics of teaching aids:** The teachings selected should be able to sustain audience's interest, motivate the thinking process and promote health-seeking behaviour.
- **Skill of the user:** The user should have technical skill to handle the A-V aids devices and check them before using them. Should maintain and keep ready for use at any time.
- **Availability of resources and facilities:** A-V aids should be selected on the basis of the availability of funds, educational material, power supply and preparation for its use.

- Always written in capital letters.
- Few and simple words should be used.
- Color combination should be attractive.
- One poster should have one message.
- Symbols and pictures should be self-explanatory.
- Should be displayed in places where people can see and realize the importance of the message conveyed. Can be displayed at railway stations, bus stands, clinics, hospitals, health camps, fairs and exhibitions, schools and other public places.

Advantages

- Easy to prepare and transport
- Less expensive
- Portable
- Attract the audience

Disadvantages

- If not displayed at the proper place, it is a mere wastage.
- Pasting and tearing make them unsuitable for long-term use.

Flip Charts

Flip charts can be prepared in advance for maximum clarity and impact. These can be hung on a special board fitted with screws. Can be rolled up for easy transport.

Preparation

- Write the title of each page
- Should be written clearly in capital letters
- Letters should be of 1-inch size so that they can be read from 10 feet distance.
- Pictures and symbols should be used to make the message attractive.

Uses

Flip charts are used for demonstration of figures, tables, pictures, maps and graphs, etc.

Advantages

- Electricity is not required for displaying.
- Can be prepared at home.
- Can be prepared in different sizes as per the requirement of the learner.

Disadvantages

- Not suitable for bigger groups
- Expensive for commercial use

Graphs, Maps and Pictures

- Size of graphics should be appropriate according to the chart.
- Attractive colors should be used.
- Pictures, maps, graphs diagrams and photographs can be pasted on chart.

Advantages

- Can be prepared in advance as per the requirement of the group.
- Easily portable

Disadvantages

- Expensive
- Cannot be used for long-term.

Charts

Charts are visual presentations of diagrams, pictures, graphs or maps. Charts can be prepared on thick paper or art paper. Charts are prepared according to the needs and interests of the group for preparation. Words should be suitable, precise and meaningful according to the topic chosen for communication and health education. Color combinations should be attractive and dark colors should be used. The size of the words should be appropriate, visible and readable by all the audience. Important points to be highlighted.

Uses

- Present data in summarized form
- Make the teaching interesting and initiate thinking process
- Sustain the attention of the learner

Advantages

- Can be prepared according to the needs of the audience.
- Easy to use
- Electricity is not required for displaying them.
- Provide an opportunity to the learner to get clarification and meaning at a glance.

Disadvantages

- Not suitable to use for large groups.
- Cannot be used for illiterate people as they find it difficult to understand tables, charts and diagrams.
- Cannot be used for long-term as they get spoiled due to pasting and tearing.

Bulletin Boards

Bulletin boards are used for displaying visual materials, for example, pictures with relevant headings or conveying health messages or important events.

Preparation of Bulletin Boards

These are made out of soft and light cardboard boxes or softwood or any such material on which paper can be made stable by pining. Then a colored cloth is pasted over the paper within the frame. Pictures or photographs are displayed on the colored cloth with related ideas and information with maps, pictures with arrows and circles to draw the attention of the audiences.

Advantages

- Health messages on current events can be conveyed to a large group by displaying picture cutting, three-dimensional objects and photographs on it.
- Beneficial for illiterate groups.

Disadvantages

- Require time for preparation
- Expensive
- Cannot be used everywhere as transportation is not so easy.

Blackboard/Chalkboard/Green Board

This is the most commonly used teaching aid and is the traditional aid. It can be easily prepared by using black or dark green paint over a wooden board or wall. Originally, the boards were made of smooth, thin sheets of black or dark-gray slate stone. Nowadays, roller boards are made of coiled sheets of plastic drawn across two parallel rollers are also used to create additional writing space.

Chalk sticks made with calcium sulfate are used for writing text. Chalk marks can be easily cleaned with a duster or with a special chalkboard eraser.

Uses

- It provides live experience.
- It creates interest in learning.
- It is reusable.
- It is used on the spot. Prior preparation is not required.
- Colored chalks can be used to explain different structures.

Advantages

- It is cheap, convenient and easy to use.
- It is not dependent on electricity.
- It can be used anywhere.
- No maintenance cost.

Disadvantages

- Produces dust and can cause allergy to some people.
- Chalk dust can cause respiratory problems.
- The written material over the board cannot be stored.
- Eye- to- eye contact is lost.
- If not used properly, the conversation between the speaker and the audience can break, become unclear, boring and create difficulty in seeing or writing.

Printed Aids

Printed aids include:

Newspaper

- Newspaper is a continuous and regular source of visual aids containing special health pages.
- People can read health messages sitting at home.
- Can preserve cutting of important health topics.
- Up-to-date information on health and health programs reach to people.

Advantages

- The written material on health can be preserved
- No preparation is required.
- No power supply is needed.

Disadvantage

Illiterate people cannot read and get the benefit.

Magazines

There are plenty of national and international health magazines available including world health magazines. These are printed monthly, quarterly half-yearly, or yearly.

Advantages

- Very useful for training institutions.
- Provide up-to-date knowledge on health-based research studies.
- Provide the latest information on health.

Disadvantages

- Expensive
- Everybody cannot have access to it.

Pamphlets

Various health organizations print health materials on pamphlets. These pamphlets are distributed to various health settings or can be circulated to the people along with newspapers.

Uses

- People can become aware of their health and health needs while sitting at home.
- Pamphlets can motivate people for health-seeking behavior.

Advantages

- No preparation required
- Students get readymade health materials
- Can be preserved
- No power supply is required to use
- Teacher can distribute pamphlets to students and explain.

Disadvantages

- Illiterate people cannot take advantage of it
- Expensive

Advertisements and Special Health Editions

These are printed from time to time and circulated to the health agencies. These can be spread through health bulletins to all the segments of the society.

Advantages

- Increase awareness
- Build goodwill
- Expand audience
- Educate audience
- Eliminates middlemen

Disadvantages

This can be an inappropriate medium for educational field.

Written Handouts

To provide written communication, the written material is circulated to the audience before taking lecture so that they can have some prior knowledge of the health topic. The written material should be clear, concise, relevant, specific, meaningful and readable. These are prepared by typing and then cyclostyling or photocopying the typed material.

Uses

- Provide additional reading material to the audience
- Bring key points in attention to participants during class

Advantages

- Participants can read before starting the lecture and can clarify their doubts.
- Enhance learning teaching activities

Disadvantages

- Expensive
- If not presented in attractive manner, students may not read it.

Three-dimensional Aids

Three-dimensional aids include the following:

Models

The models are an imitation or a copy of the real thing. These are actual representations of the real objects. The original size and shape of the actual thing can be enlarged or reduced according to the convenience of use.

Preparation

These are made from cheap and easily available material, clay, cardboard, paper, glass, sand, cutout pictures and pieces of wood can be used to prepare models.

Uses

- Models are used to explain the internal structures and functions of an object or system which is not possible with cross section.
- Minute parts of the system can be shown clearly.

Advantages

- Models can be used safely and conveniently.
- Adequate flexibility and freedom are there in the use of models.

- Models draw attention to the essentials.
- Students can be given assignments to make models of the primary health centers, sanitary wells, smokeless chulha, so that they can learn by doing.

Disadvantages

- Can easily break while handling or transporting if models are made from clay or mud.
- Can convey wrong ideas if the size of models is altered from the actual size.
- Cannot be transported from place to place.

Specimens and Objects

The real specimens and actual objects used in teaching learning activities are affective as they convey the actual appearance of an object or specimen to the senses of students. Without showing the actual specimens of certain organs like heart, liver, brain, kidney, eye, etc., the students doubts cannot be cleared.

Advantages

- Specimens and models are very effective aids in teaching.
- Students can have the correct knowledge of the structures and functions of specimens and models.

Disadvantages

- Specimens if not preserved properly can disintegrate
- Not easily available everywhere

Puppets

Health education can be imparted through puppets in rural areas. The plastic dolls are made of different characters of the play and tied with fine rope. Puppets are placed on the table and the ropes are with the artist behind the ropes screen. According to the play or story, the artist pulls the rope and makes them dance, sing, laugh or cry. The message conveyed through this play reaches, the audiences are touched, and their thinking process is stimulated to change their attitude toward their health needs.

Advantages

- Very effective means of communication in rural areas.
- Used in rural areas to attract the attention of people toward health.
- Illiterate people can understand the meaning.

Disadvantages

- Expensive
- Cannot be used frequently.

Projected Aids

Types of Projected Aids

The projected aids include the following types (Fig. 16.4):

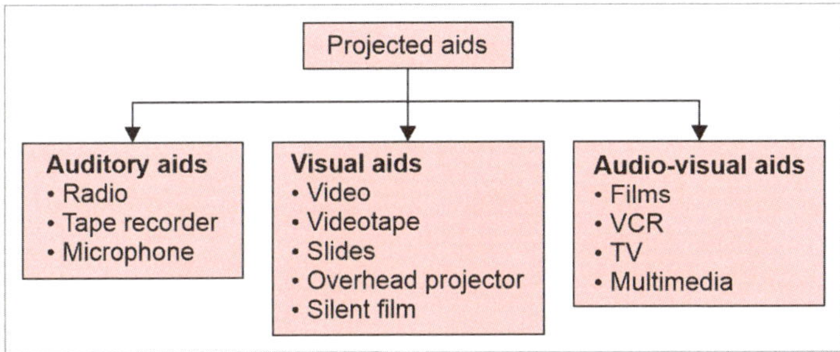

Fig. 16.4: Types of projected AV aids

Audio Aids

Auditory aids involve the sense of hearing and touch. Health education can be imparted to people by direct transmission or recorded versions of seminars, interviews, dramas and songs. These are also very useful media as there is the repetition of health messages, slogans and information, which people can hear while sitting or working at home through radio, tape recorder or microphones.

Advantages
- Useful for people with impaired vision
- Common and easily available in remote areas
- The recorded information on health can be used whenever required.

Disadvantage
Not useful for people with defective hearing. Unawareness regarding time of broadcasting.

Visual Aids

Projected visual aids include video, videotape, overhead projector, slide projector and silent films. These devices involve the sense of vision and touch in learning. These aids enhance the learning process.

Advantages
- Useful for people with hearing defects
- Enhance learning
- Useful for giving health education to illiterate people.

Disadvantage
- Expensive
- Cannot be used without electricity

Audio-visual or Combined Projected Aids

These projected AV aids are used to improve the quality of education. These make learning interesting as these involve auditory visual sensations. These are such as:
- Films
- VCR
- Television
- Multimedia

Advantages of Combined Projected Aids
- Excellent method to change people's attitude regarding health
- Suitable for all age groups
- Beneficial for auditory and visually handicapped

Disadvantages of Combined Projected Aids
- Expensive
- Require electricity to operate

HEALTH EDUCATION PLAN FOR A GROUP OF POSTNATAL MOTHERS

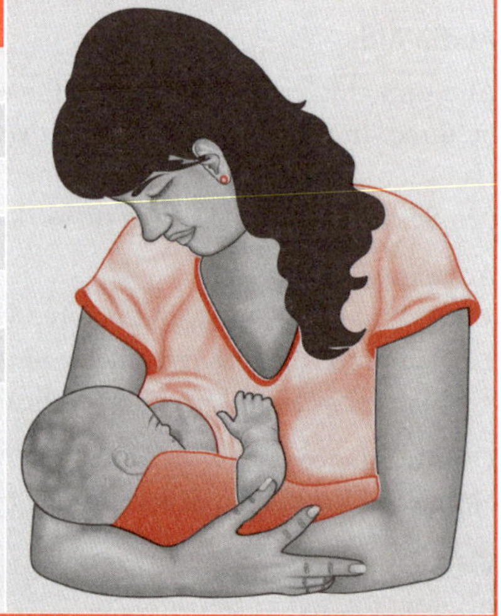

Name of the teacher:	
Subject :	Community health nursing
Topic :	Maternal and child healthcare
Subtopic :	Breastfeeding
Group :	Postnatal mothers
Date :	
Place :	Postnatal OPD at civil hospital
Time :	10 AM–10.30 AM

- **Previous knowledge of mothers:** Mothers have general information about breastfeeding through family members and exposure to mass media. A-V aids, charts and flash cards.
- **General objective:** After the health education session, the group will be able to gain knowledge regarding 'Breastfeeding' and its importance in the growth and development of baby, develop the right attitude regarding breastfeeding and will be able to adopt it in their lives.

Specific Objectives

- Define exclusive breastfeeding.
- Describe the techniques of breastfeeding.
- Explain the preparations for breastfeeding.
- Describe the instructions for breastfeeding.
- Discuss the advantages of exclusive breastfeeding.
- Enlist the facts regarding breastfeeding.
- Discuss the myths and misconceptions about breastfeeding.
- Explain difficulties in breastfeeding and their management.

The health education plan meant for health education is presented in Table 16.1.

TABLE 16.1: Health education plan for postnatal mothers

Time	Specific objectives	Content	AV Aids	Teacher learners' activity	Evaluation
1 minute	To introduce the topic	**Introduction:** When God created the human being, he also created a source of living. When a baby is born the best care provided to the baby is breastfeeding.			
1 minute	Define exclusive breastfeeding	Exclusive breastfeeding is giving nothing orally other than breast milk up to 6 months of age.	Chalkboard	Teacher defines the group with the help of chalkboard.	Define exclusive breastfeeding.
3 minutes	Describe techniques of breastfeeding.	**Techniques of breastfeeding:** • The mother and baby should be in a comfortable position. • **Feeding in sitting position (Fig. 16.5A):** The mother holds the baby in an inclined upright position on her lap, the baby's head on her forearm on the same side close to her breasts, the neck is slightly extended. • Good attachment means infant is wide open and chin touches the breast. • The mother should guide the nipple and areola into baby's mouth. For effective milk transfer is chest to chest contact between infant and mother. • The infant's hip, shoulder, and ear are in one line. Baby sucks the areola and nipple holding between tongue and palate. • **Feeding in lateral position (Fig. 16.5B)** following cesarean, delivery or with painful perineum is carried out by placing the baby along her side between the trunk and the arm.	**A** Fig. 16.5A: Feeding in sitting position **B** Fig. 16.5B: Feeding in lateral position	Teacher demonstrates breastfeeding position to the group.	What are the techniques of breastfeeding?

Contd...

Time	Specific objectives	Content	AV Aids	Teacher learners' activity	Evaluation
2 minutes	Explain the preparations for breastfeeding	**Preparations for breastfeeding are started from pregnancy:** Any abnormality in the nipple like cracked or depressed nipple (Figs 16.6 C to F) should be treated by massaging breast, and expression of colostrum and maintenance of cleanliness should be carried out during last 4 weeks of pregnancy.	**Figs 16.6C to F:** Types of nipples	Teacher explains the abnormalities of the nipple compared with normal nipple with the help of diagrams and the group listens and looks at the diagrams.	How will you prepare yourself for breastfeeding?
4 minutes	Describe the instructions for breastfeeding	**Instructions for breastfeeding:** • In the absence of anatomical and medical complications, a healthy baby is put to the breast 1/2–1 hour following normal delivery; following cesarean of 4–6 hours may be sufficient for the mother to start feeding her baby. • During the first 24 hours the mother should feed the baby at an interval of 2–3 hours. Gradually, regularity must be established at 3–4 hours' pattern by the end of the first week. Baby should be fed on demand. • **Demand feeding:** The baby should be put to the breast as soon as the baby becomes hungry. There is no restriction on feeds or the number of sucking times. • **Duration of feed:** The initial feeding should last for 5–10 minutes from each breast. Then, gradually the duration is increased according to the demand of baby.		Teacher describes the instructions for breastfeeding with the help of chalkboard.	What should be the frequency and duration of breastfeeding?

Contd...

Time	Specific objectives	Content	AV Aids	Teacher learners' activity	Evaluation
		• Baby should be fed from one breast completely so that the baby gets both the foremilk and the hindmilk. Hindmilk is richer in fat and supplies more calories to the infant. The next feed should start with the second breast. • It is important to have a drink (preferably water) at the mother's side while breastfeeding. Feeding is thirsty work at first, and water helps replenish fluids that the baby is taking from the mother. • To avoid sore nipples, feed your baby in different positions and alternate breast during feeding time. • Feeding the baby on demand helps to increase the mother's milk supply. • In case mother cannot breastfeed the baby directly, the newborn is hospitalized, unable to suck, the mother is very sick mother is working, she has to express her milk by using both hands. Gently squeeze milk from the breast as shown in Fig. 16.7G.	Fig. 16.7G: Self-expression of breast milk	Teacher explains to the group with the help of a chart how to express breast milk manually.	What are the problems with the nipple that causes difficulties in breastfeeding?
3 minutes	Discuss the advantages of breastfeeding.	**Advantages of breastfeeding:** There is no doubt that breast milk is the best milk for babies. It provides maximum emotional satisfaction to both the mother and child. **To child** • It is a wholesome food with protein, sugar, fat and vitamins that the baby needs. • It helps protect the baby against certain diseases and infections like diarrhea and allergies. • It is easier for babies to digest than buffalo or formula milk. Even premature babies digest it with ease.		The teacher discussed the advantages of breastfeeding.	Enlist the advantages of breastfeeding.

Contd...

Time	Specific objectives	Content	AV Aids	Teacher learners' activity	Evaluation
		To mother • Easy to feed, no extra labor required for cleaning bottles or preparing formula milk. • Breastfeeding makes the mother burn more calories and helps her get back to her prepregnancy weight more quickly. • Breastfeeding delays the return of the menstrual period, and so it is natural contraceptive method. • It reduces the risk of ovarian and breast cancer in women. • It is cost-effective, does not need to be prepared and is in ample supply. • As breast milk directly goes to baby's mouth, there is limited risk of infection.			
3 minutes	Enlist the facts about breastfeeding.	**Facts about breastfeeding:** • All mothers can successfully breastfeed their babies, which is the most natural way to feed babies. • Mother's milk is complete nutrition for the baby for the first 6 months and the child should be exclusively breastfed during this period of time. • No other milk, food, drink or even water is required up to 6 months. • Baby should be breastfed immediately after birth, preferably within half to one hour of birth, to give colostrum to the baby—the initial yellowish mother's milk during the first 2–3 days after birth. • Breastfeed the baby on demand without any restrictions. • No pacifiers should be given to the baby. • Mother can continue breastfeeding during sickness without any harm to the baby and herself.	 **Figs 16.4H and I:** **H.** Bottle feeding; **I.** Introducing solid food	Teacher listed the facts about breastfeeding.	Enlist the facts about breastfeeding.

Contd...

Time	Specific objectives	Content	AV Aids	Teacher learners' activity	Evaluation
		• Mother may continue breastfeeding for 2 years or beyond. • Bottle feeding (Fig. 16.8H) is not necessary and can even be harmful to your baby. It is the leading cause of loose stools in babies. • Solid foods (Fig. 16.8I) should be introduced only after 6 months of age. • Homemade, family food is better than commercial food for baby. • Commercially available powdered milk is always inferior to mother's milk.			
3 minutes	Discuss the myth and misconceptions about breastfeeding	**Myths about breastfeeding:** • **Mother has to drink a lot of milk to produce more milk:** This is not true. Any type of food and fluid taken by the mother is in adequate quantity and is sufficient to produce enough milk. The production and quality of breast milk are not dependent on the milk intake of the mother. The baby's sucking on the breast is the key factor and more sucking makes more milk. • **Small breasts will not produce enough milk:** Being able to breastfeed successfully does not depend on the size of the breast. The size of the breast depends on the amount of fatty tissue layer under the skin. • **Do not eat certain foods during breastfeeding:** No, the mother can continue eating all of her favorite foods during breastfeeding. If the mother is worried about a particular food, she should eat a small amount each time and see if it causes any problem to the baby. If it bothers the baby every time she eats it, she may consider avoiding that food. • **Failure to feed in the previous pregnancy confirms that the mother cannot feed in present pregnancy also:** The mother can be successful in breastfeeding the baby even if she was not able to breastfeed the previous baby. Confidence is important.		Teacher discussed the myths about breastfeeding and their management.	Enlist the myths and any misconceptions about breastfeeding.

Contd...

Time	Specific objectives	Content	AV Aids	Teacher learners' activity	Evaluation
5 minutes	Explain difficulties in breastfeeding and their management.	**Difficulties in breastfeeding and there failure due to mother:** • **Reluctance or not wanting to breastfeed:** Careful listening to the mother and skilful counseling can solve these problems. • **Infant's attachment to breast:** When poor, it leads to quick shallow sucks instead of slow and deep. Areola remains outside the lips. This causes nipple pain. **Management:** Skilled support from a healthcare provider can improve the technique of breastfeeding. Prelacteal feeds (honey, milk) inhibit the lactation process and should be avoided. • **Anxiety and stress:** Previous history of lactation failure or elderly primipara—the mother fails to relax during feeding and as such, the baby refuses to suck. **Management:** Reassurance and practical support are helpful. • **Difficulty with operative delivery:** Cesarean section following prolonged and exhaustive labor (so mother should be helped to feed the baby in a comfortable position as early as possible). • **Milk secretion is inadequate:** Unrestricted feeding, a well-positioned infant, practical and emotional support for the mother are all important.		The teacher explains to the group difficulties in breastfeeding and their management.	How will you overcome the difficulties in breastfeeding?

Contd...

Time	Specific objectives	Content	AV Aids	Teacher learners' activity	Evaluation
		• **Breast ailments:** Common problems related to breastfeeding include engorgement of the breast, (Fig. 16.9J) cracked nipples, depressed nipples and mastitis, which need treatment. Due to the infant's low birth weight baby—the baby is too small to suck. **Management:** ■ Hot fomentation (Fig. 16.1J) with the help of a towel can be applied on the breast to relieve engorgement. ■ Breastfeeding should be continued after engorgement is relieved. • **Sick baby:** Temporary illnesses such as respiratory tract infections, nasal obstruction, due to jaundice and oral thrush. All these conditions lead to imperfect sucking. Over distension of stomach with swallowed air. **Management** ■ Small frequent feeds, should be given. ■ Burping followed by each feed should be done. • **Congenital malformation in baby:** **Management** ■ Congenital malformation such as cleft palate needs surgical correction.	**Fig. 16.9J:** Mother relieving engorgement of breast by applying hot fomentation with the help of small towel		

Contd...

Time	Specific objectives	Content	AV Aids	Teacher learners' activity	Evaluation
2 minutes			**Conclusion:** Breast milk is the ideal food for the infant. No other food is required by the baby for 6 months duration. It is very essential to breastfeed every child. **Bibliography:** • Picciano M. "Nutrient composition of human milk". Pediatric Clin North Am 48 (1): 53–67. • Horton S, Sanghvi T, Phillips M. 1996. "Breastfeeding promotion and priority setting in health". Health Policy Plan 11 (2): 156–68. • Park K. Preventive and Social Medicine. 18th edition. Chapter 9 p 397. • Gulani K K. Principles and Practices of Community Health Nursing 1st ed 2007: Kumar Publishing House p 380.		

Summary

- Audio-visual aids are tools for imparting health education.
- The purposes of audio-visual aids are to enhance learning, initiate thinking and learning and keep the learner attentive.
- More than one sense is involved to make learning long-lasting.
- Audio-visual aids motivate learners to learn more.
- The types of audio-visual aids used are audio aids, visual aids and combined aids.
- The selection of audio-visual aids depends on the background of the audiences, age groups, level of previous knowledge, needs of the learner, their capacity to learn and the place where audio-visual aids are to be used.
- There are advantages and disadvantages of various audio-visual aids although electronic aids are very useful in conveying health messages.

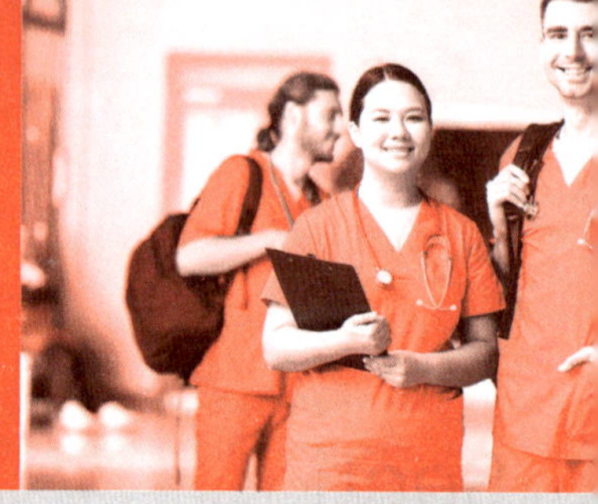

LONG ANSWER TYPE QUESTIONS

1. Explain the classification of audio-visual aids in detail.
2. Describe the guidelines for designing and using A-V aids.
3. State the criteria for the selection of A-V aids.

SHORT ANSWER TYPE QUESTIONS

1. Write short notes on:
   a. Three-dimension aids
   b. Projected aids
2. Define audio-visual aids

MULTIPLE CHOICE QUESTIONS

1. **The A-V aid which is not suitable to educate the visually handicapped group:**
   a. Audio-tape
   b. Radio
   c. Flip chart
   d. Microphone

2. **The most common A-V aid used for educating the general public is:**
   a. Radio
   b. Audio-tape
   c. CD system
   d. Tape recorder

3. **Which of the following is not an activity aid?**
   a. Role play
   b. Puppet show
   c. Field trip
   d. Graph

4. **The cheapest, oldest, easily available and commonly used A-V aid is:**
   a. LCD
   b. Bulletin board
   c. Tape recorder
   d. Blackboard

ANSWER KEY

1. c   **2.** a   **3.** d   **4.** d

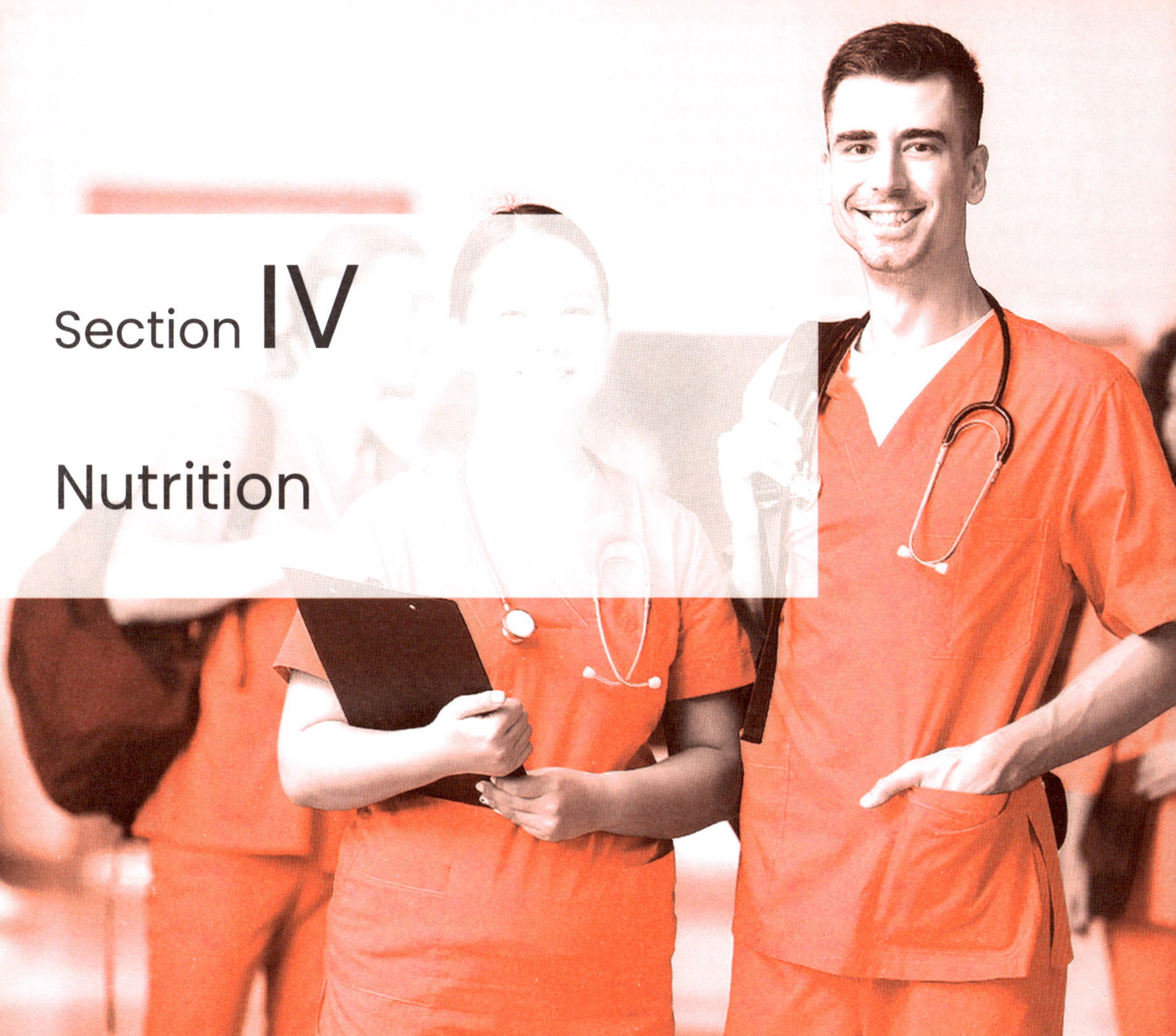

Section IV

Nutrition

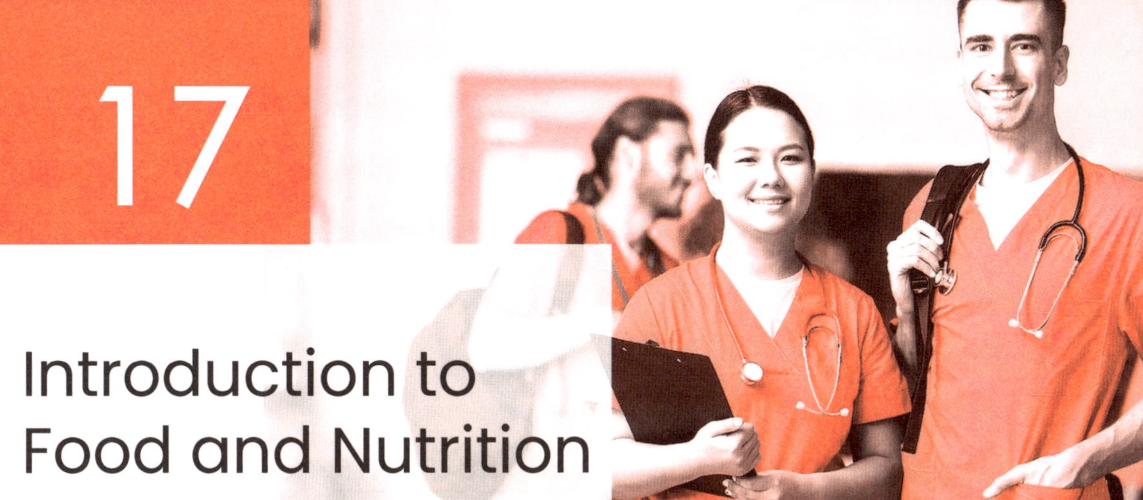

17

Introduction to Food and Nutrition

INTRODUCTION

Food and nutrition are the way that we get fuel, providing energy for our bodies. We need to replace nutrients in our bodies with a new supply every day. Food provides essential substances called nutrients. The body needs these nutrients to help it make energy; to grow, repair, and maintain its tissues; and to keep its different systems working smoothly. Nutrition is important for all organisms.

MEANINGS OF FOOD, NUTRITION AND NUTRIENTS

Food

Food is one of the basic requirements of our body. It is essential to sustain life. Our body requires food to provide energy, to carry out vital functions such as breathing, circulation, maintenance of body temperature and other body activities. Any substance used for energy, physical growth, development and repair in the body can be called food.

Definition

"Food contains substances which are digested, absorbed and transported to the different tissues and organs of the body for its growth, development, regulation and repair".

Functions of Food

- It provides energy to carry out various body activities.
- It is required for growth and development of body.
- It repairs tissues.
- It helps in maintenance and regulation of tissue functions.
- It produces enzymes and hormones to regulate body processes.

Nutrition

Nutrition is the science of food and its relationship to health. Physiology of consumption and utilization of food in our body is shown in Figure 17.1.

Definition

"Nutrition is defined as a dynamic process in which the food is ingested, digested, its nutrients are absorbed, transported and utilized by the body and their end products are disposed of".

Good health depends upon healthy eating. Our dietary habits are influenced by various factors such as religion, culture, economic state, age, climate, health and medicine.

Nutrition is the combination of processes by which all parts of body receive and utilize food.

Factors Affecting Nutrition

The factors affecting nutrition are as follows (Fig. 17.2):

- Age
- Economic status
- Religion
- Culture
- Climate
- Health
- Medicine

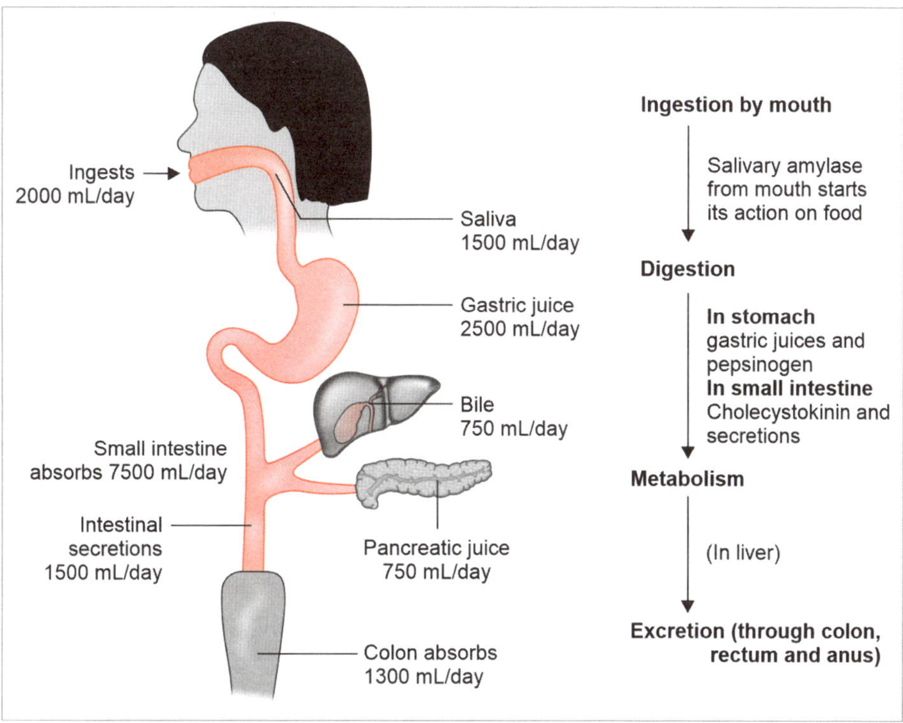

Fig. 17.1: Physiology of consumption and utilization of food in our body

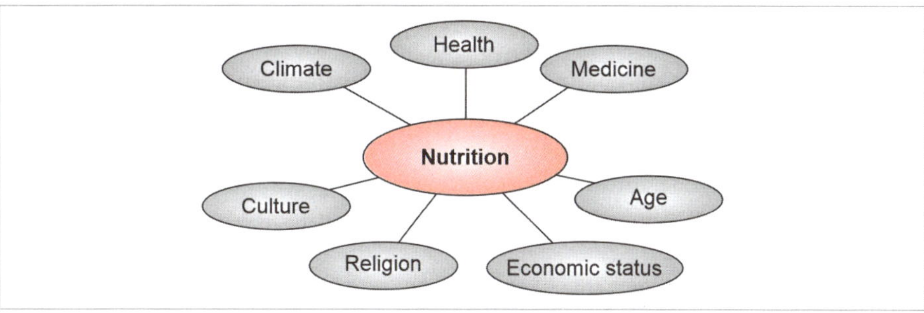

Fig. 17.2: Factors influencing nutrition

Nutrients

Nutrients are the organic and inorganic complexes contained in the food we eat daily. These include carbohydrates, proteins, fats, vitamins, minerals, and water. There are about 50 nutrients which are supplied through the food. Each nutrient has specific function in the body.

Classification of Nutrients

The nutrients required by human body are divided into two groups (Fig. 17.3):

1. **Macronutrients:** They form the major bulk of our food. Proteins, fats, carbohydrates, and water are the macronutrients. They are easily perceived by the naked eyes.

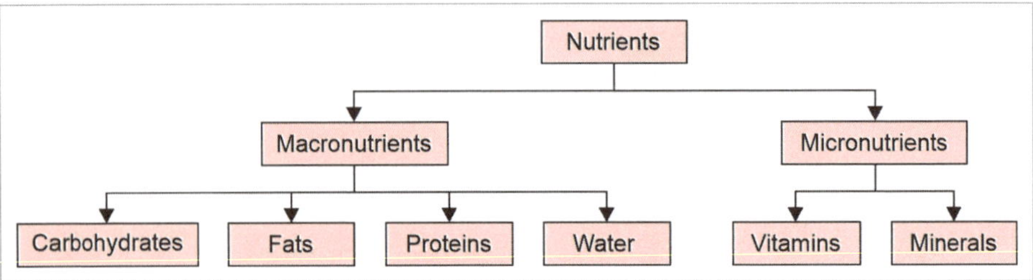

Fig. 17.3: Types of nutrients

They supply total energy to the body in the following proportion:

Carbohydrates : 60–80%

Proteins   : 20–30%

Fat   : 10–15%

2. **Micronutrients:** These are required in small quantities but essential for the body. Vitamins and minerals are the micronutrients. They do not supply energy. These are not seen with naked eyes. They play an important role in the regulation of metabolic activities and help in utilization of macronutrients.

FOOD HABITS AND CUSTOMS

We eat food according to our habits and customs. Some customs and habits have good nutritional importance. But the customs, habits and beliefs vary in different parts of the country. Some of the food habits and customs are listed as follows:

* **Cultural factors:** Different cultures have different food habits and food patterns. Food cultures for various cultural groups have been practiced for centuries. With the passage of time, various changes have taken place in culture. Culture is passed from one generation to another. For example, Gujarati uses sugar in all vegetables and pulses (dals) making its taste sweet whereas most of other southern states use plenty of tomatoes, tamarind and pepper in making curries.

* **Availability of food:** Depending upon the climate, temperature and humidity, all food items are not available in certain regions and states people get accustomed to the locally available food which is their staple food.

* **Lifestyle:** It plays an important role in shaping the food habits. A heavy worker, for example, a farmer, gardener or a player, eat heavy meals as their energy requirement demands it. On the other hand, an office worker is sedentary worker and takes light food as their activities are light and caloric requirement is less as compared to the heavy workers. So, the food patterns become according to the energy requirement.

* **Economic factors:** The menu planning of the family depends upon the financial status and capacity to spend on food. The lower income group purchases cheaper foods for their nutritional requirement. On the other hand, the high-income group selects variety of foods from all food groups. Accordingly, the selection of food items according to the financial status becomes their food habits.

* **Food fads:** Personal likes and dislikes play an important role in selection of foods. These likes and dislikes are known as **food fads**. The food fads may result in nutritional deficiencies. For

example, some people prefer only vegetables and they do not like pulses. This may result in protein deficiency diseases.

- **Nutritional education:** People with some knowledge of nutrition select foods according to the requirement of a balanced-diet even if they are from low-income group. They select cheaper foods but having nutritional importance, on the other hand, the high-income group not having nutritional knowledge may spend lot of money on the food items which carries little nutritional importance.

- **Cooking practices:** Peeling the vegetables and washing it after cutting, draining away the water from rice after cooking and prolonged boiling of food while cooking influence the nutritional values.

- **Religious factors:** Religion plays a great role in food habits of people. Muslims do not eat pork. A large section of Hindus do not eat beef. Fasting is common in almost all religion due to some or the other festival. Jains and Brahma Kumaris do not eat onion and garlic.

- **Traditional factors:** Traditional beliefs and customs also have a great role in food habits. There is a concept of hot and cold foods. Foods like nuts, jaggery, meat, fish and eggs are considered to generate heat in the body, are known as hot foods. People avoid consuming these foods in summer season. These foods are also avoided for the growing girls before puberty as there is a belief that girls will mature at early age. Some foods such as curd, banana, orange and lemon are considered cold foods. People avoid these foods in winter season. This concept of hot and cold foods leads to malnutrition. Papaya is avoided during pregnancy in some societies as it is believed to cause abortion. In male dominating families, male eats first and women eat last and poorly. In some societies, colostrum is not given to the newborn early because they believe that it is hard and not digested easily.

FACTORS AFFECTING NUTRITION

Good health depends upon healthy eating. Our dietary habits, influenced by various factors which are as follows (Fig. 17.4):

- **Age:** The requirement of food varies with age. The calorie intake increases with growing age. The teenagers from 16 to 20 years require 3500 kcal as this is the period of maximum growth. With the advancing age, when the physical activities are decreased, the basic metabolic rate falls and calorie requirement decreases.

- **Sex:** The calorie requirement for female is 20% less than the male of the same age.

- **Body size and weight:** Big body size having larger surface area and weight requires more calories.

- **Physical activity:** Calorie requirement increases with the type of physical activities, so food requirement also increases.

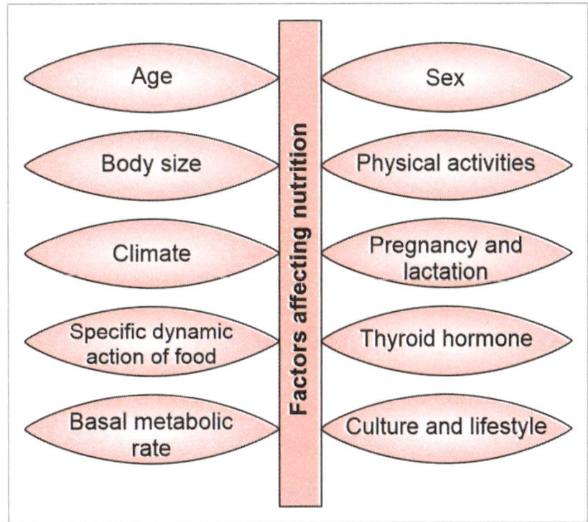

Fig. 17.4: Factors affecting nutrition

- **Climate:** In cold climate, the requirement of calories increases by 3% as more heat is required to protect the body from cold.
- **Pregnancy and lactation:** During pregnancy, the calorie requirement increases by 10% for the growing fetus, placenta and the increased basal metabolic rate. Similarly, during lactation, the calorie requirement increases 20% for the production of milk.
- **Specific dynamic action of food:** After consumption of protein foods, the more heat is produced by the body due to anabolism process.
- **Thyroid hormone:** It stimulates the metabolism process so more heat is produced as the oxygen consumption increases and BMR also increases.
- **Basal metabolic rate:** The catecholamines increase the BMR in the presence of thyroxine (T_4) and calorie requirement increases.
- **Cultural factors:** Lifestyle and food habits, affect the food and nutrition status of the people. People prefer food according to their culture, lifestyle and food habits.

CHANGING CONCEPT IN FOOD AND NUTRITION

Adequate food of good quality, i.e., having all essential nutrients, has been recognized for good health and in sickness through centuries. The science of nutrition had limited importance till the beginning of 19th century. Carbohydrates, proteins and fats had been recognized as energy producing foods.

But in the middle of the nineteenth century, the discovery of vitamins, minerals and dietary fibers, discovered that maintaining a good nutritional status is essential for proper growth and development. The nutritional science has drawn the attention of the scientist. The specific nutritional deficiency diseases were identified such as protein-energy malnutrition, nutritional anemia, blindness and endemic goiter and the means to control these diseases have been identified. The noncommunicable diseases have association with nutrition such as coronary heart disease, diabetes mellitus, cancer, hypertension, anemia.

The importance of therapeutic diet in communicable and noncommunicable diseases has engaged scientific attention. Nutrition is the corner stone of socioeconomic development. The health sector only is not responsible for nutritional problems but also these are multifactorial with its roots in other sectors of development. The intersectoral and integrated approach of development is required to tackle the present nutritional problems. Epidemiological methods are used for planning and evaluation of several nutritional programs. In the global campaigns of "Health For All", "promotion of proper nutrition", is also placed on integration of nutrition into primary health care system. Some Millennium Development Goals are directly related to nutrition. Some national and international agencies are also engaged in nutritional education and programs.

RELATION OF NUTRITION TO HEALTH

Nutrition affects human health from birth to death. Good nutrition is a basic component of human health. In developing countries like India, a fair section of population due to poverty, does not get enough food to eat. So nutritional deficiency diseases in infants and preschool children are common. Studies have revealed that extra cereals, green leafy vegetables and fortified with essential vitamins and mineral have helped to overcome malnutrition. The relation of nutrition to health is clear from the following points:

- **Growth and development:** Good nutrition maintains fetal growth and development during pregnancy, during infancy and childhood. Adequate nutrition is also needed during adult life for optimum health. In elderly people, special nutrition is required to meet their physiological and chronological changes. Pregnant and lactating mothers need more calories and protein to prevent abortion, growth retardation and low birth weight babies.
- **Specific deficiency diseases:** Malnutrition, blindness, goiter, anemia, beriberi and rickets are due to nutritional deficiencies. These are prevented and treated with diet therapy.
- **Resistance to infections:** Diet rich in protein, minerals and vitamin builds up body resistance to various infection.
- **Mortality and morbidity:** Poor nutrition lowers the expectancy of life due to ill health and infections. Prematurity and malnutrition are the main causes of infant mortality, overnutrition is responsible for obesity, diabetes, hypertension, cardiovascular, renal diseases, liver diseases and gallbladder diseases. Even the deficiency of trace elements such as zinc is considered to be the possible cause of growth retardation.

To minimize nutritional deficiency diseases, Government of India has launched several nutritional programs, e.g., Mid-Day School Meal, Integrated Child Development Scheme, Anemia Control Program and Iodine Deficiency Disease Control Program, Vitamin A Deficiency Disease Control Program.

Summary

- Food contains substances which are ingested, digested, absorbed and transported to different tissue and organs of the body for growth, development, regulation and repair.
- Food is basic necessity to sustain life.
- Food habits are determined by various cultural factors such as lifestyle, food fads, cooking practices, child-rearing practices and eating left over food by the women at last.
- Religions based food habits include vegetarian foods consumed by Hindus and nonvegetarian by Muslims and Christians.
- The factors affecting nutrition are age, sex, body, size, weight, physical activity, climate, pregnancy, thyroid hormones, specific dynamic action of food. Basal metabolic rate, culture and lifestyle.
- New concept in nutrition such as nutrition assessment, dietary survey, growth monitoring, nutritional indicators and nutritional intervention has been developed.
- A broad intersectoral and integrated approach is needed to tackle the present nutritional problems.
- The relation of nutrition to health may be viewed from its role in growth and development, specific deficiency diseases and its relation of infant's mortality due to malnutrition.
- The various diseases like obesity, cardiovascular disease and hypertension are due to malnutrition.

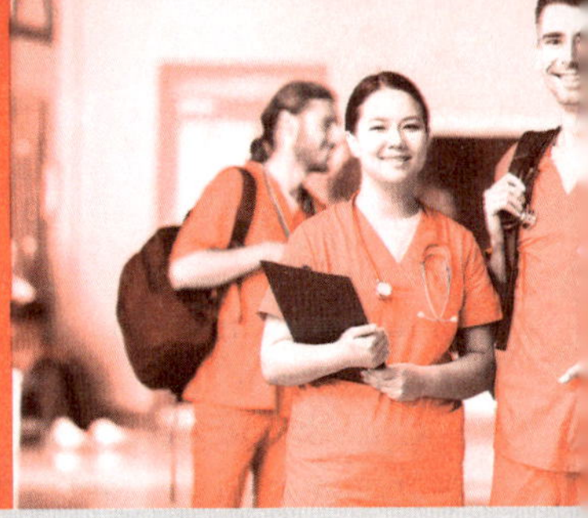

LONG ANSWER TYPE QUESTIONS

1. Describe the various factors affecting food habits and nutrition of people.
2. Explain the relationship between nutrition and health.

SHORT ANSWER TYPE QUESTIONS

1. Enlist macronutrients and micronutrients.
2. Define the following:
   a. Health
   b. Food
   c. Nutrition
   d. Malnutrition

MULTIPLE CHOICE QUESTIONS

1. **Nutrition is defined as:**
   a. Science of food
   b. Relation of food to health
   c. Role of nutrition in growth, development and maintenance of body
   d. All of the above

2. **Which of the following factors determine the food habits of society?**
   a. Religious factors
   b. Cultural factors
   c. Customs and traditions
   d. All of these

3. **Which one of the following does not fall into the group of macronutrients?**
   a. Carbohydrates
   b. Vitamins
   c. Proteins
   d. Fats

4. **Which of the following is incorrect?**
   a. The first breast milk should not be given to newborn
   b. Hot foods like egg, fish, and meat should not be given to children
   c. Papaya causes abortion
   d. All of the above

5. **Which of the following is not a macronutrient?**
   a. Proteins
   b. Minerals
   c. Fats
   d. Carbohydrates

ANSWER KEY

1. d   **2.** d   **3.** b   **4.** d   **5.** b

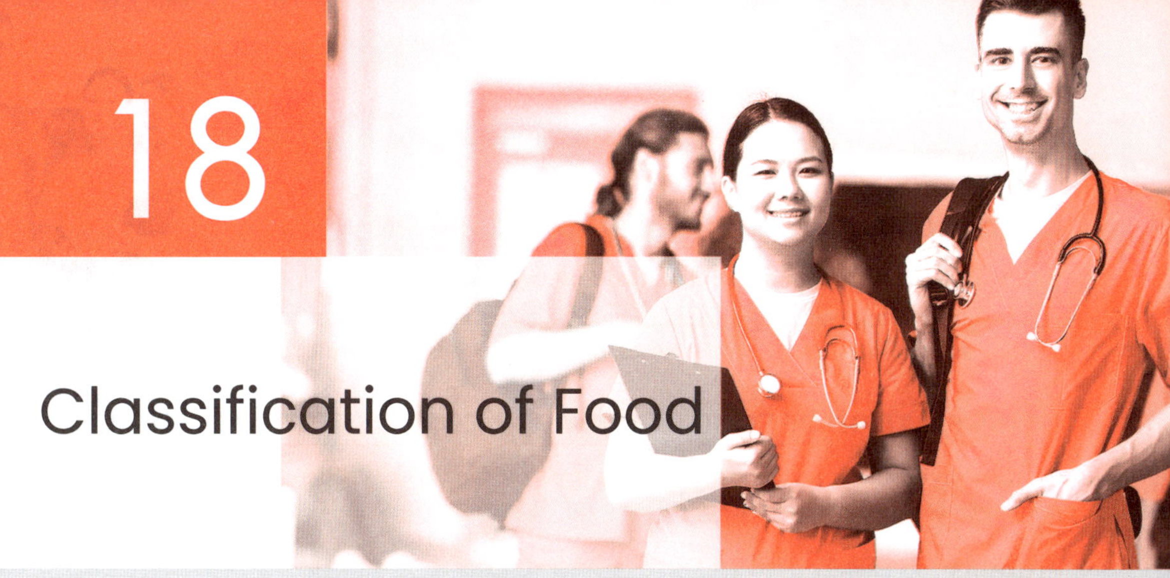

LEARNING OBJECTIVES

After the completion of the unit, the readers will be able to:
- Classify food by origin, chemical composition, functions and nutritive values.
- Describe the functions of proteins, fats, carbohydrates, minerals and vitamins.
- Classify the nutritive values of different types of nutrients.

UNIT OUTLINE

- Introduction
- Classification of Food Based on its Origin
- Classification of Food by Chemical Composition and Sources
- Classification of Food by Predominant Function
- Classification by Nutritive Values

KEY TERMS

Carbohydrates: A group of organic compounds occurring in living tissues and foods in the form of starch, cellulose, and sugars.

Lipid: Organic compounds that contain fatty acids, sterol or isoprenoid compound.

Peptides: Two or more amino acids linked by peptide bonds.

Proteins: Organic molecules that are present in living organisms. They serve a wide range of functions including organization, transportation, and defense. These are compounds of amino acids. Amino acids consist of carbon, hydrogen, oxygen, nitrogen, sulfur and phosphorous.

Vitamins: Organic compounds that are required in small quantities in diet and are essential to an organism for proper metabolic function.

INTRODUCTION

The classification of food refers to the categorization of food items or products into different groups or categories based on various criteria. Food can be classified in accordance to their origin, to their chemical composition and sources. There are >40 different kinds of nutrients in food and they can generally be classified into different groups.

CLASSIFICATION OF FOOD BASED ON ITS ORIGIN

On the basis of origin, foods are classified into two main groups:
1. **Foods of animal origin:** Meat, fish, eggs, milk, and milk products.
2. **Foods of plant origin:** Cereals, pulses, millets, oil, seeds, nuts, fruits, and vegetables.

CLASSIFICATION OF FOOD BY CHEMICAL COMPOSITION AND SOURCES

On the basis of chemical composition and sources, the food is classified as proteins, carbohydrates, fats minerals, vitamins, and water.

Proteins

Proteins are made of simpler chemical substances known as amino acids. The amino acid content of protein differs from one protein to another. The amino acids consist of carbon, hydrogen, nitrogen, oxygen, sulfur and phosphorous.

Body requires 20 amino acids. Out of which, nine are essential amino acids and the remaining are nonessential (Fig. 18.1).

- **Essential amino acids:** These are called essential amino acids as these are not synthesized by the body and have to be supplied in diet. These are given in Figure 18.1.
- **Nonessential amino acids:** Body can synthesize these amino acids in sufficient quantities and hence, called nonessential amino acids. These are required for proper growth. These are mentioned in Figure 18.1.

Essential amino acids	Nonessential amino acids
• Leucine	• Arginine
• Isoleucine	• Tyrosine
• Lysine	• Cysteine
• Histidine	• Serine
• Methionine	• Glutamic acid
• Phenylalanine	• Aspartic acid
• Threonine	• Proline
• Valine	• Glycine
• Tryptophan	• Alanine
	• Hydroxyproline

Fig. 18.1: Types of amino acids

Classification

Protein can be classified as:
- **First class proteins:** Proteins containing all essential amino acids are called first class proteins, e.g., meat, fish, pork, chicken, liver, soybean, and milk.
- **Second class proteins:** Proteins which are not having all the essential amino acids are called second class protein, e.g., pulses, cereals, and oil seeds.

Types

The proteins are of the following types (Fig. 18.2):
- Simple proteins
- Conjugated proteins
- Derived proteins

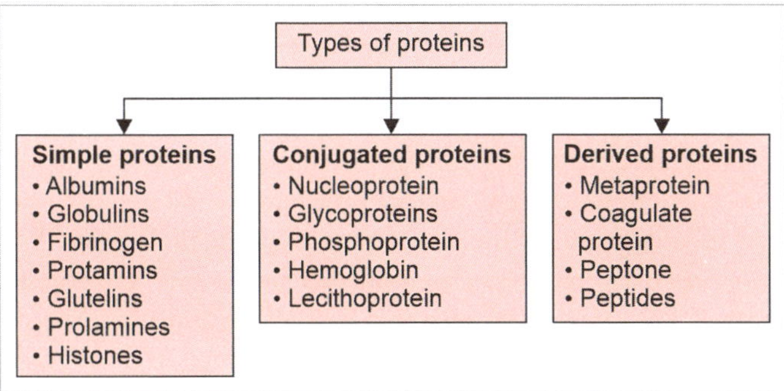

Fig. 18.2: Types of proteins

Sources

Proteins are derived from two types of foods:

1. **Animal sources:** Proteins derived from animal sources contain all essential amino acids and hence, known as first class proteins. These include meat, chicken, fish, pork, egg, and milk.
2. **Plant sources:** These proteins lack one or more essential amino acids and called second class proteins. Cereals, pulses, and oil seeds come under this category. Soybean, though, it is from plant sources but it is first class protein.

MUST KNOW

Daily nutritional requirement of proteins
Indian Council of Medical Research (ICMR) has recommended 1 g of protein/kg body weight for adult male and female.

For infants and growing children—1.5–2 g/kg body weight.

The requirement increases during pregnancy and lactation, i.e., 1.5–2 g/kg body weight. 1 g of protein provides 4 kcal of energy. About 20–30% of the total requirement of calories for the body comes from protein.

Functions

- Necessary for the growth and development of the body.
- Required for maintenance and repair of tissues.
- Provide amino acids for the synthesis of enzymes, hormones, antibodies and blood protein.
- Maintain osmotic pressure.
- Required for the growth of fetus during pregnancy and lactation after delivery.

Carbohydrates

Carbohydrates are composed of carbon, oxygen, and hydrogen. They are found in vegetable kingdom. They are synthesized from carbon dioxide present in the atmosphere in the presence of sunlight. Carbohydrates are the major source of energy in our diets. About 60–70% calories are from carbohydrates of our daily requirement 1 g of carbohydrate provides 4 kcal.

Classification

- **Monosaccharides:** These are the simplest form of carbohydrates. They contain single saccharide/ group, a single sugar molecule, e.g., glucose, galactose, and fructose.
- **Disaccharides:** These types of carbohydrates are composed of two units of monosaccharides, e.g., sucrose (cane sugar or beet sugar), lactose (milk sugar) and maltose (malt sugar).
- **Polysaccharides:** It contains many units of monosaccharide molecules. These polysaccharides first broken down into disaccharides, then monosaccharide and then digested and absorbed in the alimentary tract, e.g., starch, glycogen and cellulose and pectin. The cellulose and pectin cannot be digested by the enzyme in human body. They simply form roughage in the diet.

Sources

- **Starches:** They are present in abundance in cereals, millets, roots, fibers and fruits. Starches are found in wheat, rice, pulses, coarse, grains.
- **Sugars:** Glucose, fructose, and galactose.
- **Cellulose:** This is indigestible part of diet having no nutritional value but contains dietary fibers helps in defecation and prevents constipation. It is found in green leafy vegetables, fruits, and cereals.

> **MUST KNOW**
>
> **Daily nutritional requirement of carbohydrates**
> Carbohydrates form the main bulk of our diet. About 60–70% of calories of our daily requirement are derived from carbohydrates.

Functions

Functions of carbohydrates are as follows:
- Main source of energy for various physiological processes.
- They spare the valuable proteins.
- Necessary for oxidation of fats.
- Provide carbon structure for synthesis of nonessential amino-acids.
- They are stored in various tissues where they can be utilized whenever necessary.
- Make diet tasty and palatable.

Fats

Fats are the compounds of carbon, oxygen and hydrogen. They are the concentrated source of energy. 1 g of fat yields 9 kcal of energy. Fats are insoluble in water but soluble in biological solvents some fats are liquid at 20°C are called oils, e.g., groundnut oil. Some fats are solid at ordinary temperature, e.g., ghee, butter.

Classification

- 1st classification (Fig. 18.3)
    - Simple lipids—fats and oils
    - Compound lipids—phospholipids
    - Derived lipids—cholesterol
- 2nd classification (Fig. 18.4)
    - Saturated fats
    - Unsaturated fats

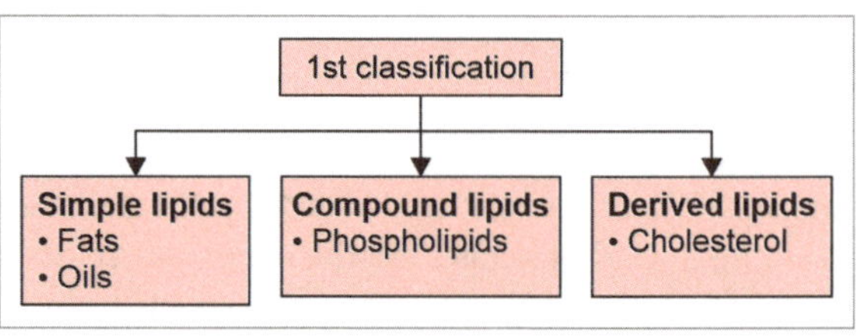

Fig. 18.3: 1st classification of fats

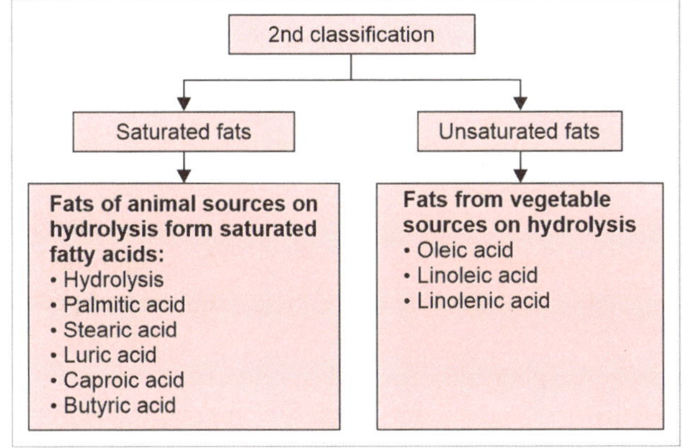

Fig. 18.4: 2nd classification of fats

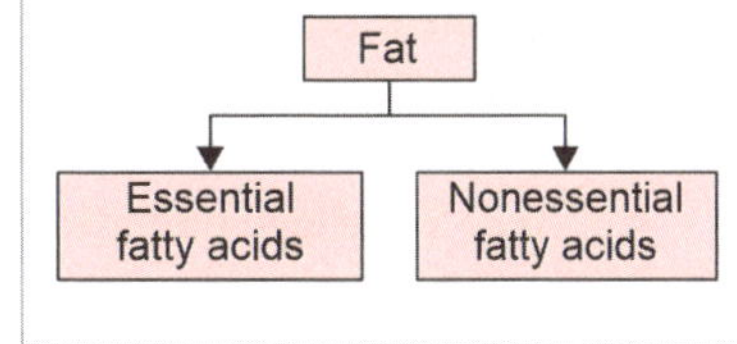

Fig. 18.5: 3rd classification of fats

- 3rd classification (Fig. 18.5)
  - **Essential fatty acids:** These are not synthesized in the body but obtained through diet, e.g., linoleic acid is one of the essential fatty acids obtained from vegetable oils.
  - **Nonessential fatty acids**: These fatty acids are synthesized in the human body. Examples are stearic acid, palmitic acid and arachidic acid, etc.

Sources

- **Animal sources:** Ghee, meat, fish, butter, eggs, fish, oil, etc.
- **Vegetable sources:** Groundnut, mustard, sesame, coconut, til, flax seeds, and dry fruits. Indirect sources are cereals, pulses and some vegetable.

> **MUST KNOW**
>
> **Daily nutritional requirement of fats**
> According to World Health Organization (WHO), daily allowance of fats should be restricted to 20–30% of total caloric requirement.

Functions

- Fats are concentrated source of energy.
- Essential for absorption of vitamin A, D, E and K.
- Fats under the skin help in maintaining body temperature.
- Fats in adipose tissue provide support to internal organs like heart, kidney and intestines, etc.
- Essential for the digestion of galactose.
- Essential fatty acids keep the tissue healthy.
- Some fats are essential components of nervous tissue, e.g., sphingomyelins, cell membrane, glycolipids.
- Essential fatty acids act as precursor of prostaglandins and are important in maintaining tissue in normal health.
- Make the food tasty and increase the palatability of food.
- Fats have satiety value of food.

Minerals

Minerals are the chemical elements which are required for growth, development and repair of tissues and conduction of various biological processes. There are about 50 minerals which the body receives through diet. Minerals do not yield energy but required for vital body functions.

Classification

- **1st classification** based on the nature of the minerals:
  - **Alkali forming elements:** They include calcium, magnesium, potassium, sodium, iron, and manganese.
  - **Acid forming elements:** They include phosphorus, sulfur, and chlorine, etc.
- **2nd classification:** It is based on the requirement and quantity of these elements present in the body and major elements are divided into two groups:
  1. **Major elements:** Calcium, phosphorus sodium, chlorine, sulfur, and magnesium, etc.
  2. **Trace elements:** They are required in minute quantities but are very essential for the body, e.g., iron, iodine, fluorine, cobalt, zinc, copper, manganese, etc.

Vitamins

Vitamins are the organic compounds fall in the category of micronutrients. They do not yield energy but act as a catalyst in many physiological reactions. They are essential for maintenance of health and development of human body. Body is unable to synthesize in sufficient quantity but must be provided by the food. A well-balanced diet usually fulfills the requirement.

Classification

- **Fat-soluble vitamins**
  - Vitamin A and carotene (Provitamin A)
  - Vitamin D
  - Vitamin E
  - Vitamin K
- **Water-soluble vitamins**
  - Vitamin B group B1 (Thiamine), B2 (Riboflavin), B6 (pyridoxine), B12 (cyanocobalamin), nicotinic acid, folic acid, biotin.
  - Vitamin C (ascorbic acid)
  - Vitamin P (bioflavonoids)

Water

Water is a liquid compound of hydrogen and oxygen. Two third of our bodies are made of water. In the body, water is divided among intracellular fluid, interstitial fluid and blood. We get water by drinking and also from many food items which contain water. Loss of water from the body takes place from kidney, skin, lungs, and intestines.

Functions

- Water maintains fluid and electrolyte balance in the body.
- Water plays an important role in maintaining body temperature.
- All the chemical processes in the body takes place in the presence of water.

- Water is necessary for digestion, absorption and metabolism of food.
- Water provides moisture in the body which is necessary for various cellular functions of the body.
- Water helps in blood circulation.
- Water is a component of blood, lymph, and cerebrospinal fluid.
- Water transports many nutrients and water-soluble vitamins, e.g., vitamin B complex and vitamin C to the target organs and tissues.
- Water leads to cooling, satisfaction and quenching thirst.
- Water breaks up indigestible parts of food and helps in their excretions. It is a major component of blood, urine, and stool.

CLASSIFICATION OF FOOD BY PREDOMINANT FUNCTION

- **Body building foods:** The foods which are responsible for growth and repair of body tissues are called body building foods. The foods which are rich in protein come under this group. This includes meat, fish, eggs, milk and milk products, pulses, nuts and oil seeds, and soybean.
- **Energy giving foods:** The foods which are consumed to provide energy are called energy giving foods. They include carbohydrates and fats. As the greater proportion of energy for daily requirement for the body comes from energy giving foods. This group includes cereals, wheat, rice, tubers, roots, sugars, jaggery, dry fruits, oils, and fats.
- **Protective foods:** The foods which are responsible for maintaining health and providing resistance against diseases are called protective foods. They include proteins, vitamins, and minerals. All fresh fruits and yellow and green leafy vegetables are rich in minerals and vitamins. Foods rich in proteins are milk, meat, eggs, fish, pulses, and nuts.

Minerals

The important minerals required for the body are calcium, phosphorus, sodium, potassium, chlorine, sulfur and magnesium are the major minerals.

Calcium

Calcium constitutes 2% of the total body weight 99% of this is present in the bones.

Sources

- Milk and milk products
- Green leafy vegetables, pumpkin
- Meat, fish and eggs
- Oil seeds, ragi, til, flax seeds, dry fruits, and cereals.

> **MUST KNOW**
>
> **Daily nutritional requirement of calcium**
> - Children and adults 400–500 mg/day
> - During pregnancy and lactation 1000 mg/day
> - Normal value of calcium in blood is 8.5 mg/deciliter

Functions

- Maintains the permeability of capillary walls
- Required for the formation and maintenance of bones and teeth
- Helps in coagulation of blood
- Essential for the contraction and relaxation of muscles

- Maintains balance between nerve center and nerves
- Activates number of enzymes such as pancreatic juice

Deficiency Diseases

- Deficiency causes rickets in children and osteomalacia in adults
- Delayed coagulation of blood
- Tetany
- Hyperparathyroidism
- Weakness of bones and teeth

Phosphorus

An adult body contains 500–800 g of organic phosphorus as phosphates. It constitutes 10% of the body weight. 80–85% of it is present in the skeleton and remaining in the intracellular compartment. The inorganic phosphorus is present as calcium phosphate in bones and teeth, as sodium and potassium phosphates in body fluids and soft tissues.

Sources

Meat, milk, egg, fish, vegetables, pulses, cereals, oil seeds, and coconut.

Functions

- Helps in formation of bones and teeth along with calcium and magnesium.
- Constituent of DNA, RNA and nucleic acid.
- Helps in the production of phospholipids necessary in the metabolism of fats, proteins and carbohydrates.
- Phospholipids are the constituents of cell membranes and regulate the transport of solutes into and out of the cells.
- Inorganic phosphates in the body fluids constitute an important buffer system maintaining the body neutrality.

> **MUST KNOW**
>
> **Daily nutritional requirement of phosphorus**
> The Food and Nutrition Board has suggested the same requirement of phosphorus as that of calcium:
> - Adults and children—400 mg/day
> - Pregnancy and lactation—1000 mg/day
> - Infants—750 mg/day
> - The normal diet meets this requirement

Deficiency Diseases

Phosphate deficiency is rare which are as follows:
- **Hypophosphatemia:** It may occur in gastrointestinal disorders such as sprue, celiac disease. It can also occur in starvation and due to vitamin D deficiency.
- **Hyperphosphatemia:** It is caused due to hypothyroidism.

Sodium Chloride

Sodium chloride is a table salt which is daily ingredient of our diet. It is found in all body fluids.

Sources

Milk, egg, meat, poultry, green leafy vegetables, beetroot, nuts, and raisins.

> **MUST KNOW**
>
> **Daily nutritional requirement of sodium chloride**
> 5–10 g/day depending upon the diet

Functions

- Regulates the acid base balance in the body.
- Maintains fluid balance and osmotic pressure between intracellular and extracellular compartment.
- Helps in muscle contraction.
- Maintains normal irritability of nerves.
- Plays a role in originating and maintaining heartbeat.

Deficiency Diseases

It can occur in cases of severe dehydration due to diarrhea, vomiting and heat strokes resulting in weakness and muscle cramps.

Potassium

The adult human body contains about 250 g potassium. Major portion is present in the cells.

Sources

Cereals, green leafy vegetables, Bengal gram, pear, cauliflower, carrot, spinach, onion, coriander, radish, sweet potatoes, raisin, almond, groundnut, apples, sweet lime and banana.

Functions

- Regulates acid-base balance
- Regulates osmotic pressure of cells
- Relaxes cardiac muscles.

MUST KNOW

Daily nutritional requirement of phosphorus
Requirement is met through ordinary diet.

Deficiency Diseases

It can occur in severe malnutrition, chronic alcoholism and surgery and in patients who are on diuretics.

Magnesium

Magnesium is also an important constituent of bones and is present in all body cells but in much smaller quantities. An adult human body contains 25 g of magnesium.

Sources

Cereals, maize, bajra, green gram, almond, groundnut, milk, green leafy vegetables, fruits eggs, meat, and fish.

MUST KNOW

Daily nutritional requirement of magnesium
200–300 mg/day for adults, children below 5 years of age 150 mg/day. Infants 50–70 mg/day.

Functions

- Necessary for the metabolism of calcium and phosphorus
- Activates many enzymes
- Involved in protein synthesis
- Regulates the nerve impulses and muscle contractions and relaxation along with calcium, sodium, and potassium
- Essential for skeletal structure.

Deficiency Diseases

- **Osteoporosis:** Magnesium is essential for bone health, and about 60% of the body's magnesium is stored in the bones.

- **Cardiovascular disease:** Magnesium deficiency can affect the electrical activity of the heart and vascular tone, increasing the risk of cardiac arrhythmias.
- **Type 2 diabetes:** Low magnesium intake can increase the risk of developing type 2 diabetes.
- **Hypertension:** Low magnesium levels have been associated with hypertension.
- **Alzheimer's dis ease:** Low magnesium levels have been associated with Alzheimer's disease.
- **Migraine headaches:** Low magnesium levels have been associated with migraine headaches.
- **Stroke:** Low magnesium levels have been associated with cerebrovascular accident (stroke)

Iron

Iron plays an important role in our body as it is a component of hemoglobin. Each gram of hemoglobin contains 3.34 mg of iron. It transports oxygen to the body tissues and cells.

Sources

Green leafy vegetables, beans, cereals, banana, guava, mango, some spices, e.g., jeera, meat, fish, egg, etc.

Functions

- Transports oxygen to all body cells and tissue
- It is an essential part of several oxidative enzymes
- Necessary for the formation of hemoglobin, brain development, regulation of body temperature and muscle activity
- It facilitates complete oxidation of carbohydrate and fats within the cell and releases energy for physical work.

MUST KNOW

Daily nutritional requirement of iron
1–12 years children	: 15–20 mg/kg
13–18 years female	: 35 mg/kg
Average adult	: 25 mg/kg
Pregnancy	: 40 mg/kg
Lactation	: 30 mg/kg

Deficiency Diseases

Iron deficiency anemia is a blood condition that occurs when the body does not have enough iron to produce healthy red blood cells. It is the most common type of anemia worldwide.

Zinc

Zinc is a component of many enzymes. Small quantity is present in body tissues, while higher amount is present in bones. An adult body contains 1.4–2.3 g of zinc.

Sources

Present in vegetables as well as in animal sources of food.

Functions

- Essential for the synthesis of insulin
- Constituent of many enzymes, e.g., alkaline phosphates
- It is a constituent of insulin hormone.

MUST KNOW

Daily nutritional requirement of zinc
- Adult—15 mg
- Infants—3–5 mg
- Children—10–15 mg
- Pregnancy and lactation—20–25 mg

Deficiency Diseases

- Impaired development
- Immaturity of female and male sex organs
- Anemia
- Dwarfism

Iodine

Iodine is a trace element required for the synthesis of thyroid hormones from the thyroid gland. Thyroid hormones, thyroxine (T4) and triiodothyronine (T3) are composed of two molecules of tyrosine combined with 3 or 4 atoms of iodine. An adult body contains 50 mg of iodine.

Sources

Found in sea salt, sea fish, cod liver oil and vegetables and iodized salt.

Functions

- Essential for physical growth and development
- Required for the synthesis of T_3 and T_4 hormones
- As it is a constituent of thyroxin, it regulates the rate of oxidation in the cells and determines the rate of metabolism

Deficiency Disease

Deficiency can lead to goiter.

Copper

Copper is also a micronutrient required in minute quantity. An adult body contains 100–150 µg of copper.

Sources

Green leafy vegetables, carrot, banana, green peas, tomatoes, and dry fruits.

Functions

- Constituent of several enzymes
- Found in red blood cells and plasma.

Deficiency Disease

It can lead to anemia.

Fluorine

Fluorine is found in bones and teeth and is the normal constituent of the body. It is always found in combined form as it is highly reactive.

Sources

Drinking water, sea fish and cheese, tea, milk, eggs.

Functions

- Essential for normal mineralization of bones.
- Required for the formation of dental enamel.

MUST KNOW

Daily nutritional requirement of iodine
- Children above 10 years and adults 150 µg
- Children 2–10 years, 100–120 µg
- Infants 40–50 µg
- In pregnancy and lactation 170–200 µg.

MUST KNOW

Daily nutritional requirement of copper
Daily requirement for an adult is 2 micrograms. An ordinary diet can provide enough of copper for daily requirement.

MUST KNOW

Daily nutritional requirement of flourine
Recommended level of fluorine in drinking water is 0.5 mg/L.

Deficiency Diseases

- Deficiency can cause dental caries.
- Excess fluorine can cause fluorosis.

Chlorine

Chlorine is present in the body in the form of chlorides. It constitutes 0.15% of the human body weight. Chlorides are present in the cerebrospinal fluid and in gastrointestinal secretions. Small amount is present in bones. It is major electrolyte present in plasma and interstitial fluid as chloride ions.

Sources

Present in common salt and small amount in vegetables, fruits, pulses and cereals.

Absorption

Absorbed from small intestine.

Excretion

Excreted in urine, sweats, vomit and diarrhea.

Functions

- It is essential for the production of hydrochloric acid in stomach.
- Maintains acid-base balance in the body fluids
- Osmosis
- Maintains fluid and electrolyte balance.

Deficiency Diseases

Deficiency of chlorine can occur due to severe loss of fluids from the body in cases of:

- Diarrhea
- Vomiting
- Excessive sweating
- Heat strokes
- Diuretic therapy

Symptoms of Deficiency

- Muscle cramps
- Exhaustion
- Low BP
- Decreased ventilation

> **MUST KNOW**
>
> **Daily nutritional requirement of chlorine**
> 5–10 g of common salt (Sodium chloride) in daily diet

Sulfur

Sulfur is an important constituent of proteins, amino acids (cysteine and methionine), thiamine, biotin, insulin, keratin and various glycoproteins.

Sources

A well-balanced diet with adequate protein, green vegetables, pulses and cereals meet the requirement.

> **MUST KNOW**
>
> **Daily nutritional requirement of sulfur**
> The recommended daily intake of sulfur is around 850 milligrams. However, the body usually gets enough sulfur from the foods people eat.

Functions

- Helps to treat gout
- Helps to treat ulcers
- Used for treating various skin diseases

Deficiency Disease

Deficiency causes cystine crystal kidney stones.

Vitamins

Vitamins are required in small quantities, vitamins come under the category of protective food as they are required for specific functions in body. They are classified into two groups (Fig. 18.6):

1. Fat-soluble vitamins are A, D, E, and K
2. Water-soluble vitamins are B group and vitamin C as given in Figure 18.6.

Fat-Soluble Vitamins

Fat-soluble vitamins are insoluble in water but soluble in fat. They require fat for their absorption and can be stored in the body. Their deficiency cannot be seen immediately. It occurs if the intake is poor as body utilizes the stored vitamins. Only the prolonged deficiency can show the signs and symptoms. These vitamins include A, D, E and K.

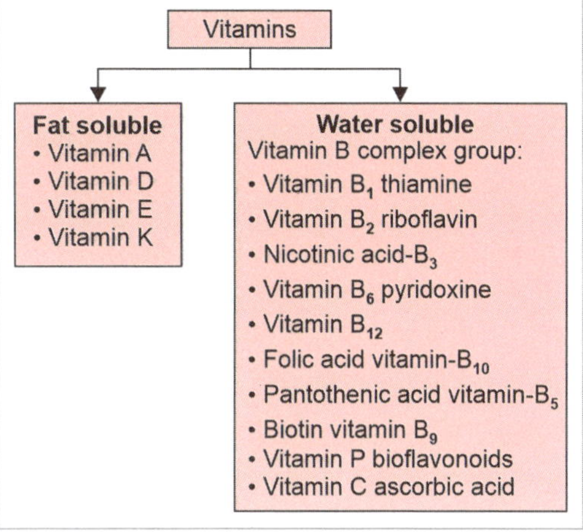

Fig. 18.6: Classification of vitamins

Vitamin A

Pure vitamin A is a pale yellow crystalline compound occurring in animal kingdom. It is measured in international units or micrograms.

- **Sources:** Found in animal foods as well as in plant foods.
    - **In animal sources** as retinol found in meat, fish, liver oil, butter, cheese, eggs (egg yolk).
    - **In plant sources** as carotene. All yellow vegetables and fruits, i.e., carrot, pumpkin, mango, papaya, peaches and apricots. All green leafy vegetables such as spinach, amaranth, curry leaves, fenugreek. All plant sources are provitamin A, i.e., carotene fortified sources are vanaspati ghee, fortified milk.
- **Functions:**
    - Necessary for the normal vision in dim light
    - Maintains the integrity of epithelial cells of skin and mucous membranes of respiratory. Gastrointestinal, genitourinary tract, throat and eyes
    - Necessary for the formation of skeletal bones

> **MUST KNOW**
>
> **Daily nutritional requirement of vitamin A**
> - **Adults:** 750 µg/day
> - **Infants:** 300–400 µg/day
> - **Children:** 10–12 years 600 µg/day.

- Protects body against infections, being an antioxidant
- Protects against epithelial cancers such as bronchial cancer.

Vitamin D

The antirachitic vitamin is vitamin D. It is a fat-soluble vitamin and synthesized in the body. The nutritionally important forms of vitamin D are vitamin D_2, i.e., calciferol and vitamin D_3, i.e., cholecalciferol.

- **Sources:**
  - **Sunlight:** The ultraviolet rays of sunlight convert cholesterol in the skin to vitamin D
  - Food sources are fish, liver, egg yolk, liver oil, butter and cheese, milk.
- **Functions:**
  - Helps the absorption of calcium and phosphates from intestine.
  - Promotes the mineralization of bones and teeth after calcium and phosphorus are absorbed
  - Permits the normal growth.
  - Increases the tubular reabsorption of phosphates in the kidneys which affects the reabsorption of calcium.

> **MUST KNOW**
>
> **Daily nutritional requirement of vitamin D**
> - **Adults:** 2.5 mg (100 IU)
> - **Infants and children:** 5 mg (200 IU)
> - **Pregnancy and lactation:** 10 mg (400 IU)

Vitamin E or Tocopherol

Vitamin E is antisterility vitamin. It is fat-soluble vitamin and stable to heat and acid.

- **Sources:** Vegetable oils, i.e., cotton seed oil, sunflower seed oil, soya and safflower oil, egg yolk, butter, wheat germ oil. Vegetables and fruits are the poor sources for vitamin E.
- **Functions:**
  - It is an antioxidant and gets oxidized and protects cell membranes from oxidative damage
  - Essential for reproductive health
  - Delays aging process
  - Prevents the oxidation of vitamin A in intestine
  - Prevents muscular dystrophy
  - Prevents skin problems acne and psoriasis
  - Prevents the hemolysis of red blood cells
- **Absorption and storage:**
  - Absorbed along with fat from intestine and stored in liver, muscles and body fat.

> **MUST KNOW**
>
> **Daily nutritional requirement of vitamin E**
> - **Children:** 10 mg/day
> - **Adolescents and adults:** 25 mg/day.

Vitamin K (Antihemorrhagic Vitamin)

Vitamin K occurs in two forms, i.e., vitamin K_1 and vitamin K_2.

- **Sources:** Vitamin K_1 is found in fresh green leafy vegetables, cow's milk and fruits, vitamin K_2 is synthesized in intestinal flora by the bacteria. Long-term use of antibiotic (more than a week) can suppress the normal intestinal flora and can cause temporarily deficiency of vitamin K.

> **MUST KNOW**
>
> **Daily nutritional requirement of vitamin K**
> **Adults:** 60–80 mg/day.

- **Functions:**
  - Vitamin K stimulates the production and releases certain coagulating factors.
  - Helps in clotting of blood during bleeding.
  - Increases the prothrombin level in blood.

Water-Soluble Vitamins

Vitamin B complex group and vitamin C are water soluble vitamins. They are not stored in the body hence, to be supplied in diet on daily basis.

Vitamin B$_1$ (Thiamine)

Vitamin B$_1$ is water-soluble vitamin destroyed by cooking in neutral or alkaline medium.
- **Sources:**
  - Whole grain cereals such as wheat, rice, grams, pulses, yeast, wheat germ, oil seeds and nuts, milk.
  - It is also synthesized by bacteria in large intestines
- **Functions:**
  - Thiamine functions as a coenzyme thiamine pyrophosphates (TPP) required in the breakdown of glucose to yield energy.
  - Thiamine helps to maintain healthy nervous system as nervous tissues use glucose as their primary source of energy.
  - Required for normal appetite and digestion.

> **MUST KNOW**
>
> Daily nutritional requirement of vitamin B$_1$
> 0.5 mg/1000 kcal of energy intake

Vitamin B$_2$ (Riboflavin)

Vitamin B$_2$ is a cofactor in a number of enzymes involved with energy metabolism. It is stable to heat and acids. Destroyed by bright light.
- **Sources:**
  - Richest source is milk, liver eggs, green leafy vegetables. Cereals and pulses are poor sources.
  - Also synthesized by bacteria in large intestines.
- **Functions:**
  - It is a cofactor in number of enzymes involved with energy metabolism.
  - Functions as a coenzyme in protein metabolism.
  - As a coenzyme in carbohydrate metabolism.

> **MUST KNOW**
>
> Daily nutritional requirement of vitamin B$_2$
> 0.6 mg/1000 kcal of energy

Vitamin B$_3$

Niacin (Nicotinic Acid) also called P–P factor or antipellagra factor.

This vitamin differs from other B complex group as an essential amino acid tryptophan serves its precursor. It is not excreted in the urine but metabolized to two major methylated derivatives.
- **Sources:**
  - Rich sources are dried yeast, liver, rice, peanut, flour.
  - **Good sources:** Meat, fish, legumes and whole grain cereals.

> **MUST KNOW**
>
> Daily nutritional requirement of vitamin B$_3$
> 6.6 mg/1000 kcal of energy intake

- Milk is poor source but its protein is rich in tryptophan which is converted in the body into niacin.
- **Functions:**
  - Essential for the metabolism of carbohydrate, protein and fat.
  - Helps in the normal functioning of skin, intestine and nervous system.
- **Deficiency:** It results in pellagra and neurological changes.
  - **Pellagra** is characterized by dermatitis, diarrhea and dementia. The gastrointestinal symptoms include anorexia, diarrhea, glossitis, gingivitis, stomatitis and achlorhydria.
  - Neurological symptoms include headache, insomnia, depression, and psychosis.

Vitamin B_6 (Pyridoxine)

Vitamin B_6 occurs in three forms, i.e., pyridoxine, pyridoxal, and pyridoxamine.

- **Sources:**
  - Dried yeast, wheat germ, corn, liver, cereals, pulses, nuts, soybean and groundnut are the good sources. Fruits and vegetables are poor sources.
- **Functions:**
  - Essential for the metabolism of amino acids, fats and carbohydrates
  - Helps in the production of antibodies
  - Required for the synthesis of heme
  - Helps in conversion of tryptophan to niacin
  - Required for the conversion of linoleic acid to arachidonic acid.

> **MUST KNOW**
>
> **Daily nutritional requirement of vitamin B_6**
> - **Adults:** 1.5–2 mg/day
> - **Children:** 1–1.5 mg/day
> - **Infants:** 0.5 mg/day
> - **Pregnant and lactating mothers:** 2.5 mg

Pantothenic Acid Vitamin B_5

Pantothenic acid has specific role in the biosynthesis of corticosteroids.

- **Sources:** Liver, wheat germ, yeast, rice, whole cereals, legumes, nuts, oil seeds and eggs are good sources.
- **Functions:**
  - It is a constituent of coenzyme A, thus necessary for the metabolic process
  - It has got specific role in the biosynthesis of corticosteroids.

> **MUST KNOW**
>
> **Daily nutritional requirement of vitamin B_5**
> - **Adult:** 10 mg/day
> - **Infants:** 1.5–2.5 mg/day
> - **Children:** 5–8 mg%/day
> - **Pregnant and lactating women:** 10–15 mg/day

Folic Acid (Folates) Vitamin B_{10} or M

Folic acid occurs in two forms:

1. Free folates
2. Bound folates

Total folates represent both, i.e., free folates and bound folates.

- **Sources:** Folate means leaf. Green leafy vegetables, fruits, cereals, dairy products,

> **MUST KNOW**
>
> **Daily nutritional requirement of vitamin B_{10}**
>
> | | | |
> |---|---|---|
> | **Adults** | : | 100 mg/day |
> | **Children** | : | 100 mg/day |
> | **Pregnancy** | : | 300 mg/day |
> | **Lactation** | : | 150 mg/day |

liver, meat and eggs, fermented foods, idli, dosa, dhokla. It is also synthesized by intestinal bacteria.

- **Functions:**
  - Required for the maturation of red blood cells (RBC) in the bone marrow.
  - Acts as a coenzyme in the synthesis of methionine and purine.
  - Plays a role in the synthesis of DNA.

Vitamin B_{12} (Cyanocobalamin)

Vitamin B_{12} is a complex organometallic compound with a cobalt atom. For its absorption from the intestine, an intrinsic factor secreted by the stomach is required. B_{12} is stored in liver in fair amount which is sufficient to tide over deficiency for 1–3 years.

- **Sources:** Liver, meat, fish, eggs, milk and cheese, It is not found in foods of vegetable origin.
- **Functions:**
  - It is required for the maturation of red blood cells in the bone marrow.
  - It is essential for the formation of platelets and white blood cells.
  - It acts as a coenzyme in the synthesis of methionine.
  - It is required for the synthesis of fatty acids in the myelin.
  - It is necessary for DNA synthesis.

> **MUST KNOW**
>
> **Daily nutritional requirement of vitamin B_{12}**
> - **Adults** : 1–0 mg/day
> - **Pregnancy and lactation** : 1.5 mg/day
> - **Infants and children** : 0.2 mg/day

Biotin (Vitamin H) or B_9

Vitamin H is synthesized in the intestinal tract. It is sparingly soluble in cold water and freely soluble in hot water.

- **Sources:** Dried yeast and liver are the richest source of biotin, found in vegetables and fruits, wheat germ, peanuts, soybean, legumes, whole cereals, milk, egg, mutton.
- **Functions:**
  - It maintains skin and nervous system in healthy conditions.
  - It is essential for normal gestation and lactation in experimental animals.

> **MUST KNOW**
>
> **Daily nutritional requirement of vitamin B_9**
> Minimum daily requirement is not known. But it may range from 30 mg to 100 mg/day.

Bioflavonoids or Vitamin P

Sources: Found in apples, carrot, cauliflower, orange and lemon juice, apricot, spinach, tomatoes, walnut, turnips, beetroot and pear

- **Functions:**
  - It reduces RBC permeability.
  - It prevents intestinal bleeding in scurvy.
  - It affects the oxidation of adrenaline.

> **MUST KNOW**
>
> **Daily nutritional requirement of vitamin P**
> Daily requirement is not known but is met with diet having sufficient fruits and vegetables.

Vitamin C (Ascorbic Acid)

Vitamin C is highly soluble in water. It is easily destroyed as compared to other water-soluble vitamins. It is readily oxidized and destroyed by heat.

- **Sources:** Amla is the richest source of vitamin C. All citrus fruits, i.e., lemon, orange and sweet lime, guava, tomato, green leafy vegetables, germinating pulses, small amount in meat and milk.

> **MUST KNOW**
>
> Daily nutritional requirement of vitamin C
> - **Pregnant women and adults** : 50 mg/day
> - **Children** : 40 mg/day
> - **Infants** : 30 mg/day
> - **Lactating women** : 80 mg/day.

- **Absorption and storage:** Readily absorbed from intestine and passed on through the portal vein to the general circulation.
- **Functions:**
  - It helps in wound healing.
  - It helps in the absorption of iron.
  - It is an antioxidant. Prevents the oxidation of vitamin A and unsaturated fatty acids.
  - It prevents bleeding from small blood vessels.
  - It helps in conversion of phenylalanine to tyrosine and in oxidation of tyrosine.
  - It increases resistance to infections.
  - Essential for the synthesis of collagens
  - It keeps the gums and teeth in healthy condition.

CLASSIFICATION BY NUTRITIVE VALUES

On the basis of nutritive values foods are classified:

- Cereals and millets
- Pulses (legumes)
- Oil seeds and nuts
- Vegetables
- Roots and tubers
- Fruits
- Fats and oils
- Milk and milk products
- Animal foods
- Sugar and jaggery
- Condiments and spices
- Miscellaneous foods

Cereals and Millets

Cereals

Cereals include rice, wheat and maize. Rice is the main staple food in India, wheat ranks second and maize is the next to rice and wheat.

Cereals are main source of energy and provide 70–80% of the total energy requirement as they are rich sources of carbohydrate. Other than carbohydrate they contain 6–12% of protein, minerals and B group vitamins. The cereal protein is poor in quality being deficient in essential amino acids.

Rice and wheat protein is deficient in lysine while maize protein is deficient in lysine and tryptophan. When the cereals are eaten with pulse protein, they complement each other and provide complete first-class protein. Nutritive values of cereals are shown in Table 18.1.

TABLE 18.1: Nutritive values of cereals per 100 g

Nutrients	Raw milled rice	Whole wheat	Dry maize
Protein (g)	6.8	11.81	11.1
Fat (g)	6.5	1.5	3.6
Carbohydrate (g)	78.2	71.2	66.2
Thiamine (mg)	0.06	0.45	0.42
Niacin (mg)	1.9	5.0	1.8
Riboflavin (mg)	0.06	0.17	0.1
Minerals (mg)	0.6	1.5	1.5
Energy (kcal)	345	346	342

Millets

Millets are the smaller grains which are grounded and eaten without removing the outer layer. They are rich in calcium and contain more protein and vitamin as compared to cereals. Nutritive values of millets are shown in Table 18.2.

TABLE 18.2: Nutritive values of millets per 100 g

Nutrients	Jowar	Bajra	Ragi
Proteins (g)	10.4	11.6	7.3
Fat (g)	1.9	5.0	1.3
Carbohydrate (g)	72.6	67.5	72.0
Minerals (g)	1.6	2.8	2.7
Calcium (mg)	25.0	42.0	344.0
Iron (mg)	4.1	8.0	3.9
Thiamine (mg)	0.3	0.3	0.2
Riboflavin (mg)	1.3	0.25	0.18
Niacin (mg)	3.1	2.3	2.3
Energy (kcal)	349	361	328

Pulses (Legumes)

Pulses are the protein foods for vegetarians and include Bengal gram (black chana), green gram (moong), red gram (Arhar), black gram (urad), lentil or masoor, moth, peas, and beans including soybean. The quality of protein is inferior to animal protein except soybean. Soybean has all essential amino acid and known as first class protein. Rest of pulses are known as second class protein as they are lacking methionine and to some extent cysteine. But when taken in diet with cereals they complement each other and provide first class protein.

In addition to protein, pulses are rich in minerals and vitamin B group. Fermentation also modifies nutritive value of pulses (Table 18.3).

TABLE 18.3: Nutritive values of pulses per 100 g

Pulses	Energy (Kcal)	Proteins (g)	Fat (g)	Calcium (mg)	Iron (mg)	Thiamine (mg)	Riboflavin (mg)	Niacin (mg)	Vitamin C (mg)
Soybean	432	43.2	19.5	240	10.4	0.73	0.39	3.2	0
Bengal gram	360	17.1	5.3	202	4.6	0.30	0.15	2.9	3
Black gram	347	24.0	1.4	154	3.8	0.42	0.20	2.0	0
Red gram	335	22.3	1.7	73	2.7	0.45	0.19	2.9	0
Green gram	348	24.5	1.2	75	3.9	0.72	0.18	2.8	0

Soybean: Soybean is the richest source of good quality of protein. It contains 40% protein, 20% fat and 4% mineral. Soybean is used in various forms; i.e., milk of soybean, paneer or tofu, soybean dal, soybean water, soya biscuits, etc.

Vegetables

Vegetables are protective foods and contain vitamin, minerals and fibers, vegetables are divided into:
- Green leafy vegetables
- Roots and tubers
- Others vegetables

Green Leafy Vegetables

Green leafy vegetables include spinach (palak), amaranth (bathua), fenugreek (methi), cabbage. They are rich in iron, calcium, carotene and some other micronutrients.

They contain 2–4% of leaf protein and good source of lysine but deficient in sulfur-containing amino acids. The oxalates and phytates present in leafy vegetables interfere with calcium absorption, vegetables supply 20–25 kcal/100 g. The daily requirement of an adult is 40 g.

Roots and Tubers

Potatoes, sweet potatoes, colocasia, tapioca, yam, onion, carrot, radish, turnip, come under this category. They are good source of carbohydrates, but poor in protein, minerals and vitamins. Carrots are rich source of beta-carotene. Daily requirement of roots and tubers is 56–60 g for an adult.

Other Vegetables

Brinjal, tomatoes, cauliflower are good source of minerals and vitamins. Daily requirement is 60–70 g for an adult.

Nuts and Oil Seeds

Ground nut, coconut, cashew nut, walnut, almond, pistachio, mustard seeds, cotton seeds, sesame seeds, sunflower seeds are good source of fat and good quality of protein. Vegetable oil is obtained from these nuts. The oils are rich in essential fatty acids. Nuts are good source of vitamin B group, calcium, phosphorus and iron. Nuts should be properly dried and stored to avoid fungus growth which produces "aflatoxin".

TABLE 18.4: **Nutritive values of fruits per 100 g of edible portion**

Name of fruits	Calories	Calcium (mg%)	Iron (mg%)	Carotene (mg%)	Vitamin C (mg)
Fresh fruits					
Banana	104	10	0.36	124	7
Grapes	71	20	1.5	0	1
Guava	54	10	0.27	0	212
Mango	74	14	1.3	2210	16
Orange	48	26	0.32	2240	68
Papaya	32	17	0.5	2740	57
Custard apple	104	17	4.31	0	37
Amla	58	50	1.2	9	600
Dry fruits					
Dates	317	120	7.3	44	3
Raisins	308	87	7.1	24	1

TABLE 18.5: **Nutritive values of meat, fish, egg, per 100 g**

Animal foods	Proteins (g)	Fats (g)	Minerals (mg)
Meat (goat)	21.4	3.6	1.1
Fish	19.5	2.4	1.5
Egg (hen)	13.3	13.3	1.0
Liver (goat)	20.0	3.0	1.3

Fruits

Fruits are protective foods and are good sources of vitamins, minerals, and fibers. Nutritive value of fruits is presented in Table 18.4.

Animal Foods

Meat, fish, eggs and milk, come under this category. Nutritive values of these items are given in Table 18.5. These foods are rich in proteins and vitamins (except vitamin C) and minerals and fats.

Sugar and Jaggery

Sugar and jaggery are produced from sugarcane and are carbohydrate foods only. No other nutrients.

Condiments and Spices

Ginger, garlic, turmeric, tamarind, chilies, cardamom, asafoetida, coriander, black pepper, jeera are used to enhance the palatability of food and stimulate appetite. The essential oils present in them contain carminative properties which aid in digestion.

Miscellaneous

Beverages and water are essential component of body fluids and body tissues.

Beverages: Coffee, tea, cocoa, fruit, juice and aerated drinks.

Alcoholic beverages: Wine, beer, whiskey, all are rich in calories not in other nutrients.

Summary

- Food has been classified on the basis of origin, chemical composition, functions and nutritive values.
- Cereals form the bulk of daily diet and supply 70–80% of total energy requirement. 100 g of cereals yield 350 kcal of energy.
- Cereal proteins are lacking one or two essential amino acids hence, labeled as second class protein. When combined with pulses, they complement and provide all essential amino acids. Soybean contain all essential amino acids, hence, is a first class protein whereas pulses like grams, chana, moong, urad, peas, lentils lack one or two amino acids.
- Vegetables have high vitamin and mineral content. Green leafy vegetables are rich in B complex (except B_{12}), carotene, calcium, iron and vitamin C.
- Roots and tubers are food sources of carbohydrates, but poor in protein, minerals and vitamin. Nuts and oils provide fat and good quality of proteins, most vegetable oils are rich in essential fatty acids.
- Fruits provide vitamins, and mineral. B_{12} is found only in animal foods.
- Milk and milk products provide calcium, proteins, minerals, but are poor in iron.
- Sugar and jaggery are carbohydrate foods and are concentrated sources of energy and contain iron. Condiments and spices stimulate appetite and enhance the food palatability.
- Beverages have stimulant properties and are appreciated for their flavor.

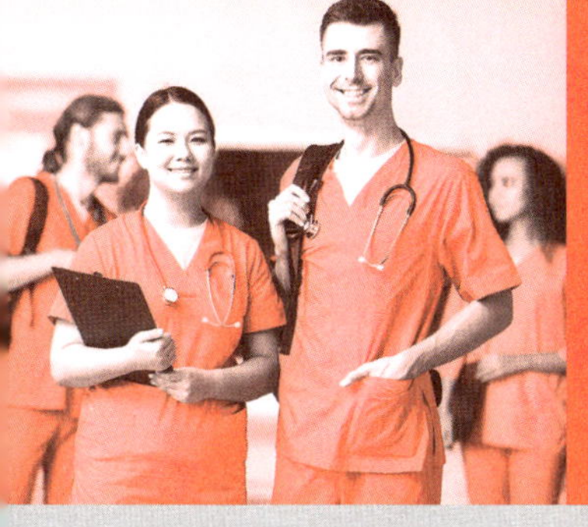

LONG ANSWER TYPE QUESTIONS

1. Describe the functions of proteins, carbohydrates and fats.
2. Describe the nutritive values of pulses and vegetables.

SHORT ANSWER TYPE QUESTIONS

1. How are the foods classified by their chemical composition?
2. Enlist essential amino acids.
3. Enlist saturated and unsaturated fatty fats.

MULTIPLE CHOICE QUESTIONS

1. **Which one of the following is a millet?**
   a. Rice
   b. Maize
   c. Jowar
   d. Wheat

2. **Energy provided by cereals per 100 g is:**
   a. 350 kcal
   b. 250 kcal
   c. 450 kcal
   d. 150 kcal

3. **Which of the following is not a millet?**
   a. Bajra
   b. Lentil
   c. Jowar
   d. Ragi

4. **Lathyrism is caused by:**
   a. Khesari dal
   b. Red grams
   c. Lentil
   d. Green grain

5. **Which of the following is not a body building food?**
   a. Meat
   b. Roots and tubers
   c. Pulses
   d. Eggs

6. **Which of the following is not a protective food?**
   a. Meat
   b. Green leafy vegetables
   c. Milk
   d. Fish

7. **Which of the following in not true about nutrient content of soybean?**
    a. Highest content of protein (43.2 g%)
    b. Highest content of fat (19.5 g%)
    c. Highest content of calcium, iron and B complex
    d. Highest content of vitamin C

19

Normal Dietary Requirements

LEARNING OBJECTIVES

After the completion of the unit, the readers will be able to:

- Explain body mass index and normal dietary requirements.
- Demonstrate skill in calculating normal food requirements.
- Plan menu considering the combination of food affecting and enhancing the nutritive value of diet.
- Understand the factors involved in budgeting of food.
- Discuss the disorders caused by the imbalance of nutrients.
- Plan diet modification in gluten, lactose and protein intolerance.

UNIT OUTLINE

- Introduction
- Energy
- Body Mass Index
- Basal Metabolic Rate
- Balanced Diet
- Nutritive Value
- Normal Food Requirement
- Balanced Diet for Adults
- Combination of Food Affecting and Enhancing the Nutritive Value of the Diet
- Budgeting for Food
- Low-Cost Meals
- Diseases and Disorders Caused by the Imbalance of Nutrients
- Diseases and Disorders Due to Imbalance of Minerals
- Minerals and their Deficiencies
- Deficiency Diseases of Trace Elements or Micro Elements
- Diseases and Disorders Due to Imbalance of Vitamins
- Food Allergy

KEY TERMS

Balanced diet: A diet containing all required nutrients needed for body.

BMI: The BMI is defined as the body mass divided by the square of the body height in meters, and is expressed in units of kg/m², resulting from mass in kilograms and height in meters.

BMR: It is Basal metabolic rate, the minimum amount of energy required to maintain vital functions at rest.

Diet: A kind of food on which a person lives.

Energy: It is capacity to do work.

Food exchange list: A list of similar foods of a food group so that specified amount of all the foods listed in that group and exchange have approximately the same nutritive value.

Joule: It is international unit of energy.

Meal planning: Application of the knowledge of food, nutrients, food habits, likes and dislikes to plan wholesome and attractive meal.

RDA: It is a recommended daily dietary allowance of food.

INTRODUCTION

Dietary requirements are the minimum amount of nutrients a person needs to maintain a healthy level of nutrition. They help prevent deficiency diseases and promote health. A healthy diet includes a variety of nutritious foods that meet your body's nutritional needs at different life stages. The recommended dietary intake (RDA) is the average daily amount of nutrients that meets the needs of almost all healthy people in a particular age group and gender.

ENERGY

Energy may be defined as the capacity to do work.

We require energy to carry out the basic body functions. It is also required to maintain vital processes, such as respiration and circulations. We get this energy from the food we eat.

Energy Value of Food

- The main energy sources in diet are carbohydrates fats and proteins.
- 1 g of protein yields 4 kcal of energy.
- 1 g of fat yields 9 kcal of energy.
- 1 g of carbohydrates yields 4 kcal of energy.
- About 60–70% of the total energy required by the body should come from carbohydrate foods, 20–30% from the fats and 15% from the protein foods.

Units of Energy

Energy needed by the body is measured in kilocalories and usually expressed as calories.

Kilocalorie is defined as the amount of heat required to raise the temperature of 1 kg of water through 1°C.

The international unit of energy is Joule denoted by J.

$$1 \text{ kilocalories} = 4184 \text{ Joules or } 4.184 \text{ kilo Joules.}$$

MUST KNOW

Energy requirements by different people

Energy recommended by nutrition expert group Indian Council of Medical Research (ICMR).

- For male of average weight 55 kg
  - An adult sedentary worker: 2,400 kcal
  - Moderate worker: 2,800 kcal
  - Heavy worker such as: (Farmer, laborer, gardener) 3,900 kcal
- For female of average weight 45 kg
  - Sedentary worker: 1,900 kcal
  - Moderate worker: 2,200 kcal

Contd...

- Heavy worker: 3,000 kcal
- During pregnancy + 300 kcal
- During lactation + 550 kcal
- For infants
  - 0–6 months 100 kcal/kg body weight
  - 7–12 months 120 kcal/kg body weight
- For children
  - 1–3 years — 1,200 kcal
  - 4–6 years — 1,500 kcal
  - 7–9 years — 1,800 kcal
  - 10–12 years — 2,100 kcal
  - 13–15 years — 2,300 kcal
  - Boys 16–19 years — 3,000 kcal
  - Girls 16–19 years — 2,200 kcal.

BODY MASS INDEX

Definition: Body mass index (BMI) may be defined as the weight in kilograms divided by the square of the height in meters:

$$\text{BMI} = \frac{\text{Weight in kg}}{(\text{Height in Meters})^2} = \frac{W}{(H)^2}$$

- Body mass index is the most effective and scientific method used to assess the obesity.
- Normal value of BMI in males is 20–25.
- Normal value of BMI in females is 19–24
- Individuals with value of 25–30 are overweight and those with values >31 are obese.

BASAL METABOLIC RATE

- **Basal metabolism:** "The energy metabolism of a subject at complete physical and mental rest and having normal body temperature and in the post absorptive state (i.e. 12 hours after the intake of last meal) is known as Basal metabolism" (Swaminathan, Vol. I).
- **Basal metabolic rate (BMR):** The minimum amount of energy required by the body to carry out the vital functions of the body (i.e. maintaining temperature, circulation and respiration) is known as the basal metabolic rate (BMR).

Determination of BMR

The estimated minimum level of energy required to sustain body's vital functions when at rest is measured after 12 hours of starvation by using the apparatus of Benedict and Rath. This, apparatus is a closed chamber in which the person is placed and he breathes in oxygen from a metallic cylinder of 6 L capacity. The carbon dioxide given off by the individual is absorbed by soda lime present in the tower.

Conditions Necessary for the Measurement of BMR

- The person should be at complete rest at least half an hour before performing the test after the overnight sleep and rest.
- Should be fasting for 12 hours, thus avoiding the effect of digestion and absorption.
- The environmental temperature should be comfortable, i.e. 20–25°C during test.
- Person should be awake in recumbent position.

The individual wears a nose clip and breathes through the mouth piece, the oxygen is present in the cylinder for six minutes. The volume of oxygen used is recorded on a graph paper.

The calorific value of 1 L of oxygen consumption is 4.8 kcal and total calories required for 24 hours can be calculated from the amount of oxygen consumed for 24 hours.

The oxygen consumed in 6 minutes is 1.1 L.

Heat produced in 6 minutes = 4.8 × 1.1 = 5.28 kcal.

$$\text{Heat produced in 24 hours} = \frac{24 \times 60 \times 5.28}{6} = 1267 \text{ kcal.}$$

Factors Affecting BMR

- **Age:** BMR is higher in case of children during the period of rapid growth, i.e. 15–20% higher and gradually declines with age at the rate of 5%.
- **Body surface area:** BMR is directly proportional to surface area. The larger is the surface area of the body, the higher is the BMR.
- **Sex:** BMR is slightly higher in male as compared to female due to larger surface area.
- **Body temperature:** For every rise of 0.5°C of internal body temperature, BMR increases by 7%.
- **Hormones:** BMR increases in hyperthyroidism due to increase in thyroid hormones and decrease in hypothyroidism due to decreased production of thyroid hormones.
- **Climate:** BMR rises in cold weather as body requires more energy to maintain normal temperature BMR decreases during warm climate.
- **Psychological conditions:** BMR increases during anxiety and worry.
- **Exercise:** There is an increased consumption of oxygen during exercise, so BMR increases.
- **Diet:** BMR increases after taking meals. Maximum rise is seen after taking protein meals and minimum with fat and carbohydrates. Protein causes increase in cellular metabolism to maximum, i.e. due to specific dynamic action of protein.
- **During pregnancy and lactation:** BMR rapidly increases due to the growth of fetus in pregnancy and due to milk secretion in lactation.

BALANCED DIET

Balanced diet is one which provides all the nutrients required for maintenance and regulation of body functions in adequate amount. The nutrients included in balanced diet are as follows:

- Carbohydrate foods to provide energy, protein foods for growth and repair of body tissues, fat to provide energy and for absorption of fat-soluble vitamins. Minerals and vitamins protective foods essential for digestion, absorption, transportation and utilization of the nutrients.

Principles

- Balanced diet must include:
  - **Staple food:** Wheat, rice, millets, carbohydrate, vegetables, potatoes and fruits like banana, etc.
  - **Protein foods:** Pulses, legumes, milk products, meat, fish, eggs, etc.
  - **Protective foods:** Green leafy vegetables, other vegetables, fruits, etc.
  - **Fats and sugars:** Cooking oil, sugar, jaggery, honey for additional calories
- Balance diet should provide protein 15–20% of daily energy requirement, i.e. 1 g/kg body weight.
- Fat should not exceed 20–30% of daily energy requirement out of total calories.
- Rest of energy should come from carbohydrates.
- Balanced diet must provide all vitamins, minerals and water in sufficient quantity.
- All factors age, sex, beliefs and working conditions should be considered while planning the menu.

Planning a Balanced Diet

- Identify the requirement of individual according to recommended dietary allowance considering the socioeconomic and religious background of the individual.
- Select food stuffs from all food groups.
- Select the total amount of food stuffs for day's menu
- Divide the total food stuffs in days, various meals 3–4 times a day
- Decide the menu
- Monitor the day's diet for correct food groups and quantity

Recommended dietary allowances (RDA) is defined as the intake of nutrient derived from diet which keeps nearly all people in good health.

NUTRITIVE VALUE

The nutritive values of various food items are given in Tables 19.1–19.8.

TABLE 19.1: Nutritive values of cereals and millets

Food items	Energy (kcal/100 g)	Proteins (g/100 g)	Carbohydrates (g/100 g)	Calcium (mg/100 g)	Iron (mg/100 g)	Fat (g/100 g)
Bajra	361	11.6	67.5	42	8.0	5.0
Barley	336	11.5	64.6	26	1.67	1.3
Jowar	349	10.4	72.6	25	4.1	1.9
Maize	342	11.1	66.2	10	2.3	3.6
Maize flour	125	4.7	24.6	9	1.1	0.9
Rice whole	345	6.8	78.2	10	0.7	0.5
Rice bran	393	13.5	48.4	67	35.0	16.2
Rice flakes	346	6.6	77.3	20	20.0	1.2
Wheat whole	346	11.8	12.0	41	5.3	1.5

Contd...

Food items	Energy (kcal/100 g)	Proteins (g/100 g)	Carbohydrates (g/100 g)	Calcium (mg/100 g)	Iron (mg/100 g)	Fat (g/100 g)
Wheat flour	341	12.1	69.4	48	4.9	1.7
Wheat flour refined	348	11.0	73.9	23	2.7	0.9
Semolina	348	10.4	74.8	16	1.6	0.8
Wheat bread	245	7.8	51.9	11	1.1	0.7
Bengal gram (whole)	360	17.1	60.9	202	4.6	5.3
Bengal gram dal	372	20.8	59.8	56	5.3	5.6
Black gram dal	347	24.0	59.6	154	3.8	1.4
Green gram whole	334	24.0	56.7	124	4.4	1.3
Green gram dal	348	24.5	59.9	75	3.9	1.2
Rajma	346	22.9	60.6	260	5.1	1.3
Soybean	432	43.2	20.9	240	10.4	19.5
Rice puffed	325	14.7	73.6	23	6.6	0.1
Lentil	343	24.1	59.0	69	7.58	07
Peas dry	315	19.7	56.5	75	7.05	1.1

TABLE 19.2: Nutritive value of fruits

Food items	Energy (kcal/100 g)	Proteins (g/100 g)	Carbohydrate (g/100 g)	Calcium (mg/100 g)	Fe (mg/100 g)	Fat (g/100 g)
Apple	59	0.2	13.4	10	0.660	0.5
Banana	116	1.2	27.2	17	0.36	0.3
Chiku	53	1.8	11.1	10	2.0	0.2
Coconut	444	6.8	13.0	10	1.7	41.6
Grapes	71	0.5	16.5	20	0.52	0.3
Leechi	61	1.1	13.6	10	0.7	0.2
Anaar	65	1.6	14.5	10	1.79	0.1
Orange	48	0.7	10.9	26	0.32	0.2
Peach	50	1.2	10.5	15	2.4	0.3
Pear	52	0.6	11.9	8	0.5	0.2
Pineapple	46	0.4	10.8	20	2.42	0.1
Plum	52	0.7	11.7	10	0.6	0.5
Papaya	32	0.6	7.2	17	0.5	0.1
Mango	74	0.6	16.9	14	1.3	0.4
Guava	51	0.9	11.2	10	0.27	0.3
Cherry	64	1.1	13.8	24	0.57	0.5

TABLE 19.3: **Nutritive value of vegetables**

Food items	Energy (kcal/100 g)	Proteins (g/100 g)	Carbohydrates (g/100 g)	Calcium (mg/100 g)	Fe (mg/100 g)	Fat (g/100 g)
Beans	150	7.4	29.8	50.0	9.6	1.0
French beans	31	3.4	6.5	–	–	–
Beet	46	1.4	4.0	380.0	16.2	0.8
Brinjal	24	1.8	4.6	18.0	0.38	0.3
Cabbage	27	5.9	7.6	39.0	0.8	0.1
Cauliflower	66	0.9	10.6	626.0	40.0	1.3
Carrot	48	0.8	7.7	33.0	1.03	0.4
Bitter gourd	25	1.6	4.2	20.0	0.61	0.2
Garlic	145	6.3	29.8	30.0	1.2	0.1
Ginger	67	2.3	12.3	20.0	3.5	0.9
Gourd	12	0.2	2.5	20.0	0.46	0.1
Lemon	16.8 to 29	1.1	9.3	26	0.6	0.3
Onion	50	1.2	11.1	46.9	0.60	0.1
Ladies finger	35	1.9	6.7	66.0	0.35	0.2
Mushroom	22.2	3.1	3.3	3	0.5	0.3
Turnip	67	4.0	9.4	710.0	28.4	1.5
Capsicum	24	1.3	4.3	10.0	0.567	0.3
Tinda	21	1.4	3.4	25.00	0.9	0.2
Peas	93	7.2	15.9	20.0	1.5	0.1
Tomato	23	1.9	3.6	20.0	1.8	0.1
Cucumber	13	0.4	2.5	60.0	0.5	0.1
Potato	17	1.6	22.6	10.0	0.48	0.1
Radish	17	0.7	3.4	35.0	0.4	0.1

TABLE 19.4: **Nutritive value of nuts, condiments and spices**

Food items	Energy (Kcal/100 g)	Proteins (g/100 g)	Carbohydrates (g/100 g)	Fat (g/100 g)	Calcium (mg/100 g)	Iron (g/100 g)
Asafoetida	297	4.0	67.8	1.1	690	39.4
Cardamom (Big)	229	10.2	42.1	2.2	130	4.6
Cardamom small	246	11	68	7	383	13.97
Chilies (dry)		15.9	31.6	6.2	160	2.3

Contd...

Food items	Energy (Kcal/100 g)	Proteins (g/100 g)	Carbohydrates (g/100 g)	Fat (g/100 g)	Calcium (mg/100 g)	Iron (g/100 g)
Cloves	286	5.2	46.0	8.9	740	11.7
Coriander	288	14.1	11.6	16.1	630	7.1
Cumin seeds	356	18.7	36.6	15.0	1080	11.7
Nutmeg	472	7.5	28.5	36.5	120	2.03
Garlic	145	6.3	29.8	0.1	30	1.2
Onion	363	17.1	24.6	21.8	1525	12.5
Cinnamon	–	–	–	–	–	–
Ginger	80	1.2	17.7	0.75	0.9	0.6
Pepper dry	304	11.5	49.2	6.8	460	12.4
Tamarind	283	3.1	67.4	0.1	170	17.0
Turmeric	349	6.3	69.4	5.1	150	67.8
Chili green	29	2.9	3.0	0.6	30	4.4
Coriander powder	288	14.1	21.6	16.1	630	7.1
Chili powder	246	15.9	31.6	6.2	160	2.2
Amchoor	–	–	–	–	–	–
Ginger dry	–	–	–	–	–	–
Methi seeds	–	–	–	–	–	–
Garam masala	–	–	–	–	–	–

TABLE 19.5: Nutritive value of milk and milk product

Food Items	Energy (kcal/100 g)	Fat (g/100 g)	Proteins (g/100 g)	Carbohydrates (g/100 g)	Calcium (mg/100 g)	Fe (mg /100 g)	Minerals (mg/100 g)
Curd	60	4.0	3.1	3.0	149	0.2	0.8
Milk	67	4.1	3.2	4.4	120	0.2	0.8
Paneer	348	25.2	24.1	0.3	790	2.1	4.2
Ghee	900	100.0	–	–	–	–	–
Cream	729	81.0	–	–	–	–	2.5

TABLE 19.6: Nutritive value of fats and oils

Food items	Energy (Kcal/ 100 g)	Fat (g/100 g)	Proteins (g/100 g)	CHO (g/ 100)	Calcium (mg/100 g)	Fe (mg/ 100 g)	Mineral (mg/100 g)	Vit A IU	Vit C (mg/ 100 g)	Thiamine (mg /100 g)
Hydrogenated oil	900	100	–	–	–	–	–	–	–	–
Sunflower oil	900	100	–	–	–	–	–	–	–	–
Mustard oil	900	100	–	–	–	–	–	–	–	–
Groundnut	567	40.1	25.3	26.1	90	2.5	2.4	–	–	–
Vanaspati ghee	900	100	–	–	–	–	–	–	–	–
Desi ghee	900	100	–	–	–	–	–	–	–	–
Dalda	729	810	–	–	–	–	–	–	–	–
Coconut oil	900	100	–	–	–	–	–	–	–	–
Nut (dry)	662	62.3	6.8	18.4	400	7.8	1.6	–	–	–
Coconut fresh	444	41.6	4.5	13.4	10	1.7	1.0	–	7	0.05
Almond	655	58.9	20.8	10.5	230	8.09	2.9	–	–	–
Cashew nut	596	46.9	21.2	22.3	50.0	5.81	2.4	–	–	–
Walnut	667	64.5	15.6	11.0	100	2.64	1.8	–	–	–
Refined oil	900	100	–	–	–	–	–	–	–	–
Ground nut oil	900	100	–	–	–	–	–	–	–	–
Watermelon seed	628	52.6	34.1	4.5	100	7.4	3.7			
Butter	570	81.0	–	–	–	–	–	3200	–	–

TABLE 19.7: Nutritive value of meat, fish and egg

Food items	Energy (kcal/ 100 g)	Fat (g/100 g)	Proteins (g/100 g)	CHO (g)	Calcium (mg)	Fe (mg/100 g)	Vit A IU	Vit C (mg/100 g)	Thiamine (mg/100 g)
Mutton	194	13.3	18.5	–	150	2.5	9	–	0.18
Egg	173	18.4	13.3	0.6	60	2.1	630	–	0.1
Fish	103	1.4	16.4	4.4	650	1.0	–	22	0.05

TABLE 19.8: Nutritive value of sugars

Food items	Energy (kcal/100 g)	Fat (g/100 g)	Protein (g/100 g)	CHO (g)	Calcium (mg)	Fe (mg/100 g)	Mineral (mg/100 g)
Sugar	396	0	0.1	99.4	12	0.155	0.1
Jaggery	383	0.1	0.4	95.0	80	2.64	0.6
Honey	319	0	0.3	79.5	5	0.696	0.2
Sago	351	0.2	0.2	87.1	10	1.3	0.3

NORMAL FOOD REQUIREMENT

Normal food requirements for different categories of people are given in Tables 19.9 to 19.11.

- Energy requirement for infants:
  - **Protein requirement:**
    - 1st 6 months 2 g/kg body weight
    - Later 6 months 1–5 g/kg body weight per day
  - **Carbohydrates:** 10 g/kg body weight/day
  - **Fluid requirement:** 100 mL/kg body weight/day

For the first 6 months, this requirement is usually met with mother's milk.

But after 6 months, the supplementary foods should be added gradually and at the age of one year, child should eat everything what elderly eat (Table 19.9).

TABLE 19.9: Recommended food stuffs for toddler and preschool child

Food items	Age group 1–3 years (1,200 kcal)	Age group 4–6 years (1700 kcal)
Cereals	175 g	270 g
Pulses	35 g	35 g
Leafy vegetables	40 g	50 g
Other vegetables	20 g	30 g
Roots and tubers	10 g	20 g
Milk	350 mL	250 mL
Oils & fats	15 g	25 g
Sugar and jaggery	30 g	40 g

Note: For nonvegetarian 20–30 g meat, 1 egg can replace 20–30 g of pulses.

- Menu plan for 1–3 years of children caloric requirement is 100 kcal/kg body weight/day, protein requirement 1.5–2 g/kg body weight/day for this growing age. The Table 19.10 will provide adequate requirement for proper growth and development.

TABLE 19.10: Menu for the day for 1–3 years' children

Time	Diet
Morning 6.30 am	Milk 100–150 mL with sugar
8.30 am breakfast	Bread 1–2 slices with butter 5 g, porridge with milk and sugar
Mid-morning 11 am	Seasonal fruit, banana, apple, papaya, guava, juice, etc.
1.00 pm lunch	Rice/chapatti 75–100 g, vegetable—one serving 30 g, pulses—one serving ghee and oil 5 g
Mid-evening 4.30 pm	Snacks, biscuits with sweetened milk
8 pm dinner	Same as lunch

- Daily requirement of later childhood/school children of age group of 6–12 years (Table 19.11).
  - This is the period of rapid growth and development. The absorption rate is also higher as compared to the school age.
  - The caloric requirement 2,000–2,400 kcal, protein requirement 36–45 g/day.
  - In girls, the requirement of protein and calories is less than boys, but they require more calcium and iron in the comparison of boys.

TABLE 19.11: Recommended requirement of food for 6–12 years age group

Food items	Age groups	
	7–9 years	10–12 years
Cereals	350 g	420 g
Pulses	40 g	45 g
Leafy vegetables	50 g	50 g
Other vegetables	40 g	50 g
Roots and tubers	25 g	30 g
Milk	250 mL	250 mL
Fats and oils	30 g	40 g
Sugar and jaggery	40 g	45 g
Seasonal fruit	100 g	100 g

Note: For nonvegetarian diet, pulses can be reduced and replaced by meat, or fish, 20–30 g, egg-1.

- **The daily requirement of adolescent** is higher than the 10–12 years of age group and almost equal to adults.

BALANCED DIET FOR ADULTS

The calories and protein requirement depends upon the type of work, body weight and age. Refer to Table 19.12.

TABLE 19.12: Balanced diet for adult male

Food items	Sedentary workers (2,400 kcal/day)	Moderate worker (2,800 Kcal/day)	Heavy worker (3,900 Kcal/day)
Cereals	460 g	520 g	670 g
Pulses	40 g	50 g	60 g
Leafy vegetables	40 g	40 g	40 g
Other vegetables	60 g	70 g	80 g
Roots and tubers	50 g	60 g	80 g
Milk	150 mL	200 mL	250 mL
Fats and oils	40 g	45 g	65 g
Sugar and Jaggery	40 g	45 g	65 g
Seasonal fruit	150 g	200 g	200 g

Note: For nonvegetarian 20–30 g meat, and an egg can be added as additional fat in place of 20–30 g of pulses.

Diet During Pregnancy

In addition to the recommended balance diet in Table 19.13 of adult females, the following requirement is added in diet during pregnancy (Table 19.14):

TABLE 19.13: Balanced diet for adult female

Food items	Sedentary workers (1900 kcal/day)	Moderate worker (2200 kcal/day)	Heavy worker (3900 kcal/day)
Cereals	410 g	440 g	575 g
Pulses	40 g	45 g	50 g
Leafy vegetables	100 g	100 g	50 g
Other vegetables	40 g	40 g	100 g
Roots and tubers	50 g	50 g	60 g
Milk	100 mL	150 mL	200 mL
Fats and oils	20 g	25 g	40 g
Sugar and Jaggery	20 g	20 g	40 g
Seasonal fruit	150 g	200 g	200 g

Note: For nonvegetarian/meat or fish 20–30 g, one egg can be included in place of 20–30 g of pulses.

TABLE 19.14: Additional diet to be added during pregnancy

Food items	300 kcal/day
Cereals	35 g
Pulses	20 g
Milk	1000 mL
Sugar	10 g

For the additional requirement of minerals and vitamins, green leafy vegetables and fruits are increased to get extra calcium and iron. These extra nutrients and calories are necessary for the growth of growing fetus, the uterus and the placenta.

Diet During Lactation

Extra requirement of calories and nutrients for the production of milk is necessary. It includes the following in addition to the requirement of an adult female (Table 19.15).

During lactation the extra requirement is 20 g protein and 2 g of extra calcium per day.

TABLE 19.15: Additional diet to be added during lactation

Food items	550 kcal/day
Cereals	60 g
Pulses	40 g
Milk	1000 mL
Fat	10 g
Sugar	40 g

Diet During Old Age

The nutritional requirement decreases with advancing age due to decrease in metabolic rate.

- The protein requirement is 1.5 g/kg body weight for the repair and maintenance of tissues.
- Fat is provided by vegetable oils.
- Calcium, iron and vitamin should be supplied in diet.
- Diet should be soft, palatable and easily digestible. Adequate amount of fruits and fibers should be supplied to prevent constipation.

COMBINATION OF FOOD AFFECTING AND ENHANCING THE NUTRITIVE VALUE OF THE DIET

The vegetable proteins, i.e., pulses and legumes are lacking one or more essential amino acid. So, to get a balance diet, the following can be done:
- Mixed pulses enhance the nutritive values of food.
- Combining cereals and pulses in menu complements the essential nutrients.
- Use of mix vegetables also enhance vitamin B_{12} and mineral content.
- Enough legumes, dried seeds and nuts to be added in diet to get iron and calcium.
- Dairy foods should be increased for calcium and vitamin B_{12} and protein.
- The sugar and visible fat should be reduced to cut down empty calories.
- Whole grain bread and cereals should be added for vitamin B group.

BUDGETING FOR FOOD

Budgeting for food is very important for the protection of health of all family members, so that the nutritional requirement of every individual in the family is considered.

Factors to be Considered in Budgeting of Food

- **Size of the family:** The number of family members, age, sex, occupation. The need for special nutrient for growing children, pregnant and lactating women, elderly and of any person with chronic disease in the family.
- **Family income:** How much money the family can spend on food purchase?

- **Choice of food** within each food group.
- **Location of market:** Super markets provide food at low cost than neighborhood market.
- **Alternative marketing choice:** To buy foods from wholesale market at low cost as nutritive value of the foods is also good.
- **Home prepared** and convenient foods are less expensive, e.g. homemade pickle, juices, chutney, papad, wadi, etc.
- **Snacks and beverages:** This group of foods can increase food expenditure without increasing the appropriate nutritive value of food.
- Availability of supplementary programs where income is limited for example mid-day meal in schools and supplementary feeding for pregnant and lactating mothers.

Ways to Save on Food Budget

- Prepare shopping list
- Always try to purchase family packs as they are economical.
- Foods, like cereals, pulses, legumes, etc., buy when they are plenty in the market according to their season. These foods will be cheap at that time. Buy according to storage space.
- Buy the seasonal vegetables and fruits as they are cheaper.
- Try low-priced brands. They may be similar in quality as compared to more expensive ones.
- Plan meals in advance and make use of food guides to ensure good nutrition.
- Limit the money to be spent on snacks and beverages. They will increase the expenditure without providing nutrients.
- Limit the use of ready to eat food and prefer home prepared food.
- Avoid food wastage at home by properly storing to maintain their freshness.
- Buy oil, spices, soya in bulk, but buy only that quantity which can be used before they get spoil.
- If possible, make butter and ghee at home from daily use of milk.

LOW-COST MEALS

In every country, there are people of varying income group from high, medium and low. The people of low-income group usually suffer from nutritional deficiency diseases. About 80% of the low-income group depend upon the cereals for energy and they do not include protective foods, like pulses, green leafy vegetables, milk, fruits and fats. Partially due to lack of nutritional knowledge in addition to lack of purchasing power.

Nutritional Education for Low-Cost Meals and Food Substitutes

- The food items selected should be cheap, but have the nutritional importance (Table 19.16).
- For protein, pulses and legumes should be added to provide requirement rather than spending on expensive nonvegetarian foods.

TABLE 19.16: An exchange list of low-cost balanced meal

Food items	Quantity
Cereals	460 g
Pulses	40 g
Green leafy vegetables	50 g
Other vegetables	60 g
Milk	150 mL
Roots and tubers	50 g
Oil and fat	40 g
Sugar and Jaggery	30 g

- Local seasonal vegetables are cheap and should be included in diet to provide minerals and vitamins rather than spending on expensive and transported vegetables from other places.
- Seasonal fruits are cheap at their peak season, and so they should be added to menu.
- About one glass of milk should be included in diet.

The above food items provide balanced meal having adequate calories from carbohydrate and fat. Adequate protective foods, i.e. protein, vitamins and minerals are present in the menu.

DISEASES AND DISORDERS CAUSED BY THE IMBALANCE OF NUTRIENTS

Carbohydrate

Deficiency of Carbohydrates

Deficiency of carbohydrate in diet results in utilization of fat for the production of energy. Incomplete oxidation of fats causes ketone bodies to accumulate in the blood thereby causing keto acidosis. Ketone bodies may appear in the urine also. Deficiency of carbohydrate can occur in:
- Prolonged starvation
- Less intake of carbohydrates in diet

Prevention

Daily diet should have sufficient carbohydrate to supply 60–70% of total energy requirement.

Excessive Intake of Carbohydrates

- Excessive intake of carbohydrates results in excess production of glucose which is converted into fat and deposited in the adipose tissue which can lead to obesity.
- Excessive fibers present in carbohydrate foods can irritate intestinal mucosa causing cramps and gas formation.
- Excessive fibers also interfere with the absorption and utilization of mineral elements such as calcium and iron.
- Deficiency of carbohydrates when accompanied with deficiency of protein in case of children causes PEM. Now known as Protein Energy under Nutrition (PEU).

Protein

Deficiency of Protein

- Protein deficiency in adults
    - Can cause loss of weight, especially muscular weight, anemia
    - Nutritional edema
    - Lowered resistance to infection
    - Poor healing of the wound
- In pregnancy
    - Protein deficiency causes intrauterine growth retardation of the fetus
    - Anemia
    - Edema

- ■ Poor resistance to infection
  - ■ Preeclampsia
  - ■ Increased risk of hemorrhage during labor and after delivery
- • During lactation
  - ■ Anemia
  - ■ Failure of lactation

In preschool children, protein deficiency results in protein energy undernutrition, i.e., PEU.

Protein Energy Malnutrition

It is a major health and nutritional problem in India.

Incidence: PEU is common in preschool children and incidence is 1–2%.

Clinical forms PEU occurs in two clinical forms (Table 19.17):

1. **Kwashiorkor:** In this, there is a deficiency of protein only. It occurs in children of age 1–3 years after arrival of next sibling. The older child is put on high carbohydrates and low-protein diet.
2. **Marasmus:** There is deficiency of protein as well as carbohydrate due to lack of protein as well as enough food to eat for meeting caloric requirement.

TABLE 19.17: Clinical presentation of kwashiorkor and marasmus

Signs and symptoms	Kwashiorkor	Marasmus
Edema	Present on lower limbs, lower arms and face, pot belly.	Not present
Muscle wasting	Muscle wasting is there but may be hidden by edema and fat.	Severe muscle wasting is present. Extreme emaciation.
Fat loss	No fat loss.	Severe loss of subcutaneous fat due to lack of calories.
Appearance of face	Moon face due to edema, cheeks may be swollen due to accumulation of fluid and fatty tissue.	Monkey-like face appearance, wrinkled face giving appearance like old man.
Appetite	Poor.	Usually good, but child does not get sufficient food to eat.

Contd...

Signs and symptoms	Kwashiorkor	Marasmus
Weight or height	Retarded growth	Severe growth retardation
Diarrhea and respiratory infections	Often present	Often present due to lack of immunity.
Anemia	Anemia is present due to deficiency of protein, iron and vit A and B Complex deficiency are also found.	Anemia present along with the deficiency of some other micro nutrients, e.g. vitamin A, and vitamin B deficiency.
Mental changes	Mental development arrested, child may lose interest, becomes irritable and apathetic.	Mental development arrested along with physical growth, child becomes irritable and apathetic.
Skin changes	Dry, flaky, peeling and pigmented skin	Skin changes rare.
Hair changes	Thin, dry, brown hair, easily plucked	Hair changes are common.
Liver	Enlarged with fatty changes	Liver mildly enlarged but no fatty changes.
Biochemical changes	Low serum albumen, low immune system response, reduced enzyme activity, moderate deficiency of potassium.	Severe potassium deficiency, normal enzyme activity, normal immune system, response slightly, decreased serum albumen.
Treatment response	Fairly good and rapid recovery with increase in protein intake in diet.	Takes longer time to recover

Prevention and Treatment of PEU

- **Nutritional education to the mothers about child's nutrition:** Mothers should be taught during the antenatal periods about the importance of exclusive breastfeeding up to 6 months of age and thereafter introduction of supplementary foods along with breastfeeding.
- **Immunization of children:** Infants and children must be immunized at prescribed age.
- **Treatment of diarrhea:** Use of oral rehydration therapy. Mothers should be taught how to prepare ORS at home and give to child in case of diarrhea to prevent dehydration.
- **Maintain growth chart at home:** Mothers should be educated to make record of height and weight according to the growth chart, so that they can recognize the signs of under nutrition.
- **Nutritional management:** Daily diet in case of PEU should contain:
    - **Protein:** 3–4 g/kg body weight. Foods. Eggs, milk, pulses, soybean and nuts, cereal and fats should be included in diet.
    - **Energy:** 170–200 kcal/kg body weight/day.
    - **Fats:** 15–20% of total calories should be from fats such as milk, butter, coconut, oil, etc.
    - Vitamin and mineral should be given liberally.

Fat

Deficiency of Fat

Deficiency of essential fatty acids in diet causes phrynoderma or toad's skin.

Signs and Symptoms

Horny papular rashes on the posterior and lateral aspects of thighs and on the back and buttocks.

Recent studies have shown that phrynoderma in adults and children can be cured by administration of safflower seed oil along with vitamin B complex in diet. Safflower seed oil is rich in essential fatty acids.

Deficiency in fat may also result in deficiency of fat-soluble vitamins thereby affecting the growth and weight of children.

Management

20–30% of energy should come from fat in diet, foods added in diet are butter, ghee, and cooking oil.

Excessive Intake of Fat

- **Obesity:** Excess fat is stored in the adipose tissue. Normal storage of fat in adipose tissue is 10–15% of the body weight. When fat storage is >15%, it causes obesity. Most of the fat is in the form of triglycerides which can be synthesized by the human body.
- **Hypercholesterolemia and coronary heart disease:** Excess intake of fat increases blood cholesterol level which leads to atherosclerosis, i.e. narrowing of the arteries due to deposition of cholesterol in them. This causes diminished blood supply. This condition can lead to hypertension and coronary heart disease.
- **Fat and cancer:** Studies have shown that high intake of fat has association of colon, breast and uterine cancer.
- **Management:** Fat in diet should be reduced to 20 g/day. Red meat should be avoided. Daily exercise, low fat diet is advised.

Micronutrients

The micronutrients include minerals and vitamins.

DISEASES AND DISORDERS DUE TO IMBALANCE OF MINERALS

Deficiency of Calcium

Rickets

Deficiency of calcium can occur due to deficiency of Vitamin D, as deficiency of Vitamin D decreases the absorption of calcium. This leads to Rickets in children and osteomalacia in adults. Rickets develop in growing children due to defective mineralization of bones. This condition found normally in overcrowded areas where sunlight does not penetrate through fog or smoke. There is combined deficiency of vitamin D, calcium and phosphorus.

Signs and symptoms:

Failure to grow normally

- Bone deformities
- Large head
- Softened cranial bones
- Delayed closure of anterior fontanels
- Pigeon's chest, i.e., retraction of chest
- Deformities of weight-bearing joints

- Bowing of legs
- Knock knee
- Wrist, knees and ankles become prominent
- Widening of the ends of long bones
- Pot belly
- Lack of muscle tone
- Poorly developed muscles
- Delayed walking
- Restlessness and nervous irritability
- Raised level of serum alkaline phosphatase.

Management:

- Increasing the intake of milk and milk products. About 250 mL of fat free buffalo's milk is sufficient to correct the deficiency.
- Oral calcium supplements.
- Foods rich in calcium, e.g., ragi, banana, cereals and millets can be added in diet.
- Exposure to sunlight for 10–15 minutes daily helps in absorption of calcium and phosphorus from diet.
- Health education to the mothers regarding diet of the child to prevent from rickets.

Osteomalacia

It is also known as adult rickets. It occurs mostly in women who are not exposed to sunlight. As a result, calcium and phosphorus is not absorbed. There is decreased deposition of calcium and phosphorus on the bones.

Signs and symptoms:

- There is rheumatic type of pain in bones of legs
- Spine and pelvis bend into deformities
- Generalized weakness
- Difficulty in walking and climbing stairs
- Spontaneous multiple fractures may occur

Treatment:

The following are the preventive measures:

- Exposure to sunlight for 10–15 minutes daily.
- Adequate intake of calcium in diet, i.e. milk and milk products, millets, cereals, pulses, legumes, soybean turnips, reddish, cauliflower and amaranth are the richest sources of calcium.
- Taking supplement calcium and vitamin D under the guidance of physician.

Osteoporosis

It is a chronic disease that commonly affects the menopausal women and associated with aging also. In this complication, there is deficiency of vitamin D and decreased estrogen level. Calcium and phosphorus level decreased from the bones and bones become fragile and easily breakable. The onset of the disease is gradual and initially patient is asymptomatic.

Signs and symptoms:

As the disease progresses, bone deformities occur, and symptoms of pain, difficulty in walking and performing daily activities become painful.

Treatment:

This condition is irreversible but can be prevented. The treatment should be started before the menopause. Increase in daily intake of calcium and moderate exercise can prevent the occurrence of the disease. Nowadays, hormonal therapy along with estrogen and vitamin D is practiced to prevent osteoporosis.

Tetany

In this disease, there is a condition of diminished ionized serum calcium. There may be lack of calcium in diet.

Signs and symptoms:
- Muscle twitching, spasm
- Uncontrolled muscle contractions
- Convulsions may occur

Treatment:
As the condition is mostly due to hypoparathyroidism, the condition improves if parathyroid hormones are administered.

Hypercalcemia

It is due to increased level of blood calcium, which could be >10 mg%. In this calcium, level may be increased up to 15 mg%.

Normal value of blood calcium is 8 mg%.

Causes:
- Hyperactivity of parathyroid glands
- Overdose of vitamin D
- Milk alkalis syndrome hypocalcemia in cases when peptic ulcer is treated with soluble alkalis.

Signs and symptoms:
The most common complaints include dehydration and polyuria.

Treatment:
Calcitonin hormone reduces calcium level by inhibiting the bone resorption.

MINERALS AND THEIR DEFICIENCIES

Phosphorus

Deficiency of Phosphorus

Hypophosphatemia

Deficiency of phosphorus is rare as diet rich in calcium, vitamin and protein is also rich in phosphorus.

Symptoms:
- Poor mineralization of bones
- Poor growth
- Rickets in children
- Osteomalacia in adults. Management is same as that of calcium deficiency.

Magnesium

Deficiency Diseases

It may occur in chronic alcoholic, cirrhosis of liver, PEU and Malabsorption syndrome. Dietary deficiency is not known. Experimental study showed symptoms of deficiency in some patients causes:

- Depression
- Muscular weakness
- Nervous irritability
- Tremors
- Vertigo
- Delirium and liability to convulsion

Serum level of magnesium 1 mg%. Normal serum magnesium is 1.5–1.8 mg%, symptoms were cured within 4 hours after giving magnesium chloride.

High Intake

- Extreme thrust
- Feeling of excessive warmth's
- Drowsiness
- The condition is corrected by giving calcium gluconate.

Sodium

Deficiency Diseases

Sodium deficiency is seen in hot climate as due to sweating and excessive loss of water from the body, sodium is lost. Sodium is also lost from the body in the following conditions:

- Diarrhea
- Vomiting
- Severe dehydration
- Heat strokes
- Symptoms weakness muscle cramps.

Management:

- Plenty of lime juice with salt
- Fluids containing excess salt such as lassi or curd with salt.
- Soup containing plenty of salt
- If patient is not able to take orally, intravenous therapy of normal saline is given.

High intake:

Predisposes to edema and hypertension. It should be avoided.

Potassium

Deficiency Diseases

It is very rare and may occur in the following conditions:

- Severe malnutrition
- Chronic alcoholism
- Surgery
- In patients who are on diuretics and do not take oral potassium.

> **MUST KNOW**
>
> Normal serum level of potassium is 3.5–5 mEq/L

Symptoms:

- Weakness
- Muscular cramps
- Mental apathy
- Cardiac arrhythmias

Treatment:

- Potassium supplement, 1 g of potassium in fruit juice to patients who are on diuretics daily.
- Potassium chloride supplement intravenous after surgery, if potassium serum levels low.
- Malnutrition and alcoholic are treated with oral potassium with *Mausami or mosambi* juice, bananas, orange, apple and foods containing potassium, i.e., cereals, vegetables, fish and chicken.

DEFICIENCY DISEASES OF TRACE ELEMENTS OR MICRO ELEMENTS

Iron

Deficiency of Iron

Anemia

Anemia results due to the deficiency of iron. There is a decreased concentration of circulating hemoglobin <10 g%.

Signs and symptoms:

- Hemoglobin level is <10 g%
- Pallor of skin and conjunctiva and tongue
- General fatigue
- Breathlessness on exertion
- Edema of the ankles
- Reduced resistance to infection
- Decreased capacity of work performance.

Prevention and treatment:

- Supplementary iron tablets to growing children, menstruating girls and pregnant women.
- Nutritional education to the families regarding selections of food having rich iron content in the diet.
- Government of India launched a program on prevention of nutritional anemia, according to this program, young children, menstruating girls and pregnant women are given free iron tablets through all health centers. One tablet of iron and folic acids containing 60 mg elementary iron (180 mg of ferrous sulfate) and 0.5 mg folic acid should be given daily for 100 days.

Iodine

Deficiency of iodine causes goiter and cretinism. Iodine deficiency is found in hilly areas and areas where the soil content of iodine is low. In India, it is found in Kangra in the Himalayan belt.

Deficiency of Iodine

Goiter

Goiter is a condition resulted due to the deficiency of iodine in diet at places where the soil content of iodine is low and the foods and vegetables grown there have poor content of iodine. Due to lack of iodine, the size and number of epithelial cells of thyroid gland get enlarged. This condition is known as endemic goiter.

Signs and symptoms:

- Enlargement of thyroid
- Mental retardation
- Dwarfism
- Lethargy
- Congenital disorders
  - Cretinism
  - Deaf mutism
  - Spastic diplegia
- Abortion
- Stillbirth

Management:

- **Iodized table salt:** Government of India launched national iodine deficiency disease control program in 1986 by providing table salt fortified with iodine to control the deficiency.
- Iodine present in see fish, cod liver oil and traces in meat, milk and vegetables.

Cretinism

This condition occurs in infants when the pregnant women suffer from iodine deficiency.

Signs and symptoms:

- Low BMR
- Weakness
- Enlarged tongue
- Retarded skeletal growth
- Muscular flabbiness
- Thick lips
- Severe mental retardation.

Treatment:
Thyroid hormone given to infants in early stage improves the condition.

Fluorine

Deficiency of Fluorine

Dental Caries

It causes dental caries where water contains <0.5 mg of fluorine/L.
- **Treatment:** Addition of fluorine to drinking water containing 1 mg/L fluorine can reduce the incidence.
- **High intake**: It causes dental and skeletal fluorosis when the fluorine content is high in drinking water.

Dental Fluorosis

- Teeth lose their lustrous appearance
- Enamel becomes weak and there is loss of enamel leaving teeth dull and chalky.
- Yellow or brown staining of teeth occurs

Skeletal Fluorosis

Due to high content of fluorine in drinking water for a prolonged period results in pathological changes in the bones.

- Bone density increases due to hyper calcification of spine, pelvis and limbs.
- Ligament of spine gets calcified resulting into "poker back".
- Joints become stiff.
- Bending and squatting becomes impossible.

Prevention:

By removing the excess fluorine from drinking water by treatment with activated carbon or by some other suitable means reduces the incidence.

Zinc

Deficiency of Zinc

A diet with high phytate and fiber can interfere with zinc absorption by chelating and can cause zinc deficiency.

Signs and symptoms:

- Retarded growth
- Delayed wound healing
- Alopecia
- Skin lesions
- Loss of taste

Management:

Deficiency can be treated with oral zinc supplements in addition to balanced diet under the guidance of physician.

High Intake

Zinc supplements toxicity: High intake of zinc supplement interferes with copper absorption. Welders may inhale zinc toxic fumes while welding.

Signs and symptoms:

Signs and symptoms of zinc toxicity are:
- Vomiting
- Cramps
- Diarrhea

Management:

During welding, proper precautions should be taken to prevent inhaling toxic zinc fumes. Zinc supplements should be taken only under the supervision of physician.

Copper

Deficiency of Copper

It is very rare but can occur in infants as anemia who are exclusively fed on milk diet.

Deficiency is also seen in nephrosis PEU and in Wilson's disease.

DISEASES AND DISORDERS DUE TO IMBALANCE OF VITAMINS

Fat Soluble Vitamins

Deficiency of Vitamin A

It can occur due to insufficient intake of vitamin A and protein in diet.

Signs and symptoms:

- Night-blindness
- Xerophthalmia (Drying of eyeball)
- Bitot's spot (Dirty, foamy raised spots on conjunctiva)
- Dermatitis
- Growth failure
- Corneal ulcers
- Keratomalacia (Softening of cornea)

Prevention and control:

- Nutritional education to parents.
- Effective implementation of national vitamin A prophylaxis program.
- Protection of children from PEU, diarrhea measles and respiratory tract infection.
- Administration of 200,000 IU of vitamin A, every 6 months to children up to age of 6 years. First dose of supplement is given at 12 to 23 months of age.
- During serious deficiency administration of Vitamin A, 5,000 to 10,000 microgram for several weeks.

Hypervitaminosis A

Excess vitamin A causes headache, nausea, vomiting, drowsiness, loss of appetite and pains in the bones.

Vitamin D Deficiency

Vitamin D deficiency causes reduced absorption of calcium and phosphors from small intestine and leads to incomplete mineralization of bones and teeth. Bones become unable to bear the weight and skeletal deformities occur due to:

- Inadequate use of vitamin D.
- Overcrowded and dark places where sunlight does not penetrate.
- Drugs that interfere with the activity of vitamin D.

Vitamin D deficiency disease in children is known as rickets and in adult as osteomalacia. These diseases are discussed under the deficiency diseases of calcium.

Vitamin E Deficiency

Effects of vitamin E deficiency are:

- Sterility
- Severe deficiency increases hemolysis of red cells and causes anemia
- May lead to muscular dystrophy

Prevention and treatment:

Vitamin E 10 mg/day for children. 25 mg/day for adolescents and adults. Nutrients containing adequate vitamin E are egg yolk, butter, wheat germ oil, sunflower seed and sunflower seed oil, should be supplied in diet.

Vitamin K Deficiency

Vitamin K deficiency is uncommon in adults. Newborn babies may have this deficiency due to immaturity of liver, sterile intestinal flora and minimum stores of prothrombin. As preventive measure 1mg of vitamin K is given to all newborn babies.

In adults it may occur due to use of antibiotics and sulfur drugs for a long time. The patient can have prolonged bleeding. If injury takes place due to lack of prothrombin, bleeding and clotting time is increased. Patients suffering from vitamin K deficiency, if going for surgery, then Vitamin K 10 mg IM is given to him/her before surgery. The condition improves after discontinuing antibiotic and sulfa drugs as these drugs destroy the normal intestinal flora.

Water Soluble Vitamins

Vitamin B Deficiency

- Vitamin B$_1$ (Thiamine) deficiency can occur due to inadequate intake of calories
- Severe diarrhea
- Vomiting
- Alcoholics are also susceptible to deficiency.

Beriberi

The deficiency of thiamine causes beriberi and Wernick's encephalopathy. Beriberi is of two types: dry beriberi and wet beriberi.

- **Symptoms of dry beriberi**
  - Fatigue and loss of strength
  - Lack of interest
  - Emotional instability
  - Depression
  - Anger and fear
  - Loss of appetite
  - Loss of weight
  - Wasting of muscles
  - Difficulty in walking
  - Polyneuritis
  - Numbness of extremities
  - Cramps
- **Symptoms of wet beriberi**
  - In addition to the symptoms of dry beriberi the other features are:
  - Severe edema
  - Cardiomegaly
  - Palpitation
  - Breathlessness
  - Mental confusion.
- **Infantile beriberi:** This condition occurs in 2–4 months' old infants who are breastfed by mothers having thiamine deficiency.

Wernick's Encephalopathy

This is seen in alcoholics.

- Symptoms
  - Ophthalmoplegia
  - Polyneuritis
  - Ataxia
  - Mental deterioration

- Prevention
  - Nutritional education to the people about the importance of well-balanced diet.
  - Supplement of thiamine to high-risk group.

Deficiency of Riboflavin (Vitamin B$_2$)

Riboflavin deficiency occurs in association with other B complex vitamins. It is seen in people whose staple food is rice.

Signs and symptoms:
- Cracking of lips at the corner (cheilosis).
- Angular stomatitis, i.e. cracking in the skin at the corners of month.
- Tongue becomes swollen and purple, i.e. glossitis.
- Itching, burning and watering of eyes.
- Loss of visual acuity
- Corneal vascularization
- Greasy eruptions of the skin and nasal angles
- Scrotal dermatitis

Treatment:
- 5 mg of riboflavin orally to children for one month.
- 10 mg riboflavin is given orally to adults for one month.

Prevention:
Nutritional education to the families

Deficiency of Nicotinic Acid or Niacin

- **Initial signs and symptoms:**
  - Muscular weakness
  - Anorexia
  - Indigestion
  - Rough skin
- **Severe deficiency leads to pellagra and characterized by:**
  - Diarrhea
  - Dermatitis
  - Dementia
- **Treatment:**
  - Injectable nicotinic acid 50 mg BD for one weak followed by 100 mg BD for 3 weeks orally.
  - Soft and balanced diet.
  - Nutritional education.

Deficiency of Pyridoxine (Vitamin B$_6$)

Deficiency is more common in Tuberculosis patients who are on isoniazid and not taking supplementary pyridoxine orally. This is also found in women who are on oral contraceptives.

- **Signs and symptoms:**
  - Hypochromic anemia
  - Peripheral neuritis in case of tuberculosis patients on isoniazid
  - Nervous irritability and convulsions in children
  - Seborrhea, like skin lesions around the eyes and nose
- **Treatment:**
  - Oral pyridoxine
  - Nutritional education
  - Balanced diet

Deficiency of Pantothenic Acid

This deficiency is very rare.

- **Symptoms include:**
  - Fatigue
  - Nausea
  - Vomiting
  - Tremors of out-stretched hands
  - Burning feet
  - Depression and insomnia
- **Treatment and prevention:**
  - Nutritional education
  - Diet supplements

Deficiency of Folate (Folic Acid)

This kind of deficiency is found in pregnancy and lactation.

Signs and symptoms:

- Megaloblastic anemia
- Diarrhea
- Distension and flatulence
- Lethargy and tiredness
- Infertility

Prevention:

- Folic acid supplements during pregnancy, lactation and during rapid growth of children.
- Under national nutritional anemia prophylaxis program, supplements of iron and folic acid tablets containing 60 mg of iron, 180 mg ferrous sulfate, 0.5 mg of folic acid are distributed in all health centers to the adolescent girls, pregnant and lactating women.

Deficiency of B_{12} (Cyanocobalamin)

Dietary deficiency is rarely found in nonvegetarian. Deficiency of vitamin B_{12} causes pernicious anemia.

Pernicious Anemia

The deficiency of vitamin B_{12} causes pernicious anemia. In pernicious anemia, vitamin B_{12} is not absorbed due to the absence of intrinsic factor in stomach.

- **Signs and symptoms:**
    - Pallor of the skin and eyes
    - Raw and red tongue
    - Mouth ulcers
    - Numbness and tingling sensations in the fingers
    - Anorexia
    - Dysphonia
    - Abdominal discomfort
    - Mental depression
- **Treatment:** Injection B_{12} throughout life as oral doses cannot be absorbed due to lack of intrinsic factor.

Deficiency of Ascorbic Acid (Vitamin C)

Deficiency of Vitamin D Causes Scurvy

Scurvy

- **Signs and symptoms of scurvy:**
    - Poor wound healing
    - Increased susceptibility to infection
    - Bleeding gums
    - Easy bruising and pin point bleeding under the skin
    - Painful joints
    - Anemia.

Scurvy is of two types:
1. **Infantile scurvy is characterized by:**
    - Loss of appetite
    - Listlessness
    - The infant cries when his arms and legs are moved due to swollen joints.
    - Bleeding from gums and gums are swollen.
    - Bleeding under the skin
    - Convulsions may occur in advanced cases.
2. **Scurvy in adults is characterized by:**
    - General weakness
    - Spongy bleeding gums
    - Joints swollen and tender
    - Hemorrhage under the skin
    - Loose teeth with desorbed dentine

Treatment
- **Adults:** Injection vitamin C 500 mg IV once a day for one week followed by tablet of vitamin C 500 mg OD for 1 month.
- **Infants:** Injection vitamin C 100 mg IV OD for 1 week followed by tablet of vitamin (100 mg 01) for 1 month.
- **Diet:** Rich in vitamin C

FOOD ALLERGY

Food allergy (Fig. 19.1) is defined as an abnormal immune response to food when the body's immune system sees a certain food as harmful and reacts by causing symptoms.

Allergens: Foods that cause allergic reactions are called allergens.

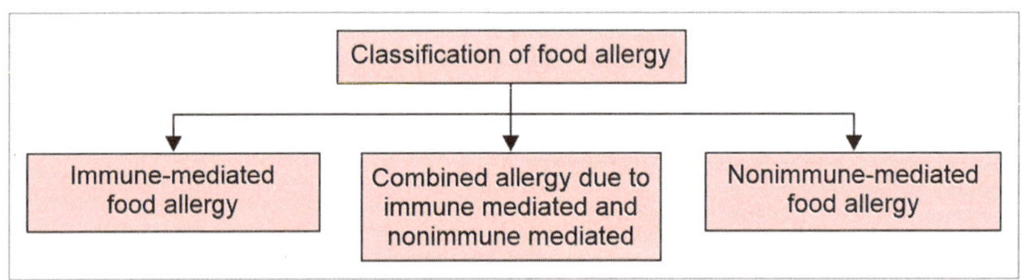

Fig. 19.1: Classification of food allergy

Immune-Mediated Food Allergy

In this type of food allergy, body's immune system reacts with food allergens and produces immunoglobulin antibodies lgE

The most common food allergens are:

- Eggs   — mostly in children
- Fish   — children and adults
- Milk   — cause allergy in all age groups
- Soybean — mostly in children
- Wheat   — people of all age groups

Symptoms

As food allergy is immune mediated, the symptoms may vary from mild to severe life-threatening condition.

- Urticaria
- Itching of the mouth, throat, eyes, skin
- Abdominal cramps, nausea, vomiting, diarrhea
- Nasal congestion
- Running nose
- Swelling of eyelids, face, lips, tongue
- Headache, cold, asthma
- Tightness in the chest
- Shortness of breath
    - Angioedema
    - Severe bronchospasm
    - Choking and fainting

Management

- Immediate resuscitation of the patient includes the following treatments:
  - Antiallergic drugs
  - Bronchodilators
  - Steroids
  - Oxygen inhalation
  - Clear airway by gentle suctioning of throat
  - Maintenance of vital parameters
- Stop all food allergens
- Careful history of allergy
- Patient should be referred to allergist for careful evaluation and management.

Nonimmune-Mediated Food Allergy

In this type of food allergy, other parts of the body's immune system react to certain foods. This reaction causes symptoms but immunoglobulin IgE antibodies are not formed.

Symptoms

The symptoms are similar to immune-mediated food allergy, but less severe:

- Urticaria
- Severe itching
- Abdominal discomfort
- Nausea, vomiting, diarrhea
- Nasal congestion
- Eczema

Combined Food Allergy

It is due to immune-mediated and non-immune-mediated response.

In this type, there may be immune-mediated food allergy along with nonimmune-mediated response to the allergen.

Symptoms

Combined

Diagnosis

It is very difficult to distinguish between the three types of foods allergy. Diagnosis can be made from:

- History of allergy after taking specific foods
- Allergy test

Gluten Intolerance

Gluten is found in variety of food items and processed foods, such as roti, rava, crackers, cookies, cakes pasta, bread and cereals, wheat is also minor ingredients in condiments, marinades soya sauce, hard candies, low-fat products, etc.

Patient is put on gluten-free diet, all products containing wheat flour or wheat are eliminated from the diet, as wheat is the staple food in many states of north India. Patient is advised to have the following varieties to compensate wheat.

- Besan chapatis
- Maize, Bajra and Jowar roti
- Can have rice

Rest of the nutrients, i.e., vegetables, fruits protein and other carbohydrates can be taken as usual. Only wheat is replaced by maize, bajra, jowar and rice for life-long period. Gluten-free diet is low in vitamin B, calcium, vitamin B_6 riboflavin niacin, folic acid iron and zinc, magnesium, and fibers. Diet should be supplemented with nutrients rich in vitamin B, calcium iron, zinc magnesium and fibers. There are many wheat-free products made from alternative flours. The availability of gluten-free foods can also benefit people with wheat allergy.

Cause

There is an abnormal immune reaction to gluten and affects 1% of the population. The inflammatory reaction of mucosa of intestine interferes in the absorption of nutrients.

Symptoms

- Nausea
- Vomiting
- Fever
- Pain abdomen
- Diarrhea
- Urticaria

Management

- Careful history from the patient about foods, which cause these symptoms.
- **Allergy test:** After confirmation of the allergy test, patient is placed on elimination diet.

Diet Modification in Gluten Intolerance

Diet modification in gluten intolerance. Gluten intolerance is non-IgE mediated food allergy. It is common in adults and children with celiac disease.

A list of gluten-free diet is given in Table 19.18 for adult and children.

TABLE 19.18: Gluten free-diet

Food items	4–6 years child		Adult	
	Vegetarian	Nonvegetarian	Vegetarian	Nonvegetarian
Rice or corn	100 g	100 g	300 g	300 g
Dal split (legume)	20 g	–	40 g	–
Milk (half fat)	1000 mL	600 mL	1000 mL	600 mL
Meat and liver	–	50 g	–	100 g
Egg	–	30 g	–	50 g
Cheese	30 g	–	50 g	–
Fleshy fruit: Banana, mango, apple, papaya	150 g	150 g	200 g	200 g
Fruit juice	100 mL	100 mL	200 mL	200 mL
Tender vegetables	30 g	30 g	50 g	50 g
Sugar	30 g	30 g	40 g	40 g

Gluten-Free Diet for Children 4–6 Years and Adults

There is allergy to gluten, so wheat and commercial products that contain wheat flour or maida, are completely eliminated from diet.

- In case of lactose intolerance, milk is eliminated and soya milk may be substituted.
- In case of protein intolerance, according to the allergy test, that specific protein is eliminated and substituted by other protein or synthetic protein.

Food Intolerance—Inborn Errors of Metabolism

The Inborn errors of metabolism can result due to:

- Anatomical abnormalities of small intestine
- Deficiency or complete absence of some digestive enzymes

As a result of inborn errors of metabolism, the absorption of one or more nutrients is poor or not absorbed.

Signs and Symptoms

- Diarrhea (Steatorrhea, i.e., loss of excess fat in stool)
- Abdominal distension
- Loss of weight
- Anemia
- Hypoproteinemia
- Deficiency of vitamins and minerals.

Other features: Stomatitis, glossitis, dermatitis, paresthesia and pain in loins

Food intolerance due to inborn errors of metabolism can be:

- Gluten intolerance
- Lactose intolerance
- Protein intolerance

Management

After proper diagnosis and the type of foods that are not digested due to lack or absence of particular enzymes, those foods are eliminated and substituted by other varieties to provide those nutrients.

Lactose Intolerance

This occurs mostly in children.

Symptoms

- Abdominal discomfort
- Flatulence
- Distension of abdomen
- Nausea, vomiting
- Diarrhea

Management

Elimination of milk, i.e. cow/buffalo milk from his diet and all milk products.

Diet Modification in Lactose Intolerance

Substitute for cow's milk: Soya milk and its products, i.e. curd, soya, paneer and sweets made out of soya milk can be added in the diet in place of cow's milk, children are likely to face the deficiency of calcium, Vitamin D, and vitamin A, riboflavin, so the food containing above nutrients are added in the diet, i.e. ragi, carrot and green leafy vegetables.

Protein Intolerance

It is a disorder that results from an adverse effect of the ingestion of food proteins. It develops through immunological, nonimmunological, metabolic, genetic, and pharmacological mechanisms.

Signs and Symptoms

It is often associated with gastrointestinal symptoms.

Diet Modification in Protein Intolerance

After allergy test about the type of protein, which causes allergy is eliminated from diet. The synthetic preparation of protein is added to diet to meet protein requirement.

Summary

- Energy is the capacity to do work. It is measured in kilocalories. Joule is the international unit of energy.
- Energy requirement varies according to the age group and type of work.
- Body mass index **is** the ratio of weight in kg to the square of height in meters.
- Basal metabolic rate is the minimum amount of energy required to carry out vital functions at rest. It depends upon age, sex, body surface, area, hormones, exercise, diet, body temperature, climate, pregnancy and lactation.
- Balanced diet is one which contains all the nutrients for growth, development and maintenance of body functions.
- Budgeting of food is the financial planning for food, i.e., how much money can be spent on food and utilization of that money in such a way that all important nutrients essential for body are included in diet.
- Diseases and disorders caused by imbalance of nutrients are either due to deficiency or excess.
- Food allergy is an abnormal immune response to food.
- Food allergy can be immune-mediated and nonimmune-mediated.
- Those food substances that cause allergy has to be completely eliminated and substituted by alternative foods.

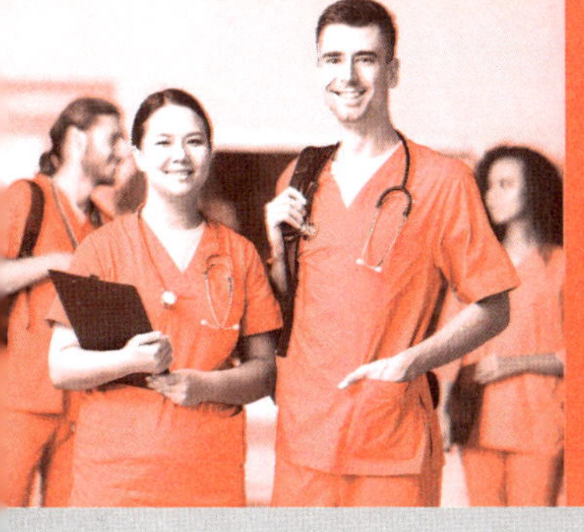

LONG ANSWER TYPE QUESTIONS

1. Explain about the energy requirement of different age groups.
2. Explain the deficiency diseases of protein.

SHORT ANSWER TYPE QUESTIONS

1. Write short notes on:
   a. Body mass index
   b. Basal metabolic rate
   c. Balanced diet
2. Define budgeting of food. Explain the factors to be considered in budgeting of food.
3. Write the signs/symptoms and management of iron deficiency.
4. Write the modification in gluten intolerance.

MULTIPLE CHOICE QUESTIONS

1. **The amount of heat required to raise the temperature of 1 kg of water through 1°C is called:**
   a. Kilocalorie
   b. Calorie
   c. Joule
   d. Kilojoule

2. **One of the following is not an energy yielding food:**
   a. Carbohydrate
   b. Fat
   c. Protein
   d. Vitamins and minerals

3. **A woman weighing 65 kg, height 155 cm will have BMI:**
   a. 21
   b. 23
   c. 27
   d. 29

4. **The amount of protein in daily energy intake should be:**
   a. 10–15%
   b. 15–20%
   c. 20–25%
   d. 25–30%

5. **Which of the following is essential for food guides:**
   a. Knowledge of RDA
   b. Knowledge of food groups
   c. Knowledge of food exchanges system
   d. All of the above

6. **Which of the following is not the aim of meal planning?**
   a. To meet the nutritional needs of the normal persons and the patients
   b. To plan meal according to food cost
   c. To subdue the appetite so that minimum diet is consumed
   d. To provide variety and to improve the quality of food

7. **Diabetes mellitus is caused when glucose level exceeds:**
   a. 140 mg%   b. 160 mg%
   c. 180 mg%   d. 200 mg%

8. **Fat soluble vitamins are:**
   a. ADEK   b. ABEK
   c. ABDK   d. CDEK

9. **Which of the following does not belong to B complex group?**
   a. Ascorbic acid   b. Nicotinic acid
   c. Folic acid   d. Thiamine mine

10. **One of the following is not a major mineral:**
    a. Sodium   b. Potassium
    c. Zinc   d. Magnesium

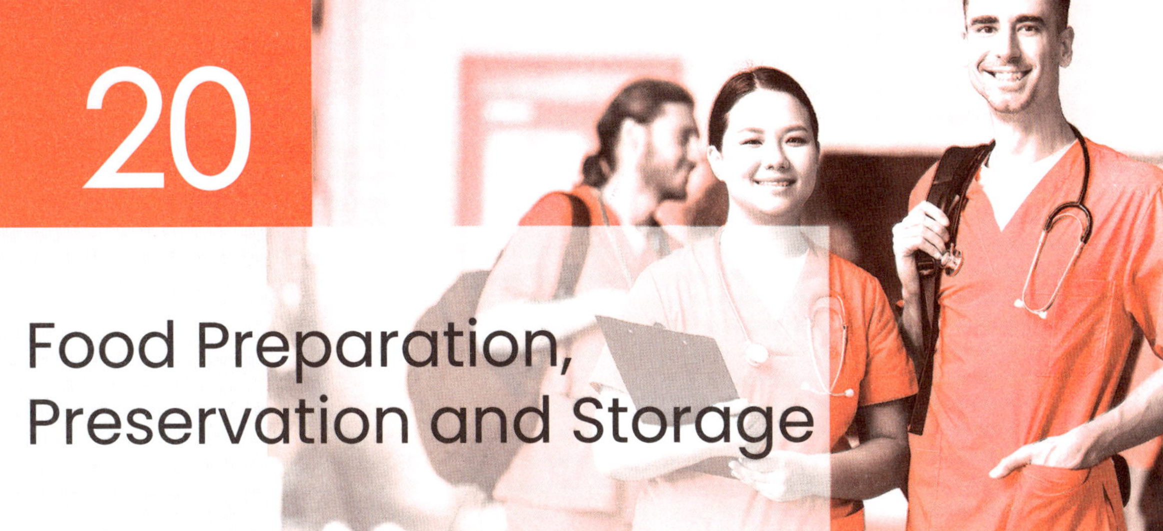

20

Food Preparation, Preservation and Storage

LEARNING OBJECTIVES

After the completion of the unit, the readers will be able to:
- Enlist the principles of cooking.
- Describe various methods of cooking.
- Identify the effects of cooking on various nutrients.
- Describe the methods of food preservation and storage.
- Explain food adulteration and acts related to it.

UNIT OUTLINE

- Introduction
- Cooking
- Safe Food Handling and Health of Food Handlers
- Food Preservation
- Food Storage
- Methods of Food Storage
- Ill Effects of Poorly Stored Food
- Food Adulteration and Related Act

KEY TERMS

Adulteration: Addition or subtraction of anything from the food by unfair means which affects its nutritional value or quality.

Aflatoxins: A group of mycotoxins produced by *Aspergillus flavus* and *Aspergillus parasiticus*.

Baking: Cooking by dry heat in hot air oven.

Blanching: A process in which foods are immersed in hot boiling water for a few minutes prior to processing (freezed, dried or canned).

Food additives: Non-nutritious substances which are intentionally added to food in small quantities to improve its appearance, texture and storage properties.

Grilling: Cooking by direct heat either in a grill or on flame.

Pasteurization: A process in which packaged and nonpackaged foods (such as milk and fruit juice) are treated with mild heat (<100°C) to eliminate pathogens and extend shelf-life.

Simmering: Cooking below the boiling point.

Sprouting: Allowing the soaked whole grains to germinate.

Stewing: Simmering near boiling point in less water for a prolonged period.

INTRODUCTION

Food maintenance involves the care and treatment of food so that it stays in good condition for a long time. Food storage is the storage of food stored or purchased in a safe and suitable environment. Food preservation is a more advanced process that requires learning and experience to master. In this chapter there is discussion on the different aspects of food preparation, preservation and storage.

COOKING

Cooking is an art in itself and can be defined as the process of preparing food with any method of heat application. It is done in many ways depending upon the availability of food stuffs, culture, religion and food habits. But cooking eventually fulfills the nutritional needs.

Purposes of Cooking

- Cooking improves flavor and palatability of food.
- It makes the food easily digestible.
- Cooking kills the microorganisms, parasites, ova, and eggs, thereby making food safe for consumption
- Cooking increases the availability of some nutrients. Trypsin inhibitor present in protein food is destroyed by cooking which makes trypsin freely available to the body
- Cooking in different ways provides variety in the diet
- Cooking eliminates indigestible material
- Cooking increases appetite and acceptability of food.

Principles

- Cooking should be done at a hygienic place. There should be sufficient light.
- Cooking area should be at a reasonable distance from sanitary area.
- Handling and storing of food should be near the cooking area.
- Always wash the vegetables and fruits before peeling and cutting to prevent the loss of water-soluble vitamins.
- Always cook in minimal water to preserve the vitamins.
- Cook in a covered pan except green vegetables.
- Foods must not be overcooked or undercooked to prevent the loss of vitamins and later to control the microbial count.
- Do not add alkalis like sodium bicarbonate to the food while cooking as alkalis destroy vitamin B and vitamin C.
- Always cook in pressure cooker. It will help in retaining the vitamins.
- Avoid cutting into small pieces as more surface area is exposed.
- Soak pulses and rice in water before cooking. It reduces the cooking time.
- Store foods in a refrigerator, covered with a lid or aluminum foil to retain nutrients.
- The persons involved in cooking should maintain cooking hygiene by keeping the foods clean and covered.

Methods of Cooking

Different methods of cooking are used as per the requirement (Fig. 20.1). Some of them are as follows:

- **Boiling:** In this method, the foods are cooked in water at 100°C. Rice, grams, pulses, roots and tubers are cooked by this method. Boiling should be done in minimum amount of water to prevent the loss of vitamins.
- **Simmering:** This method involves cooking below the boiling point of water, i.e., at about 84°C. It helps in preserving the essential vitamins. Fish and meat are cooked by this method as higher temperature causes hardening of fibers of such foods.
- **Steaming:** This method is used to cook food in direct heat steaming. The temperature attained is >100°C. Pressure cooker is used to cook foods by steam under pressure. This method is very effective as it saves fuel, time and preserves the nutrients.
- **Stewing:** It is the method of cooking vegetables, fruits, and other foods in small quantity of water at a lower temperature than boiling, usually at 80°C. The foods to be cooked are covered with little water in a pan and then covered with lid. Cooking is done for prolonged low degree heat. The nutrients are not lost, but are present in the liquid. This stewing of fruits and vegetables is used for small children and old people with dentures. Stewing ensures high nutrition.
- **Frying:** It refers to cooking food in oil. It is of two types:
    i. **Deep fry:** In deep frying, foods are immersed in a large amount of hot oil. This method is used for making pakoras, samosa, puri, cutlet, kachori, etc. The principle of deep frying is that oil must be hot enough to prevent absorption of oil in the food.

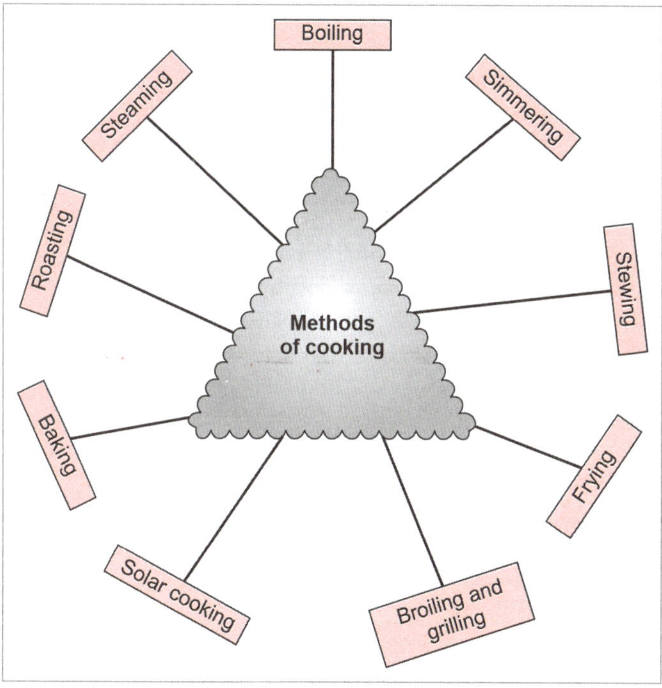

Fig. 20.1: Methods of cooking

ii. **Shallow fry:** It requires less quantity of oil and suitable for making omlet, dosa, parantha, and precooked food.

- **Roasting:** In this method, the foods are directly exposed to heat or flame after smearing with little fat. This makes the food tender. Chicken and tender meat are cooked by this method. This is also called "Barbeque". This is the best method to cook as it reduces the risk of cardiovascular disorders, obesity and hypertension.
- **Baking:** In this method, the foods are cooked by dry heat in hot air oven. Food is enclosed in hot air in an oven and heat from all sides is utilized for cooking. Temperature for baking is 250–500°F. Baking is an expensive and slow process. Foods cooked by this method are cakes, pastry, patties, bread and biscuits.
- **Broiling and grilling:** It refers to cooking by direct heat. Grill pans are used to cook on direct flame. It is a quick method of cooking for tender foods like cheese, brinjal, tomatoes, kabab, etc.
- **Solar cooking:** This method is used in areas where direct sunlight is available. In this method, solar energy is utilized for cooking foods. Solar cookers and closed containers are used, which absorb maximum solar energy. This is a very simple and economical method, but takes longer time for cooking.

Effects of Cooking on Food

- Cooking softens the texture of food, thereby increasing its taste.
- It makes the food easily digestible.
- It helps in the destruction of microorganisms present in food.
- There is a loss of some water-soluble vitamins during cooking.
- Fat-soluble vitamins have no effect of heat; so, they are not lost.
- Antitrypsin substance present in pulses is destroyed to make the trypsin available for digestion.
- Complex proteins are broken down into simple proteins.
- Overcooking destroys essential nutrients.
- Undercooking prevents killing of microorganisms present in the food.

Effects of Cooking on Different Types of Foods

- Effects of cooking on different types of foods are as follows:
  - **Effects of cooking on cereals:** Cereals and millets contain starch with little protein enclosed within the cell wall of cellulose. Cereals are the chief staple food and cooked before consumption. Boiling causes gelatinization process in cereals in which starch grains swell and burst the cellulose. Rice is cooked in double quantity of water. Excessive use of water during cooking results in loss of thiamine. If sodium bicarbonate is used in cooking, it destroys thiamine.
    After gelatinization, cereals become easily digestible as the protein content on their coating coagulates. Cooking cereals with pulses improves the quality of nutrients and prevents the protein deficiency diseases.
  - **Effects of cooking on pulses:** Antitrypsin substance present in pulses inhibits complete digestion of proteins. On cooking, antitrypsin substance is destroyed. Pulses must be thoroughly cooked before consumption.
  - **Effects of cooking on green leafy vegetables:** If green vegetables like spinach are cooked in excess water, the minerals and vitamins are lost. If baking soda is used, it destroys thiamine.

Vitamin A is not lost during cooking in water. To preserve minerals and vitamins, vegetables should be cooked in pressure cooker using less water.

- **Effects of cooking on roots and tubers:** Roots and tubers like potatoes and yam contain abundant starch as compared to other vegetables. These must be thoroughly cooked for complete gelatinization. These vegetables must be boiled slowly as rapid boiling breaks the mineral rich skin; less water should be used for cooking to avoid the loss of minerals.

- **Effects of cooking on fruits:** Fruits mainly contain water, vitamins and minerals; and protein and fat content is less. Carbohydrates, in the form of sugars, are present in varying amount in fruits. Citrus fruits are rich in vitamin C and potassium. Majority of fruits are eaten raw and supply good amount of nutrients. But during preparation of fruit stews, vitamin C and little amount of sugar are lost. Fruits contain plenty of fibers and cooking reduces this level and increases the digestibility.

- **Effects of cooking on meat, fish and liver:** Animal foods contain fat and protein. On cooking, fat melts, and the protein and fibers are lost to some extent in soup. On grilling the meat, the protein on surface coagulates and seals all juices inside the meat. During boiling or stewing, minerals are lost. Prolonged cooking makes its texture hard and indigestible. Meat soup is rich in minerals, vitamins and protein. Fish loses its flavors on cooking but digestibility improves. Liver, kidney and other organs are rich in minerals and protein but difficult to digest.

- **Effects of heat on milk:** On heating, a layer of fat forms on the surface. Taste also changes on heating. If cream is removed from surface after boiling, it reduces casein (protein) and fat content of milk. Thiamine and vitamin C are lost. The microorganisms are killed; and enzymes and lactic acid bacteria are not destroyed present in milk. On boiling, vitamin K is conserved.

Effects of Cooking on Various Nutrients

Effects of cooking on various types of nutrients are discussed as follows (Fig. 20.2):

- **Effects on carbohydrates:** Cereals and starch granules absorb water and swell up to burst finally. This process is known as gelatinization. Cooked starch is digested more easily than raw starch. As the carbohydrates are the main source of energy, they must be cooked properly for effective digestion in the gut.

- **Effects on protein:** Proteins coagulate and shrink in moist heat. Cooked proteins are digested easily, proteins are a valuable body building food and secondary source of energy in carbohydrate deficiency. Overheating of protein foods result in destruction of their nutritive values. They should be properly cooked for effective digestion.

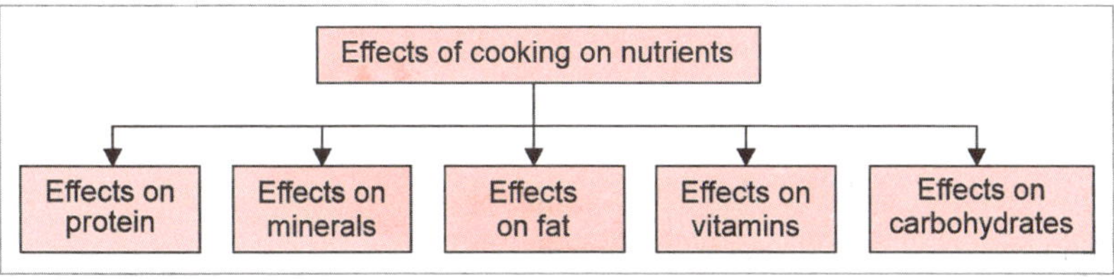

Fig. 20.2: Effects of cooking on various nutrients

- **Effect on fats:** When fats are cooked at normal temperature, they do not undergo any change in their chemical composition during cooking. However, on overheating while deep frying, they lose some of their essential fatty acids; and some polymerized harmful substances are produced which have harmful effect on body.
- **Effect on vitamins:** Water-soluble vitamins B groups and vitamin C are lost during cooking and loss from dissolved water. Vitamins are destroyed if alkalis are used in cooking like sodium bicarbonate. Fat-soluble vitamins are slightly destroyed due to oxidation by air, when foods cooked in water. But frying or roasting vegetables causes enough loss of vitamin A and carotene.
- **Effects on minerals:** Minerals present in foods like calcium, phosphorus, iron, sodium, potassium, magnesium and trace elements are lost when cooked in excess water for prolonged period. But some of the minerals are incorporated back while cooking in hard water, calcium is incorporated back and iron is incorporated by cooking in iron vessels.

SAFE FOOD HANDLING AND HEALTH OF FOOD HANDLERS

Safe food handling is the basic step to prevent foodborne diseases in the food industry as well as at household level. Food can get contaminated at any stage right from storage, cooking, preservation and distribution. The contaminated food can cause various foodborne diseases and food poisoning.

Points to be Kept in Mind for Safe Food Handling

The following points must be observed for safe food handling:
- **Clean storage place:** The place for storing food should be clean and properly sanitized.
- **Food hygiene:** The perishable foods start deteriorating immediately if not properly preserved. Fruits, vegetables, milk and meat should be kept at a low temperature in refrigerator.

The food handlers suffering from any infectious disease should be excluded from food handling.
- **Control of rats, rodents and insects:** They should not have access to food storage or preparation places.
- Sanitation of all work surfaces, utensils and equipment should be ensured.
- Use separate equipment, utensils, knives and cutting board for raw foods.
- All raw vegetables and fruits should be thoroughly washed before use.
- Periodical medical examination of the food handlers should be conducted to exclude the carriers of the disease.
- After cooking food, it should be covered and kept at a safe place.
- Safe water should be used for cooking food.
- Milk, milk products and eggs should be pasteurized.
- Food must be thoroughly cooked. Most of the food poisoning organisms are killed at 60°C.
- Foods not eaten immediately should be kept in cold storage to prevent bacterial contamination.
- Cooking and eating on the same day is a golden rule.

Health Education to Food Handlers

- Food handlers should be educated regarding personal hygiene, clean habits and food hygiene. They should be made to practice the following:
  - Hands should be scrubbed and washed with soap and water immediately after going to toilet.

- Finger nails should be trimmed to make them free from dirt.
- Hair should be covered with cap.
- Apron and gloves should be used while preparing food and serving. Smoking, coughing and sneezing in the food premises should be forbidden.

Health of Food Handlers

Health of food handlers is of paramount importance as the diseases, such as typhoid and paratyphoid fever, viral, hepatitis, diarrhea, dysentery and worm infestations and tuberculosis, are spread through them if they are carriers of the diseases or suffering from these diseases. The following practices are to be carried out to prevent the spread of diseases through them:

- At the time of employment, complete medical examination has to be carried out including blood, urine and stool test and chest X-ray to exclude the respiratory tract diseases.
- Any person with a previous history of typhoid, fever, chronic dysentery should not be employed in eating establishment.
- Persons suffering from skin diseases, ear discharge or infected wound should not be permitted to handle food or utensils.
- Health education regarding personal hygiene should be frequently reinforced. Healthy habits should be inculcated.
- Every 3 months, their medical examination has to be carried out including urine, stool and blood test to rule out any infection.
- Coughing, sneezing and cigarette smoking should be prohibited in the premises of area where food is prepared and distributed.
- Any person suffering from diseases that can be transmitted through food and coughing, sneezing should be treated immediately and excluded from place of work till he/she is clear of infection.
- Periodical immunization during the outbreak of cholera, viral hepatitis, typhoid and paratyphoid should be done for all the workers engaged in food preparation and distribution.
- Hand washing after toilet, covering hair with cap and use of apron and gloves should be strictly implemented.

FOOD PRESERVATION

Food preservation can be defined as the science involving application of scientific and engineering principles to the practical control of food destruction.

Purposes of Food Preservation

- To have all types of foods available throughout the year, i.e., to make non-seasonal foods also available.
- Readymade canned foods save time and energy.
- Variety of foods are available for consumption.
- To prevent wastage of food, due to spoilage or destruction.
- To preserve foods for future use.
- To make commercial profit.
- To export the surplus foods.
- To preserve the taste, odor and flavor of food.

Methods of Food Preservation

Methods of food preservation are shown in Figure 20.3.

- **Chemical preservation:** In this method, certain chemicals are added to the food products to prevent the growth of microorganisms. The chemical preservatives include benzoic acid, citric acid, ascorbic acid, sulfur dioxide, sodium benzoate, nitrates, etc. These chemicals extend the shelf life of the foods.

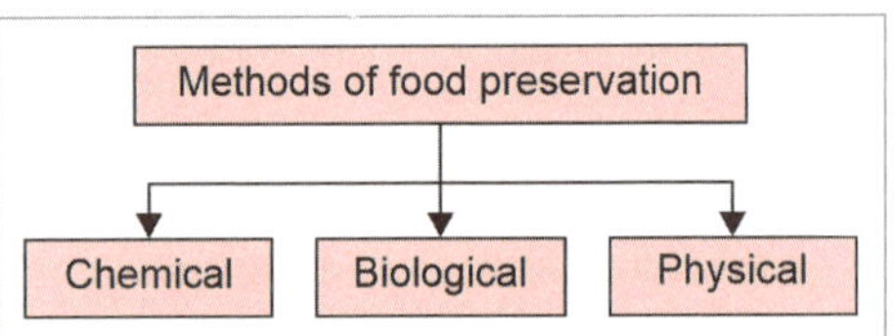

Fig. 20.3: Methods of food preservation

  Some preservatives, e.g., antioxidants, ascorbic acid, butylated hydroxyanisole, are used in fats and oils to prevent rancidity. Smoking process in meat contains formaldehyde and phenols as preservatives. Some foods are pickled or fermented for long-term use. Jams, murabbas, dried vegetables, salted fish, squash and fruit juice are examples of chemical preservation.

- **Biological preservation:** In this method, the enzymatic action involves alcoholic or acidic fermentation. In this type of preservation, microorganisms are used to increase the palatability, nutritive value and shelf life of foods such as bread, wine, tea, coffee, alcoholic drinks.

- **Physical preservation:** This is the traditional method, most commonly used at household level. This is a simple and economical method. It involves the basic skills as follows:
  - Increasing energy level, temporarily by heating and irradiation.
  - Controlling reduction of water content by air drying and freeze drying.
  - Use of protective packages.

  Using heat for preservation includes the following methods:
  - Cooking
  - Blanching
  - Pasteurization
  - Sterilization
  - Irradiation
  - Dehydration

Household Methods of Food Preservation

- **Cooking:** It is done by various methods like boiling, frying, stewing, simmering, roasting and baking. The cooked foods can be stored for prolonged time than uncooked ones. Cooking at different temperatures kills microbes and destroys toxins in the food.

- **Sun drying:** Sun drying is used to dry many foods for long-term preservation, for example, potato chips, macaroni, vermicelli, vegetables such as spinach, methi, cauliflower, carrots, turnips, curry patta, tejpatta, ginger. This method is simple and economical where there is an abundant sunlight, such as by drying in sun, moisture is removed and the microorganisms cannot grow.

- **Refrigeration:** Temperature of 1°C–4°C prevents foods from spoiling for a short time. Fruits, vegetables and cooked foods are preserved in the refrigerator for a few days. The frozen foods kept at –18°C are preserved for a year.

- **Salting and pickling:** Salt is a good preservative. By adding certain condiments and spices along with a lot of salt, certain foods are preserved. Mango pickle, lime and vegetable pickles, chutney and fish can be stored for a long time as microorganisms cannot grow in high concentration of salt. Similarly, sugar with certain spices is used to preserve fruits. Murabbas of various fruits like apple, amla and jams are also prepared on the same basis.

- **By adding chemicals:** Certain chemicals like citric acid, benzoic acid and sodium benzoate are used for pickling vegetables such as cauliflower, radish, green chilies, ginger, etc.

Commercial Methods of Food Preservation

- **Canning:** Some foods such as fruit juices, milk, baby foods, soups and soft drinks are preserved by canning. The food is sterilized first at a temperature of 135°C–175°C for a short time, i.e., for only a few seconds and then cooked and filled in presterilized containers in a sterile atmosphere. There is some loss of heat labile vitamins during the process of canning.

- **Creating a vacuum:** This process is just like canning, only difference is that oxygen is removed from the top so that food can be packed in air tight container. Oxygen removal can stop the growth of microorganisms. Packing of prepared food in vacuum packs of special plastic pouches is an excellent means of preserving food. Vacuum packed food does not get oxidized. There is minimal weight loss. Once packed, chances of cross contamination are reduced. Packs should be stored at room temperature and well labeled.

- **Freezing:** A number of fruits and vegetables, meat and fish are preserved by freezing techniques. Vegetables can be preserved for 8–10 months and meat for 3 months.

- **Irradiation:** Gamma rays of various frequencies ranging from low to high frequency are being used to preserve various foods. Ultraviolet radiation is the most widely used in food industry. It is an invisible form of light and is used to control mold growth on the surface of bakery products and to prevent spoilage of meat while tendering. Treating water for beverages is another use of ultraviolet rays. These are also used to inhibit sprouting of potatoes and onions, garlic, ginger and to control insect infestations of rice, wheat, pulses and dry fruits.

- **Drying:** Drying of milk at large scale in milk plants by mechanical dryers is done to keep it for a long time in air tight containers.

- **By adding preservatives:** Preservatives are used for long-term storage of foods as the preservatives retard the deterioration of food. Preservatives are :
  - **Class-I preservatives:** This class includes sugar, common salt, glucose, fructose, alcohol, spices, vinegar and honey. There is no restriction by law on the addition of these substances in food.
  - **Class-II preservatives:** This class includes chemicals which inhibit microbial growth, but are added to certain foods only in permitted quantities. The chemicals are added at the end of processing operation and their presence and concentration have to be mentioned on the label. These are benzoic acid, nitrites, acetic acid, sodium benzoate and sulfurous acid.

- **Sugar:** A high concentration of sugar prevents molds, yeast and bacterial growth. High concentration of sugar is used to preserve jams, jellies and candied fruits.

- **Using high temperature:** High temperature destroys microorganisms by denaturation of cells, proteins and inactivation of enzymes required for the metabolism of bacterial growth. Heat used may be dry heat, wet heat and pasteurization. The following methods make use of high temperature for preserving food:
  - **Blanching:** It is a process in which foods are immersed in hot boiling water for a few minutes prior to processing (frozen dried or canned). It helps in removal of peels, inactivation of enzymes that oxidize vitamin and removal of gas.

- **Pasteurization:** It is used to control microorganisms in milk, fruit juices and wines. Foods are pasteurized by any of the 3 methods:
  - Low temperature holding method at 62°C for 30 minutes
  - High temperature short time at 92°C for 15 minutes
  - Extra high temperature above 135°C for 2 seconds. This method makes food commercially sterile.

Precautions During Food Preservation

- The area of food preservation should be located at clean zone. It should be free from rodent and insects.
- Before starting the process of preservation, the absolute cleanliness of the place should be maintained.
- Workers engaged in preservation of food should have strong knowledge of personal hygiene and food hygiene.
- Workers should wear gown, mask, cap and gloves before entering the area of food preservation.
- Any worker having infection of respiratory tract or any other infection or communicable disease should not be allowed to enter the area of food preservation.
- Rules of preservation should be strictly and religiously followed.
- All food stuffs should be properly cleaned before starting the process of preservation.
- All labels should be correctly prepared as per the composition of preserved foods. Before labeling the containers with date of manufacturing, expiry date and other instructions for use, a thorough check should be performed.
- Clean chain should be maintained right from production, marketing, purchasing, storing, preserving and transporting the foods to prevent contamination.
- The supervisors should strictly observe the food hygiene of the workers to prevent the contamination of food.
- Periodically, medical examination of workers engaged in food preservation should be done.
- Safety measures should be observed while dealing with heating process.

FOOD STORAGE

Certain food items are not consumed immediately after preparation. These food items should be stored carefully to prevent their spoilage and foodborne diseases.

Purposes of Food Storage

- To preserve taste, odor and flavor of food.
- To acquire all types of foods, i.e., fruits and vegetables and other edible foods regardless of season.
- To transport food to other parts of the country or to export the surplus.
- To preserve food for future use.
- To make commercial profit.
- To preserve the quality and nutritive values of food as far as possible.

METHODS OF FOOD STORAGE

Two major methods of food storage are household methods and chemical methods. Methods of food storage are given in Figure 20.4.

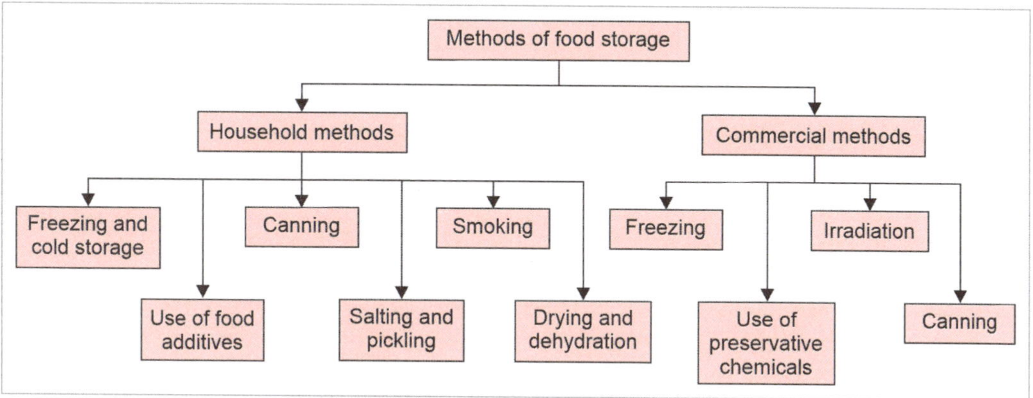

Fig. 20.4: Methods of food storage

Household Methods of Food Storage

Household methods of food storage are explained as follows:

- **Freezing and cold storage:** Refrigerator is the best storage device for cooler temperature. In refrigerator, cool air circulates evenly on the stored variety of foods. Before storing fruits and vegetables, clean and healthy vegetables are separated from damaged, soft and bruised ones and washed dried and stored in plastic bags in refrigerator except green leafy vegetable. Green leafy vegetables should not be washed but should be cleaned and kept in bags in refrigerator.
  - Potatoes and onions are kept at cool temperature in well-ventilated space.
  - Canned vegetables and fruits should be stored at room temperature in a dry place.
  - Frozen ones should be placed at lowest temperature in refrigerator.
- **Drying and dehydration:** Moisture is favorable for the growth of microorganisms. So, removal of water by drying prevents the growth of microbes. Some fruits, vegetables and fish can be stored after drying in the sun.
- **Smoking:** Smoke contains phenols as preservatives. Meat can be stored in smoky environment to preserve the loss of nutrients and stop the growth of microorganisms.
- **Canning:** This is a storage method for prolonged use. Foods are seasoned and canned for a longer time. But at home, this method is not in much use as food is prepared in limited quantity.
- **Use of food additives:** Saffron, turmeric, cardamom, saccharine, citric acid, etc., are food additives which can be used in domestic preservation of food. Sugar, oil and salt can preserve food for a longer time.
- **Salting and pickling:** Salt is a good preservative. Seasoning of food stuffs with salt, spices and condiments help their preservation for a longer time, e.g., pickles of mangoes and vegetables, and meat, etc.

Commercial Methods of Food Storage

Commercial methods of food storage are described as follows:

- **Freezing:** Freezing technique is used for storing food at commercial area for a prolonged period. The foods stored by freezing are pastries, bread, cakes, ice creams and meat in industry for a maximum of 3 months.
- **Canning:** In this method, the foods are first sterilized at temperature of 275°F–350°F for a short period of time, followed by cooling and filling in presterilized containers in a sterile environment. The food stuffs stored by this method are fruit juices, vegetables, dals, soups, fish and meat.
- **Use of preservative chemicals:** Chemicals like benzoic acid and sodium benzoate are used for preservation. The contents of preservatives should be up to the standard limits as per the recommendation of the food standard acts. Preservatives are mainly used to protect food from microbes. Antioxidants are added to ghee and oil.
- **Irradiation:** This method of storage includes the use of gamma rays in storing certain foods like wheat, rice, pulses, onions, potatoes, etc.

Principles of Correct Food Storage

- Refrigerator must be defrosted once a week. All spillage must be cleaned immediately.
- All cupboards and pantries must be kept spotlessly clean.
- Keep regular check for signs of mice, cockroach, ants and rodents and take proper action.
- All perishable foods like eggs, milk, meat, cheese, etc., should be stored in refrigerator.
- Rotate all supplies properly. The supplies first received should be used first.
- No drainage pipes or water pipes should run through the storage places where food or utensils are being stored.
- All raw and unclean vegetables must be kept separately at the bottom of the storage area in baskets.
- All cleaning agents and chemicals should be kept out of food storage under lock and key as they can contaminate the food.

ILL EFFECTS OF POORLY STORED FOOD

Bad effects of poorly stored food are due to:
- Improper handling of food
- Faulty food preparation
- Inadequate food storage
- Poor preservation of food stuffs
- Poor hygienic practices
- Lack of sanitation
- Unsafe packaging
- Careless transportation
- Injudicious use of chemicals

During storage, food can get contaminated and cause foodborne diseases and foodborne intoxications. Ill effects of poorly stored food are given in Figure 20.5.

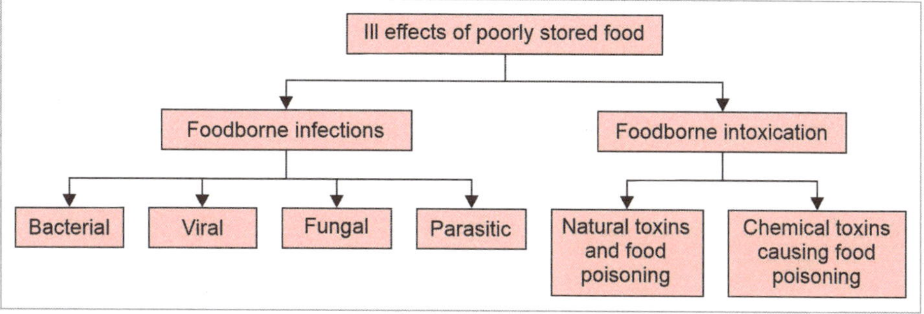

Fig. 20.5: Ill effects of poorly stored food

Foodborne Infections

- **Bacterial infections:**
  - Botulism due to infection by *Clostridium perfringens*.
  - Salmonellosis caused by *Salmonella*.
  - Bacillus cereus food poisoning due to *Bacillus cereus*.
  - Staphylococcal food intoxication caused by *Staphylococcus aureus*.
  - Typhoid fever, paratyphoid fever caused by *Salmonella typhi* and *Typhoid bacillus*.
- **Fungal infection:**
  - Ergotism
  - Alimentary toxic aleukia
  - Liver diseases (Aflatoxin aspergillus flavus).
- **Viral infection:**
  - Viral hepatitis due to hepatitis A virus.
  - Gastroenteritis due to viral infection.
- **Parasitic infections:**
  - Amebiasis due to infection of *Entamoeba histolytica*.
  - Ascariasis caused by Ascaris lumbricoides.
  - Trichinosis caused by *Trichinella spiralis*.

Foodborne Intoxications

- **Natural toxins and food poisoning:**
  - Neurolathyrism caused by beta oxalyl amino alanine.
  - Watery diarrhea due to phalloidin, toxic mushrooms
  - GIT disturbances due to cyanogen.
  - Diarrhea, vomiting, abdominal pain due to solanine.
  - Dropsy due to Argemone seeds.
- **Chemical toxins causing food poisoning:**
  - **Pesticides:** DDT, BHC
  - **Fertilizers:** Nitrates, nitrites

- Hormones
- **Heavy metals:** Lead, mercury, cadmium
- **Oils:** Petroleum products
- Antibiotics

Some of the foodborne diseases cause mild symptoms, whereas others may cause severe symptoms resulting in emergency hospitalization due to food poisoning.

- **Food poisoning:** Signs and symptoms of food poisoning:
  - Vomiting and nausea
  - Severe diarrhea resulting in severe dehydration
  - Rapid pulse
  - Low BP
  - Sunken eyes and dry coated tongue
  - Low urinary output
  - Cold and clammy skin
  - Shock may be present

Management

- Replacement of fluids and electrolyte by intravenous therapy.
- Antiemetic drugs to stop vomiting
- Antibiotic to treat infection

FOOD ADULTERATION AND RELATED ACT

Food adulteration is the addition or subtraction of anything from the food which affects its nutritional value for unfair economic gains.

Methods of Adulteration

- Mixing up food products with edible or nonedible substances.
- Substitution of the quality nutrients with substandard adulterants.
- Abstraction of nutrients, i.e., removing something from the original food article.
- Misbranding
- Concealing the quality
- Mislabeling
- Adding toxic substances
- Excessive use of food additives

Adulteration on commercial scale plays with people's health. Adulteration of mustard oil with *Argemone mexicana* seeds results in dropsy. In 1998, about 60 people died in Delhi due to dropsy and many were hospitalized after using adulterated mustard oil in cooking.

Adulteration varies with different food items. Some of the examples of food adulteration are given in Table 20.1.

TABLE 20.1: List of food adulterants

Food stuffs	Adulterants
Milk	Removal of fat, addition of water, extraction of cream, mixing arrowroot, urea, etc.
Ghee	Pure ghee is adulterated with dalda and animal fat, such as pig's fat
Vegetable oil	Mineral oil, inedible oil
Cereals	Mixing with soil, pieces of stones, powder, infested cereal and broken food grains
Pulses	Mixing with colored stone pieces, khesari dal, coal tar, dyes
Bengal gram flour	Starch powder, maize flour.
Tea	Used tea leaves, other colored leaves, black gram husk, saw dust
Black pepper	Mixing with papaya seeds
Clove	Oil extraction of cloves.
Dhania	Saw dust—horse or donkey's dung
Red chili powder	Saw dust, powdered red bricks
Turmeric powder	Yellow soil, colored maize
Honey	Sugar, water boiled with empty beehives
Ice cream	Cellulose starch, nonpermitted colors

Prevention of Food Adulteration Act

To prevent the adulteration of food, the Government of India passed the **"Prevention of Food Adulteration Act" (PFA Act)** in 1954 and it was implemented in June 1955. To rectify its drawbacks, some amendments were made in 1964, 1976, 1986, 2001 and 2002 to make the Act more stringent. The Prevention of Food Adulteration Act, 1954 was later replaced by the Food Safety and Standards Act, 2006 (FSS Act 2006). The FSS Act 2006 consolidates multiple acts and orders related to food, including the Prevention of Food Adulteration Act, 1954.

The FSS Act 2006 establishes the Food Safety and Standards Authority of India (FSSAI) to regulate the manufacture, storage, distribution, sale, and import of food. The FSSAI also lays down science-based standards for food to ensure the availability of safe and wholesome food for human consumption.

Amendments in 1986

- The consumer and the voluntary organizations have been empowered under the Act to take samples of food and checking adulteration.
- Marinating the quality of food stuffs
- Establishing public analysis, consumer tests and food testing laboratories and training of workers
- For cases of proven adulteration, a minimum imprisonment of 6 months with a minimum fine of ₹1000 is envisaged under the Act, whereas for the cases of adulteration which may render the food injurious to cause death or such harm, which may amount to grievous hurt (within the meaning of Section 320 IPC), the punishment may go up to life imprisonment and a fine which shall not be less than ₹5000.

Food Adulteration (7th Amendment) Rules, 2006

The Prevention of Food Adulteration (7th Amendment) Rules, 2006 came into force on August 20, 2007, with the exception of rule 9, which came into force on November 20, 2006. These rules amended the Prevention of Food Adulteration Rules, 1955. Training is an important component of the Act for Prevention of Food Adulteration.

In 2007, the government planned to amend the Prevention of Food Adulteration Rules, 1955. The amendments included a condition for the sale of package food without staple pins. The Prevention of Food Adulteration (7th Amendment) Rules, 2006 came into force on August 20, 2007.

Replacement of The Food Adulteration Act with Food Safety and Standards Act, 2006

The Prevention of Food Adulteration Act, 1954 was repealed on August 5, 2011. The Food Safety and Standards Act, 2006 replaced the Prevention of Food Adulteration Act.

It is an Act to consolidate the laws relating to food and to establish the Food Safety and Standards Authority of India for laying down science-based standards for articles of food and to regulate their manufacture, storage, distribution, sale and import, to ensure availability of safe and wholesome food for human consumption and for matters connected therewith or incidental thereto.

Rules are framed which after time-to-time revision by expert body called the "Central Committee for Food Standards", which is constituted by the Central Government under the provision of the Act.

Main points of Food Safety and Standards Act, 2006

The Act covers many aspects of food safety, including:

- **Food products:** The Act covers additives, contaminants, pesticides, GMOs, packaging, labeling, advertising, and fair-trade practices.
- **Food safety authority:** The Act establishes the Food Safety and Standards Authority of India (FSSAI) and outlines its duties and authority.
- **Food safety principles:** The Act is anchored by principles like risk assessment, precaution, transparency, and consistency.
- **Enforcement:** The Act establishes designated authorities to enforce the Act, issue licenses and registrations, and use improvement notices, prohibition orders, and investigative powers.
- **Food analysis:** The Act establishes recognized and accredited labs to handle food analysis.
- **Penalties:** The Act clearly defines offenses and penalties for substandard, misbranded, unsafe, or adulterated food.
- **Food safety training:** The Act provides training programs for people involved in food businesses.
- **Food safety awareness:** The Act promotes general awareness about food safety and food standards.

MUST KNOW

Food Adulteration

Any food that does not confirm to the minimum standard is said to be adulterated.

Food items	Adulterants
Red chilli powder	Saw dust, powdered red bricks, rhodamine B dye, red lead,
Turmeric powder	Yellow soil. Colored maize
Honey	Sugar, water boiled with empty beehives, molasses, dextrose, sugar and corn syrups
Ice cream	Cellulose starch, non-permitted colors, pepper oil, ethyl acetate, butyraldehyde, nitrate, washing powder, and gum is added which is prepared by boiling different animal parts including the tail, udder, nose, etc.

FOOD ADULTERATION STANDARDS

PFA Act is responsible to lay down minimum standard for various categories of food. The standards are:

- **Fruit Product Order (FPO) Standard (1961):** This order specifies the standards for qualities of fruits and vegetables products. The manufacturer is required to obtain license to meet the required standard. The main aim of FPO is to maintain minimum level of quality during farming, manufacturing and retailing (Fig. 20.6).

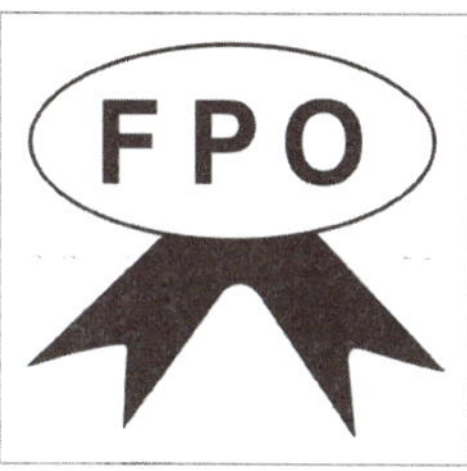

Fig. 20.6: Certification mark of fruit product order standard

- **AGMARK Standard (Fig. 20.7):** The Directorate of Marketing and Inspection gives this standard. The foods under this standard are vegetable oils, ghee, butter, rice, jaggery, eggs, ground nut, spices, potatoes and pulses. It also specifies various foods according to quality:

Grade I   — special

Grade II   — good

Grade III — fair

Grade IV — ordinary

- **Indian Standard Institution (ISI):** The ISI mark (Fig. 20.8) symbolizes quality. Foods covered under this are vegetable and fruit products, spices, condiments, meat products, processed foods such as biscuits, sweets, flour, soya products, tea, coffee, beverages, etc.

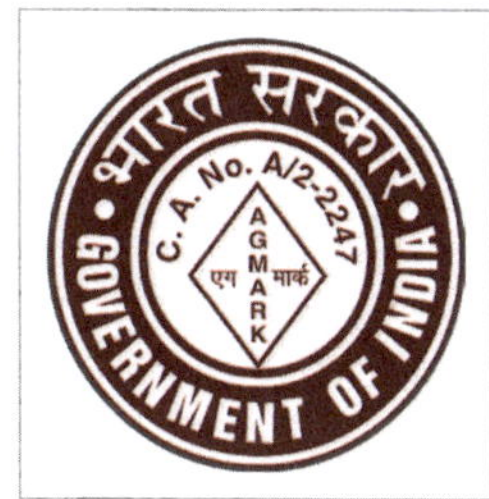

Fig. 20.7: AGMARK standard logo

- **Codex Alimentarius Commission standard:** This is one of the international standards. It is active in India for this purpose.

- **Vegetarian and nonvegetarian standard:** According to this standard, on each packet of food stuff or edible product, if it is vegetarian, a green mark should be there and brown mark on foods containing nonvegetarian products.

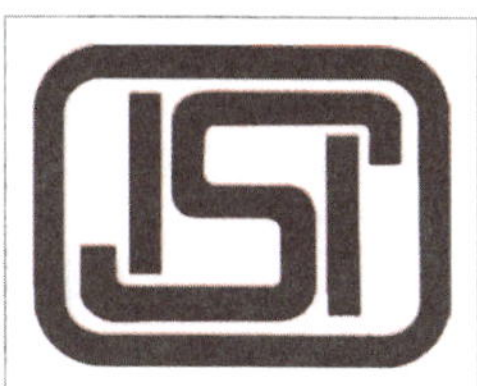

Fig. 20.8: ISI mark

Summary

- The purpose of cooking is to increase palatability, digestibility, shelf life, flavor, acceptability, sterilization and improve appearance of food.
- The methods of cooking include boiling, simmering, steaming, stewing, roasting, frying, baking and grilling.
- Effects of cooking food include gelatinization of starch, coagulation of proteins, hydrolysis and oxidation of fats and loss of vitamins.
- The methods of food storage are household and commercials methods. Household methods include cold storage, drying and dehydration, canning, etc. Commercial methods are canning, freezing, irradiation and use of preservatives.
- Food hygiene and health of food handler are very important.
- Proper storage of food at house, and at a commercial level is done by freezing, drying, canning, pickling and by the use of food additives.
- The ill effects of poorly stored foods result in various foodborne diseases.
- Food adulteration is the addition or subtraction of anything from the food by unfair means to affect the nutritional value of food.
- There are various acts related to food adulteration which safeguard the nutritive values of food.

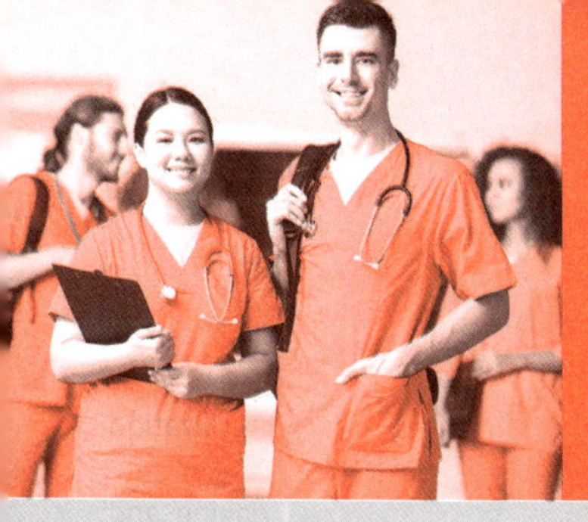

STUDENT ASSIGNMENT

LONG ANSWER TYPE QUESTIONS

1. Describe the methods of cooking.
2. Explain the methods of food preservation.
3. Classify foodborne diseases. How do you deal with suspected foodborne illness?

SHORT ANSWER TYPE QUESTIONS

1. Enlist the purposes of cooking.
2. Write a short notes on:
   a. Prevention of Food Adulteration (PFA) Act 1954
   b. Food preservation
   c. Safe food handling
   d. Health of food handlers

MULTIPLE CHOICE QUESTIONS

1. **Cooking below the boiling point is called:**
   a. Simmering
   b. Stewing
   c. Roasting
   d. Baking

2. **Which of the following is not much changed by heat?**
   a. Vitamins
   b. Carbohydrate
   c. Fats
   d. Proteins

3. **Which of the following should be boiled thoroughly?**
   a. Cereals
   b. Pulses
   c. Green leafy vegetables
   d. Fish

4. **What should we do not to preserve maximum vitamins?**
   a. Wash fruits and vegetables after peeling
   b. Cooking in minimum quantity of water
   c. Use shortest cooking method
   d. Avoid soaking in water

5. **Which of the following is not a household method of food preservation and storage?**
   a. Cold storage
   b. Salting and pickling
   c. Irradiation
   d. Smoking

6. **Which of the following milk-borne diseases come indirectly from human handlers?**
   a. Typhoid and paratyphoid
   b. Brucellosis
   c. Anthrax
   d. Streptococcal infections

7. **Which of the following is not a food toxin?**
   a. Beta oxalyl amino alanine
   b. Aflatoxin
   c. Ergot
   d. Sodium benzoate

8. **Which of the following is not true regarding fruit storage?**
   a. Over ripened and bruised fruits should not be stored
   b. Fruits like strawberries, cherries and grapes should not be washed prior to storage
   c. Frozen fruits should be stored in freeze for not more than a week
   d. Canned fruits should not be stored in refrigeration

9. **Which of the following is not a food additive?**
   a. Saffron
   b. Vanilla essence
   c. Argemone oil
   d. Saccharin

ANSWER KEY

1. a	2. c	3. b	4. a	5. c	6. a	7. d	8. d

9. c

21

Therapeutic Diet

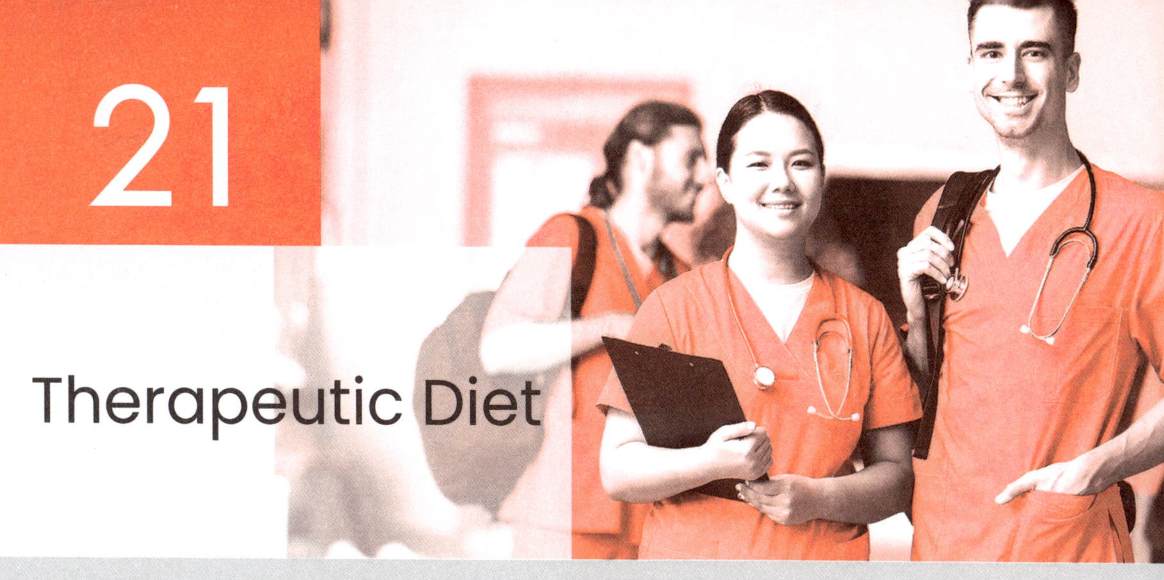

LEARNING OBJECTIVES

After the completion of the unit, the readers will be able to:

- Define diet therapy and identify the need of diet therapy in various disorders and conditions.
- Describe the methods of diet modification and health education on nutrition needs.
- Discuss the factors affecting diet acceptance.
- Demonstrate feeding the helpless patients.

UNIT OUTLINE

- Introduction
- Diet Modification
- Therapeutic Diet Planning
- Bland Diet
- High-Protein Diet
- Low-Protein Diet
- Low-Calorie Diet
- Geriatric Diet
- Iron-Rich Diet
- Liquid Diet
- Semisolid Diet
- Soft Diet
- High Fiber Diet
- Factors Affecting Diet Acceptance
- Nurse's Responsibility in Food Serving
- Health Education on Nutritional Needs and Methods in Diet Modification
- Nutrition Counseling

KEY TERMS

Bland diet: A diet consisting of foods that are generally soft, low in dietary fiber, cooked rather than raw, and not spicy.

Gastrostomy feeding: Food is given through a tube which is introduced into the stomach wall by making a surgical opening in case of obstruction in the esophagus.

Intravenous feeding: Parenteral nutrition. Fluids and nutrients are directly infused into the blood circulation. It is used when the digestive tract cannot adequately absorb nutrients, as occurs in severe malabsorption disorders.

Therapeutic diet: A meal plan that controls the intake of certain foods or nutrients in the treatment or management of certain diseases, illnesses or medical conditions.

Tube feeding: A way of giving medicines and liquids, including liquid foods, through a small tube placed through the nose or mouth into the stomach or small intestine.

INTRODUCTION

Dietary modifications are changes made during food preparation, processing, and consumption to increase the bioavailability of micronutrients—and reduce micronutrient deficiencies. A modified diet is any diet altered to include or exclude certain components, such as calories, fat, vitamins and minerals. Diets are modified for consistency, nutrition and new methods of making regular dishes.

DIET MODIFICATION

Definition

Diet modification in relation to medical and surgical conditions of the individual such as, protein-energy malnutrition (PEM), diabetes, cardiovascular diseases, hepatitis, renal gout, irritable bowel syndrome (IBS), obesity, colostomy, gastrostomy, bariatric surgery, etc. Diet modification involves some changes in the normal diet for the patients who cannot tolerate normal diet but do not require therapeutic diet. These modifications include soft diet, semisolid diet or fluid diet. These modifications are done keeping in consideration of patient's normal requirement of energy and nutrients.

Purposes

- Modification of diet are the therapeutic agents along with medical treatment in some metabolic disease, e.g., diabetes mellitus type-2.
- Therapeutic diet supports many diseases such as elimination of gluten in celiac disease and restriction of sodium in hypertension.
- Therapeutic diet is also advised as preventive measures in some diseases, e.g., fat restricted diet in liver disorders and heart disease.
- Low-calorie diet with low carbohydrate and low fat content is advised to control obesity.
- High fiber diet to prevent constipation.

Objectives

- To correct nutritional deficiencies and to maintain good nutritional status of the patient
- To formulate the diet according to patient's needs considering his/her personal preferences and dislikes

Principles of Diet Modification

- The nutritional requirement of each patient should be kept in mind while planning for modification.
- The changes made in modification may be temporary for few days or months for the duration of illness or lifelong.
- Diet modification should be based on facts and finding and it should be rational.
- Diet modification is permanent in cases of chronic disease.
- Patients should be told about the reason, objectives and usefulness of the modification.
- Disease and drugs affect body functions hence, diet modification should be done accordingly.
- Diet modification refers to the changed behavior of the patient.

Methods of Diet Modification

The methods of modification in diet are given in Figure 21.1.

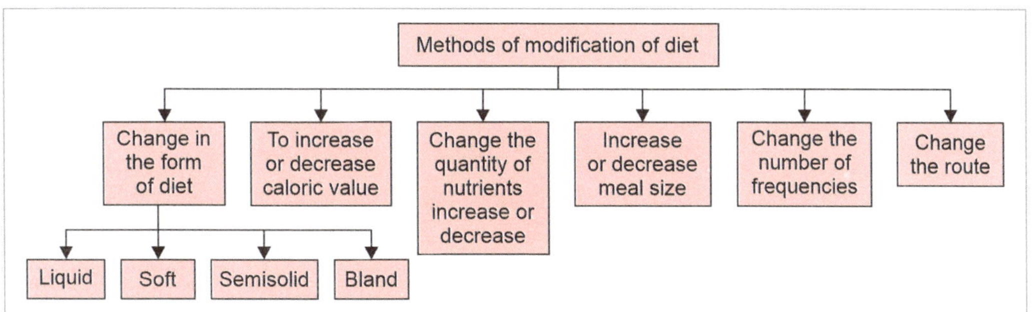

Fig. 21.1: Methods of diet modification

Classification of Diet Modification

To modify the form of diet: Change in the form of diet modification includes liquid diet, soft diet, semisolid diet, full fluid diet and bland diet (Fig. 21.2).

- **Liquid diet:** It is advised in febrile condition, postoperative cases and the patients who cannot tolerate soft diet and semisolid diet. Liquid diet is of two types:
  1. **Clear fluid:** This diet is advised to minimize the bowel activity in case of diarrhea and vomiting, it includes clear soup, barley water, coconut water, sago kanji, rice kanji, arrowroot water, fruit juice, tea, coffee, lime juice and aerated water.
  2. **Full fluid diet:** This diet is prescribed for those who are not able to chew, swallow the solid food. It is given after clear fluid diet and before starting solid diet. It is planned to meet the nutritional needs of individuals. It contains fruit juice without straining, milk with Bournvita, Horlicks, Complan, cereals, soups, dal soup, egg flip, egg yolk, milk shakes, rice, gruel, cocoa and lassi.
- **Soft diet:** It is given during acute infections after surgery and during convalescence.
- **Semisolid diet:** This diet is given to patients who are having chewing problems. In case of old people or small children, or patients who are recovering from acute illness. The diets include khichdi, dalia, suji, upma, poha, soft cooked rice, curd, sago, cornflakes, poached egg, milk base preparation, stewed vegetables, fluid can be given.
- **Bland diet:** This diet includes low-fiber content. Refined cereal, gram, butter, boiled and baked vegetables and fruits, pulses without husks, curd, stewed meat and fish. This diet is recommended in cases of gastric or duodenal ulcer, gastritis and ulcerative colitis. These foods are nonirritating.

To increase and decrease the calories in diet:

- **High-calorie diet:** It is recommended to malnourished, underweight, tuberculosis patients and other condition where metabolism is increased in case of prolonged fever and hyperthyroidism. It is also the normal requirement of heavy workers.
- **Low-calorie diet:** It is advised in cases of obesity, diabetes mellitus and hepatic coma.

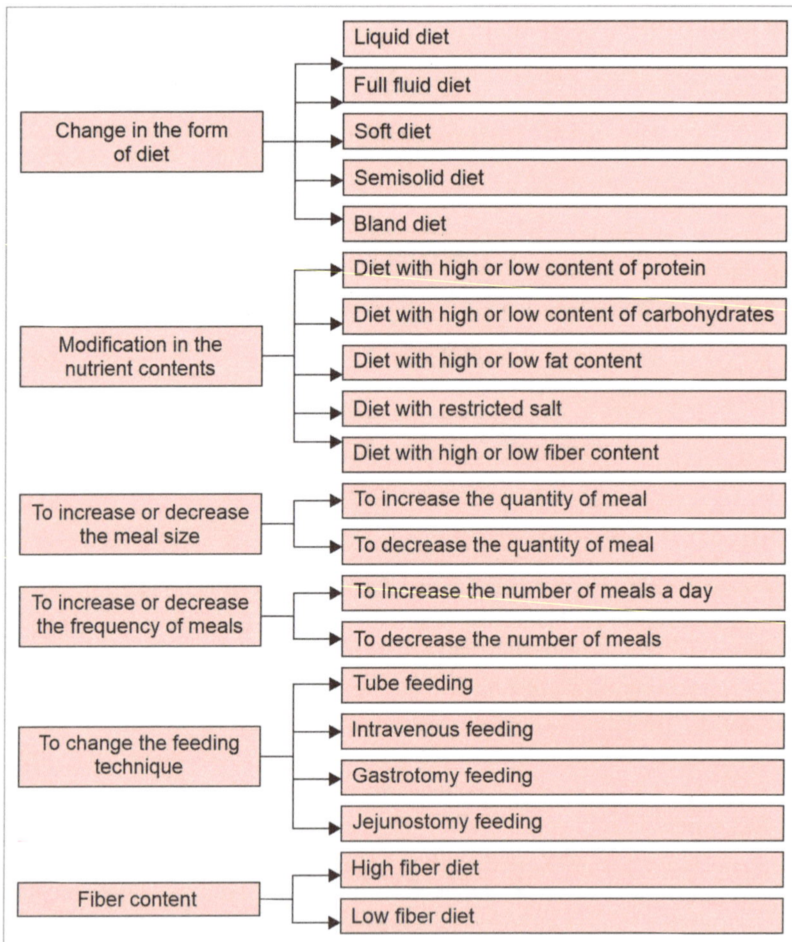

Fig. 21.2: Classification of diet modification

Modification in the Nutrient Content

The modifications in the nutrients of the diet are presented in Figures 21.3 to 21.7.

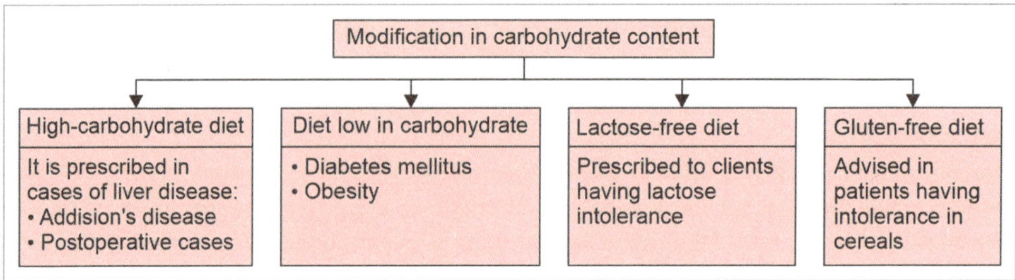

Fig. 21.3: Modification in carbohydrate content

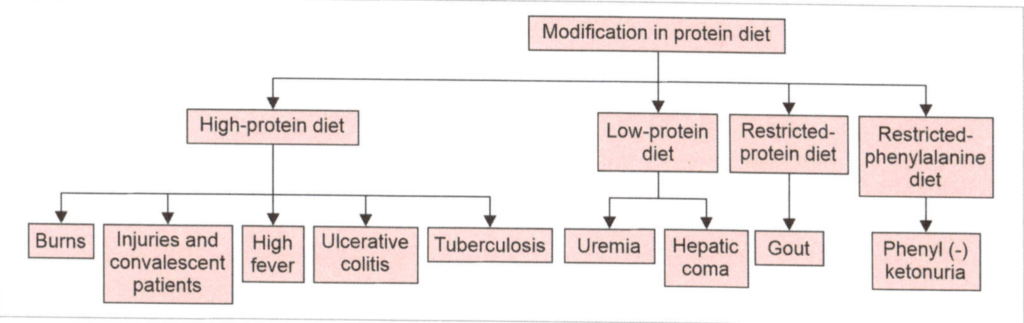

Fig. 21.4: Modification in protein diet

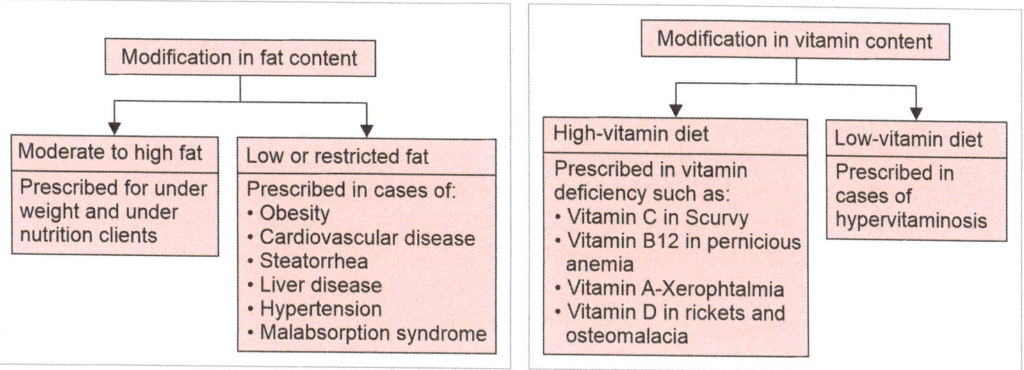

Fig. 21.5: Modification in fat content

Fig. 21.6: Modification in vitamin content

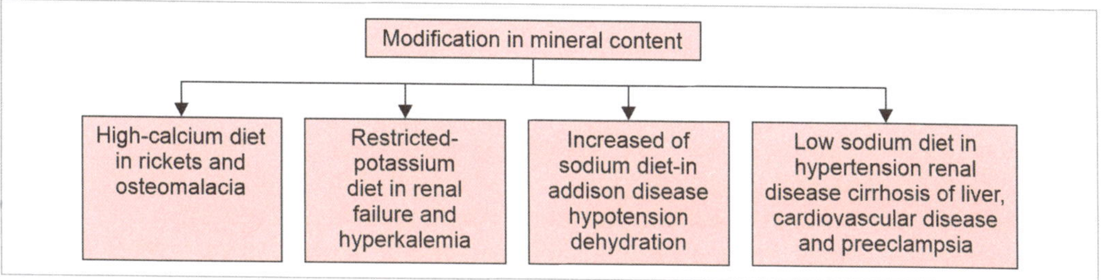

Fig. 21.7: Modification in mineral content

Modification in Fiber Content

- **High fiber diet:** It is advised in cases of constipation. Diet should contain plenty of roughage, i.e., green leafy vegetables, fruits and raw vegetables to form bulk to the diet. The diet leaves large undigested bulk in the intestinal tract which helps to relieve constipation. It has been shown in some studies that fibers in diet interfere with absorption of fat and lower the cholesterol level in blood. Fibers retain water which makes the stool soft bulky and eliminated easily. Fibers also dilute the toxic substances.

- **Low fiber diet:** This is indicated in cases of diarrhea, dysentery, peptic ulcer, ulcerative colitis and abdominal distension.

Modification in Feeding Technique

The different techniques of feeding depending upon the patient's condition are as follows:

- **Tube feeding:** It is given through nasogastric tube. An appropriate size of nasogastric tube is passed after lubricating its tip through the nose into the stomach. The length of the tube to be passed is measured from the tip of nose to the lobe of the ear and from the ear lobe to the lower end of the xiphisternum. Patient in semi sitting or Fowler's position, in case of unconscious patient head is elevated above the pillow. After ensuring that tube is in stomach, clamp it and fix it.

  Indications:
    - Unconscious patients.
    - Head injuries with injury to the jaw bone.
    - Patients who have undergone surgery of mouth, tongue or face.

  Type of feeds: Full fluid, milk, egg flip, dal, soup, fruit juice, kanji water, Bournvita, Horlicks, Complan, etc.

  Feed is prepared after calculating the requirement:
    - Always have written order of nasogastric feed.
    - Prepare the feed at temperature slightly above room temperature.
    - Place the patient in appropriate position.
    - Aspirate the gastric content before starting food.
    - Measure the quantity of food and give with 20 mL syringe slowly. It should go itself by gravity. No force to be applied on piston, taking care of air should not go into stomach.
    - After giving feed, push little plain water to clean the tube and clamp it and secure it.
    - Place the patient in left lateral position.
    - Observe for any abdominal distension.
    - Record and report the time and amount of feed given.

- **Gastrostomy feeding:** In this type, the rubber tube is inserted into the stomach through an opening made in the stomach wall. The indication of gastrostomy feed is esophageal or stomach carcinoma or esophageal surgery. Diet must have all the nutrient supplements with predigested proteins and carbohydrates. Feed is given through the funnel and tube.

- **Jejunostomy feeding:** When surgery is performed on the upper alimentary tract, then an opening made into the jejunum and tube is passed. Feed is given through the funnel and tube. Feed must be homogenized with vitamin and minerals as there are no salivary and gastric secretions. The feed should be given in smaller quantities at frequent intervals.

- **Intravenous feeding:** Intravenous feeding is indicated in postoperative cases, in severe dehydration, nausea, vomiting, burns, and coma due to any cause, i.e., diabetic coma, uremia, hepatic coma, severe head injury and cancers of upper alimentary canal.
    - The main aim is to maintain fluid and electrolyte balance.
    - To provide enough calories to meet the daily requirement.
    - To prevent dehydration.
    - The fluids used are 5–10% dextrose, normal saline, Ringer's lactate, isotonic glucose saline, amino acids, emulsified fat and whole plasma.

THERAPEUTIC DIET PLANNING

The diet planned for individual suffering from specific diseases is known as therapeutic diet. The therapeutic diet is modified according to disease condition, digestive and absorptive capacity, stage of the disease and alleviation and arrest of the disease process.

Therapeutic Diet in Protein-Energy Undernutrition

Protein-energy undernutrition (PEU) is a disease of children 1–3 years age group, it is due to the deficiency of protein or protein and calories both. PEU has its two forms:

1. **Kwashiorkor:** This is due to the deficiency of protein only. Caloric requirement is not affected.
2. **Marasmus:** This is due to the deficiency of protein as well as calories in diet.

Recommended Dietary Allowances (RDA) of Age Group 1–3 Years

Energy requirement: 1,240 kcal

Protein: 22 g

Since there is a severe deficiency of protein, so protein requirement has to be increased above the normal. Protein intake is increased from 22 g/day to 35 g/day.

Menu should be planned according to the child's preference for foods keeping in mind the nutritional value of food (Tables 21.1 and 21.2). Menu should be frequently changed to provide variety.

TABLE 21.1: Recommended dietary allowances in case of PEU

Food items	Quantity
Egg	1
Cereals	175 g
Pulses	35 g
Leafy vegetables	40 g
Other vegetables	20 g
Roots and tubers	10 g
Milk	300 mL
Oil and fat	15 g
Sugar and jaggery	30 g
Nuts	20 g

TABLE 21.2: Menu plan for PEU

Meals	Food items
6.30 am	Milk with sugar—100 mL
8.30 am breakfast	Porridge with milk, bread with butter—1 slice, egg boiled/fried—1
11 am mid-morning	Boiled vegetables/fruits—banana/mango/guava papaya, etc.
1 pm lunch	Rice—1/2 cup, chapatti—1/2, dal—1/2 cup, vegetables—1/2 cup, curd—1/2 cup
4.30 pm evening	Milk with sugar 100 mL, roasted nuts 20 g/biscuits/snacks.
8 pm dinner	Rice—1/2 cup, chapatti—1/2, dal—1/2 cup, vegetables—1/2 cup. Sweet dish custard/kheer—1/2 cup.

Therapeutic Diet in Diabetes Mellitus

Diabetes mellitus is a metabolic disorder in which the beta cells of pancreas either do not produce enough insulin or the quality of insulin produced is not effective, as a result the cells and tissues cannot utilize glucose. The level of glucose increases in the blood, when it increases >180 mg% then it is excreted in the urine.

Signs and Symptoms

- Glycosuria (passage of sugar in urine)
- Polyuria (increased urination)
- Polyphagia (increased appetite)
- Polydipsia (excessive thirst)
- Laboratory tests reveal hyperglycemia
- Abnormal glucose tolerance test

If diabetes mellitus is not controlled, it can result in:

- Blurred vision
- Weakness
- Renal failure
- Poor wound healing
- Ketoacidosis
- Coma

Management

Dietary management is an integral part of the treatment of the disease.
Disease can be controlled with:

- Diet and exercise only
- Diet, exercise and drugs
- Diet exercise and insulin.

Dietary Consideration of Diabetic Diet

- Calories to be restricted depending upon the blood glucose level and the requirement of individual according to the type of work (Table 21.3).
- The percentage of protein, fat and carbohydrate in the diet:
  - Protein: 20% of the total calories
  - Fat: 15–25%.
  - Carbohydrates: 50% it should be complex carbohydrate.
- Foods like jaggery, sugar, honey, sweets, cakes, chocolate, ice cream, should be avoided.

TABLE 21.3: The food stuffs for 1500 kcal diabetic diet

Food items	Quantity
Cereals and millets	175 g
Pulses and legumes	50 g
Milk and milk product	600 mL (for nonvegetarian 300 mL)
Green leafy vegetables	200 g
Other vegetables	200 g
Paneer/egg	30 g, egg—1 for nonvegetarian
Fruit	200 g
Oil	15 g
Fish/chicken	100 g (for nonvegetarian)

- Roots, tubers, banana, mangoes, grapes, rice, should be avoided.
- Aerated water, fruit juice with sugar should not be consumed.
- Raw vegetables and salads should be added plenty as fillers to satisfy hunger because the calories are restricted.
- Patients liking, disliking, religious belief and cultural background should be considered while planning diet.
- Minerals and vitamins should be added in liberal quality and quantity.
- Green leafy vegetables, tomatoes, cucumber, radish, lemon, clear soup coffee/tea without sugar
- Polyunsaturated fats should be used in preference to saturated fats.
- Multigrain flour should be used for chapattis.
- All fried foods like puri, kachori, samosa, pakora should be avoided.
- Schedule for the meals for a diabetic patient is enlisted in Table 21.4.

TABLE 21.4: Sample menu of diabetic diet 1500 Kcal

Meal	Food items with quantity	
Early morning	Bed tea—1 cup without sugar	
Breakfast	Cornflakes with milk 100 mL Toast with butter—2 Tea/coffee (without sugar)—1 cup	For vegetarian cheese—30 g For nonvegetarian Boiled egg—1
Mid-morning	Fruit juice without sugar—1 glass	
Lunch	Multigrain chapatti—2 (small) Rice—1 serving Salad—no restriction Green vegetables—1 bowl medium Curd—200 g Dal—1 bowl medium Fruit citrus—1	For nonvegetarian, chicken/fish—100 g
Mid-evening	Tomato soup/vegetable soup—1 cup Salty biscuits 2–3	
Dinner	Tomato soup/vegetable soup—1 cup Multigrain chapatti small size—2 Rice—1 serving Dal—1 bowl medium Another vegetable—1 bowl Salad	
Bedtime	Milk without sugar—1 glass	

Variety of menu and color combination of vegetables and salad has to be frequently changed.

Therapeutic Diet in Cardiovascular Disease

Cardiovascular diseases include hypertension, angina pectoris, ischemic heart disease and myocardial infarction. These diseases are due to increased deposition of fat in the walls of blood vessels.

Diet plan and sample menu for cardiac patient are given in Tables 21.5 and 21.6.

TABLE 21.5: Sample of daily diet for cardiac patient 1600 kcal

Food Items	Quantity
Skimmed milk and milk products	750 mL for vegetarian 500 mL for nonvegetarian
Egg white	1
Paneer/fish/chicken	30 g/50 g
Fruits	200 g
Vegetables • Green 200 g • Other 200 g	400 g
Cereals	200 g
Oils unsaturated	15 g
Sugar	20 g
Pulses	60 g

TABLE 21.6: Sample menu for cardiac patient 1600 kcal diet

Meals	Food items with quantity
Early morning	Bed tea with sugar—1 cup
Breakfast	Bread with jam—1 slice Cornflakes with milk—200 mL White of an egg—1
Mid-morning	Fruit juice with sugar—1 glass
Lunch	Salad Multigrain chapatti small size—2 Rice—1 serving Dal—1 small bowl
	Green vegetables—1 small bowl Curd—200 g Paneer/chicken—30/50 g Fruit—1
Mid-evening	Weak tea with sugar—1 cup with biscuits—2–3
Dinner	Vegetable/Tomato soup—1 cup Multigrain chapatti small size—2 Rice—1 serving Dal—1 small bowl Other vegetable—1 small bowl Sweet dish-custard/jelly—1/2 small bowl
Bedtime	Toned milk with sugar—200 mL

Dietary Management

Dietary management includes the following:
* To decrease fat intake to minimum.
* Saturated fats to be avoided.
* Low calorie diet to provide rest to the diseased heart.
* High fiber diet including green leafy vegetables, other vegetables and salad in liberal quantity.
* Low sodium intake.
* Alcohol and smoking have to be avoided.
* Regular walk and avoid sedentary lifestyle.

Foods to be Included in Diet

* Whole grain cereals and pulses
* Vegetables and fruits
* Skimmed milk
* White of egg, paneer from skimmed milk
* White lean meat, i.e., fish or chicken.

Foods to be Avoided

* Cholesterol-rich diet
* Whole milk, butter, cream, cheese (processed)
* Indian sweet meals, i.e., puddings and bakery products
* Organ meats (liver, kidney, etc.)
* Egg yolk
* Nuts, oil seeds, pickles

Therapeutic Diet in Hepatitis

Hepatitis is a communicable disease and occurs due to infection of hepatitis A, B, C, D, E and G virus. There is inflammation of the liver cells. Fatty changes, fibrosis and necrosis of the liver cell and the diseased liver is not able to metabolite the nutrients. The symptoms are anorexia, nausea vomiting, fever, abdominal pain and discomfort, urine, discoloration, diarrhea may be there. Enlargement of liver and yellow discoloration of skin eyes, and sclera.

Objectives

* To relieve symptoms
* To provide rest and aid in regeneration
* To prevent further damage.

Dietary Considerations

* Calories are restricted as liver is diseased and not able to metabolize the nutrients.
* In severe cases, 1,600 kcal and in mild case, 2000 kcal diet are recommended.
* Carbohydrates are easily digested and provide energy, so its requirement has to be increased.
* Proteins are decreased as they release nitrogenous products which are excreted and get accumulated and may lead to hepatic coma. Once the condition improves proteins are increased

- **Fats** are also decreased as the digestion and absorption of fat is affected due to impaired bile secretion. But emulsified fat is not restricted such as milk and eggs as bile is not required for their emulsification.
- **Mineral and vitamins** need to be increased, calcium, iron are increased in diet, vitamin A, D, E, K, B group and C are to be supplemented.
- **Foods to be advised:** Sugar, glucose, sugarcane juice, honey jam, chocolate, pulses and cereals, milk and milk products eggs, fruits and vegetables.
- **Foods to be avoided:** Fried, fatty foods, oils, nuts, oil seeds, saturated fat, intake of alcohol and cigarette.
- A sample diet of high carbohydrate, moderate fat and low protein diet in viral hepatitis of 1600 kcal is given in Table 21.7 and menu plan in Table 21.8

TABLE 21.7: Sample menu for hepatitis patient (1,600 kcal diet)

Food items	Quantity
Cereals	200 g
Skimmed milk	500 mL
Potatoes	100 g
Leafy vegetables	50 g
Apple/mango/papaya and banana	200 g
Fruit Juice	400 mL
Sugar and jam	60 g
Fats and oils	15 g
Multivitamin and vitamin C.	

TABLE 21.8: Menu plan for hepatitis client (1600 kcal diet)

Meals	Food items with quantity
Early morning	1 cup light tea with sugar or lime juice with sugar–1 glass
Breakfast	Bread with jam–1 slice Sago/cornflake, 30 g Milk skimmed 150 mL
Mid-morning 10 am	Fruit juice/sugarcane juice, 1 glass
Lunch	Rice–1 serving, chapatti (multigrain)–1, Dal–1 serving, curd 100 g, Green vegetables—1 serving, Citrus fruit—1.
Mid-evening 4 pm	Banana—1, weak tea with sugar—1 cup
Dinner	Multigrain chapatties—2, Vegetable well-cooked—1 serving, Dal—1 serving Mixed fruit—250 g
Bedtime	Skimmed milk with sugar—200 mL

Therapeutic Diet for a Patient with Gout

Gout is a condition characterized by the inflammation of smaller joints known as rheumatoid arthritis. It is due to the accumulation of uric acid into the smaller joints leading to the inflammatory condition of joints. The normal level of uric acid is 2–4 mg% but when the level is increased above the normal, it starts getting crystallized and deposited in the smaller joints. The uric acid level rises either due to excessive production as a result of purine synthesis or its diminished excretion by the kidney. The purine-rich foods are organs meat and fish which should be avoided. Menu plan for gout patient is given in Table 21.9.

Aims

- To limit the exogenous source of uric acid. The organ meats, i.e., liver, kidney, heart and fish should be excluded from diet.
- Fat decreases the excretion of water by the kidneys, so it should be decreased.
- Carbohydrates enhance the secretion of water; it should be increased in diet.
- Protein intake should be moderate and organ meat should be avoided.
- Plenty of fluids and fibers should be included in diet.
- Alcohol should be restricted.
- Body weight should be maintained to ideal level in case of obese person.
- Foods with low purine content should be used.

List of Low Purine Contents

- Washed pulses except lentil
- All fruits
- Nuts and oil seeds
- Eggs
- All vegetables except spinach, mushrooms and asparagus
- Wheat, rice, suji, maida, maize.
- Tea, coffee, aerated beverages.

TABLE 21.9: **Menu plan for gout patient**

Meals	Food items with quantity
Early morning	Bed tea with sugar–1 cup or lemon tea
Breakfast	Porridge with milk 200 mL Bread with Jam/slice-1 Egg boiled/poached (for vegetarian Cheese 2 slices)
Mid-morning	Fruit Juice/lime juice/butter/milk-1 glass (200 mL)
Lunch	Rice—1 serving, chapatties-2, salad, vegetable-1 serving, dal without peels (Washed) 1 serving, curd–100 g, fruit-1
Mid-evening	Tea with sugar-1 cup, biscuits-2
Dinner	Vegetable soup, Rice—1 serving, chapatties—2, milk pudding—small bowl Cooked vegetables—one serving, dal—one serving
Bedtime	Milk–150 mL

Foods to be Avoided

- Whole pulses, i.e., rajma, chana, green gram, black gram, masoor, lobia.
- Organ's meat and fish.
- Spinach, asparagus, mushrooms, dried peas and lentil.

Therapeutic Diet in Renal Diseases

- **Acute renal failure:** It occurs due to acute infection mainly bacterial. During this stage, the nutritional requirement is met by glucose 400 g/day through nasogastric tube. Once the urine flow is resumed, fluids are given in the form of milk, fruit juice, etc., gradually edema decreases, blood urea comes to normal then normal fluid intake and normal diet is given.
- **Chronic renal failure:** It is a condition resulting from slowly progressive destruction of the kidney. The waste products are not eliminated from kidneys due to decreased filtration rate and urinary output decreased causing edema. List of food items to be followed in chronic renal failure is given in Table 21.10.

TABLE 21.10: Low protein, low sodium diet for chronic renal failure

Nutritive content	Nutritive value
Protein	20 g
Calories	2000 kcal
Sodium	180 mg
Potassium	1226 mg
Phosphorus	491 mg

Aims

- To restrict protein intake since the end product of protein metabolism are not excreted by the kidney.
- To restrict sodium and potassium intake.
- To restrict the fluid intake.
- To provide caloric requirement by carbohydrate.
- To maintain normal nitrogen balance so as to avoid wasting of body tissue.
- To supply vitamins to maintain nutritional status.

Dietary Consideration

- Since the protein intake is restricted, the fat and carbohydrates are increased to meet the energy requirement.
- Protein intake is restricted depending upon the blood urea level.
- Cereals, pulses, beans should be taken in prescribed amounts.
- If sodium and potassium are restricted, then the green vegetables are boiled and water should be thrown to decrease sodium potassium content.
- Starch foods, sugar, ghee, etc., are used to increase the palatability of food.
- Spices and condiments are to be used in limited quantity.
- Fruits and fruit juices can be given to supply vitamin and minerals (if potassium is not restricted).

Foods to be Avoided

- Dry fruits like almonds, cashew nuts, walnut, peanuts, etc.
- Meat poultry and fish

- Aerated drinks
- Bakery products
- Green leafy vegetables (If potassium is restricted)
- Butter, salt.

Sample of daily diet and sample menu in case of renal disease are given in Tables 21.11 and 21.12

TABLE 21.11: Sample of daily diet in case of renal disease

Food items	Quantity
Milk and milk products	250 mL
Egg/Paneer	1/30 g
Cereals	75 g
Potatoes	100 g
Other vegetables	100 g
Fruit	100 g
Sago	100 g
Arrowroot powder	100 g
Butter without salt	25 g
Cooking oil	25 g
Sugar/glucose	50 g

TABLE 21.12: Sample menu for chronic renal failure patients

Meals	Food items
Breakfast	Bread – 1 slice Egg/paneer – 1/10 g Milk with porridge – 1 cup
Mid-morning	Fruit – 1
Lunch	Fried rice – 1 serving Chapatti – 1 Fried potato – 100 g Vegetable – 1 serving Curd – 1/2 katori
Evening	Light tea with sugar – 1 serving Sweet sago – 1 serving
Dinner	Sweet rice – 1 serving Chapatti 1 Mashed potato – 100 g Vegetable – 1 katori Dal – 1 katori

Therapeutic Diet for a Patient with Nephrotic Syndrome

Nephrotic syndrome is characterized by severe edema, albuminuria and hypoalbuminemia. Urine output and blood urea may be normal but albumin protein is lost in the urine and albumin content of blood protein falls. Menu plan for nephrotic syndrome is given in Table 21.13.

TABLE 21.13: Menu plan for nephrotic syndrome client

Meals	Food items
Breakfast	Bread 2 slices with butter and jam, cheese 2 slices, tea/coffee with sugar 1 cup
10 am	Milk with sugar—1 cup. Fruit– Banana/Apple/Mango/Orange.
Lunch	Rice—1 serving, chapattis—2 Dal—1 Bowl (medium), cooked vegetables-1 serving Curd— 200 g, paneer 50 g/chicken – 50 g, Fruit—1
4 pm	Milk—1 cup with Proteinex 2 tsp, nuts—30 g, biscuits—3 to 4
Dinner	Chapattis—2, Dal—1 Bowl, cooked vegetables one serving, curd—200 g, paneer—50 g/meat—50 g, rice kheer—1/2 bowl
Bedtime	Milk with sugar—1 cup

Aims

- To replace the albumin protein by increasing dietary protein intake. High protein of good quality has to be given.
- Salt intake is restricted to prevent aggravation of edema.
- Fluid intake 100 mL/day in addition to fluid loss from body.
- Carbohydrates and fat in moderate quantity.

Therapeutic Diet for Renal Calculi Cases

Stones are formed in kidneys due to excessive consumption of diet containing oxalates, calcium, phosphorus and nucleoproteins. To prevent the formation of stones, diet containing less calcium, phosphorus, oxalates and nucleoprotein should be given. Patients should drink plenty of water.

Foods to be Avoided

Aerated water, butter, chocolate, cheese, liver, kidney, peas, spinach, tomatoes, soyabean, turnip, radish and spices containing calcium. Recommended foods are given in Table 21.14.

Therapeutic Diet in Irritable Bowel Syndrome

Irritable bowel syndrome is chronic gastrointestinal disorder of unknown origin. The patient complains of flatulence, abdominal cramps, constipation and altered bowel habits. Patient is motivated to change diet and lifestyle.

Dietary Advice to the Patient

- Take smaller meals, easily digestible at frequent intervals to reduce the cramps.
- To drink plenty of water.
- Light exercises for relaxation and diversion.
- Diet should have high carbohydrates contents for easy digestion.
- Fats to be decreased
- Proteins as per the requirement.

TABLE 21.14: Sample of daily diet in case of renal calculi

Meals food item	Quantity
Milk	200 mL/day
Egg/cheese	1/day, cheese—2 slices for vegetarians
Fish/meat/peeled pulses (without skin)	100 g/day, peeled pulses— 30 g for vegetarian
Fruits	100 g
Fat	As per the requirement
Green and Yellow vegetables	200 g/day
Cereals, rice, sugar, honey, salt, tea/coffee, mild spices.	
Caloric requirement: Normal according to the weight and type of work.	

- Fibers should be in liberal quantity to relieve constipation.
- Variety of menu should be frequently changed.

Foods to be Avoided

- Cauliflower, cabbage, beans, broccoli, sprouts.
- Aerated drinks and squashes, tinned fruits and juices.
- Stimulating drinks like, coffee, alcohol, dairy.
- Products and fried foods should be avoided.

Therapeutic Diet for Obesity Client

Obesity is the abnormal growth of the adipose tissue either due to the enlargement of fat cell size or due to increase in fat cell number. The degree of grading of the obesity can be calculated by body mass index.

$$\text{Body mass index (BMI)} = \frac{\text{Weight in kg}}{(\text{Height in meters})^2}$$

$$\text{BMI} = 25 \text{ no obesity.}$$

- If it is between 25 and 29.9 grade, I obesity.
- If it is between 30 and 40 grade, II obesity.
- Above 40 is grade III obesity.

Aims

The main aims of dietary management are as follows:
- To bring down the weight gradually to the normal level
- To find out the cause of obesity and rectify
- To correct the faulty food habits

Dietary Management

- Weight reducing diet
- Weight maintenance diet
- Physical exercises to utilize stored fat in adipose tissue.

Dietary Considerations

- Calories to be reduced
- Protein intake slightly increased
- Fat should provide 20% of the energy requirement.
- Unsaturated fats should be used.
- Fried foods should be avoided.

A reduction of 500 kcal reduces the weight about ½ kg/week. Reduction in calories should be brought gradually. A sample menu for obese patient is given in Table 21.15.

TABLE 21.15: **Sample menu plan in case of obesity**

Meals	Food item with quantity
Morning 6 am	Lemon tea, lime juice with little sugar—1 glass
Breakfast	Bread with 1/2 tsp, butter, boiled egg—2 slices or—1 Multigrain chapatti—1 With curd—100 g Dalia, porridge—30 g Toned milk—200 mL
Mid-morning	Weak tea with 1/4 tsp sugar or—1 cup Butter milk without sugar—1 glass Fruit-apple—1
Lunch	Multigrain roti—1 Rice—1 serving Green leafy vegetables—1 katori Curd—100 g Salad—No restriction Citrus fruit—1
Evening tea 4 pm	Tea/coffee with 1/4 tsp sugar—1 cup Salty biscuit—2 Or Roasted or sprouted gram—30 g
Dinner	Vegetable soup—1 cup Multigrain chapatti—1 Other vegetables—1 katori Salad - No restriction Dal or paneer—1 katori/30 g For nonveg (no dal or paneer) Chiken/fish—100 g

Foods to be Avoided

- Butter, cheese, chocolates, cream, ice cream, fatty meats, nuts, dry fruits, cake, pastries, paratha, purees, pakora, kachori, samosa, bhatura, etc., should be strictly avoided.
- Sweets, potatoes, fried rice, jam, honey and rich puddings should be avoided.
- Carbonated beverages, squashes, and preserved fruit juices, alcoholic drinks to be avoided.
- Saturated fats to be avoided.

The following measures must be taken for weight reduction:

- Diet should provide low calories, high protein and high fiber content.
- Low fat, low sugar and refined carbohydrates.
- White meat instead of red meat to be consumed.
  - Three small meals during the day and in between the meals plenty of salad and raw vegetables can be taken as fillers.
  - Vegetables, soup, salad, lime juice without sugar, lassi from skimmed milk can be taken.
  - Cereals, pulses, beans, egg, poultry and milk should be included in diet.

Therapeutic Diet in Cholecystectomy

Cholecystectomy is the surgical removal of gallbladder due to formation of stones in it. As the gallbladder acts as a reservoir for bile which is essential for absorption of fat, after surgery, the fatty foods are avoided for few days. Once the patient is allowed to eat after surgery, start with oral fluids and gradually to semisolids and solid foods. It takes about one month to return to the normal diet. But during this period, the fatty foods are avoided and gradually introduced, except the fried foods.

Foods to be Avoided

- All fried foods puri, paratha, samosa, pakora, potato chips, etc.
- Dairy products such as paneer, cream, ice cream and whole milk.
- Creamy soups and sauces.
- Spicy foods.
- High-fiber food and gas-forming vegetables like cabbage, cauliflower, beans and cucumber, etc.
- Meat, pizza and coconut oil.

Therapeutic Diet for a Patient with Partial Gastrectomy

In partial gastrectomy, a portion of the stomach is removed due to carcinoma or peptic ulcer. The patient is kept on intravenous fluid till the wound heals properly except small quantities of fluids introduced after 3rd day of operation orally. When the patient starts tolerating oral fluids, IV fluids are stopped.

First few days, the fluid diet is given and gradually semisolids easily digestible foods are added.

Objectives

- Since a part of stomach is removed and hence, the capacity of digestion and holding food is reduced, so the foods are to be given:
    - In small quantities
    - At frequent interval
    - Easily digestible foods.
- To maintain adequate caloric requirement.
- The enzymes acting on protein foods may be reduced due to operation, so protein should be given just to meet daily requirement and it should be well-cooked and easily digestible.
- Fried and fatty foods to be avoided as it delays the emptying of the stomach.
- Counseling of the patients and family regarding the limitations and capability of stomach to hold due to operation.
- All vitamin supplements should be given as absorption of B_{12} is affected.

Foods to be Avoided

- Fried foods, puri, paratha, samosa, pakora, etc.
- Saturated fats to be avoided
- Spicy foods
- Dairy products
- Gas-forming vegetables like, cauliflower, cabbage, broccoli, cucumber, beans, etc.

- Hard meat
- Bakery products
- All junk foods, cream, ice cream, pizza.

Foods to be Advised to Reduce the Churning Efforts

- Toned milk
- Half-boiled egg
- Soft-cooked chicken and fish
- Stewed vegetables, fruits like, papaya, watermelon, muskmelon, mangoes, citrus fruits, banana, apple
- Soft-cooked puddings

Diet for Gastrotomy Patients

Gastrotomy is surgical opening made directly into the stomach in case of obstruction in the esophagus, either due to carcinoma, injury, burns or strictures.

It may be temporary or permanent.

In permanent gastrotomy, patient has to be on gastrostomy feeds throughout the life.

In gastrectomy, a feeding tube is passed directly into the stomach through the opening made on its wall and secured properly and kept clamped except when feed has to be given (Fig. 21.8). This type of feed is called enteral feed.

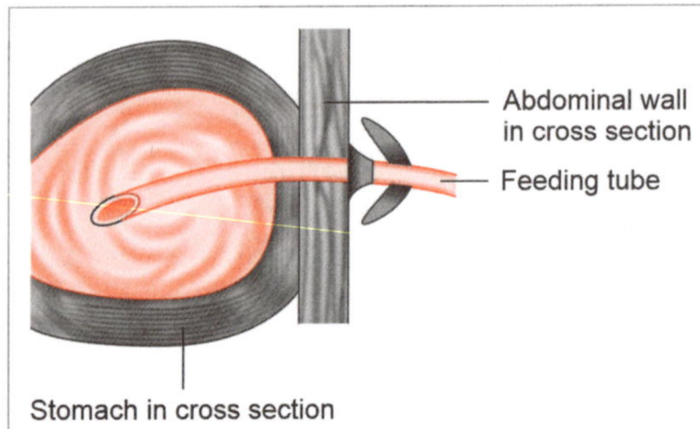

Fig. 21.8: Cross section of stomach showing feeding tube

Objectives

- To meet the caloric requirement of the patient.
- To provide balanced nutrition and meet the requirement of fluid intake.
- To observe the satiety value of food for the patient.
- To provide nutrition education to the patient and family.
- To supplement vitamins and minerals.

Types of Food to be Given

- Homogenized milk
- Partially digested proteins, carbohydrates, vitamins and minerals.

Foods Included

Soups, fruit, juices, well-cooked thin liquids, dals, custards, fruits shakes, egg flips, milk with Bournvita, Horlicks, kanji, coconut water, etc., can be given through the tube.

Feed is given either through 50 mL syringe or a funnel. Feed should be given in small quantities not >350 mL at a time initially and gradually as per the tolerance it can be increased. Feed should be given slowly, i.e., 50 mL/minute. Time interval depends upon the requirement usually 3–4 hours interval is adequate. At the end of feed, little water is passed to clean the tube.

Therapeutic Diet for Patients with Bariatric Surgery

Bariatric surgery is an operation performed on the stomach that helps the extreme obese patients to lose weight when the other means of losing weight do not succeed.

Dietary Consideration

- Total caloric intake should not exceed 1000 kcal.
- Extra water and calorie free fluids should be taken in between the meals.
- Since the caloric intake is reduced, additional vitamin, supplement is to be given regularly.

General Guidelines

- Balanced diet with small quantities should be given.
- Diet should have low fat, and low calories.
- In the beginning, clear fluids should be started like fruit juice in small quantities.
- Rice, bread, raw vegetables, fresh fruits and meat should be avoided.
- Patient is advised to have small bites and chew slowly.
- Sugar and sugar containing foods are to be avoided.
- All soft drinks, aerated drinks are to be avoided.
- Initial two months, calories intake should be 400–600/day and gradually increased to 1000 kcal.
- Daily chart of the food intake should be made.
- One cup of fluid between each small meals at least 8 times a day has to be taken to avoid dehydration.
- Use of straw and chewing ice may cause discomfort, so it should be avoided.
- All supplement vitamin tablets should be crushed before taking.

Therapeutic Diet for Patient with Colostomy

Colostomy is an opening made on the colon through the abdominal wall after bowel surgery or to relieve obstruction to prevent remaining bowel from contamination by the fecal matter. This opening of the colon is called stroma. It may be temporary or permanent.

Dietary Considerations

- Diet should be adequate in nutrients, minerals and vitamin to meet the requirement.
- Fluid intake should be sufficient.

The fibrous foods, leafy vegetables and gas-forming foods should be restricted to control the stool patterns.

Special Considerations

- Meals should be taken in small quantities at regular intervals at least 4–6 smaller meals to promote regular bowel pattern.
- Main meals should be taken at breakfast, lunch and small meals in the evening to reduce the stool output at night.

- Foods should be chewed completely to help the digestion. Large pieces of leafy vegetables can block stroma so it should be avoided.
- Sufficient water should be taken.
- Fibers and bran should be avoided.
- Gas-forming foods like cabbage, cauliflower, legumes, banana, beverages, excessive milk should be avoided.
- Daily dietary chart should be maintained.

Special Diet

- **Low-sodium diet:** It is prescribed in cases of:
  - Renal diseases
  - Hypertension
  - Cardiovascular diseases
  - Cirrhosis of liver
  - Preeclampsia.

Sodium causes retention of water and aggravates edema, raises blood pressure and overloads the heart.

Dietary Management

Aim: Reduce the salt intake to minimum.

Foods to be Avoided

- Table salt should not be used in cooking food.
- Salted butter, bread and all bakery products should be avoided.
- Aerated water, squashes, canned juices should be avoided.
- Fish and green leafy vegetables should be avoided as they contain more sodium.
- Commercial cheese should be avoided.
- Saturated fat, oil, ghee, butter.
- Meat, eggs, whole milk, commercial cheese.

Dietary Counseling

Dietary counseling is very difficult to adjust salt restricted food. Though the cooking salt is not used but most of foods contain some amount of sodium. Foods cooked without salt should be garnished with lemon, onion or vinegar to make it palatable and acceptable by the patient. A pinch of salt can be given making the food tasty. Patient and family should be educated about the importance of salt-restricted diet.

Fat-Free Diet

Fat-free diet is advised in cases of:
- Obesity
- Liver diseases
- Malabsorption syndrome
- Steatorrhea

Foods to be Taken

Cereals, pulses, vegetables, green leafy vegetables, fruits, white meat, i.e., fish, chicken and foods is cooked without oil but garnished with onion, lemon, coriander leaves and vinegar to make it palatable.

Dietary counseling and nutrition education to the patient and family about restriction of fat in diet, how to cook and serve fat-free food.

BLAND DIET

Bland diet or nonirritating diet is advised in cases of:

- Peptic ulcer
- Malabsorption syndrome
- Ulcerative colitis

Bland diet is easily digestible as it has low roughage content free from mechanical and chemical irritants.

Foods to be Avoided

- Fruits with cellulose, skin of vegetables, seeds and fibers.
- Chilies, black pepper, ginger and strong spices should be avoided.
- Fat is restricted to minimum quantity.
- Beverages containing excessive sugar.
- Tea, coffee, soup, curry, alcohol.

Foods to be Included

Vegetables without skin, bulk of fruits, milk, half -boiled egg, lean meat, well-cooked.
The foods are cooked by boiling, steaming and roasting.

HIGH-PROTEIN DIET

High-protein diet is recommended in cases of:

- Protein-energy undernutrition
- Burns
- Tuberculosis
- Postoperative cases
- Injuries
- Nephrotic syndrome
- Peptic ulcer
- Cirrhosis of liver
- High fever
- Ulcerative colitis.

Normal intake of protein is 1 g/kg body weight/day. In case of high-protein diet, the protein requirement is 2–3 g/kg, body weight/day. For 3000 kcal diet for 50 kg body weight.

- Protein requirement — 150 g
- Fat   — 60   g
- Carbohydrates   — 300 g
- Milk   — 1000 mL

The protein foods include milk, egg, meat, chicken, fish, cheese, curd, soyabean, pulses, legumes, grams, nuts and dry fruits.

The type of protein, i.e., vegetarian or nonvegetarian and preparation of menu is made as per the acceptance and digestibility of the client according to the disease condition.

LOW-PROTEIN DIET

Low-protein diet is prescribed for patients suffering from:

- Chronic renal failure
- Viral hepatitis

For caloric requirement 2,000 kcal and 50 kg body weight

The protein requirement is reduced to minimum as the nitrogenous waste products are accumulated in the blood and the diseased kidney is not able to excrete it.

- Protein intake — 20–25 g
- Fat   — 60 g
- Carbohydrates — 250 g
- Milk   — 500 mL

The energy requirement is mainly from the carbohydrates and fats. The protein intake should be of good quality to provide essential amino acids, i.e., fish, chicken or soft cooked meat. Salt intake is avoided in renal failure and fat is restricted in viral hepatitis. Protein food should be well-cooked and easily digestible. The menu plan is already described under the heading of therapeutic diet.

LOW-CALORIE DIET

The low-calorie diet is prescribed in cases of obesity, and also for patients with diabetes mellitus. **In obesity:** The aim of providing low calorie diet is to reduce the weight by making the stored body fat to burn during exercise. Initially for first week, 500 kcal are reduced, and then gradually the reduction is made up to 1000 kcal from the existing intake of calories. Diet of 1300 kcal will reduce 0.5–1 kg weight per week.

Dietary Considerations

- Fat and carbohydrate are reduced.
- Protein intake is slightly increased.
- Salad and green leafy vegetables are increased.
- Menu plan for obesity is already described in this chapter.

GERIATRIC DIET

Due to improvement in healthcare facilities, nutrition, environmental hygiene and sanitation, the life expectancy at birth in India has increased after independence.

Aging is irreversible biological change that occurs throughout an individual's, life until death. The changes associated with aging are physiological changes and psychological changes.

Physiological Changes

Physiological changes include:

- Reduced BMR.
- Osteoporosis due to demineralization of bones.
- Changes in gastrointestinal tract result in decreased saliva, decreased gastric juice and decreased digestive enzymes and decreased absorption of nutrients from intestine.
- Cardiovascular changes resulting into decreased efficiency of heart muscles.
- Decreased renal function.
- Diminished activity of endocrine glands.
- Decreased neuromuscular coordination.
- Diminished vision.
- Impaired hearing.
- Falling of teeth and change in taste.
- Changes in the skin.

Psychological Changes

Psychological changes include:

- Depression
- Anxiety
- Loneliness
- Less income
- Loss of self-esteem and independence.

All these problems affect the nutrition related health problems, i.e., undernutrition, obesity, diabetes mellitus, cardiovascular diseases and osteoporosis.

Nutritional Requirement

Nutritional requirements depend upon the ability to ingest, digest, absorb and utilize the nutrients and hence, it may differ for same age and same body weight.

Generally, the calorie requirement is assumed to be 10% less than the sedentary workers. It also depends upon the physical activities, and various physiological changes in the body.

ICMR has given 1768 kcal for male of weight 50 kg and for female of same weight 1704 kcal however, the nutritional need of the elderly can be modified according to the specific requirements.

- Protein requirement is 1 g/kg body weight
- Calcium   – 500–800 mg
- Fat   – 30 g
- Carbohydrates – 250 g
- Milk   – 750 mL

Dietary Considerations

- Adequate intake of calcium and exposure to sunlight to prevent bone deformities.
- Unsaturated fat to prevent the risk of cardiovascular disease.
- Liberal amount of protective foods, i.e., fruits, milk and vegetables and protein of good quality.
- Meals should be soft, well-cooked requiring minimum mastication.

- Frequent change in variety of menu to maintain palatability and interest in food.
- Meals should be small at shorter intervals for easy digestion.
- The green leafy vegetables should be well-cooked.
- Plenty of fluid intake to prevent constipation vitamin supplements should be given.

Foods to be Avoided

All fried foods and baked foods should be avoided.

IRON-RICH DIET

Iron-rich diet is prescribed in cases of iron deficiency anemia.

Iron deficiency anemia may result due to decreased intake of iron in diet, deficient absorption due to lack of hydrochloric acid in the stomach or due to chronic loss of small quantity of blood daily in cases of bleeding piles, peptic ulcer, etc. In adolescent girls, it may be due to excessive loss of blood during menstruation.

Dietary Management

- To find out the cause of anemia and its appropriate treatment.
- But the most common cause of iron deficiency anemia in India is nutritional anemia.
- Balanced diet containing adequate amount of cereals, pulses, green leafy vegetables, beans, tomatoes, citrus fruits, almonds, walnuts, grams and lemon should be given.
- For nonvegetarian: Liver, kidney, meat, beef and eggs should be given.
- Supplement iron.
- Vitamin B_{12}, folic acid and vitamin C should be given.
- Iron-rich foods are spinach, amaranth, drum sticks, curry leaves, coriander leaves, beans, pomegranate, groundnut, jaggery, organ meats, liver, and kidney.
  These foods must be included in diet in sufficient quantity.

LIQUID DIET

Liquid diet is indicated in the patients who are not able to tolerate semisolid diet or normal diet. It is prescribed in the following cases:
- Postoperative cases
- Preoperative cases for surgery of gastrointestinal tract
- Fever cases
- Diarrhea
- Dehydration cases to replace the fluids
- Patients who are on nasogastric feeds such as unconscious patients, coma and certain head injury cases.

Types

- **Clear fluid diets:** It is given in cases where the patient cannot tolerate roughage specially in postoperative cases after discontinuing intravenous fluid. The fluids included are light tea with little milk, clear soups, coconut water, lime juice and soft drinks. This diet has little calories and can be given only 2–3 days.

- **Full fluid diet:** It is given in cases which are not able to chew or tolerate solid or semisolid foods. It usually is prescribed after clear fluid diet when the patients are able to tolerate. It can be given for a longtime as more nutrients are added to the fluids. It is advised during infection, gastritis, fever, and diarrhea.
- **Full fluid diet includes the following:**
  - Dal soup and vegetable soups without straining
  - Milk shakes
  - Soya milk
  - Milk with Horlicks, Bournvita, Complan, chocolate, etc.
  - Egg flip
  - Kanji water
  - Lassi, whey water, blended curd
  - Tea, coffee, barley water
  - Fruit juices without straining

SEMISOLID DIET

Semisolid diet is given to the patients who are recovering from acute stage. After full fluid diet they are put on semisolid diet. Variety of foods can be given in semisolid diet. It provides adequate nutritional values for recovery. The foods included in this type of diet are as follows:

- Khichdi
- Dalia
- Suji
- Curd
- Half-boiled egg and poached egg, cornflakes
- Puddings, i.e., custard, kheer, vermicelli, raw fruits without skin, e.g., papaya, banana, grapes, orange, pears, peaches, and apples.

SOFT DIET

Soft diet is comparable with the normal diet but the foods are prepared in such a way that it is easily chewed, swallowed and digested, soft diet is prescribed in cases of:

- Convalescent patients who are recovering from acute illness or surgery
- With weak digestive power
- Old patients who have difficulty in chewing food
- Acute infections
- Gastrointestinal disorders.

This diet provides adequate calories vitamins and minerals. The foods are prepared in such a way that they are soft in texture and consistency, easy to chew and digest with little fibers, spices and condiments. All variety of foods can be selected from basic food groups so that a nutritionally adequate diet can be planned. The foods are cooked well, till become soft. The cooking methods used to prepare soft foods are boiling, steaming, stewing or poaching, fruits with fibers and vegetables with strong flavors or spices should be avoided.

HIGH FIBER DIET

High fiber diet contains a lot of roughage in the diet which provides bulk to the diet. The roughage contains lot of fibers. High fiber diet is indicated in cases of:

- Constipation
- Obesity, as the patient on low calorie diet, fibers act as filler to satisfy hunger
- Cardiovascular diseases to avoid straining during constipation
- Old people where the intestinal motility is slow
- To avoid constipation in such cases high fiber diet is given.

The high fiber diet leaves large amount of undigested bulk in the intestinal tract which help to relieve constipation. High fiber diet is also thought to be interfering with absorption of cholesterol and decrease its level in the blood. Fibers hold water so that stools become soft, bulky and readily eliminated. It also dilutes the toxic substances. The foods included in high fiber diet are whole, grain cereals and pulses, legumes, dal, milk, meat, egg, green leafy vegetables, fruits, sugar and jaggery, roots and tubers and other vegetables.

Food Items with High Fiber for Adults

The food items with high fiber content are tabulated in Table 21.16.

- Total calories   — 2400 kcal
- Protein   — 60 g
- Fats   — 50 g
- Carbohydrates   — 350 g

FACTORS AFFECTING DIET ACCEPTANCE

During illness, patient's appetite and digestion may be affected due to altered physiology and anxiety during the disease process. Patient may show aversion to food. It is very important for the nurse to know the factors which affect the acceptance of meal. Some of the factors discussed as follows:

Environmental Factors

- Excessive noise due to shouting and crying in the unit during meal timings.
- Unpleasant surroundings.
- Lack of cleanliness of the dining place, presence of undesirable articles, scenes.

TABLE 21.16: Amount of the food taken by an adult to meet the energy requirement for both vegetarian and nonvegetarian category

Food items	Vegetarian	Nonvegetarian
Whole grain cereals	300 g	300 g
Whole legumes	80 g	50 g
Dals	50 g	30 g
Milk	600 mL	400 mL
Meat	–	40 g
Egg	–	1
Green leafy vegetables	200 g	200 g
Other vegetables	100 g	100 g
Roots and tubers	100 g	100 g
Fruits	150 g	150 g
Sugar and jaggery	50 g	50 g
Oils and fats	50 g	50 g

- Lack of ventilation and lighting.
- Excessive humidity and unsuitable temperature of the dining place.
- Improper dress of the patient and the people who serve food.

Cultural Factors

- Change in the style of eating.
- Not getting time to pray before food.
- Timings not suitable with religious belief.
- Vegetarian people may not like nonvegetarian food served at the same place.
- Irregular timings or excessive punctuality.
- Methods of cooking not according to religious beliefs.

Psychological Factors

- Meals not prepared according to liking and taste of the patient.
- Unattractive flavor and color of meals.
- Physical and mental exhaustion.
- Undesirable behavior of the doctors, nurses, and those serving meals with the patients.
- Patient may be worried and remembering his/her home problems during meals.
- Unclean and unprotected serving utensils.

Other Factors

- Physical weakness of the patient
- Loss of appetite
- May be scared to eat due to digestive problems.

The patient can show untoward behavior or can create problems in accepting the diet. The nurse should understand and skillfully motivate and encourage the patient to accept the food by removing undesirable factors.

NURSE'S RESPONSIBILITY IN FOOD SERVING

- **Diet planning:** Diets should be planned according to physical and mental conditions of the patient, his/her social and cultural background, treatment requirements, availability of food and economic aspects.
- **Preparation of environment during meals:** Dinning place should be clean and well-ventilated while serving food on bed or dining table.
    - There should be fixed meal hours.
    - No dressing or painful procedure should be performed during meal timings.
    - No sweeping or mopping to be done during meal timings.
    - Proper lighting and temperature of the dining place.
    - Make the patient feel fresh by giving mouth wash, combing hair, changing clothes and washing his/her hands before meals.
    - The undesirable articles should be removed from the dining place like urinals, kidney tray and bed pan, etc.

- **Serving food:**
    - Proper and comfortable position of the patient, if food to be served on bed, Fowler's position with cardiac table or trolley for keeping food tray should be arranged.
    - Small flower vas may be arranged in the dining unit.
    - Food should be served in an attractive manner.
    - Food hygiene should be maintained.
    - The color combination of vegetables and salads in menu should be given importance to make the serving tray attractive.
    - Food should be served in covered tray at appropriate temperature.
    - Help the patient in adjusting the tray if required and direct him/her to use spoon.
    - Give water along with food.
    - Sufficient time should be allowed for proper mastication of food.
- **Aftercare of the patient:**
    - Remove the feeding tray
    - Help patient in washing hands and rinse mouth.
    - Make patient comfortable
    - Note the quantity and quality of food consumed by the patient.
    - While serving food, appreciate the foods and their nutritive value should be explained to the patient.
- **Feeding the helpless patient:** Helpless patients are unable to eat their meals due to diseased conditions such as, bedridden patients with fractures of upper limbs, very weak patients, head injury patients or patients on complete bed rest. While feeding helpless patients the following points are to be kept in mind:
    - To assess the patient's inability or weakness, requirement of diet, likes and dislikes and instructions about diet.
    - The articles required for feeding should be kept ready near patient before starting feed.
    - Patient's surrounding should be clean and pleasant before serving meal.
    - Comfortable position should be given to the patient and nurse also should assume appropriate position during feeding to avoid spilling of food.
    - In case of lying in patients, a small mackintosh and towel is spread around neck to protect patients' clothes from spilling of food articles.
    - Patient is shown the tray and asked the choice, what food he/she likes to eat first.
    - While spoon-feeding care should be taken not to spill food on bed.
    - Sufficient time should be given for mastication. Dry foods can be consumed by the patient himself if upper limbs are not affected.
    - Patient should be engaged in interesting conversation during feed.
    - Never show anger or disinterest while feeding the patient.
    - Patient should be encouraged to eat all the food served and the importance of the prescribed diet should be explained to the patient.
    - Do not force the patient to overeat or eat against his/her wishes.
    - Weak patients should be motivated and encouraged to eat with their own hands as far as possible, but needs to be helped in making them to sit and serve and adjust proper position for comfortable eating.
    - After feed, wash patient's hands and help him/her in rinsing mouth, serve water to drink.

- Nutrition education should be provided during conversation with patient while feeding.
- Remove feeding tray. Place the patient in comfortable position.
- Note the quantity and type of feed consumed and enter in feeding chart.
- Semiconscious and unconscious patients are given nasogastric feeds.

HEALTH EDUCATION ON NUTRITIONAL NEEDS AND METHODS IN DIET MODIFICATION

The main objective of health education on nutrition is to raise the health status of the individual, family and community.

Objectives

- To avoid wrong concept, idiosyncrasy prejudices and unhealthy food habits regarding diet.
- To educate individual, family and community regarding balanced diet, the nutritive values of different foods and proper methods of cooking.
- To explain the means of balanced diet based on the availability and financial budgets for the food.
- To educate about food substitutes and modification in diet.
- To educate various methods of cooking to preserve the nutrients.
- To teach about the symptoms of dietary deficiency diseases and means to prevent and treat it.
- To educate about the methods of storage and preservation of food.
- To teach about food hygiene.

Opportunities for Nutrition Education

- During home visits.
- While conducting antenatal clinic, postnatal clinic, well baby clinics, under-five clinic and family welfare clinics.
- While conducting school health program.
- In outdoor and indoor clinics.
- In ladies club meetings, during nutrition demonstration.
- In industries to the industrial workers.

Methods of Providing Education on Nutrition

- **Individual nutrition education:** During pregnancy, lactation and to the mothers of malnourished children, nutrition education is more effective when imparted with school education.
- For men, individual and group education to inform about the importance of nutrition in health and disease.
- Cooking demonstration is useful to groups of mothers.
- The methods of nutrition education used are, role play, demonstration, nutrition drama, puppet show, music, folk dance, posters, pictures, radio, tape recorder, journals, computers, etc., television, films.
- Kitchen gardens are also effective medium of health education.

Principles of Nutrition Education

- To bring a charge in the dietary habits, one should know the:
  - Educational level of individual or community.
  - Religion, culture, dietary habits and idiosyncrasies.
  - Local availability of food stuffs.
- Any change in food habits should be advised according to the individual's religion and cultural practices.
- Sufficient time should be given to adopt new ideas and habits.
- Locally available foods should be advised.
- The individuals are made to understand the importance of nutrition education regarding health.
- Foods which are beyond the individual's financial power to purchase should not be advised to include in diet.
- People should be encouraged to ask questions and clear their doubts and misconceptions regarding diet habits.
- Nutrition education should be continuous process and must be combined with reproductive and child health.

Responsibilities of Nurse in Nutrition Education

- To assess the health status of the individual, family and community.
- Making early diagnosis of nutritional deficiency diseases and intervention in dietary habits to treat deficiencies.
- Special attentions should be paid to the vulnerable groups, i.e., children, pregnant and lactating mothers, elderly people and poor community.
- To emphasize on kitchen gardens to grow vegetables for the requirement.
- To impart education on Anganwadi and midday school meals.

NUTRITION COUNSELING

The goal of nutrition counseling is to help people to establish good nutrition habits and assist them to modify their behavior regarding healthy food habits.

Steps in Nutrition Counseling

- Establishing rapport with good communication in a friendly environment.
- Taking history and assessing their nutritional needs.
- Assessing the person's financial resources, emotional maturity, living standard and ability to learn.
- Assessing the nutritional problem and setting priorities.
- Determining the time and kind of nutrition counseling.
- Discussing with individual to solve his/her mutually defined nutrition problems and suggesting alternative solutions to select and solve the problem.
- Continuous evaluation is required to identify the person's progress, reassess, replan the type and technique of nutrition counseling.

Summary

- Therapeutic diet is the diet planned for individual suffering from a specific disease.
- The objectives of diet therapy are to meet the nutritional needs of the client and correct the nutritional deficiencies.
- The method of modification is planned according to the requirement of the diseased condition of the client.
- Modification in carbohydrate, i.e., low carbohydrate diet in obesity and diabetic patient, high carbohydrate diet in Addison's disease and postoperative cases lactose-free diet in lactose intolerance and gluten-free diet in cases of intolerance to cereals.
- High-protein diet is indicated in burns, injuries, fever, anemia, ulcerative, colitis and PEU.
- Low protein diet is indicated in uremia gout and phenyl ketone urea.
- Modisfication in fat is done, i.e., high-fat diet in undernutrition and low-fat diet in obesity, cardiovascular diseases, hypertension and malabsorption syndrome.
- High mineral content diet is in various deficiency disease, e.g., calcium in rickets and osteomalacia, restricted potassium in renal failure. Rich-iron diet in case of anemia and low-sodium diet in hypertension.
- Modification in feeding technique, tube feeding is given to unconscious patients and patients who have undergone surgery of mouth, tongue or Jaw.
- Gastrostomy and jejunostomy feeds are given through tubes passed into the stomach and jejunum due to diseased condition.
- Liquid diet is prescribed in postoperative cases, fever, diarrhea, dehydration and in patients who are on nasogastric feeds.
- Semisolid diet prescribed in patients recovering acute stage. Food includes Khichdi, Dalia, Suji, custard, curd, half-boiled egg, etc.
- Soft diet in cases of convalescent patients with weak digestive power and in acute infections.
- High-fiber diet indicated in constipation, obesity and cardiovascular diseases. Factors accepting diet are environmental factor, cultural factors, and psychological factors.
- Nurses' responsibility is in serving food, in diet planning, preparation of environment during meals, i.e., serving meals and after care of patients and feeding helpless patients.
- Nurses' responsibility is to provide nutrition education and nutrition counseling.

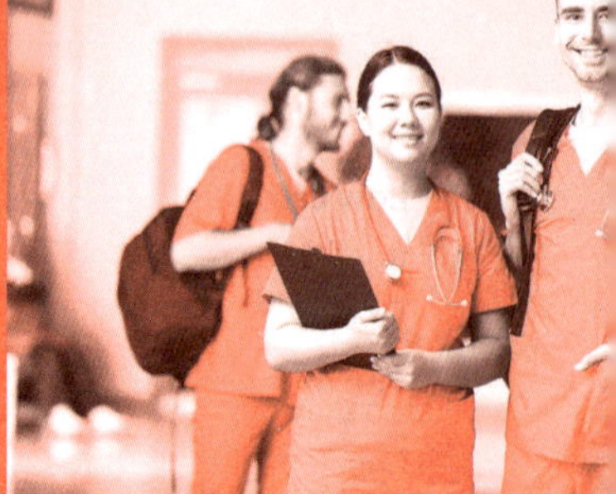

LONG ANSWER TYPE QUESTIONS

1. Describe the modification in various contents of nutrients.
2. Describe various modification in consistency of diets.
3. Describe various therapeutic modifications.

SHORT ANSWER TYPE QUESTIONS

1. Write briefly about diet modification.
2. Enlist various types of modifications.
3. Why is it essential for a nurse to study principles of nutrition?

MULTIPLE CHOICE QUESTIONS

1. **Liquid diets are prescribed in:**
   a. Febrile condition
   b. Postoperative case
   c. Gastritis and diarrhea
   d. All of these

2. **Which of the following is a full fluid diet?**
   a. Fruit juices
   b. Clear vegetables and Dal soups
   c. Milk shakes
   d. Beverages

3. **Which of the following diet is given in case of PEU, before and after surgery and burns?**
   a. High-protein diet
   b. Low-protein diet
   c. Low-calorie diet
   d. High-vitamin diet

4. **Low carbohydrate diet is prescribed in case of:**
   a. Hypertension
   b. Diabetes mellitus
   c. Obesity
   d. Both (B and C)

5. **Khichdi, Dalia, Suji, Kheer, and custard have the consistency of:**
   a. Semisolid diet
   b. Soft diet
   c. Full fluid diet
   d. Both a and b

6. **Which of the following method is used for feeding for unconscious patient?**
   a. Intravenous patient
   b. Tube feeding
   c. Gastrostomy feeding
   d. Jejunostomy feeding

7. **Low calorie diet is given in case of:**
   a. Tuberculosis
   b. Hepatic coma
   c. Malnourished and underweight
   d. High fever

8. **The diet recommended in cases of jaundice and chronic renal failure is:**
   a. Low calorie
   b. High protein
   c. Low protein
   d. High fat

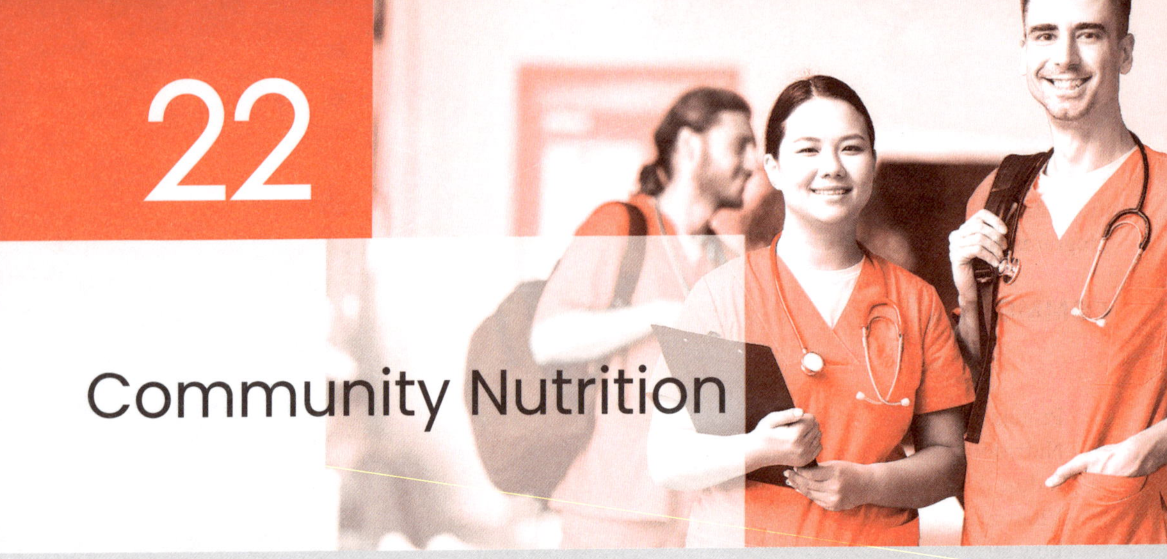

22

Community Nutrition

LEARNING OBJECTIVES

After the completion of the unit, the readers will be able to:

- Describe the concept of community nutrition.
- Discuss community food supply and food hygiene.
- Describe the nutrition program in India, national and international food agencies.
- State the food safety and standard authority of India.

UNIT OUTLINE

- Abbreviations
- Introduction
- Common Nutritional Problems in India
- Nutrition Programs in India
- Community Food Supply
- National and International Food Agencies

KEY TERMS

Fluorosis: It is fluoride toxicity resulting in white or brown speckles on teeth.

Goiter: Enlargement of thyroid gland due to deficiency of iodine.

Lathyrism: Paralyzing disease of human and animals by consuming khesari dal.

Nutritional Problems: A range of conditions that can occur when a person's diet is deficient or excessive in nutrients, or when the body has trouble absorbing nutrients.

ABBREVIATIONS

ICDS: Integrated Child Development Services
MDM: Mid-Day Meal Program
NNP: National Nutritional Policy
SNP: Special Nutrition Program

BNP: Balwadi Nutrition Program
NRHM: National Rural Health Mission
NIN: National Institute of Nutrition
IDD: Iodine Deficiency Disorder

INTRODUCTION

The National Nutrition Policy (NNP) was adopted in 1993 under the Department of Women and Child Development. The mission of NNP was to achieve optimum state of nutrition for all sections, but with special priority to the mothers, women and children. The policy recognized the multifaceted problems of malnutrition and advocated multisectoral approach for controlling the nutrition problems of India. To solve the nutritional problems of India, various nutritional programs were started.

COMMON NUTRITIONAL PROBLEMS IN INDIA

Problems due to Undernutrition

- Protein energy undernutrition due to deficiency of proteins and carbohydrates
- Nutritional anemia due to iron deficiency
- Iodine deficiency diseases, endemic goiter and cretinism
- Vitamin A deficiency diseases
- Low birth weight babies
- Endemic fluorosis
- **Lathyrism:** Spastic paralysis of lower limbs due to consumption of khesari dal

Problems due to Overnutrition

- Obesity
- Diabetes mellitus
- Hypertension
- Cardiovascular diseases

NUTRITION PROGRAMS IN INDIA

Integrated Child Development Scheme (ICDS)

The ICDS was launched in 1975 by the Government of India in the Ministry of Social and Women's Welfare in pursuance of the national policy for children. It provides an integrated package of early childhood services:

- Supplementary nutrition
- Immunization
- Health check-up
- Medical referral services
- Nutrition and health education for women
- Nonformal education of children up to 6 years of age and of pregnant and nursing mothers of rural, urban and tribal areas.

Objectives

- To improve the nutritional health status of children in the age group of 0–6 years.
- To decrease the morbidity and mortality rate due to nutritional deficiency diseases.
- To prevent the drop out of children from school.
- To lay the foundation of proper psychological, physical and social development.
- To achieve effective coordination of the policy and implementation among various departments, working for promotion of child development.
- To enhance the capability of mothers for nutritional needs of child through nutritional education.

Beneficiaries of the Programs and Services

The beneficiaries of programs and services are given in Table 22.1.

TABLE 22.1: Beneficiaries of programs and services

• Pregnant women	Health check-up, immunization, supplementary nutrition and health education
• Children 3–6 years	Supplementary nutrition, immunization, health check-up, referral services, nonformal education
• Children <3 years	Supplementary nutrition, immunization, health check-up and referral services
• Nursing mothers	Supplementary nutrition, health check-up, health education
• Women 15–45 years	Nutrition and health education

These services are provided through Anganwadi workers.

Mid-day School Meal Program

Mid-day School Meal Program is a centrally sponsored scheme from 1962–1963 in all the states. CARE, UNICEF and many international governmental voluntary agencies give their contribution to this program.

Objectives

- To improve nutritional status of school children.
- To create interest about school and education among children.
- To reduce absenteeism of children in school.
- To motivate poor communities for children education.

There is free supply of food grains through Food Corporation of India (FCI) to states. The center through FCI, provides 100 g of grains/student/day and 12 g of protein/student/day to provide at least 300 calories.

Principles

- The meal should be a supplement and not a substitute to the home diet.
- It should supply 1/3rd of the total calories and half the protein requirement/day of the child.
- The cost of meal should be reasonably low and should be prepared easily at school.
- As far as possible, locally available foods should be used to minimize the cost of meal.
- Menu should be frequently changed.
- Food hygiene should be observed and utensils can be procured with local support.

Sample menu of Mid-day School Meal as suggested by National Institute of Nutrition, Hyderabad is tabulated in Table 22.2.

According to National Institute of Nutrition, the Mid-day School Meal Program should be organized for 250 days in an educational calendar year. Teachers have an important role in supervision and distribution.

TABLE 22.2: Sample menu of mid-day school meal

Food nutrients	g/day/child
Cereals and millets	75 g/day/child
Pulses	30 g/day/child
Green leafy vegetables	30 g/day/child
Oil	8 g/day/child

Mid-day Meal Scheme

Mid-day Meal Scheme was launched on 15 August 1995, a central sponsored scheme which was revised in 2004. Mid-day Meal Scheme is also called National Program of Nutritional Support to Primary Education.

Objectives of the Scheme

- Increasing the enrolment of primary classes
- Reducing the absenteeism

There is a free supply of food grains through Food Corporation of India (FCI) to states. The center through FCI provides 100 g of grains/student/day and 12 g of protein/student/day to provide at least 300 calories.

Special Nutrition Program

Special Nutrition Program was started in 1970–71. It provides supplementary feeding to preschool children, i.e., about 300 calories and 10 g of protein and 500 calories and 20 g of protein to the expectant and nursing mothers for 300 days in a year. At present, it is combined with ICDS program at state level. It is funded by States and Union Territories from SNP budget.

Balwadi Nutrition Program

Balwadi Nutrition Program was implemented by the Central Social Welfare Board in the year 1970–71. National level organization gives active support to Balwadi Nutrition Program and provides help to the voluntary agencies for implementation. According to this scheme, 12–15 g of protein and 300 calories/child/day are to be provided to satisfy basic nutritional requirement for children of 3–5 years of age for 270 days in a year. With the implementation of ICDS scheme, Balwadis are being phased out.

Nutritional Anemia Prophylaxis Program

Nutritional Anemia Prophylaxis Program was started in 1970, by the Government of India under the IVth Five-Year Plan. Under this program, the pregnant women, lactating women and adolescent girls, as well as women acceptors of family planning are given one tablet of iron containing 60 mg of elementary iron, 180 mg of ferrous sulfate and 0.5 mg of folic acid daily for a period of 100 days who all are having hemoglobin <10 g%. Children within the age group of 1–12 years are given iron tablets containing 20 mg of elementary iron, 60 mg of ferrous sulfate and 0.1 mg folic acid daily for 100 days who are having hemoglobin <10 g% to prevent nutritional anemia.

Vitamin A Prophylaxis Program

India was the first country in the world to start this program in 1970 to prevent vitamin A deficiency diseases in India. According to World Health Organization (WHO), this program is targeted toward children under 6 months of age, as this group is more exposed to night blindness, Bitot's spot, corneal ulcer, xerosis, etc. Under this program, the children are given vitamin A solution every 6 months interval, up to 5 years of age, 1st dose of vitamin A, 100,000 IU (1 mL) at the age between 6 months to 11 months of age. The subsequent doses are given every 6 months up to the age of 5 years so that child receives 9 doses of vitamin A solution. Along with this, vitamin A rich food is also necessary.

Two policies are carried out for implementation of this program.

1. **Short-term policy:** To give heavy doses of vitamin A solution to children under 5 years of age.
2. **Long-term policy:** To promote consumption of foods rich in vitamin A.

This program is being implemented in the Maternal and Child Health Wing of Health and Family Welfare Department as well as in ICDS Program.

Goiter Control Program (Iodine Deficiency Disorder Control Program)

The Government of India launched the National Goiter Control Program (NGCP) in 1962. The aim is to control goiter by supplying iodized salt to the susceptible group. Since April 1992, NGCP has been replaced by National Iodine Deficiency Disorder Control Program (NIDDCP).

Objectives

- To supply iodized salt in place of common salt to all, especially to goiter endemic regions
- To conduct survey to assess the effect of supply of iodized salt

Salt Department is the principal agency for production, distribution, monitoring and quality control of iodized salt. The State Government takes the responsibility to distribute iodized salt through Public Distribution System or through open market.

National Diarrheal Diseases Control Program

National Diarrheal Diseases Control Program was started in 1981 to reduce the mortality in children below 5 years of age due to diarrheal diseases by introducing oral rehydration therapy. The services of this program are rendered through MCH program which was started in 1980–1985 and now it has been strengthened extensively. Anganwadi centers under ICDS scheme are active in providing ORT supply to prevent dehydration caused by diarrhea to the children.

COMMUNITY FOOD SUPPLY

Community food supply is a new concept and it is attracting the attention of the health industries. All the consumable foods are locally available during harvesting season at cheaper rates. People should purchase in bulk according to their storage capacity. The commercially prepared foods should be made available locally, and should be safe according to the laid down standards and principles of Indian Standard Institute. The commercially prepared foods should have ISI label with instructions and ingredients, their nutritional value, effects on health and the side effects. The contents of the preservatives and additives should be clearly described on the label. The time of manufacturing, date of expiry and time of consumption and opening the pack should also be mentioned.

The foods are made available at controlled rates in government depots, stores, wholesalers, retailers and local ration stores from where the community can purchase. The prices should be reasonable and affordable for daily consumable foods like, cereals, pulses, vegetables and milk, etc. The quality of food should be safe. There should be no adulteration. It is the duty of the authorities of FSSAI department to ensure standard of community food supply.

Food Hygiene

Food hygiene refers to cleanliness in production, storage, transportation, preservation, cooking, serving and consumption of foods. Food can be contaminated at any stage from production to consumption by microorganisms and can cause disease to the consumer. Food hygiene is very important aspect of community nutrition. The following facts, to be observed in food hygiene, are:

- Contaminated sewerage water should not be used in the irrigation of the land for production of fruits and vegetables.
- Transportation of food should be done in a safe packing at appropriate temperature.
- During storage and preservation, all precautions have to be taken to prevent infection.
- Special hygiene is to be observed for milk, meat, fish, fruits and vegetables, as these foods are involved in spreading of infection.
- Milk and meat of diseased animals should not be used.
- Sterilization of milk by boiling on domestic scale and by pasteurization on commercial scale should be done.
- Fruits and vegetables should be fresh and properly washed before use; cut or rotten fruits and vegetables should not be used.
- Hygiene of slaughter houses and meat market should be observed closely.
- All food articles should be covered to protect from flies and dust.
- There should be sufficient ventilation in stores for storing of vegetables and fruits.
- Absolute cleanliness of kitchen, dining hall and pantry has to be maintained.
- Personal hygiene of the personnel preparing and serving food has to be observed.
- Food hygiene is of utmost important in nutrition education.

Commercially Grown and Prepared and Food Available Locally

Commercially prepared foods are:
- Fruit juices
- Soft drinks
- Milk
- Baby foods, nutritious foods, such as, Horlicks, Protinex, Bournvita, Complan and Viva, etc.
- Soups
- Snacks, bread, biscuits, ice creams
- Tinned fruits and vegetables
- Tinned meat and fish

Vegetable oils, sugar, jaggery, flours of cereals, spices, etc., and other consumable foods which are prepared at large scale in industries are made available locally.

For all these foods, food safety should be ensured right from manufacturer to the consumer. To maintain the quality of food stuffs and edible substances, the following points should be strictly observed:

- Adulteration should be strictly prevented and if found, strict punishment to be given to defaulters
- Special rights to be given to consumers and voluntary organizations, so that they can plan an effective role in checking adulteration
- Checking the quality of imported edible stuff
- Supporting the state government for accepting PFA Act
- Establishing public analysis, consumer test and food testing laboratories and training their workers
- Fixing the standards for foods

NATIONAL AND INTERNATIONAL FOOD AGENCIES

Central Food Technological Research Institute

The Central Food Technological Research Institute (CFTRI) is situated at Mysore. This institute was started in 1956 and deals with food science and technology. The main scientific disciplines of the institute are:

- Biochemistry and nutrition
- Rice and pulse technology
- Flour milling, baking and confectionary
- Food engineering
- Packaging
- Fruits and vegetable technology
- Industrial research, consultancy and extension
- Infestation control and pesticides control
- Meat, fish and poultry technology
- Microbiology
- Protein technology
- Spices and flavor technology is one of the largest in the world and conducts fundamental and applied research work on the various aspects of food research science and technology.
- The institution also conducts a postgraduate course in food technology leading to MSc degree of Mysore University. It also conducts short courses on various subjects useful to the food industry in collaboration with Food and Agriculture Organization (FAO).
- International center located at the campus of the institution also offers technical help to the food industry.
- The institute has several technological achievements, the important ones are infants' food from vegetable protein, weaning food, high protein food and food from buffalo milk, durofume process for the fumigation of grains, improvement in the dehydration of fish and canning of fruits, popular journals and research papers are also published.

Food and Agriculture Organization

Food and Agriculture Organization (FAO) is an international agency and was founded in Quebec, Canada in 1945.

Aims of FAO

- To help raise the standard of living
- To improve the nutrition of all countries
- To increase the efficiency of farming, forestry and fisheries
- To improve the condition of rural people and through these means, to widen the opportunity of all people for production work

Structure of FAO

The Headquarters of FAO is in Rome. There is a council of 49 member nations to act as an interim governing body. The conference elects the director general to head the agency. There are 8 departments of FAO:

1. Administration and Finance
2. Agriculture
3. Economic
4. Social
5. Fisheries
6. Forestry
7. General Affairs and Information
8. Sustainable Development and Technical Cooperation

Since its inception, FAO has worked to alleviate poverty and hunger by promoting agricultural development, improved nutrition and access of all people at all times to the food they need for an active and healthy life.

In India

The FAO has been partnering in India's development from food deficit country to net food exporting country. Its focus in India is mainly on plant production activities, forestry, fisheries, nutrition and food quality and safety.

National Institute of Nutrition

National Institute of Nutrition (NIN), Hyderabad was founded by Sir Robert McCarrison in the year 1918 as Beri-Beri enquiry unit in a single room in Coonoor, Tamil Nadu and was shifted in 1928 to Hyderabad and became a nutrition research laboratory. It deals with all aspects of food and nutrition and works under the agencies of Indian Council of Medical Research (ICMR) Ministry of Health and Family Welfare, Government of India.

Objectives

- To identify various dietary and nutrition problems prevalent among different segments of the population.
- To monitor diet and nutrition situation of the country.
- To evaluate effective methods of management and prevention of nutritional problems.
- To advise government and other associations on issues relating to nutrition.
- To conduct operational research connected with planning and implementation of national nutrition programs.
- To educate and train young scientists and health workers in nutrition for the medical institution.
- To carry out research on clinical aspects of nutrition.
- To disseminate nutrition information.

Mission

To enable food and nutrition security conducive to good health, growth and development and increase productivity through dedicated research, so as to achieve the national nutrition goals set by the Government of India in the National Nutrition Policy.

Food Safety and Standard Authority of India

Food Safety and Standard Act, 2006 (FSSA) consolidates the laws relating to foods and ensures safe food products to consumer by providing quicker solution of cases within the state. Punishment offered are severe which would make the retailer or wholesaler cautious in their dealings.

The standards laid down for quality and safety in Food Safety and Standard Act, 2006 are harmonized standards and applicable throughout the country.

All types of food stuffs, genetically modified foods, organic foods, functional foods, nutraceuticals and proprietary foods, etc. are regulated by this Act. In packaged foods, labeling requirement and advertising needs are also adequately covered along with import regulation of food.

The FSSAI is an autonomous institute under the Ministry of Health and Family Welfare, Government of India, it was established in 2008. It works as a statutory body for laying down science-based standards for articles of foods and regulating manufacturing, processing, distribution, sale and import of food so as to ensure safe and wholesome food for human consumption.

General Principles of Food Safety

The general principles to be followed by Central Government, State Government and FSSAI, while implementing the provision of this act, shall be guided by the following seven principles:

1. Achieving appropriate level of protection to human life and health, safety of consumer's interest including fair practices in food related matters.
2. Carrying out risk management after assessing the risks.
3. Adopting measures for risk management necessary to ensure appropriate levels of health protection.
4. Measures adopted shall be proportionate and no more trade restrictions shall be imposed than required.
5. Measures adopted shall be revised within a reasonable period.
6. In case of suspected risk of the public consuming contaminated food, the FSSAI shall take appropriate steps to inform the general public.
7. If any lot of food fails to comply with food safety requirements, it shall be presumed that the whole consignment fails to comply with these requirements.

Main Features of FSSAI

- Establishment of FSSAI will act under the Ministry of Health and Family Welfare.
- Provision for FSSAI to establish various scientific panels on food additives, flavors processing techniques, pesticides and antibiotic residues, food labeling, analysis and food sampling, contaminants, and all types of food.
- FSSAI and state food authorities shall be responsible for the enforcement of FSSA.

- Provision for appointment of the state food safety commissioner, designated officer (not below the rank of SDM), food safety officers, adjudicating officers and other functionaries as required under the Act.
- Provision of establishment of food safety appellate tribunal.
- Recognition and accreditation of food laboratories, research institutions, food safety audit agencies.
- Provisions of penalty and punishment for:
  - Substandard, misbranded, unhygienic, unsafe foods.
  - Misleading advertisement, possessing adulterants.
  - Interfering with seized items, false information, obstructing or impersonating a food safety officer.
  - Carrying a business without license.
- Provision for compensation in case of injury or death of consumer.
- Provision and power of search, seizure, investigations and prosecution.

Food Standards

- **Bureau of Indian Standards (ISI standard):** Various committees including representatives from government, consumer and industry formulate the Indian Standards (ISI) for vegetables, fruits, spices, condiments, animal products and processed foods. Once the standards are accepted then only manufacturers are allowed to use ISI label, which confirms the guarantee of their product of good quality.
- **The AGMARK Standard:** These standards are set up by Directorate of marketing and inspector of the Government of India by introducing Agricultural Produce Act 1937 and defines the quality of cereals, spices, oil seeds, oils, butter, ghee, legumes, etc.
- **Codex Alimentarius Commission Standard:** This is one of the international standards, National Codex Committee is active in India for this purpose.
- **PFA Standard:** These standards are determined under the Provision of Food Adulteration Act.
- **Standards of Weight and Measures Act 1985:** This Act contains provision for effective legal control on weight, measures and weighing and measuring instruments used in industry.
- **Misbranding:** It is forbidden by law. If it gives misleading or false information about product, it is considered misbranding.
- **Export Inspection Council:** Council has been formed to check the quality of food materials and products for export. Council has the power to reject the product if it does not fulfill the standards prescribed for the food.

Cooperative for American Relief Everywhere

Cooperative for American Relief Everywhere (CARE) is one of the world's largest private international humanitarian organizations committed to help families in poor communities. It was founded in 1945 to provide relief to survivors of World War II.

The CARE is a broad-spectrum relief, humanitarian and developmental, nongovernment organization which fights global poverty. It is a nonpolitical, nonsectarian organization.

The main activities of CARE are:
- To eradicate poverty by women's empowerment
- To deliver emergency relief funds to survivors of war and natural calamities

- To strengthen capacity for self-help
- To provide economic opportunity
- To influence policy decision at all levels
- To address discrimination at all forms

The ongoing programs in India receiving help from CARE are:
- Mid-day Meal Program
- Preschool Feeding Program
- Nutrition Education
- Mass Communication Project
- Various national and state sponsored nutrition programs for young children and mothers

National Institute of Public Cooperation and Child Development

National Institute of Public Cooperation and Child Development (NIPCCD) is an autonomous organization with its headquarters in New Delhi. It is actively involved in training and research in the area of public cooperation and child development.

Objectives

- To develop and promote voluntary action in social development.
- To take comprehensive view of child development and to develop and promote programs in pursuance of the national policy for children.
- To develop measures for coordination of governmental and voluntary action in social development.
- To evolve framework and perspectives for organizing children's programs through government and voluntary efforts with a view to achieve the above objectives in the institute:
    - Conducts research and evaluation studies.
    - Organizes training programs, seminars, workshops and conferences.
    - Provides documentation and information services in the field of public cooperation and child development.

The institute is the apex body for training of functionaries of the ICDS Program.

Activities and Programs

- Organizes regular training programs for representatives of voluntary organization and government officials engaged in implementation of MCH, child development and women's empowerment.
- Conducts training programs under Udisha Project.
- Conducts research and documentation in the area of public cooperation and child development and other projects.

Summary

- The National Nutrition Policy was adopted in 1993 and it is recognized that nutrition is a multisectoral issue and needs to be tackled at various levels. Nutrition affects the growth and development.
- The policy recognized the multifaceted problems of malnutrition and advocated multisectoral approach for controlling the nutritional problems of India.
- To solve the nutritional problems, the various nutritional programs started are Integrated Child Development Scheme, Mid-day Meal Scheme, Mid-day Meal, Special Nutrition Program, Balwadi Nutrition Program, Nutritional Anemia Prophylaxis Program, Vitamin A Prophylaxis Program, and Goiter Control Program.
- Community food during the harvesting season is cheaper and people should purchase from government depots and wholesale retailers as the foods are cheap on these stores.
- The prices of food should be reasonable and affordable by the community.
- Food safety should be observed during preservation strictly abiding by the laws and acts of food safety. The various national and international agencies engaged in food and nutrition are Central Food Training Research Institute, Food and Agricultural Organization, National Institute of Nutrition, Hyderabad.
- To observe food safety, the Acts are Food Safety and Standard Act 2006, Bureau of India Commission Standard, PFA Standard, Standards of Weight and Measures Act, 1985.
- International agencies are Cooperative for American Relief Everywhere (CARE) and National Institute of Public Cooperation and Child Development (NIPCCD). They have contribution in nutrition programs and training and research programming regarding nutrition programs.

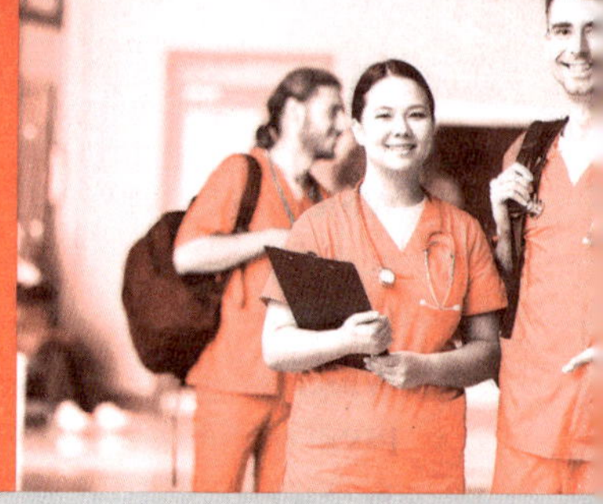

LONG ANSWER TYPE QUESTIONS

1. Describe ICDS Program.
2. Discuss the Mid-day Meal Program.
3. Elaborate Food Safety and Standard Authority of India.

SHORT ANSWER TYPE QUESTIONS

1. Enlist the common nutrition problems in India.
2. Name the nutrition programs functioning in India.
3. Write short notes on:
   a. National and international food agencies
   b. Goiter control program
   c. Nutritional anemia prophylaxis program

MULTIPLE CHOICE QUESTIONS

1. **The National Nutrition Policy was adopted by the government of India in the year:**
   a. 1997
   b. 1993
   c. 1991
   d. 1995

2. **NNP was adopted under the department:**
   a. Health and Family Welfare
   b. Food and Nutrition Board
   c. Food and Civil Supplies
   d. Department of Women and Child Development

3. **Undernutrition results in:**
   a. PEU
   b. Low birth weight
   c. Deficiency of vitamin A, iron and iodine
   d. All of the above

4. **About 90% of infant death occur with birth weight below:**
   a. 2 kg
   b. 1.9 kg
   c. 2.2 kg
   d. 2.1 kg

5. **Mission of NNP was to achieve optimum state of nutrition for all but special priority was given to:**
   a. Women
   b. Children
   c. Mothers
   d. All of these

6. Which of the following essential food is planned to be fortified with iodine and iron?
    a. Salt   b. Sugar
    c. Wheat flour   d. All of these

7. Which of the following micronutrient deficiencies should be covered under prophylaxis program among vulnerable group (children, pregnant women and lactating mothers)?
    a. Vitamin A   b. Iron and folic acid
    c. Iodine   d. All of these

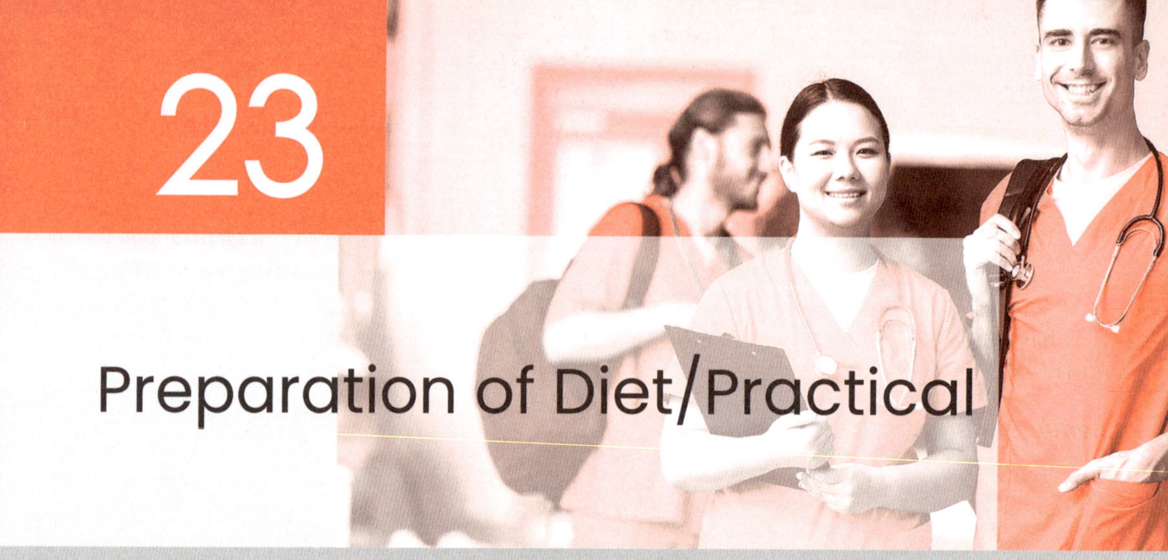

23

Preparation of Diet/Practical

LEARNING OBJECTIVES

After the completion of the unit, the readers will be able to:
- Develop skills in preparation of diet.
- Demonstrate the various preparations of diet.
- Practice the preparation of diet according to the needs of the clients.

UNIT OUTLINE

- Introduction
- Preparation of Hot Beverages
- Preparation of Cold Beverages
- Preparation of Soups
- Preparation of Eggs
- Light Diet
- Kanji
- Boiled Vegetables
- Salads
- Custards
- Low Cost High Nutrition Diet: Chikki, Multigrain Roti

KEY TERMS

Beverages: Any potable liquid, especially one other than water such as tea, coffee, beer, or milk hot and cold, juice, shakes, soups, lassi, barley water.

Gruel: A thin food made by boiling cereal in water or milk such as Khichdi, rice water, oatmeal or cornmeal.

Rice kanji: Rice water

Vanilla: A flavoring agent

INTRODUCTION

A healthy diet is essential for good health and nutrition. It protects you against many chronic noncommunicable diseases, such as heart disease, diabetes and cancer. Eating a variety of foods and consuming less salt, sugars and saturated and industrially-produced trans fats, are essential to remain healthy. In this chapter you will know about practically applicable recipes which are not only healthy but are tasty too.

PREPARATION OF HOT BEVERAGES

Tea

- It is an antioxidant.
- It has a stimulating effect on the body.
- The stimulating effect is due to the presence of caffeine in it.

Chemical Composition

- Caffeine 2–6%
- Tannic acid 6–12%
- Theophylline–traces
- Essential volatile oils 5%.

Varieties

- **Green tea:** It is more astringent than black tea. It is popular in China, Japan and Assam in India.
- Black tea

Preparation

- **Green tea/black tea without milk and sugar:** Boil one cup of water. Add one teaspoon of black tea leaves or green tea leaves, and keep it for 2–3 minutes. Strain it and serve hot.
- **Tea with lime and sugar:** Boil water, and warm the teapot with hot water. Add one teaspoon of tea leaves in a pot. Pour boiling water into the teapot. Keep it for 2–3 minutes. Strain it in a cup and add the juice of one lemon. Add sugar according to taste and serve hot.
- **Tea with sugar and milk:** Boil water and milk separately. Warm the teapot with hot water, add one teaspoon ful (tsf) of black tea leaves in a teapot, and pour one cup of boiling water. Keep it for 2–3 minutes, strain it. Add sugar and hot milk according to taste and serve hot.

Hot Coffee

Coffee

- It is also an antioxidant.
- It has a stimulating effect on the nervous system.
- It raises the blood pressure when given to a patient with low BP.

Chemical Composition

- Caffeine 0.6–2%
- Volatile oil: Caffeol
- Tannic acid

Ingredients—for Instant Coffee

- Water: 1 cup
- Coffee powder: 1/2 – 3/4 tsf
- Milk and sugar to taste

Method

- Pour boiling water over coffee powder in a cup
- Add sugar and milk according to the taste.
- Mix and serve hot.

Espresso Coffee

Ingredients

- Milk: 1 cup
- Coffee powder: 1/2 – 3/4 tsf
- Sugar: 1–1½ tsf
- Drinking chocolate to sprinkle

Method

- Beat coffee and sugar in a cup using a few drops of water.
- Pour boiling milk over it and mix well.
- Sprinkle drinking chocolate powder over it and serve hot.

Note: Do not take out coffee from the container with a wet spoon, close the lid of the container tightly, immediately after taking out coffee.

PREPARATION OF COLD BEVERAGES

Cold Coffee

Ingredients

- Milk — 1 cup
- Coffee powder — 1/2 – 3/4 tsf
- Sugar — 1½–2 tsf
- Cream — 1–2 tsf
- Ice cubes — 2–3
- Drinking chocolate powder to sprinkle.

Method

- Blend milk and sugar in a blender.
- Add coffee powder, cream and ice cubes and blend again.
- Pour into a glass, sprinkle drinking chocolate, keep the straw pipe in glass and serve cold.

Lime Juice

Ingredients

- Lemon — 1
- Common salt — 1/4 tsf
- Sugar — 2 tsf
- Cold water — 1 glass
- Ice cubes — 2–3

Method

- Squeeze the lime and take out the juice in a container.
- Add sugar and salt.
- Mix well.
- Add one glass of water, strain into a glass and add ice cubes.
- Serve

Indication

Lime juice is given in case of dehydration due to diarrhea, vomiting, fever, or heat strokes to replace fluids and electrolytes.

Fruit Shake

Ingredients

- Mango or Banana — 100 g
- Sugar   — 3 tablespoons
- Milk   — 200 mL
- Ice cubes   — 2–3

Method

- Blend the fruit pulp with sugar in a blender.
- Add milk and blend again.
- Add ice cubes and best served chilled.

Lassi (Buttermilk)

Ingredients

- Curd   — 200 g
- Sugar   — 1 tablespoon
- Salt   — 1/4 tablespoon
- Ice cubes — 2–3

Method

- Churn the curd
- The butter will float over it.
- Remove the butter, then add sugar or salt according to taste to the remaining curd.
- Mix well and add ice cubes.
- Serve in a glass.

Indication

Lassi contains protein, minerals and all vitamins except vitamin A, which is present in butter. It is given in case of dehydration due to any cause to replace fluids and electrolytes.

PREPARATION OF SOUPS

Mixed Vegetable Soup

Ingredients

- **For vegetable stock**
  - Carrot   — 50 g
  - Cauliflower   — 50 g
  - Lauki   — 50 g
  - Tomatoes   — 50 g
  - Cloves   — 2–3 g
  - Cinnamon powder — 1 pinch
  - Water   — 1 L
- **For soup**
  - Onion   — 1
  - Carrot   — 20 g
  - Cauliflower   — 20 g
  - Cabbage   — 20 g
  - French bean   — 20 g
  - Tomato sauce   — 2 tsf
  - Salt and pepper — to taste
  - Cheese   — 20 g
  - Butter   — 20 g

Method

- Add vegetables and spices for preparing stock to 1 L of water in a pressure cooker and cook for 8–10 minutes in the pressure cooker.
- Mash the vegetables lightly and strain.
- Wash the vegetables for soup and cut them into small pieces of even size.
- Fry chopped onion in melted butter in a pan and add chopped vegetables. Cook for a few minutes.
- Now add vegetable stock in a pan and cook until vegetables are done.
- Add salt, pepper and tomato sauce in it.
- Pour the soup into the soup bowl, garnish with grated cheese and serve hot.

Tomato Soup

Ingredients

Tomatoes	— 250 g		Cinnamon	— 1 small piece
Carrot	— 25 g		Cloves	— 2–3
Onion	— 1		Tomato sauce	— 2 tsf
Ginger	— 20 g		Cream	— 2 tsf
Garlic	— 4–5 pieces		Bread	— 1 slice
Butter	— 20 g		Salt	— 1/2 tsp
Maida	— 1 tsf		Black pepper	— 2–3 (grinded)
Brown elaichi	— 1		Water	— 2 cups

Method

- Wash and cut tomatoes and carrots into small pieces, chop ginger, garlic and onion.
- Cook the tomatoes, carrot, ginger, garlic, onion, cloves, cinnamon and elaichi in a pressure cooker for 7–8 minutes.
- Mash and sieve items.
- Fry small cubes of bread slice and keep aside.
- Roast maida with butter in a pan, add sieved soup and cook until thick.
- Add salt pepper powder and tomato sauce.
- Pour the hot soup into a soup bowl, add fried bread cubes and garnish with 1 tsf of whipped cream.
- Serve hot.

Dal Soup

Ingredients

Chana/moong/masoor dal	— 50 g		Salt	— 1/2 tsf
Onion	— 1		Black pepper	— 1 pinch
Ginger	— 20 g		Tomato	— 1
Garlic	— 3–4 cloves		Water	— 4 cups

Method

- Wash tomato, ginger, garlic, onion and cut into small pieces.
- Pressure cook along with dal for 7–8 minutes in 4 cups (400 mL) of water.
- Mash and sieve them.
- Pour the sieved soup into a soup bowl.
- Add salt and black pepper. Serve hot. It is for 2 people.

Barley Water

Ingredients

- Barley pearl — 30 g
- Water — 500 mL
- Sugar as per taste
- Lime juice of one lime for taste.

Method

- Blanch the barley by covering with cold water.
- Simmer the barley with 500 mL of water till it gets reduced to 300 mL.
- Strain, then cool it.
- Add sugar as per taste and juice of one lime.
- Stir well and serve.

PREPARATION OF EGGS

Egg Flip

Ingredients

- Egg   — 1
- Milk — 200 mL
- Sugar — 20 g
- Vanilla essence for flavor or any flavor

Method

- Beat egg with egg beater.
- Boil milk and keep aside.
- Mix sugar to the milk and add beaten egg to the milk, when it is lukewarm, stir well.
- Add a few drops of vanilla essence.
- Serve hot or cold.

Note: Milk should not be very hot otherwise egg white will coagulate.

Scrambled Egg

Ingredients

- Egg   — 1
- Oil   — 10 g
- Salt and pepper — for taste
- Milk   — 1 tablespoon

Method

- Beat the egg, add salt, pepper and milk, stir well.
- Put oil in a pan.
- Pour egg and cook on a slow flame, stir lightly to prevent sticking of egg to the pan.
- When it becomes soft and creamy serve immediately.

Omelette

Ingredients

- Egg   — 1
- Oil   — 5–10 g
- Onion   — 1 small size
- Green chili   — 1 small size
- Salt and pepper — to taste
- Tomato sauce   — to taste

Method

- Chop the onion and green chili into fine pieces.
- Beat the egg.
- Mix the onion and green chili, salt and pepper in a beaten egg.
- Mix thoroughly, and put oil in the saucepan. Place it on a slow fire till it becomes hot.
- Pour the beaten egg into it slowly and cook it on a slow fire till the white of the egg coagulates.
- Remove from the pan.
- Fold and serve hot with tomato sauce.

Boiled Egg

Ingredients

- Egg
- Pepper
- Salt for taste

Method

- **For quarter boil:** Boil the egg for 3 minutes, break content into egg cup, add salt and pepper, serve hot.
- **For half-boiled egg:** Boil for 5–7 minutes. Break content in egg cup, add salt and pepper, serve hot.
- **For full boil:** Boil for 10 minutes. Remove shell, serve hot with salt and pepper.

Poached Egg

Ingredients

- Egg–1
- Water
- Salt and pepper for taste

Method

- Heat the water in a pan to the simmering temperature.
- Slide the content of the egg slowly into a pan of water.
- Heat the pan until the white of the egg is coagulated completely.
- Remove quickly from water.
- Serve hot with salt and pepper.

LIGHT DIET

Light diet such as suji porridge, dalia porridge, khichdi, dalia, etc.

Suji Porridge

Ingredients

- Suji   — 50 g
- Water — 100 mL
- Sugar — to taste
- Milk   — 200 mL

Method

- Wash suji and add water in a pan along with suji.
- Cook it on a fire while stirring.
- Mix milk and sugar.
- Remove from fire. Serve as per the need of the person.

Dalia Porridge

Ingredients

- Dalia — 50 g
- Water — to cook
- Milk   — 100 mL
- Sugar — 20 g

Method

- Wash dalia and add enough of water to cook it.
- Put it on the fire, cook on a slow flame.
- Mix milk and sugar. Serve hot.

Gruel (Khichdi)

Ingredients

- Rice — 50 g
- Green, Moong dal — 25 g
- Onion — 50 g
- Oil — 10 g
- Jeera — ½ tsf
- Salt — to taste
- Water — enough to cook

Method

- Clean and wash rice and dal.

- Chop onion, fry jeera and chopped onion in oil.
- Add rice, dal and enough water to cook.
- Add salt. Then, cook it in a pressure cooker for 10 minutes.
- Serve hot with curd.

Dalia

Ingredients

- Broken wheat — 50 g
- Mung dal   — 50 g
- Sugar/Jaggery — 80 g
- Water   — enough to cook

Method

- Roast wheat flour and moong dal.
- Add sufficient water to cook in a pressure cooker, till it is soft-cooked.
- Dissolve jaggery in water, strain and add in cooked mixture and again cook it till it mixes well.
- Serve hot.

Note: Dalia can be made without moong dal in the same way. Sugar can be used in place of Jaggery.

KANJI

Rice Kanji

The kanji water contains vitamin B_1. Kanji water is given to replace fluids in diarrhea and dehydration.

Ingredients

- Rice   — 50 g
- Water   — 300 mL
- Salt and pepper — to taste

Method

- Clean and wash rice.
- Add water and rice in a pressure cooker, cook well in pressure cooker for 10 minutes.
- Sieve it and remove the rice. The sieved water is rice kanji.
- Add pepper and salt for taste and serve it either hot or cold.

Ragi Kanji

Ingredients

- Ragi   — 50 g (Powdered)
- Water   — 300 mL
- Cold water — 1 tablespoon
- Salt   — to taste
- Milk — 150 mL

Method

- Add cold water to the ragi powder and mix it well, then gradually add milk and water and a pinch of salt.

- Boil for 15 minutes.
- Serve hot.

BOILED VEGETABLES

Boiled vegetables are indicated in a fat-free diet in cases of:
- Obesity, to provide a low-caloric diet and as a filler.
- Hypertension
- Cardiovascular diseases.
- Peptic ulcer, for easy digestion.

Ingredients

- Vegetables according to season 100 g
- Coriander leaves — to garnish
- Onion   — 1
- Salt and pepper   — to taste
- Lemon   — 1 to flavor
- Water   — 1/2 cup

Method

- Vegetables and onions are washed and chopped.
- The chopped vegetables and onion are boiled in 1/2 cup of water in a pressure cooker until they become soft.
- Add a pinch of salt and pepper and garnish with coriander leaves and lemon pieces.

Note:
- To increase the nutritional value, vegetables can be mixed and boiled.
- If salt is contraindicated, use lime only.

SALADS

Salads added to the menu, make the food appealing and appetizing. It provides roughage which is necessary to provide:

- Bulk to the food
- Reduce fat absorption
- Increase digestive power
- Prevent constipation

Salads are generally uncooked raw vegetables.

Vegetable Salads

Ingredients

- Green leafy vegetables: Lettuce, spinach, coriander leaves.
- Other vegetables: Cabbage, cauliflower, beetroot, cucumbers, onion
- Radish, pineapple, carrot, tomatoes, kakadi
- Flavoring agent: lemon, vinegar

Method

- According to the season, two to three vegetables are washed properly, chopped into various designs, (i.e., round, square or cylindrical pieces), and decorated on a plate with tomatoes and onions.
- Garnish with salad leaves, coriander leaves and pieces of lemon.

Ways of Serving

- As an appetizer along with the meal.
- As a dessert in between meals.

Fruit Salads

Fruit salads can be made from any seasonal fruit. Fruit salads can be served as:
- Sweet dish after meals.
- As a dessert in between meals.
- As a high fiber diet.

Ingredients

- Apple — 50 g
- Orange — 100 g
- Banana — 100 g
- Grapes — 50 g
- Mango — 100 g
- Sugar — 15 g
- Lime juice — a few drops

Method

- Wash and dice all fruits except grapes and oranges.
- Remove seeds from orange, peel mango and dice.
- Mix all fruits except banana.
- Add sugar and lime, mix together
- Keep in the refrigerator to cool.
- Before serving, add banana slices. Serve chilled.

CUSTARDS

Custards are served as a soft diet to small children and persons who are on a soft diet or as a sweet dish after meals.

Ingredients

- Custard powder — 30 g
- Sugar — 2 tablespoons
- Cold water — to blend the custard powder
- Milk — 200 mL
- Flavoring agents — a few drops of vanilla or powdered, one small cardamom

Method

- Add cold water to custard powder and blend it to prevent lump formation.
- When mixed properly, add milk and heat it while stirring constantly till its consistency changes.
- Add sugar while cooling and keep on stirring.
- Add essence.
- Then serve hot or cold.

Egg Custard

Ingredients

- Egg — 1
- Sugar — 2 tablespoons
- Milk — 1 cup
- Flavoring agent

Method

- Break the egg to get the contents from shell.
- Blend the contents.
- Add sugar and milk, blend again.
- Heat it in a water bath, while constantly stirring the mixture till its consistency changes.
- Add a few drops of vanilla.
- Serve hot or cold.

LOW COST HIGH NUTRITION DIET: CHIKKI, MULTIGRAIN ROTI

Chikki

Chikki is rich in protein, iron, carbohydrates and vitamin A. It is recommended for growing children. It can also be preserved.

Ingredients

- Peanuts — 200 g
- Jaggery — 200 g
- Coconut — 30 g
- Saunf — 20 g
- Oil — 30 g

Method

- Roast the peanuts in a pan and remove their peels; keep aside.
- Chop the coconut into small thin pieces.
- Beat the jaggery, melt it and keep it aside.
- Put oil in a pan and heat it.
- Add coconut, saunf, roasted peanuts, and melted jaggery.
- Stir well until it is thoroughly mixed.
- Transfer the mixture to a flat tray and allow it to cool.
- Shape it into round or square pieces and serve.

Multigrain Roti

Multigrain roti itself is a balanced diet, rich with all the nutrients. It is rich in all the nutrients, i.e., protein, carbohydrates, minerals and vitamins with high fiber content.

- It provides a perfect balanced diet for all age groups.
- It prevents nutrition deficiency diseases.
- Its high fiber content prevents constipation.
- Especially, recommended for cases of cardiovascular diseases, arthritis, osteoarthritis, and obesity.

Ingredients

- Wheat flour   — 500 g
- Millet (Bajra) flour — 100 g
- Soybean flour   — 100 g
- Maize flour   — 100 g
- Black chana flour   — 100 g
- Barley flour   — 100 g

Method

- All these flours are mixed to make a dough.
- Rotis are made out of it in the same way as that of wheat flour.
- Serve with vegetables, dal, salad, etc.

Summary

- Beverages, soups, salads, soft diets and nutritious diets are recommended for patients in hospitals with various disease conditions.
- Beverages include hot tea and coffee, cold coffee, lime juice, fruit juice, fruit shakes, buttermilk, barely water, soups and kanji, etc.
- Soups can be made from vegetables, dals, and tomatoes. Salads include raw vegetables and fruits.
- Soft diets include porridges of suji, dalia, sago, khichdi, custard, rice, kheer, vermicelli, boiled vegetables and stewed fruits.
- The nutritious diet includes high protein, high carbohydrate, rich iron and vitamin diets. It includes multigrain chapatis, chikki, etc.

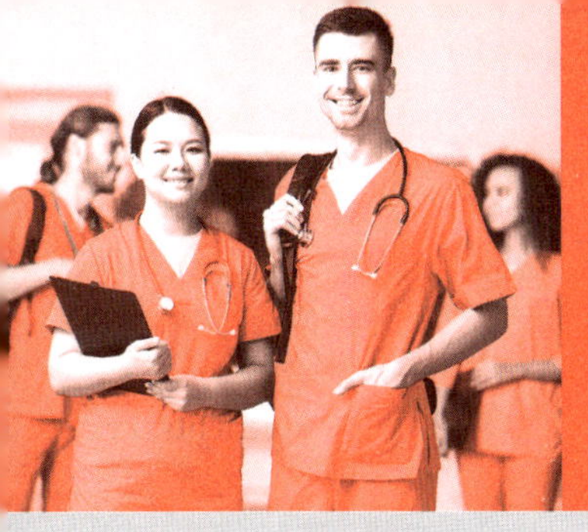

STUDENT ASSIGNMENT

LONG ANSWER TYPE QUESTIONS

1. What are the ingredients of mixed vegetable soup? Describe the method of its preparation.
2. Explain the procedure of making egg custard.
3. Describe the preparation of fruit salad.

SHORT ANSWER TYPE QUESTIONS

1. Write short notes on:
   a. Ingredients of khichri
   b. Preparation of lime juice
   c. Ingredients of tomato soup
2. Write about the light diet.

MULTIPLE CHOICE QUESTIONS

1. **The fluids given to treat dehydration are:**
   a. Lime juice
   b. Buttermilk
   c. Kanji water
   d. All of these

2. **Salads on the menu are provided:**
   a. To prevent constipation
   b. To increase digestive power
   c. To reduce digestive power
   d. All of these

3. **Chikki is rich in:**
   a. Protein
   b. Iron and vitamin A
   c. Carbohydrate
   d. All of these

4. **The ingredients of multigrain roti are:**
   a. Flour of wheat, maize, millet, soybean, black chana
   b. Flour of wheat, maida, suji, gram dust
   c. Flour of black chana, maize and soya
   d. Flour of rice, maize, barley and soybean

ANSWER KEY

1. d   2. a   3. d   4. a

Note

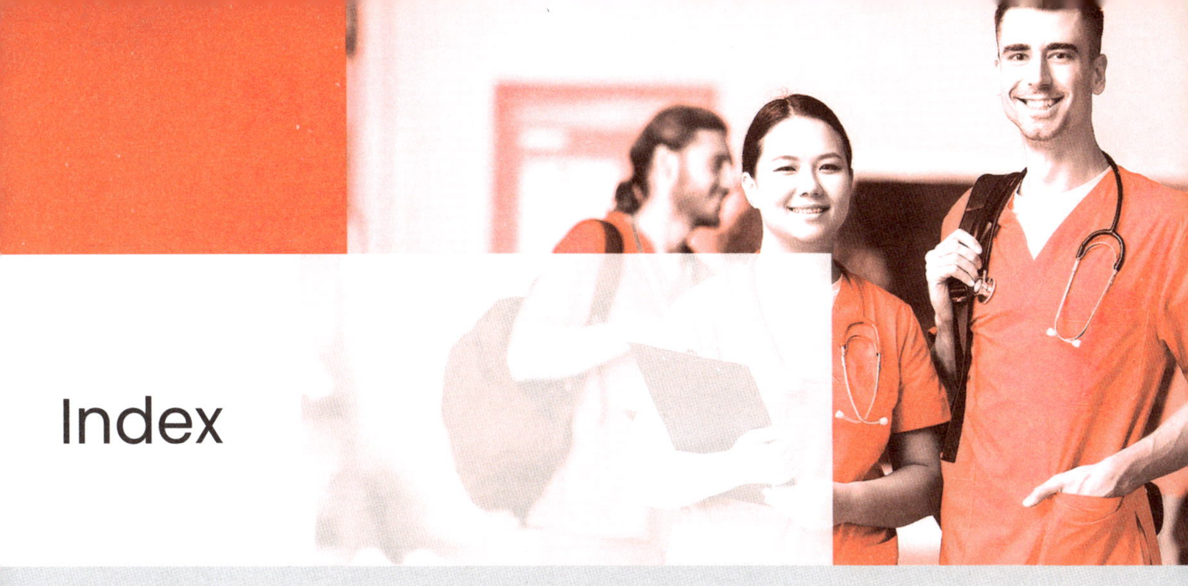

Index

Refer 'f' for figure and 't' for table respectively.

N

O

S

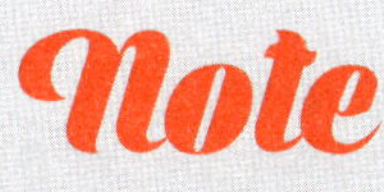

Note

Note